POCKET COMPANION

Robbins and Cotran

PATHOLOGIC
BASIS OF DISEASE

POCKET COMPANION TO
Robbins and Cotran
PATHOLOGIC
BASIS OF DISEASE
Seventh Edition

Richard N. Mitchell, MD, PhD
Associate Professor, Department of Pathology
Harvard Medical School and Health Sciences and Technology
Director, Human Pathology
Harvard-MIT Division of Health Sciences and Technology
Staff Pathologist, Brigham and Women's Hospital
Boston, Massachusetts

Vinay Kumar, MBBS, MD, FRCPath
Alice Hogge and Arthur Baer Professor
Chairman, Department of Pathology
The University of Chicago, Pritzker School of Medicine
Chicago, Illinois

Abul K. Abbas, MBBS
Chair, Department of Pathology
University of California, San Francisco
San Francisco, California

Nelson Fausto, MD
Chairman, Department of Pathology
University of Washington School of Medicine
Seattle, Washington

With Illustrations by James A. Perkins, MS, MFA

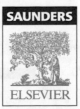

SAUNDERS

ELSEVIER

SAUNDERS
ELSEVIER

1600 John F. Kennedy Blvd.
Ste. 1800
Philadelphia, Pennsylvania 19103-2899

POCKET COMPANION TO ROBBINS AND COTRAN
PATHOLOGIC BASIS OF DISEASE, 7/E   ISBN 10 0-7216-0265-7
ISBN 13 978-0-7216-0265-3
International Edition ISBN 978-0-8089-2307-7

Notice

Knowledge and best practice in this field are constantly changing. As new
research and experience broaden our knowledge, changes in practice,
treatment, and drug therapy may become necessary or appropriate. Readers
are advised to check the most current information provided (i) on
procedures featured or (ii) by the manufacturer of each product to be
administered, to verify the recommended dose or formula, the method and
duration of administration, and contraindications. It is the responsibility of
the practitioner, relying on their own experience and knowledge of the
patient, to make diagnoses, to determine dosages and the best treatment for
each individual patient, and to take all appropriate safety precautions. To the
fullest extent of the law, neither the Publisher nor the Editors assumes any
liability for any injury and/or damage to persons or property arising out or
related to any use of the material contained in this book.

Previous editions copyrighted 1999, 1995, 1991

Library of Congress Cataloging-in-Publication Data

Pocket companion to Robbins and Cotran pathologic basis of disease / Richard
N. Mitchell . . . [et al.].— 7th ed.
   p. ; cm.
   Includes index.
   Rev. ed. of: Pocket companion to Robbins pathologic basis of disease /
Stanley L. Robbins . . . [et al.]. 6th ed. c1999.
   Companion v. to: Robbins and Cotran pathologic basis of disease. 7th ed.
c2005.
   ISBN 0-7216-0265-7
   1. Pathology—Handbooks, manuals, etc.
   [DNLM: 1. Pathology—Handbooks. QZ 39 P73921 2006]   I. Mitchell,
Richard N.   II. Pocket companion to Robbins pathologic basis of
disease.   III. Robbins and Cotran pathologic basis of disease.

RB111.R62 2006 Suppl.
616.07—dc22   2005057675

Publishing Director: *William Schmitt*
Managing Editor: *Rebecca Gruliow*
Design Director: *Ellen Zanolle*

Working together to grow
libraries in developing countries
www.elsevier.com | www.bookaid.org | www.sabre.org

ELSEVIER   BOOK AID International   Sabre Foundation

Printed in the United States of America

Last digit is the print number: 9 8 7 6 5 4 3 2 1

Contributors

Charles E. Alpers, MD
Professor of Pathology, Adjunct Professor of Medicine, University of Washington School of Medicine; Pathologist, University of Washington Medical Center, Seattle, WA
The Kidney

Douglas C. Anthony, MD, PhD
Professor and Chair, Department of Pathology and Anatomical Sciences, University of Missouri, Columbia, MO
Peripheral Nerve and Skeletal Muscle; The Central Nervous System

Jon C. Aster MD, PhD
Associate Professor of Pathology, Harvard Medical School; Staff Pathologist, Brigham and Women's Hospital, Boston, MA
Red Blood Cell and Bleeding Disorders; White Blood Cells, Lymph Nodes, Spleen, and Thymus

James M. Crawford, MD, PhD
Professor and Chair, Department of Pathology, Immunology and Laboratory Medicine, University of Florida College of Medicine; Professor and Chair, Shands Hospital at the University of Florida, Gainesville, FL
The Gastrointestinal Tract; Liver and Biliary Tract

Christopher P. Crum, MD
Professor of Pathology, Harvard Medical School; Director, Women's and Perinatal Pathology, Brigham and Women's Hospital, Boston, MA
The Female Genital Tract

Umberto De Girolami, MD
Professor of Pathology, Harvard Medical School; Director of Neuropathology, Brigham and Women's Hospital, Boston, MA
Peripheral Nerve and Skeletal Muscle; The Central Nervous System

Jonathan I. Epstein, MD
Professor of Pathology, Urology, and Oncology; The Reinhard Professor of Urologic Pathology, The Johns Hopkins University School of Medicine, Baltimore; Director of Surgical Pathology, The Johns Hopkins Hospital, Baltimore, MD
The Lower Urinary Tract and Male Genital System

Robert Folberg, MD
Frances B. Greever Professor and Head, Department of
    Pathology, University of Illinois at Chicago, Chicago, IL
The Eye

Matthew P. Frosch, MD, PhD
Assistant Professor of Pathology, Harvard Medical School;
    Assistant Pathologist, C.S. Kubik Laboratory for
    Neuropathology, Massachusetts General Hospital, Boston,
    MA
*Peripheral Nerve and Skeletal Muscle; The Central Nervous
    System*

Ralph H. Hruban, MD
Professor of Pathology and Oncology, The Johns Hopkins
    University School of Medicine; Attending Pathologist, The
    Johns Hopkins Hospital, Baltimore, MD
The Pancreas

Aliya N. Husain, MBBS
Professor, Department of Pathology, Pritzker School of
    Medicine, University of Chicago, Chicago, IL
The Lung

Agnes B. Kane, MD, PhD
Professor and Chair, Department of Pathology and
    Laboratory Medicine, Brown University Medical School,
    Providence, RI
Environmental and Nutritional Pathology

Susan C. Lester, MD, PhD
Assistant Professor of Pathology, Harvard Medical School;
    Chief, Breast Pathology, Brigham and Women's Hospital,
    Boston, MA
The Breast

Mark W. Lingen, DDS, PhD
Associate Professor, Department of Pathology, University of
    Chicago, Chicago, IL
Head and Neck

Chen Liu, MD, PhD
Assistant Professor of Pathology, University of Florida
    College of Medicine, Gainesville, FL
The Gastrointestinal Tract

Anirban Maitra, MBBS
Assistant Professor, Department of Pathology, The Johns
    Hopkins University School of Medicine; Pathologist, The
    Johns Hopkins Hospital, Baltimore, MD
Diseases of Infancy and Childhood; The Endocrine System

Alexander J. McAdam, MD, PhD
Assistant Professor of Pathology, Harvard Medical School;
    Medical Director, Infectious Diseases Diagnostic
    Laboratory, Children's Hospital Boston, Boston, MA
Infectious Diseases

Martin C. Mihm, Jr., MD
Clinical Professor of Pathology, Harvard Medical School;
  Pathologist and Associate Dermatologist, Massachusetts
  General Hospital, Boston, MA
The Skin

Richard N. Mitchell, MD
Associate Professor, Department of Pathology, Harvard
  Medical School and Health Sciences and Technology;
  Director, Human Pathology, Harvard-MIT Division of
  Health Sciences and Technology; Staff Pathologist,
  Brigham and Women's Hospital, Boston, MA
*Cellular Adaptations, Cell Injury, and Cell Death; Acute and
  Chronic Inflammation; Tissue Renewal and Repair:
  Regeneration, Healing, and Fibrosis; Hemodynamic
  Disorders, Thromboembolic Disease, and Shock; Genetic
  Disorders; Diseases of Immunity; Neoplasia*

George F. Murphy, MD
Professor of Pathology, Harvard Medical School; Director of
  Dermatopathology, Brigham and Women's Hospital,
  Boston, MA
The Skin

Andrew E. Rosenberg, MD
Associate Professor of Pathology, Harvard Medical School;
  Associate Pathologist, James Homer Wright Laboratories,
  Department of Pathology, Massachusetts General Hospital,
  Boston, MA
Bones, Joints, and Soft Tissue Tumors

Frederick J. Schoen, MD, PhD
Professor of Pathology and Health Sciences and Technology,
  Harvard Medical School; Director, Cardiac Pathology and
  Executive Vice Chairman, Department of Pathology,
  Brigham and Women's Hospital, Boston, MA
Blood Vessels; The Heart

Klaus Sellheyer, MD
Assistant Professor of Pathology, Thomas Jefferson
  University; Attending Dermatologist, Jefferson Medical
  College, Philadelphia, PA
The Skin

Arlene H. Sharpe, MD, PhD
Professor of Pathology, Harvard Medical School; Chief,
  Immunology Research Division, Department of Pathology,
  Brigham and Women's Hospital, Boston, MA
Infectious Diseases

Preface

The publication of the 7th (and newest) Edition of *Robbins and Cotran Pathologic Basis of Disease* clearly necessitates a concordant update of its *Pocket Companion*. Extensive revisions of the material in the "Big Book" have required significant changes in this *Pocket* version to capture the new material in a succinct and focused manner. However, as always, the *Pocket Companion* is also intended to be much more than a simple topical outline; indeed, it was prepared with three important goals in mind:

- To facilitate the reading and comprehension of the more detailed presentations in the parent book by providing introductory overviews along with relevant page numbers referenced to *Robbins and Cotran Pathologic Basis of Disease*, 7th Edition.

- To help students identify the core material that requires their primary attention.

- To serve as a useful tool for the review of a large body of information.

We have worked hard to rein in the final size of the *Pocket Companion* (to insure that it still actually fits in a pocket); this was particularly challenging given the wealth of updated writing in the parent volume. Consequently, tables and illustrative figures have been used whenever possible to help limit the sheer verbiage (and truly, one picture *is* worth at least a thousand words). Moreover, the *Pocket* does not routinely summarize the discussions on normal anatomy and physiology that occupy the opening of each chapter on diseases of organ systems, and most of the new "boxes" on cutting edge science are—unfortunately—given only scant attention. To maintain a usable size, the many beautiful gross and histologic figures that adorn the parent volume have also not been reproduced. Nevertheless, we feel that the *Pocket* retains much of the flavor and excitement of the Big Book, and truly is a suitable "companion". In large part, this has been made possible by the efforts and diligence of the many Contributors, who have willingly summarized their elegant (and much longer) opuses in the parent volume, and trimmed them down to their most basic elements. It is always easier to write more; to write less is actually hard work.

Although the harried medical student or over-taxed house officer—with too much to do and too little time to do it—might be inclined to use this as the sole source of knowledge about pathology, we must caution against it. While the *Pocket Companion* does contain the salient facts, it omits the discussions and expositions that enrich the fuller presentations. We hope, therefore, that this abbreviated overview of pathology will be

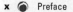

used as a companion to the parent book, enhancing the pleasure and the value of both. As for previous versions, the *Pocket Companion* is entirely and exhaustively cross-referenced to the parent book; when a reader is so inclined, the complete story can be easily found in the Big Book.

Rick Mitchell

Vinay Kumar

Abul Abbas

Nelson Fausto

Contents

Please Note

Unless otherwise specified, all page references, including those following headings and those within the text matter, refer to *Robbins and Cotran Pathologic Basis of Disease,* 7th ed.

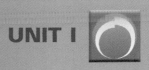

GENERAL
PATHOLOGY

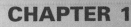

CHAPTER 1

Cellular Adaptations, Cell Injury, and Cell Death

INTRODUCTION (p. 4)

Pathology is the study of the structural and functional causes of human disease. The four aspects of a disease process that form the core of pathology are

- The cause of a disease (*etiology*)
- The mechanism(s) of disease development (*pathogenesis*)
- The structural alterations induced in cells and tissues by the disease (*morphologic change*)
- The functional consequences of the morphologic changes (*clinical significance*)

OVERVIEW (p. 4)

Normal cell function requires a balance between physiologic demands and the constraints of cell structure and metabolic capacity; the result is a steady state, or *homeostasis*. Cells can alter their functional state in response to modest stress to maintain the steady state. More excessive physiologic stresses, or adverse pathologic stimuli (*injury*), result in (i) adaption, (ii) reversible injury, or (iii) irreversible injury and cell death (Table 1–1). These responses may be considered a continuum of progressive impairment of cell structure and function.

- *Adaptation* occurs when physiologic or pathologic stressors induce a new state that changes the cell but otherwise preserves its viability in the face of the exogenous stimuli. These changes include

  Hyperplasia (increased cell number, p. 6)
  Hypertrophy (increased cell mass, p. 7)
  Atrophy (decreased cell mass, p. 9)
  Metaplasia (change from one mature cell type to another, p. 10)

TABLE 1–1   **Cellular Responses to Injury**

Nature and Severity of Injurious Stimulus	Cellular Response
Altered physiologic stimuli:	Cellular adaptations:
• Increased demand, increased trophic stimulation (e.g., growth factors, hormones)	• Hyperplasia, hypertrophy
• Decreased nutrients, stimulation	• Atrophy
• Chronic irritation (chemical or physical)	• Metaplasia
Reduced oxygen supply; chemical injury; microbial infection	Cell injury:
• Acute and self-limited	• Acute reversible injury

• Progessive and severe (including DNA damage)	• Irreversible injury → cell death
	  Necrosis
	  Apoptosis

• Mild chronic injury	• Subcellular alterations in various organelles
Metabolic alterations, genetic or acquired	Intracellular accumulations; calcifications
Prolonged life span with cumulative sublethal injury	Cellular aging

- *Reversible injury* denotes pathologic cell changes that can be restored to normalcy if the stimulus is removed or if the cause of injury is mild.
- *Irreversible injury* occurs when stressors exceed the capacity of the cell to adapt (beyond a *point of no return*) and denotes permanent pathologic changes that cause cell death. The two morphologic and mechanistic patterns of cell death are *necrosis* and *apoptosis* (Fig. 1–1 and Table 1–2). Although necrosis always represents a pathologic process, apoptosis may also serve a number of normal functions (e.g., in embryogenesis) and is not necessarily associated with cell injury:

TABLE 1–2   **Features of Necrosis and Apoptosis**

Feature	Necrosis	Apoptosis
Cell size	Enlarged (swelling)	Reduced (shrinkage)
Nucleus	Pyknosis → karyorrhexis → karyolysis	Fragmentation into nucleosome size fragments
Plasma membrane	Disrupted	Intact; altered structure, especially orientation of lipids
Cellular contents	Enzymatic digestion; may leak out of cell	Intact; may be released in apoptotic bodies
Adjacent inflammation	Frequent	No
Physiologic or pathologic role	Invariably pathologic (culmination of irreversible cell injury)	Often physiologic, means of eliminating unwanted cells; may be pathologic after some forms of cell injury, especially DNA damage

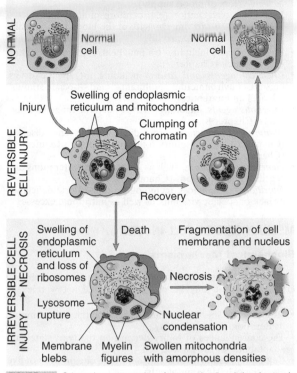

FIGURE 1-1 Schematic representation of a normal cell and the changes in reversible and irreversible cell injury. Reversible injury is characterized by generalized swelling of the cell and its organelles; blebbing of the plasma membrane; detachment of ribosomes from the endoplasmic reticulum; and clumping of nuclear chromatin. Transition to irreversible injury is characterized by increasing swelling of the cell; swelling and disruption of lysosomes; presence of large amorphous densities in swollen mitochondria; disruption of cellular membranes; and profound nuclear changes. The latter include nuclear condensation (pyknosis), followed by fragmentation (karyorrhexis) and dissolution of the nucleus (karyolysis).

- *Necrosis* is the more common type of cell death, involving severe cell swelling, denaturation and coagulation of proteins, breakdown of cellular organelles, and cell rupture. Usually, a large number of cells in the adjoining tissue are affected.
- *Apoptosis* occurs when a cell dies by activation of an internal "suicide" program, involving an orchestrated disassembly of cellular components; there is minimal disruption of the surrounding tissue. Morphologically, chromatin condensation and fragmentation occur.

CAUSES OF CELL INJURY (p. 11)

- *Oxygen deprivation (hypoxia)* affects aerobic respiration and therefore ability to generate adenosine triphosphate (ATP). This extremely important and common cause of cell injury and death occurs as a result of:

Ischemia (loss of blood supply)
Inadequate oxygenation (e.g., cardiorespiratory failure)
Loss of oxygen-carrying capacity of the blood (e.g., anemia, carbon monoxide poisoning)

- *Physical agents,* including trauma, heat, cold, radiation, and electric shock (Chapter 9)
- *Chemical agents and drugs,* including therapeutic drugs, poisons, environmental pollutants, and "social stimuli" (alcohol and narcotics)
- *Infectious agents,* including viruses, bacteria, fungi, and parasites (Chapter 8)
- *Immunologic reactions,* including autoimmune diseases (Chapter 6) and cell injury following responses to infection (Chapter 2)
- *Genetic derangements,* such as chromosomal alterations and specific gene mutations (Chapter 5)
- *Nutritional imbalances,* including protein–calorie deficiency or lack of specific vitamins, as well as nutritional excesses

MECHANISMS OF CELL INJURY (p. 14)

Biochemical Mechanisms

The biochemical mechanisms responsible for cell injury are complex but may be organized around a few relevant principles:

- Responses to injurious stimuli depend on the type of injury, its duration, and its severity.
- The consequences of injury depend on the type, state, and adaptability of the injured cell.
- Cell injury results from abnormalities in one or more of five essential cellular components:

    Aerobic respiration, involving mitochondrial oxidative phosphorylation and ATP production
    Maintenance of cell membrane integrity, critical for cell and organellar ionic and osmotic homeostasis
    Protein synthesis
    Intracellular cytoskeleton
    Integrity of the genetic apparatus

Intracellular Mechanisms

The intracellular mechanisms of cell injury fall into one of five general pathways (Fig. 1–2). It is worth emphasizing that structural and biochemical elements of the cell are so closely interrelated that regardless of the locus of initial injury, secondary effects rapidly propagate through other elements.

ATP Depletion (p. 14)

Decreased ATP synthesis and ATP depletion are common consequences of both ischemic and toxic injury. ATP is generated through glycolysis (anaerobic, inefficient) and oxidative phosphorylation in the mitochondria (aerobic, efficient). Hypoxia will lead to increased anaerobic glycolysis with glycogen depletion, increased lactic acid production, and intracellular acidosis. ATP is also critically required for membrane transport, maintenance of ionic gradients (particularly Na^+, K^+,

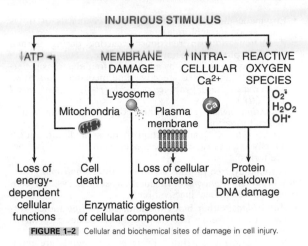

FIGURE 1–2 Cellular and biochemical sites of damage in cell injury.

and Ca^{2+}), and protein synthesis; reduced (inefficient) ATP synthesis will dramatically impact those pathways.

Mitochondrial Damage (p. 15)

Mitochondrial damage may occur directly due to hypoxia or toxins, or as a consequence of increased cytosolic Ca^{2+}, oxidative stress, or phospholipid breakdown. Damage results in formation of a high-conductance channel (*mitochondrial permeability transition,* or *MPT*) that leaks protons and dissipates the electromotive potential that drives oxidative phosphorylation. Damaged mitochondria also leak cytochrome *c*, which can trigger apoptosis (see below).

Influx of Intracellular Calcium and Loss of Calcium Homeostasis (p. 15)

Cytosolic calcium is maintained at extremely low levels by energy-dependent transport; ischemia and toxins can cause Ca^{2+} influx across the plasma membrane and release of Ca^{2+} from mitochondria and endoplasmic reticulum. Increased cytosolic calcium activates phospholipases that degrade membrane phospholipids; proteases that break down membrane and cytoskeletal proteins; ATPases that hasten ATP depletion; and endonucleases that cause chromatin fragmentation.

Accumulation of Oxygen-Derived Free Radicals (p. 16)

These partially reduced, highly reactive, unstable oxygen molecules, once induced, cause additional free radical formation in an autocatalytic chain reaction (called *propagation*). Free radicals damage lipids (peroxidation of double bonds with chain breakage), proteins (oxidation and fragmentation), and nucleic acids (single strand breaks). Free radical generation occurs by

• Absorption of radiant energy (e.g., ultraviolet light, x-rays); ionizing radiation can hydrolyze water into hydroxyl ($OH\cdot$) and hydrogen ($H\cdot$) free radicals.

- Enzymatic metabolism of exogenous chemicals or drugs (e.g., carbon tetrachloride).
- Reduction-oxidation reactions occurring during normal metabolic processes. In normal respiration, sequential reduction of oxygen to water by addition of four electrons generates small amounts of reactive intermediates: *superoxide anion radical* (O_2^-), *hydrogen peroxide* (H_2O_2), and *hydroxyl ions* $(OH \cdot)$
- *Transition metals* (e.g., iron and copper) can catalyze free radical formation.
- *Nitric oxide* (NO), an important chemical mediator, can act directly as a free radical or be converted to other highly reactive forms.

Fortunately, free radicals are *inherently unstable and generally decay spontaneously.* In addition, several systems contribute to free radical inactivation:

- *Antioxidants* either block the initiation of free radical formation or scavenge free radicals; these include vitamins E and A, ascorbic acid, and glutathione.
- Reactive forms generated by transition metals are minimized by binding to storage and transport proteins (e.g., *transferrin, ferritin, lactoferrin,* and *ceruloplasmin*).
- Free radical–scavenging *enzyme* systems catabolize hydrogen peroxide (*catalase, glutathione peroxidase*) and superoxide anion (*superoxide dismutase*).

Defects in Membrane Permeability (p. 18)

Membranes can be damaged directly by toxins, physical and chemical agents, lytic complement components, and perforins, or indirectly as described by the preceding events. Increased plasma membrane permeability affects intracellular osmolarity as well as enzymatic activity; altered organellar membrane activity will affect their function.

REVERSIBLE AND IRREVERSIBLE CELL INJURY
(p. 19)

Within limits, all the changes of cell injury described above can be offset and cells can return to normal after injury abates (*reversible injury*). However, persistent or excessive injury causes cells to pass a threshold into *irreversible injury* (see Fig. 1–1) associated with extensive cell membrane damage, lysosomal swelling, and mitochondrial vacuolization with deficient ATP synthesis. Extracellular calcium enters the cell and intracellular calcium stores are released, leading to activation of enzymes that catabolize membranes, proteins, ATP, and nucleic acids. Proteins, essential coenzymes, and ribonucleic acids are lost from hyperpermeable plasma membranes, and cells leak metabolites vital for the reconstitution of ATP.

The transition from reversible to irreversible injury is difficult to identify, although two phenomena consistently characterize irreversibility:

- *Inability to reverse mitochondrial dysfunction* (lack of ATP generation) even after resolution of the original injury
- Development of profound disturbances in membrane function

Leakage of intracellular enzymes or proteins across abnormally permeable plasma membranes into the bloodstream provides important clinical markers of cell death. Cardiac muscle contains a specific isoform of the enzyme creatine kinase and of the contractile protein troponin; hepatocytes contain transaminases, and hepatic bile duct epithelium contains a temperature-resistant isoform of alkaline phosphatase. Irreversible injury in these tissues is consequently reflected by increased circulating levels of such proteins in the blood.

MORPHOLOGY OF CELL INJURY AND NECROSIS (p. 19)

Injury leads to loss of cell function long before damage is morphologically recognizable. Morphologic changes become apparent only some time after a critical biochemical system within the cell has been deranged; the interval between injury and morphologic change depends on the method of detection (Fig. 1–3). However, once developed, reversible injury and irreversible injury (*necrosis*) both have characteristic features.

Reversible Injury (p. 19)

- *Cell swelling* appears whenever cells cannot maintain ionic and fluid homeostasis (largely due to loss of activity in plasma membrane energy-dependent ion pumps).
- *Fatty change* is manifested by cytoplasmic lipid vacuoles, principally encountered in cells involved in or dependent on fat metabolism (e.g., hepatocytes and myocardial cells).

Necrosis (p. 21)

Necrosis is the sum of the morphologic changes that follow cell death in living tissue or organs. Two processes underlie the basic morphologic changes:

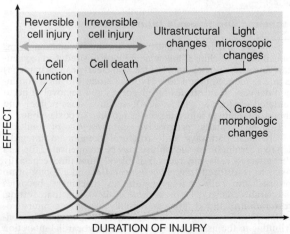

FIGURE 1–3 Timing of biochemical and morphologic changes in cell injury.

- Denaturation of proteins
- Enzymatic digestion of organelles and other cytosolic components

There are several distinctive features: necrotic cells are more *eosinophilic* (pink) than viable cells by standard hematoxylin and eosin (H&E) staining. They appear "glassy" owing to glycogen loss and may be vacuolated; cell membranes are fragmented. Necrotic cells may attract calcium salts; this is particularly true of necrotic fat cells (forming fatty soaps). Nuclear changes include *pyknosis* (small, dense nucleus), *karyolysis* (faint, dissolved nucleus), and *karyorrhexis* (fragmented nucleus). General tissue patterns of necrosis include

- *Coagulative necrosis* (p. 21) is the most common pattern, predominated by protein denaturation with preservation of the cell and tissue framework. This pattern is characteristic of hypoxic death in all tissues except the brain. Necrotic tissue undergoes either *heterolysis* (digestion by lysosomal enzymes of invading leukocytes) or *autolysis* (digestion by its own lysosomal enzymes).
- *Liquefactive necrosis* (p. 22) occurs when autolysis or heterolysis predominates over protein denaturation. The necrotic area is soft and filled with fluid. This type of necrosis is most frequently seen in localized bacterial infections (*abscesses*) and in the brain.
- *Caseous necrosis* (p. 22) is characteristic of tuberculous lesions; it appears grossly as soft, friable, "cheesy" material and microscopically as amorphous eosinophilic material with cell debris.
- *Fat necrosis* (p. 22) is seen in adipose tissue; lipase activation (e.g., from injured pancreatic cells or macrophages) releases fatty acids from triglycerides, which then complex with calcium to create soaps. Grossly, these are white, chalky areas (*fat saponification*); histologically, there are vague cell outlines and calcium deposition.

EXAMPLES OF CELL INJURY AND NECROSIS
(p. 23)

Ischemic and Hypoxic Injury (p. 23)

Ischemia and hypoxic injury are the most common forms of cell injury in clinical medicine. Hypoxia is reduced oxygen-carrying capacity; ischemia (which also clearly causes hypoxia) is due to reduced blood flow. Hypoxia alone will allow continued delivery of substrates for glycolysis and removal of accumulated wastes (e.g., lactic acid); ischemia does neither and therefore tends to injure tissues faster than hypoxia alone.

Ischemia causes progressive compromise of multiple biochemical pathways and structural component integrity. Up to a certain point, such injury may be compensated for, and the affected cells can recover if blood flow (and especially oxygen) is restored (*reversible injury*). Beyond a "point of no return," the cells' energy-generating machinery becomes irreparably damaged (*irreversible injury*). In that setting, restoration of blood flow can actually exacerbate injury, so-called *reperfusion injury*; this is clinically important in contributing to the tissue damage following myocardial infarction and stroke.

Reversible Injury

Hypoxia leads to loss of ATP generation by mitochondria; ATP depletion has multiple, initially reversible effects (Fig. 1–4):

- Failure of Na⁺/K⁺-ATPase membrane transport causes sodium to enter the cell and potassium to exit; there is also increased Ca^{2+} influx as well as release of Ca^{2+} from intracellular stores. The net gain of solute is accompanied by isosmotic gain of water, *cell swelling*, and endoplasmic reticulum dilation. Cell swelling is also increased owing to the *osmotic load* from accumulation of metabolic breakdown products.

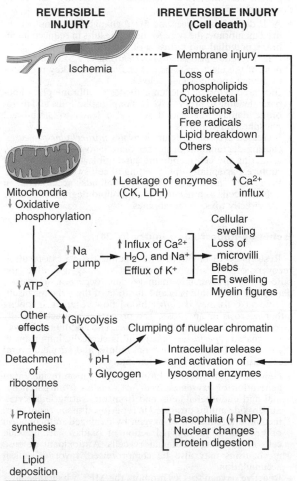

FIGURE 1–4 Postulated sequence of events in reversible and irreversible ischemic cell injury. Although reduced ATP levels play a central role, ischemia can also cause direct membrane damage. CK, creatine kinase; ER, endoplasmic reticulum; LDH, lactate dehydrogenase; RNP, ribonucleoprotein.

- *Cellular energy metabolism* is altered. With hypoxia, cells use *anaerobic glycolysis* for energy production (metabolism of glucose derived from glycogen). Consequently, *glycogen stores are rapidly depleted*, with lactic acid accumulation and *reduced intracellular pH*.
- Reduced protein synthesis results from detachment of ribosomes from rough endoplasmic reticulum.

Irreversible Injury

All the aforementioned changes are reversible if oxygenation is restored. If ischemia persists, irreversible injury ensues, a transition largely dependent on the extent of *ATP depletion* and *membrane dysfunction*, particularly mitochondrial membranes.

- ATP depletion induces the *MPT* change in the mitochondrial membrane; the pore formation results in reduced membrane potential and diffusion of solutes.
- ATP depletion also *releases cytochrome c*, a soluble component of the electron transport chain that is a key regulator in driving apoptosis (see below).
- Increased cytosolic calcium activates membrane phospholipases, leading to progressive loss of phospholipids and membrane damage; decreased ATP also leads to diminished phospholipid synthesis.
- Increased cytosolic calcium *activates intracellular proteases*, causing degradation of intermediate cytoskeletal elements, rendering the cell membrane susceptible to stretching and rupture, particularly in the setting of cell swelling.
- Free fatty acids and lysophospholipids accumulate in ischemic cells as a result of phospholipid degradation; these are directly toxic to membranes.

Ischemia-Reperfusion Injury (p. 24)

Restoration of blood flow to ischemic tissues can result in recovery of reversibly injured cells, or may not affect the outcome if irreversible damage has occurred. However, depending on the intensity and duration of the ischemic insult, additional cells may die *after* blood flow resumes, involving either necrosis or apoptosis. The process is characteristically associated with neutrophilic infiltrates. The additional damage is designated *reperfusion injury* and is clinically important in myocardial infarction, acute renal failure, and stroke. Several mechanisms underlie reperfusion injury:

- New damage may occur during reoxygenation by increased generation of *oxygen-derived free radicals* from parenchymal and endothelial cells, and from infiltrating leukocytes. Superoxide anions produced in reperfused tissue result from incomplete reduction of oxygen by damaged mitochondria or because of the normal action of oxidases from tissue cells or invading inflammatory cells. Antioxidant defense mechanisms may also be compromised, favoring radical accumulation.
- Reactive oxygen species promote the MPT, which precludes mitochondrial recovery and leads to cell death.
- Ischemic injury causes *Inflammation*, the recruitment of circulating polymorphonuclear leukocytes (Chapter 2). Result-

ing from increased cytokine and adhesion molecule expression by hypoxic parenchymal and endothelial cells, the ensuing inflammation causes additional injury. By restoring blood flow, reperfusion may actually *increase* local inflammatory cell infiltration.
- Activation of *complement* may also contribute; the complement system is normally involved in host defense (Chapter 6). Some IgM antibodies deposit in ischemic tissues; when blood flow is resumed, complement proteins bind to the antibodies, are activated, and cause cell injury and inflammation.

Chemical Injury (p. 25)

Chemical injury occurs by two general mechanisms:
- *Directly,* by binding to some critical molecular component (e.g., mercuric chloride binds to cell membrane protein sulfhydryl groups, inhibiting ATPase-dependent transport, and causing increased permeability).
- *Indirectly,* by conversion to reactive toxic metabolites. Toxic metabolites, in turn, cause cellular injury either by direct covalent binding to membrane protein and lipids or, more commonly, by the formation of reactive free radicals. Two examples are carbon tetrachloride and acetaminophen.

APOPTOSIS (p. 26)

Programmed cell death (*apoptosis*) occurs when a cell dies through activation of a tightly regulated internal suicide program. The function of apoptosis is to eliminate unwanted cells selectively, with minimal disturbance to surrounding cells and the host. The cell's plasma membrane remains intact, but its structure is altered so that the apoptotic cell becomes an avid target for phagocytosis. The dead cell is rapidly cleared, before its contents have leaked out, and therefore cell death by this pathway does not elicit an inflammatory reaction in the host. Thus, apoptosis is fundamentally different from necrosis, which is characterized by loss of membrane integrity, enzymatic digestion of cells, and frequently a host reaction (see Table 1–2). However, apoptosis and necrosis sometimes coexist, and they may share some common features and mechanisms.

Causes of Apoptosis (p. 26)

Apoptosis may be physiologic or pathologic.

Physiologic Causes

- Programmed destruction of cells during embryogenesis
- Hormone-dependent involution of tissues (e.g., endometrium, prostate) in the adult
- Cell deletion in proliferating cell populations (e.g., intestinal crypt epithelium) to maintain a constant cell number
- Death of cells that have served their useful purpose (e.g., neutrophils following an acute inflammatory response)
- Deletion of potentially harmful self-reactive lymphocytes
- Cell death induced by cytotoxic T cells (to eliminate virally infected or neoplastic cells)

Pathologic Causes

- Cell death produced by a variety of injurious stimuli. If DNA repair mechanisms cannot cope with the damage caused (e.g., by radiation or cytotoxic drugs), the cell kills itself by apoptosis rather than risk mutations or translocations that could result in malignant transformation. A variety of mild injurious stimuli (including heat and hypoxia) can induce apoptosis; however, larger doses of the same stimuli result in necrosis. Increased MPT due to any cause induces apoptosis. Endoplasmic reticulum stress induced by the accumulation of unfolded proteins also triggers apoptosis (see below).
- Cell death in certain viral infections (e.g., hepatitis).
- Pathologic atrophy in parenchymal organs after duct obstruction (e.g., pancreas).
- Cell death in tumors.

Morphologic Features (p. 27)

Morphologic features of apoptosis (see Table 1–2) include cell shrinkage, chromatin condensation and fragmentation, cellular blebbing and fragmentation into apoptotic bodies, and phagocytosis of apoptotic bodies by adjacent healthy cells or macrophages. Lack of inflammation makes it difficult to detect apoptosis histologically.

Biochemical Features of Apoptosis (p. 27)

- Protein cleavage occurs by a family of proteases called *caspases*. These may also activate DNAases to break down nuclear DNA.
- Internucleosomal cleavage of DNA into fragments about 200 base pairs in size gives rise to a characteristic ladder pattern of DNA bands on agarose gel electrophoresis.
- Plasma membrane alterations (e.g., flipping of phosphatidylserine from the inner to the outer leaf of the plasma membrane) allow recognition of apoptotic cells for phagocytosis.

Mechanisms of Apoptosis (Fig. 1–5) (p. 28)

Apoptosis is induced by a cascade of molecular events that start in distinct ways but ultimately culminate in caspase activation. The mechanisms of apoptosis are phylogenetically conserved; in fact, our basic understanding of them derives in large part from experiments with the nematode *Caenorhabditis elegans*, whose development proceeds by a highly reproducible pattern of cell growth followed by cell death. Studies of mutant worms identified specific genes (called *ced* genes, for *C. elegans death*; these have human homologues) that initiate or inhibit apoptosis.

The process of apoptosis is divided into an *initiation phase* (caspases become active) and an *execution phase*, when the enzymes cause cell death. Initiation of apoptosis occurs through two distinct but convergent pathways: the *extrinsic*, or receptor-initiated, pathway and the *intrinsic*, or mitochondrial, pathway.

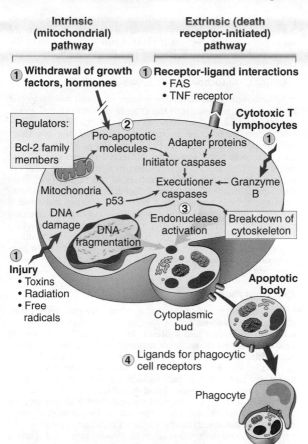

FIGURE 1–5 Mechanisms of apoptosis. Some of the major inducers of apoptosis (1) include specific death ligands (tumor necrosis factor [TNF] and Fas ligand), withdrawal of growth factors or hormones, and injurious agents (e.g., radiation). Some stimuli (such as cytotoxic cells) directly activate executioner caspases (*right*). Others act by way of adapter proteins and initiator caspases, or by mitochondrial events involving cytochrome *c*. Control and regulation (2) are influenced by members of the Bcl-2 family of proteins, which can either inhibit or promote the cell's death. Executioner caspases (3) activate latent cytoplasmic endonucleases and proteases that degrade nuclear and cytoskeletal proteins. This results in a cascade of intracellular degradation, including fragmentation of nuclear chromatin and breakdown of the cytoskeleton. The end result (4) is formation of apoptotic bodies containing intracellular organelles and other cytosolic components; these bodies also express new ligands for binding and uptake by phagocytic cells.

Initiation Phase

Extrinsic (Death Receptor) Pathway

Death receptors are members of the tumor necrosis factor (TNF) receptor family (e.g., type 1 TNF receptor and Fas); they have a cytoplasmic *death domain* involved in protein-protein interactions. Cross-linking by external ligands causes these receptors to multimerize to form binding sites for adapter proteins that in turn bring multiple inactive caspase-8 molecules into close proximity. Low-level enzymatic activity of these pro-caspases eventually cleaves and activates one of the assembled group, rapidly leading to a downstream cascade of caspase activation.

Intrinsic (Mitochondrial) Pathway

Mitochondrial permeability is increased, and pro-apoptotic molecules are released into the cytoplasm; death receptors are not involved. More than 20 proteins of the Bcl-2 family of proteins normally function to regulate apoptosis; the two main anti-apoptotic proteins are Bcl-2 and Bcl-x. When cells are deprived of survival signals or subjected to stress, Bcl-2 and Bcl-x are lost from the mitochondrial membrane and are replaced by pro-apoptotic members of the family (e.g., Bak, Bax, and Bim). With decreasing Bcl-2/Bcl-x levels, mitochondrial membrane permeability increases, leaking out several proteins that can activate caspases. For example, released cytochrome *c* binds to Apaf-1 protein (apoptosis activating factor-1) and the complex triggers caspase-9 activation. *The essence of the intrinsic pathway is a balance between pro-apoptotic and protective molecules that regulate mitochondrial permeability.*

Execution Pathway

The proteolytic caspases that mediate the execution phase are highly conserved across species: in the term *caspase,* "c" refers to an active site cysteine and "aspase" refers to the unique ability to cleave after aspartic acid residues. Caspases are divided into two basic groups—initiator and executioner—depending on the order in which they are activated during apoptosis. Initiator caspases include caspase-8 and -9; several caspases, including caspase-3 and -6, serve as executioners. Caspases exist as inactive proenzymes and must undergo an activating cleavage; the cleavage sites can be hydrolyzed by other caspases or autocatalytically. Once an initiator caspase is activated, the death program is set in motion by rapid and sequential activation of other caspases. Executioner caspases act on many cell components; they cleave cytoskeletal and nuclear matrix proteins, disrupting the cytoskeleton and leading to nuclear breakdown. In the nucleus, caspases cleave proteins involved in transcription, DNA replication, and DNA repair; in particular, caspase-3 activates a cytoplasmic DNAase resulting in the characteristic internucleosomal cleavage of DNA.

Examples of Apoptosis (p. 31)

Growth Factor Deprivation

Growth factor deprivation affects hormone-sensitive cells deprived of the relevant hormone, lymphocytes not stimulated by antigens or cytokines, and neurons deprived of nerve growth factor. Apoptosis is triggered by the intrinsic (mitochondrial) pathway due to a relative excess of pro-apoptotic versus anti-apoptotic members of the Bcl family.

DNA Damage

Radiation or chemotherapeutic agents induce apoptosis via mechanisms triggered by DNA damage. When DNA is damaged, the tumor-suppressor gene *p53* accumulates; this results in cell cycle arrest (at the G_1 phase) to allow time for repair (Chapter 7). If DNA repair cannot take place, p53 triggers apoptosis through increased transcription of several pro-apoptotic members of the Bcl family, notably Bax and Bak, as well as Apaf-1. When p53 is absent or mutated (i.e., in certain cancers) apoptosis does not occur and cell survival is favored.

TNF Family Receptors

As discussed above, the cell receptor Fas (CD95) induces apoptosis when cross-linked by Fas ligand (FasL or CD95L), a protein produced by cells of the immune system. Fas-FasL interactions are important for eliminating lymphocytes that recognize self-antigens; mutations in Fas or FasL result in autoimmune diseases (Chapter 6).

TNF is an important mediator of the inflammatory reaction (Chapter 2), and can also induce apoptosis; the pathway is summarized above. The major inflammatory functions of TNF are mediated by activation of the transcription factor nuclear factor-κB (NF-κB). TNF-mediated signals accomplish this by stimulating degradation of the inhibitor of NF-κB (IκB), which promotes cell survival. Whether TNF signals induce cell death or promote cell survival probably depends on which adapter protein attaches to the TNF receptor after TNF binding.

Cytotoxic T Lymphocytes

Cytotoxic T lymphocytes (CTLs) recognize foreign antigens on the surface of infected host cells (Chapter 6) and secrete *perforin*, a transmembrane pore-forming molecule that allows entry of the CTL-derived serine protease *granzyme B*. Granzyme B cleaves proteins at aspartate residues and thereby activates multiple caspases. Thus, CTLs bypass the upstream signaling events and directly induce the effector phase of apoptosis. CTLs also express FasL on their surfaces and kill target cells by ligation of Fas receptors.

Dysregulated Apoptosis

Dysregulated ("too little or too much") apoptosis underlies multiple diseases.

- *Disorders with defective apoptosis and increased cell survival*. Inappropriate low rates of apoptosis may prolong the survival or reduce the turnover of abnormal cells. The accumulated cells may lead to (1) *cancers*, especially tumors with *p53* mutations, or hormone-dependent tumors, such as breast, prostate, or ovarian cancers (Chapter 7); and (2) *autoimmune disorders*, which could arise if autoreactive lymphocytes are not eliminated (Chapter 6).
- *Disorders with increased apoptosis and excessive cell death*. Characterized by a marked loss of normal cells, these disorders include (1) *neurodegenerative diseases*, with loss of specific sets of neurons (e.g., the spinal muscular atrophies, Chapter 27); (2) *ischemic injury* (e.g., myocardial infarction, Chapter 12; and stroke, Chapter 28); and (3) *death of virus-infected cells* (Chapter 8).

SUBCELLULAR RESPONSES TO INJURY (p. 32)

Certain conditions are associated with distinctive alterations in cell organelles or cytoskeleton. Some of these alterations fall under the category of adaptive responses (maintaining homeostasis), others occur in more chronic forms of reversible cellular injury, and still others are seen in the setting of irreversible injury.

Lysosomal Catabolism (p. 32)

Primary lysosomes are membrane-bound organelles containing a variety of hydrolytic enzymes; they fuse with membrane-bound vacuoles containing ingested material to form *phagolysosomes* (or *secondary lysosomes*). Lysosomal catabolism degrades materials from two distinct sources:

- *Heterophagy* involves uptake and degradation of materials from the *external* environment by phagocytosis. Examples include ingestion of bacteria by leukocytes, removal of necrotic debris by macrophages, and reabsorption of protein by the proximal tubules.
- *Autophagy* involves the lysosomal degradation of degenerating *intracellular* organelles, including mitochondria and endoplasmic reticulum. Autophagy is particularly pronounced in cells undergoing atrophy.

Lysosomal enzymes can degrade most proteins and carbohydrates, although some lipids remain undigested; undigested debris or abnormal substances that cannot be completely metabolized may persist within cells as *residual bodies* or may be extruded. *Lipofuscin pigment* granules represent undigested material derived from intracellular lipid peroxidation. Certain indigestible pigments, such as carbon particles inhaled from the atmosphere, can persist in secondary lysosomes of macrophages for decades. Hereditary *lysosomal storage disorders*, caused by deficiencies of enzymes that degrade certain macromolecules, result in the accumulation of these compounds in lysosomes; this is particularly problematic in neurons, and leads to severe neurologic abnormalities (Chapter 5).

Induction (Hypertrophy) of Smooth Endoplasmic Reticulum (p. 33)

Smooth endoplasmic reticulum (SER) is the intracellular site for metabolizing a variety of exogenous agents, typically involving the mixed-function oxidase (P-450) pathway; prolonged exposure to such agents will induce SER adaptive hypertrophy. Thus, chronic ingestion of certain drugs (e.g., phenobarbital) leads to increased SER volume; such hypertrophy results in more rapid breakdown and increased tolerance to the drug, as well as increased capacity to metabolize other drugs handled by the same system.

Mitochondrial Alterations (p. 33)

Besides playing critical roles in acute cellular injury and apoptosis, changes in mitochondria also occur in some pathologic conditions:

- In cell hypertrophy and atrophy, there is a corresponding increase or a decrease in mitochondrial number.
- Mitochondria may assume extremely large and abnormal shapes (*megamitochondria*, seen in hepatocytes in alcoholic liver disease or nutritional deficiencies).
- In *mitochondrial myopathies* (an hereditary form of muscle disease), mitochondrial metabolic defects are associated with increased numbers of morphologically abnormal mitochondria.
- *Oncocytomas* are benign tumors consisting of cells with abundant enlarged mitochondria.

Cytoskeletal Abnormalities (p. 34)

The cytoskeleton consists of microtubules, thin actin filaments, myosin thick filaments, and various classes of intermediate filaments. Cytoskeletal abnormalities may cause defects in cell function, such as cell locomotion or the movement of intracellular organelles (e.g., microtubule defects cause immotile cilia or Kartagener syndrome). Alternatively, cytoskeletal changes may be caused by cellular injury; for example, metabolic derangements in alcoholic liver disease lead to abnormal intracellular accumulations of intermediate filaments (Mallory bodies)

INTRACELLULAR ACCUMULATIONS (p. 34)

Cells may accumulate abnormal amounts of various substances.
- A *normal* endogenous substance (water, protein, carbohydrate, lipid) is produced at a normal (or even increased) rate, but the metabolic rate is inadequate to remove it (e.g., fat accumulation in liver cells).
- A *normal or abnormal* endogenous substance accumulates because of genetic or acquired defects in the *metabolism, packaging, transport, or secretion* of these substances (e.g., lysososmal storage diseases, or α_1-antitrypsin disease, in which α_1-antitrypsin accumulates in the endoplasmic recticulum of liver cells that produce it).
- *Abnormal exogenous substances* may accumulate in normal cells because they lack the machinery to degrade such substances (e.g., macrophages laden with environmental carbon).

Lipids (p. 35)

Triglycerides (the most common), cholesterol and cholesterol esters, and phospholipids can accumulate in cells.

Steatosis (Fatty Change)

Steatosis occurs when a normal constituent (triglycerides) accumulates, leading to an absolute increase in intracellular lipids. It occurs occasionally in almost all organs, but is most common in the liver. Fatty change in the liver is reversible, but in excess may lead to cirrhosis.

In the liver, causes include alcohol abuse (most common in the United States), protein malnutrition, diabetes mellitus, obesity, hepatotoxins, and anoxia. Grossly, fatty livers are

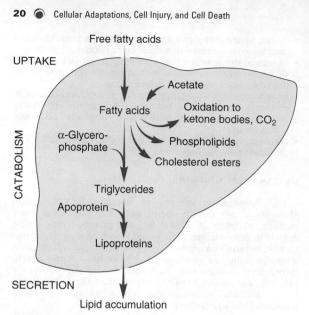

Free fatty acids

UPTAKE

Fatty acids

Acetate

Oxidation to
ketone bodies, CO_2

α-Glycero-
phosphate

Phospholipids

Cholesterol esters

CATABOLISM

Triglycerides

Apoprotein

Lipoproteins

SECRETION

Lipid accumulation

FIGURE 1–6 Schematic diagram of the possible mechanisms leading to accumulation of triglycerides in fatty liver. Defects in any of the steps of uptake, catabolism, or secretion can result in lipid accumulation.

enlarged, yellow, and greasy; microscopically, the fat is seen as small, intracytoplasmic droplets or as large vacuoles. The condition is caused by one of the following mechanisms (Fig. 1–6):

- Excessive entry of free fatty acids into the liver (e.g., starvation, corticosteroid therapy)
- Enhanced fatty acid synthesis
- Decreased fatty acid oxidation (anoxia)
- Increased esterification of fatty acids to triglycerides due to increased α-glycerophosphate (e.g., secondary to alcohol)
- Decreased apoprotein synthesis (e.g., carbon tetrachloride poisoning, starvation)
- Impaired lipoprotein secretion from the liver (alcohol, orotic acid administration)

Cholesterol and Cholesterol Esters

Cholesterol is normally required for cell membrane or lipid-soluble hormone synthesis; production is tightly regulated but accumulation (seen as intracellular cytoplasmic vacuoles) can be present in a variety of pathologic states:

- *Atherosclerosis:* Cholesterol and cholesterol esters accumulate in arterial wall smooth muscle cells and macrophages (Chapter 11). Extracellular accumulations appear microscopically as cleftlike cavities formed when cholesterol crystals are dissolved during normal histologic processing.
- *Xanthomas:* In acquired and hereditary *hyperlipidemias*, lipids accumulate in clusters of "foamy" macrophages and mesenchymal cells.
- *Inflammation and necrosis:* Lipid-laden (foamy) macrophages result from phagocytosis of membrane lipids derived from injured cells.

- *Cholesterolosis:* Focal accumulations of cholesterol-laden macrophages occur in the lamina propria of gallbladders.
- *Niemann-Pick disease, type C:* This type of lysosomal storage disease is due to mutation of an enzyme involved in cholesterol catabolism.

Proteins (p. 37)

Intracellular protein accumulation may be due to excessive synthesis, absorption, or defects in cellular transport. Morphologically visible accumulations appear as rounded, eosinophilic cytoplasmic droplets. Classic examples of *intracellular* protein deposition include protein in proximal convoluted tubular epithelium due to chronic reabsorption in the setting of proteinuria, and immunoglobulin distending the endoplasmic reticulum of plasma cells due to exuberant synthesis (forming so-called *Russell bodies*). In some disorders (e.g., *amyloidosis*, Chapter 6), abnormal proteins deposit primarily in the *extracellular* space.

Defects in *protein folding* underlie some protein depositions. After synthesis, partially folded intermediates can form intracellular aggregates that entangle multiple proteins. To prevent this, unfolded intermediates are typically stabilized by interactions with molecular *chaperones*; chaperones are also involved in transporting proteins into organellar destinations (Fig. 1–7). Altered protein folding causes disease by

- *Defective intracellular transport and secretion of critical proteins.* Examples include α_1-*antitrypsin deficiency*, in which mutations slow protein folding; partially folded intermediates accumulate in the endoplasmic reticulum of hepatocytes. Loss of secreted α_1-antitrypsin leads to emphysema (Chapter 15). In *cystic fibrosis*, the most common mutation delays dissociation of the chloride channel protein from its chaperones, resulting in abnormal folding and subsequent degradation.
- *Toxicity of aggregated, abnormally folded proteins.* Aggregation of abnormally folded proteins (e.g., due to genetic mutations, aging, or environmental factors) is characteristic of *neurodegenerative disorders*, including the Alzheimer, Huntington, and Parkinson diseases, as well as amyloidosis.

Hyaline Change (p. 39)

Hyaline change refers to any alteration within cells or in the extracellular spaces that imparts a homogeneous, glassy pink appearance in routine H&E-stained histologic sections. Examples of *intracellular hyaline change* include proximal tubule epithelial protein droplets, Russell bodies, viral inclusions, and aggregated intermediate filaments (Mallory bodies). *Extracellular hyaline change* occurs, for example, in damaged arterioles (e.g., due to chronic hypertension), presumably due to extravasated proteins.

Glycogen (p. 39)

Glycogen is a readily available cytoplasmic energy store. Excessive intracellular deposits (seen as clear vacuoles) are seen with abnormalities of glycogen storage (so-called

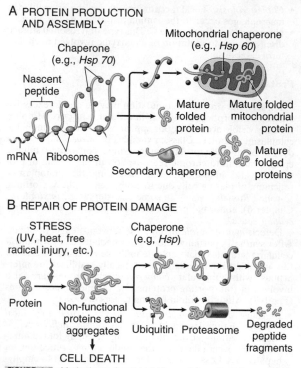

FIGURE 1-7 Mechanisms of protein folding and the role of chaperones. *A,* Chaperones, such as heat shock proteins (Hsp), protect unfolded or partially folded proteins from degradation and guide proteins into organelles. *B,* Chaperones repair misfolded proteins; when this process is ineffective, proteins are targeted for degradation in the proteasome. If misfolded proteins accumulate, they trigger apoptosis. UV, ultraviolet.

glycogenoses, Chapter 5) and glucose metabolism (*diabetes mellitus*)

Pigments (p. 39)

Accumulated materials are frequently *pigments,* which may be exogenous (e.g., coal dust) or endogenous, such as melanin or hemosiderin.

- Exogenous pigments include carbon or coal dust (most common); these deposits are called *anthracosis* when they accumulate in pulmonary macrophages and lymph nodes. Pigments from *tattooing* are taken up by macrophages and persist for the life of the cell.
- Endogenous pigments include

  Lipofuscin, the so-called "*wear-and-tear*" pigment, is usually associated with cellular and tissue atrophy (*brown atrophy*). This is seen microscopically as fine yellow-brown intracytoplasmic granules. The pigment is composed of complex lipids, phospholipids, and protein, probably derived from cell membrane lipid peroxidation.

Hemosiderin is a hemoglobin-derived, golden yellow-brown, granular intracellular pigment composed of aggregated ferritin. Accumulation may be localized (due to macrophage-mediated metabolism of a focal hemorrhage, such as in a bruise). Systemic accumulation may be due to increased dietary iron absorption (*primary hemochromatosis*), impaired utilization (e.g., thalassemia), hemolysis, or chronic transfusions (Chapter 18).

Melanin, an endogenous, non–hemoglobin-derived, brown-black pigment, is formed by enzymatic oxidation of tyrosine to dihydroxyphenylalanine in melanocytes.

PATHOLOGIC CALCIFICATION (p. 41)

Pathologic calcification occurs in two forms and is the abnormal tissue deposition of calcium salts. *Dystrophic calcification* occurs in nonviable or dying tissues in the presence of normal calcium serum levels. *Metastatic calcification* occurs in viable tissues and is associated with hypercalcemia.

Dystrophic Calcification (p. 41)

Although it may simply reflect sites of prior injury, it can also be a source of significant pathology. Dystrophic calcification occurs in arteries in atherosclerosis, in damaged heart valves, and in areas of necrosis (coagulative, caseous, and liquefactive). Calcium can be intracellular and extracellular. Deposition ultimately involves precipitation of a crystalline calcium phosphate similar to bone hydroxyapatite:

- *Initiation* (*nucleation*) occurs extracellularly or intracellularly. *Extracellular* initiation occurs on membrane-bound vesicles from dead or dying cells that concentrate calcium due to their content of charged phospholipids; membrane-bound phosphatases then generate phosphates that form calcium-phosphate complexes; the cycle of calcium and phosphate binding is repeated, eventually producing a deposit. Initiation of *intracellular* calcification occurs in mitochondria of dead or dying cells.
- *Propagation* of crystal formation depends on the concentration of calcium and phosphates, the presence of inhibitors, and structural components of the extracellular matrix.

Metastatic Calcification (p. 41)

Calcium deposits are seen as amorphous basophilic densities that may occur widely throughout the body. Typically, these have no clinical sequelae, although massive deposition can cause renal and lung deficits. Metastatic calcification results from hypercalcemia (four principal causes):

- *Increased secretion of parathyroid hormone* (e.g., in hyperparathyroidism from parathyroid tumors or ectopic secretion of parathyroid hormone by malignant tumors)
- *Destruction of bone tissue*, as in primary marrow malignancies (e.g., multiple myeloma) or by diffuse skeletal metastasis (e.g., breast cancer), by accelerated bone turnover (*Paget's disease*), or immobilization
- *Vitamin D–related disorders*, including vitamin D intoxication and systemic sarcoidosis

- *Associated with renal failure*, which causes secondary hyperparathyroidism due to phosphate retention

CELLULAR AGING (p. 42)

With age, physiologic and structural alterations occur in almost all organ systems. Aging in individuals is affected by genetic factors; diet; social conditions; and the occurrence of age-related diseases, such as atherosclerosis, diabetes, and osteoarthritis. In addition, age-induced alterations in cells, potentially reflecting the accumulated effects of sublethal cellular and molecular damage, are important in the aging of the organism (Fig. 1–8).

Functional and Morphologic Changes

A number of functional and morphologic alterations occur in aging cells:

Diminished Metabolic Functions

- Reduced mitochondrial ATP generation
- Diminished synthesis of structural, enzymatic, and regulatory proteins
- Decreased capacity for nutrient uptake
- Increased DNA damage and diminished repair
- Accumulation of oxidative damage in proteins and lipids (e.g., lipofuscin pigment)
- Accumulation of advanced glycation end products, causing protein cross-linking

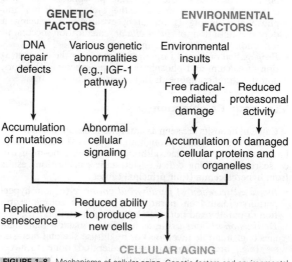

FIGURE 1–8 Mechanisms of cellular aging. Genetic factors and environmental insults combine to produce the cellular abnormalities characteristic of aging. IGF-1, insulin-like growth factor-1.

Morphologic Alterations

- Irregular and abnormally lobed nuclei
- Pleomorphic and vacuolated mitochondria
- Decreased endoplasmic reticulum
- Distorted Golgi apparatus

Mechanisms of Cellular Aging

Three interrelated processes likely account for cellular aging: (i) *replicative senescence*, that is, cells have a limited capacity for replication; (ii) genes that influence the aging process; and (iii) progressive accumulation of metabolic and genetic damage due to continuous exogenous influences.

Replicative Senescence (p. 42)

Cellular senescence is inferred from in vitro studies showing that normal human diploid fibroblasts have finite life spans in culture, with population doublings that are age dependent (i.e., they have *clocks* [the Hayflick theory]). Many changes in gene expression accompany cellular senescence, including those that inhibit cell cycle progression. *Telomere shortening* (incomplete replication of chromosome ends) is also a likely mechanism underlying cell senescence. Telomeres are short repeated sequences of DNA that compose the linear ends of chromosomes; they are important to ensure complete replication of chromosome ends and to protect chromosomal termini from fusion and degradation. When cells replicate, a small section of the telomere is not replicated. As cells repeatedly divide, telomeres become progressively shortened, ultimately signaling a growth checkpoint, and cells become senescent. In some cancer cells, telomerase seems to be reactivated, suggesting that telomere elongation might be important in conferring cell immortality (Fig. 1–9).

Genes that Influence the Aging Process (p. 43)

Studies in *C. elegans* suggest that individual genes can affect longevity; thus, decreased signaling through the insulin-like growth factor-1 (IGF-1) receptor (due to mutations or decreased caloric intake) can result in prolonged life span; signals downstream of the IGF-1 receptor may lead to gene silencing that promotes aging.

Accumulation of Metabolic and Genetic Damage (p. 43)

Cellular aging may result from a balance between damage due to metabolic events within the cell and the counterbalancing molecular responses that can repair injury. For example, reactive oxygen metabolites (byproducts of normal oxidative phosphorylation) cause covalent modifications of proteins, lipids, and nucleic acids. The amount of oxidative damage increases with age and may be an important component of senescence. Increased production of these reactive species (e.g., because of a high-calorie diet or exposure to ionizing radiation) correlates with a shortened life span. Protective cellular responses counterbalance the progressive damage. These systems include:

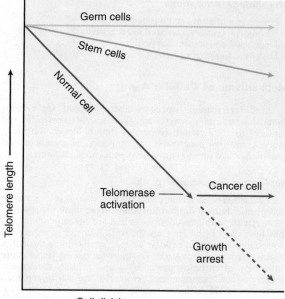

FIGURE 1-9 The telomere hypothesis and proliferative capacity. Telomere length is plotted against the number of cell divisions. In normal somatic cells, there is no telomerase activity, and telomeres progressively shorten with increasing cell divisions until growth arrest, or senescence, occurs. Germ cells and stem cells both contain telomerase activity, but only the germ cells have levels of the enzyme that are sufficient to stabilize telomere length completely. Telomerase activation in cancer cells inactivates the telomeric clock that limits the proliferative capacity of normal somatic cells. (Modified and redrawn from Holt SE, et al: Refining the telomere-telomerase hypothesis of aging and cancer. Nat Biotech 14:836–839, 1996.)

- *Antioxidant defense mechanisms.* A reduction in antioxidant defense mechanisms (e.g., vitamin E) correlates with shortened life span.
- *Recognition and repair of damaged DNA.* The importance of DNA repair in the aging process is illustrated by patients with *Werner syndrome*, who show premature aging. A defect in *DNA helicase* causes this syndrome and results in rapid accumulation of chromosomal damage, mimicking the injury that normally accrues with aging. Genetic instability is also characteristic of other disorders associated with premature aging.

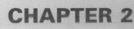

CHAPTER 2

Acute and Chronic Inflammation

GENERAL FEATURES OF INFLAMMATION (p. 48)

Inflammation is the response of vascularized living tissue to injury. It may be evoked by microbial infections, physical agents, chemicals, necrotic tissue, or immune reactions. Inflammation is intended to contain and isolate injury, to destroy invading microorganisms and inactivate toxins, and to prepare the tissue for healing and repair (Chapter 3). Although it is fundamentally a protective response, inflammation may also be harmful; it can cause life-threatening hypersensitivity reactions, or relentless and progressive organ damage from chronic inflammation and subsequent fibrosis (e.g., rheumatoid arthritis, atherosclerosis). Inflammation is generally characterized by:

- Two main components, a vascular wall response and an inflammatory cell response.
- Effects mediated by circulating plasma proteins and by factors produced locally by vessel wall or inflammatory cells.
- Termination when the offending agent is eliminated and the secreted mediators are removed; active anti-inflammatory mechanisms are also involved.

Inflammation has *acute* and *chronic* patterns:

- *Acute inflammation:* early onset (seconds to minutes), short duration (minutes to days), involving fluid exudation (*edema*) and polymorphonuclear cell (neutrophil) emigration
- *Chronic inflammation:* later onset (days) and longer duration (weeks to years), involving lymphocytes and macrophages, and inducing blood vessel proliferation and scarring

There are four classic clinical signs of inflammation (most prominent in acute inflammation):

- Heat (Latin: *calor*)
- Redness (Latin: *rubor*)

- Edema (Latin: *tumor*)
- Pain (Latin: *dolor*)

Loss of function (Latin: *functio laesa*) may also be considered a clinical sign of inflammation.

Definitions

Edema Excess fluid in interstitial tissue or body cavities; may be either an exudate or a transudate

Exudate An inflammatory extravascular fluid that has a high protein concentration and cellular debris; specific gravity above 1.020

Exudation Extravasation of fluid, proteins, and blood cells from vessels into the interstitial tissue or body cavities

Pus A purulent inflammatory exudate rich in neutrophils and cell debris

Transudate An extravascular fluid with low protein content and specific gravity below 1.012; essentially an ultrafiltrate of blood plasma resulting from elevated fluid pressures or diminished osmotic forces in the plasma

ACUTE INFLAMMATION (p. 49)

Acute inflammation has three major components that contribute to causing the clinical signs:

- Alterations in vascular caliber leading to increased blood flow (heat and redness)
- Structural changes in the microvasculature permitting plasma proteins and leukocytes to leave the circulation to produce inflammatory *exudates* (edema)
- Leukocyte emigration from blood vessels and accumulation at the site of injury (edema and pain)

Vascular Changes (p. 50)

Normal fluid exchange in vascular beds depends on an intact endothelium and is modulated by two opposing forces (Fig. 2–1*A*):

- Hydrostatic pressure causes fluid to move out of the circulation.
- Plasma colloid osmotic pressure causes fluid to move into the capillaries.

Beginning immediately after injury the vascular wall develops changes in caliber and permeability that affect flow; the changes develop at various rates depending on injury severity.

- *Vasodilation* (with or without prior transient vasoconstriction) causes increased flow into areas of injury, and thereby *increases hydrostatic pressure.*
- Increased vascular permeability causes exudation of protein-rich fluid and decreases plasma osmotic pressure (see below).

The combination of increased hydrostatic pressure and decreased osmotic pressure causes a marked net outflow of fluid and edema formation (Fig. 2–1*B*). *Stasis* occurs when fluid loss causes concentration of red cells and increased blood viscosity, slowing the blood flow. With stasis, white cells (mostly

A. NORMAL

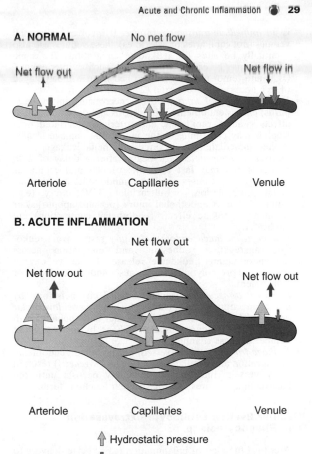

FIGURE 2-1 Blood pressure and plasma colloid osmotic forces in normal and inflamed microcirculation. *A,* Normal hydrostatic pressure is about 32 mm Hg *(open upward arrows)* at the arterial end of the capillary and 12 mm Hg at the venous end *(open downward arrows).* The mean colloid osmotic pressure of tissues is approximately 25 mm Hg. Although fluid tends to leave the precapillary arteriole, it is returned in equal amounts via the postcapillary venule. Under these conditions, net flow *(black arrows)* in or out of the vessel is zero. *B,* Acute inflammation. Arteriolar dilation causes the mean capillary pressure to increase to 50 mm Hg, and the venous pressure increases to approximately 30 mm Hg. At the same time, osmotic pressure is reduced (averaging 20 mm Hg) because of protein leakage across the venule. The net result is an excess of extravasated fluid.

neutrophils) accumulate along the endothelium (*margination*) and begin to emigrate through the vessel wall.

Increased vascular permeability can be induced by several different pathways (p. 51, Fig. 2–4):

- *Formation of venule intercellular endothelial gaps* is the most common mechanism underlying increased vascular permeability; endothelial cells are induced to contract, thereby opening intercellular gaps. Contraction is elicited by chemical mediators (e.g., histamine), occurs rapidly after injury, and is reversible and transient (15 to 30 minutes); hence, it is an *immediate-transient response*. It involves only small venules (not capillaries or arterioles); these venules will also eventually be sites for leukocyte emigration. The same response may be caused by *cytokines*, such as interleukin 1 (IL1) and tumor necrosis factor (TNF), but will be delayed (4 to 6 hours) and protracted (24 hours or more).

- *Direct endothelial injury*. Severe necrotizing injury (e.g., burns) causes endothelial cell necrosis and detachment that affects venules, capillaries, and arterioles; recruited neutrophils may contribute to the injury. The damage usually evokes immediate and sustained endothelial leakage.

- *Delayed prolonged leakage* begins after a delay of 2 to 12 hours and may last for days; venules and capillaries are affected. Causes include mild-moderate thermal injury, x-irradiation, or ultraviolet (UV) injury (e.g., sunburn). Direct endothelial injury (perhaps apoptosis) or secondary cytokine effects (endothelial contraction) are implicated.

- *Leukocyte-mediated endothelial injury* results from leukocyte aggregation, adhesion, and emigration across the endothelium. Leukocyte release of reactive oxygen species and proteolytic enzymes causes endothelial injury or detachment.

- *Increased transcytosis*. Transendothelial channels form by interconnection of vesicles from the *vesiculovacuolar organelle*. Certain factors (e.g., vascular endothelial growth factor, VEGF) induce vascular leakage by increasing the number of these channels.

- *Leakage from new blood vessels*. During repair, endothelial proliferation and capillary sprouting (*angiogenesis*) result in leaky vessels. Increased permeability persists until the endothelium matures and intercellular junctions form.

Cellular Events: Leukocyte Extravasation and Phagocytosis (p. 53)

A critical function of inflammation is leukocyte delivery to sites of injury. The sequence of events is called *extravasation*, and is divided into three steps (Fig. 2–2):

- Margination, rolling, and adhesion of leukocytes to the endothelium
- Transmigration across the endothelium (also called *diapedesis*)
- Migration in interstitial tissues toward a chemotactic stimulus

Leukocyte Adhesion and Transmigration (p. 54)

Adhesion and transmigration occur by interactions between complementary adhesion molecules on leukocytes and endothelium. The major adhesion molecule pairs are shown in Table 2–1:

- *Selectins (E, P, and L)* bind via lectin (sugar-binding) domains to oligosaccharides (e.g., sialylated Lewis X) on cell surface glycoproteins.
- *Immunoglobulin family molecules* on endothelial cells include *ICAM-1* (intercellular adhesion molecule 1) and *VCAM-1* (vascular cell adhesion molecule 1); these bind *integrins* on leukocytes.

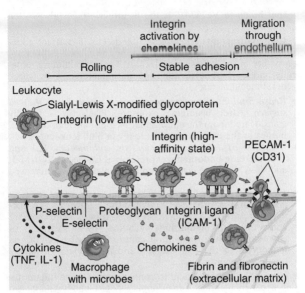

FIGURE 2–2 The multistep process of leukocyte migration through blood vessels, shown here for neutrophils. The leukocytes first roll, then (in sequence) become activated and adhere to endothelium, transmigrate across the endothelium, pierce the basement membrane, and migrate toward chemoattractants emanating from the source of injury. Different molecules play predominant roles in different steps of this process—selectins in rolling; chemokines in activating the neutrophils to increase avidity of integrins; integrins in firm adhesion; and CD31 (PECAM-1) in transmigration.

TABLE 2–1 Endothelial/Leukocyte Adhesion Molecules

Endothelial Molecule	Leukocyte Receptor	Major Role
P-selectin	Sialyl-Lewis X PSGL-1	Rolling (neutrophils, monocytes, lymphocytes)
E-selectin	Sialyl-Lewis X	Rolling, adhesion to activated endothelium (neutrophils, monocytes, T cells)
ICAM-1	CD11/CD18 (integrins) (LFA-1, Mac-1)	Adhesion, arrest, transmigration (all leukocytes)
VCAM-1	α4β1 (VLA4) (integrins) α4β7 (LPAM-1)	Adhesion (eosinophils, monocytes, lymphocytes)
GlyCam-1	L-selectin	Lymphocyte homing to high endothelial venules
CD31 (PECAM)	CD31	Leukocyte migration through endothelium

ICAM-1, VCAM-1, and CD31 belong to the immunoglobulin family of proteins; PSGL-1, P-selectin glycoprotein ligand 1.

- *Integrins* on leukocytes bind to members of the immunoglobulin family molecules and to the extracellular matrix. The principal integrins that bind to ICAM-1 are the so-called β_2 integrins LFA-1 and Mac-1 (also called CD11a/CD18 and CD11b/CD18); the principal integrin that binds to VCAM-1 is the β_1 integrin $\alpha_4\beta_1$ (also called VLA4).

Chemoattractants (*chemokines*) and cytokines affect adhesion and transmigration by modulating the surface expression or avidity of the adhesion molecules. These modulating molecules induce leukocyte adhesion in inflammation by three general mechanisms:

- *Redistribution of preformed adhesion molecules to the cell surface.* After histamine exposure, P-selectin is rapidly translocated from the endothelial Weibel-Palade body membranes to the cell surface, where it can bind leukocytes.
- *Induction of adhesion molecules on endothelium.* IL1 and TNF increase endothelial expression of E-selectin, ICAM-1, and VCAM-1; such *activated* endothelial cells have increased leukocyte adherence.
- *Increased avidity of binding.* This is most important for *integrin* (LFA-1 and Mac-1) binding. These integrins are normally present on leukocytes in a low-affinity form; they are converted to high-affinity binding by a variety of chemokines. Such activation causes firm adhesion of the leukocytes to the endothelium and is required for subsequent transmigration.

Neutrophil adhesion and transmigration in acute inflammation occur by a series of overlapping steps (see Fig. 2–2):

- *Endothelial activation:* Mediators present at inflammatory sites increase the expression of E- and P-selectin by endothelial cells.
- *Leukocyte rolling:* Because of increased vascular permeability and the resulting blood stasis, leukocytes fall out of the vessel laminar flow and roll along endothelium. An initial rapid and relatively loose adhesion results from selectin interactions with their carbohydrate ligands.
- *Integrin activation and stable adhesion:* Leukocytes become activated by chemokines (or other agents) to increase integrin avidity, becoming firmly bound and spread over the endothelium.
- *Transmigration (diapedesis):* This is mediated by homotypic (like-like) interactions between PECAM-1 (platelet-endothelial cell adhesion molecule 1 or CD31) on leukocytes and endothelial cells.

The type of leukocyte that ultimately emigrates into a site of injury depends on the age of the inflammatory response and the original stimulus. In most forms of acute inflammation, *neutrophils predominate during the first 6 to 24 hours, then are replaced by monocytes after 24 to 48 hours.* There are several reasons for this sequence: neutrophils are more numerous in blood than monocytes, they respond more rapidly to chemokines, and they attach more firmly to the particular adhesion molecules that are induced on endothelial cells at early time points. After emigration, neutrophils are also short-lived; they undergo apoptosis after 24 to 48 hours, whereas monocytes survive longer.

Chemotaxis (p. 56)

Adherent leukocytes emigrate through interendothelial junctions, traverse the basement membrane, and move toward sites of injury along gradients of chemotactic agents. For neutrophils, these agents include exogenous bacterial products and endogenous mediators (detailed below) such as complement fragments, arachidonic acid metabolites, and chemokines.

Chemotaxis involves binding of chemotactic agents to specific leukocyte surface G protein–coupled receptors; these trigger activation of phospholipase C, phophoinositol-3-kinase, and protein kinases, generating phosphoinositol second messengers (Chapter 3). These changes cause increased cytosolic calcium and GTPase activities that polymerize actin and facilitate cell movement. Leukocytes move by extending pseudopods that bind the extracellular matrix and can then pull the cell forward.

Leukocyte Activation (p. 57)

Besides cell locomotion, chemotactic agents also cause leukocyte activation including:

- Production of arachidonic acid metabolites
- Degranulation and secretion of lysosomal enzymes
- Cytokine secretion
- Increased adhesion molecule expression and increased integrin avidity

Besides the chemokine G protein–coupled proteins, other surface molecules involved in leukocyte activation include the family of *toll-like receptors (TLRs)* that mediate innate leukocyte responses to different classes of microbes (Chapter 6, Box 6-1, p. 195), various cytokine receptors, and receptors for complement fragments and immunoglobulin that promote phagocytosis.

Phagocytosis (p. 59)

Phagocytosis and enzyme release by neutrophils and macrophages constitute the major benefits accruing from leukocyte accumulation at inflammatory sites. Phagocytosis involves three steps:

- *Recognition and binding.* Microorganisms may be coated with *opsonins* that enhance phagocytosis efficiency by binding to leukocyte receptors. Two major opsonins are the immunoglobulin Fc fragment and the complement fragment C3b. *Macrophage mannose and scavenger receptors* (mannose is expressed as a terminal sugar on many microbes) are also important recognition proteins for phagocytosis.
- *Engulfment* by encircling pseudopods (involving actin polymerization) and enclosure of the particle within an intracellular *phagosome.* Phagocytic vacuoles then fuse with lysosomes, resulting in enzyme discharge into the resulting *phagolysosome.*
- *Killing and degradation* of phagocytosed particles is most efficient in activated leukocytes, and *is accomplished largely by oxygen-dependent mechanisms.* Phagocytosis stimulates a burst of oxygen consumption and production of reactive oxygen metabolites (Fig. 2–3). This occurs via activation of nicotinamide-adenine dinucleotide phosphate (NADPH) oxidase, converting oxygen to superoxide anion (O_2^-) and eventually producing hydrogen peroxide (H_2O_2). Lysosomal *myeloperoxidase* (MPO) then converts H_2O_2 and Cl^- into the highly bactericidal HOCl (hydrochlorite—essentially forming bleach). Although the MPO system is the most efficient mechanism, other reactive oxygen species of the oxidative burst can also kill bacteria.

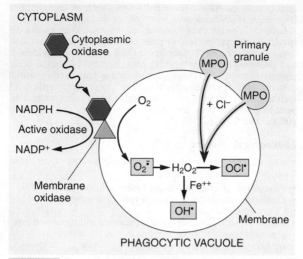

FIGURE 2-3 Summary of oxygen-dependent bactericidal mechanisms within phagocytic vacuoles.

Microbial killing can also occur via oxygen-independent pathways that largely work by increasing membrane permeability. These include *bactericidal permeability increasing protein, lysozyme, lactoferrin, major basic protein* of eosinophils, and *defensins*. Killed organisms are then degraded by a variety of lysosomal enzymes.

Release of Leukocyte Products and Leukocyte-Induced Tissue Injury (p. 61)

During activation and phagocytosis, leukocytes release products not only within the phagolysosome but also potentially into the extracellular space where they can cause tissue injury. These products include:

- *Lysosomal enzymes*, regurgitated during *frustrated phagocytosis* (large indigestible materials), premature fusion of lysosomes with forming phagosomes, or when lysosomes are damaged by ingested material (e.g., urate crystals)
- Oxygen-derived active metabolites
- Products of arachidonic acid metabolism

Defects in Leukocyte Function (p. 61)

Defects in leukocyte function (at any stage from endothelial adherence to microbicidal activity) interfere with inflammation and dramatically increase infection susceptibility. Defects may be either genetic or acquired and include:

- *Genetic deficiencies in adhesion molecules*: *leukocyte adhesion deficiency type I* is due to defective synthesis of β_2 integrins (LFA-1 and Mac-1); *type II deficiency* is due to a defect in fucose metabolism causing loss of sialyl Lewis X (ligand for E- and P-selectin).
- *Genetic defects in phagolysosome formation*: in *Chédiak-Higashi syndrome*, neutrophils have aberrant organellar

fusion with defective lysosomal enzyme delivery to phagosomes.

- *Genetic defects in microbicidal activity:* in *chronic granulomatous disease,* there are inherited defects in NADPH oxidase, leading to a defect in the respiratory burst, H_2O_2 production, and the MPO bactericidal mechanism.
- *Acquired deficiencies of neutrophils:* called *neutropenia,* this is the most common clinical cause of leukocyte defects; it may be caused by cancer chemotherapy or by metastatic tumor replacing normal bone marrow.

Termination of the Acute Inflammatory Response (p. 62)

In part, inflammation declines because mediators are only produced in quick bursts and have short half-lives. However, because of its inherent capacity to cause tissue damage, inflammation must also be tightly and actively regulated. As inflammation develops, the process therefore also triggers stop signals. These include switching production of pro-inflammatory arachidonate metabolites to anti-inflammatory forms (described below) and production of anti-inflammatory cytokines such as transforming growth factor-β (TGF-β).

CHEMICAL MEDIATORS OF INFLAMMATION (p. 63)

- The vascular and cellular events of inflammation are mediated by numerous molecules derived either from plasma or from cells (Fig. 2–4) and induced primarily by microbial products.
- Most mediators act by binding to specific receptors, although some have direct enzymatic activity (e.g., proteases), and others mediate oxidative damage (e.g., oxygen metabolites).
- Mediators can act in amplifying or regulatory cascades to stimulate the release of other downstream factors.
- Once generated, most mediators are short-lived, either quickly decaying or becoming inactivated by enzymes or inhibited by inhibitors.
- A system of checks and balances exists in the regulation of mediator action because *most mediators also have potentially harmful effects.*

Vasoactive Amines (p. 63)

Histamine and serotonin from preformed cellular stores are among the first mediators in inflammation; *they cause vasodilation and increased vascular permeability.* Mast cells, basophils, and platelets are all sources. Mast cell release is caused by physical agents (e.g., trauma, heat), immune reactions involving IgE (Chapter 6), complement fragments C3a and C5a (*anaphylatoxins*), cytokines (e.g., IL1 and IL8), and leukocyte-derived histamine-releasing factors. Platelet release is stimulated by contact with collagen, thrombin, adenosine diphosphate (ADP), antigen-antibody complexes, and platelet-activating factor (PAF).

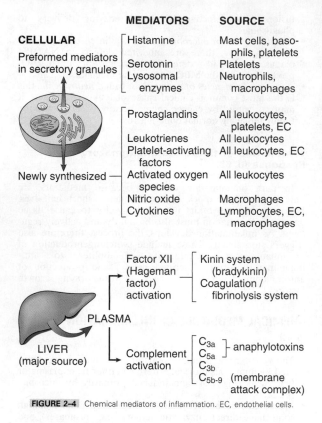

	MEDIATORS	SOURCE
CELLULAR Preformed mediators in secretory granules	Histamine	Mast cells, basophils, platelets
	Serotonin	Platelets
	Lysosomal enzymes	Neutrophils, macrophages
Newly synthesized	Prostaglandins	All leukocytes, platelets, EC
	Leukotrienes	All leukocytes
	Platelet-activating factors	All leukocytes, EC
	Activated oxygen species	All leukocytes
	Nitric oxide	Macrophages
	Cytokines	Lymphocytes, EC, macrophages

LIVER (major source)	PLASMA	Factor XII (Hageman factor) activation	Kinin system (bradykinin) Coagulation / fibrinolysis system
		Complement activation	C_{3a} C_{5a} } anaphylotoxins C_{3b} C_{5b-9} (membrane attack complex)

FIGURE 2–4 Chemical mediators of inflammation. EC, endothelial cells.

Plasma Proteins (p. 64)

Three interrelated plasma-derived mediators play key roles in inflammation: complement, kinin, and clotting systems.

Complement System (p. 64) (Fig. 2–5)

- Complement proteins are present as inactive plasma forms numbered C1 through C9; these are typically activated to become proteases that cleave other complement proteins in an amplifying cascade.
- The most important step for the biologic functioning of complement is activation of the third component, C3. C3 cleavage occurs by *C3 convertase* formed via the *classical pathway,* after fixation of C1 to antigen-antibody complexes; the *alternative pathway,* triggered by microbial surface molecules (e.g., endotoxin) and complex polysaccharides; and the *lectin pathway,* whereby plasma mannose-binding lectin binds to microbe carbohydrate and activates C1.
- C3 cleavage results in two functionally distinct fragments, C3a and C3b. C3a is released and C3b becomes covalently attached to the cell or molecule where complement is being activated. C3b and other complement fragments combine to

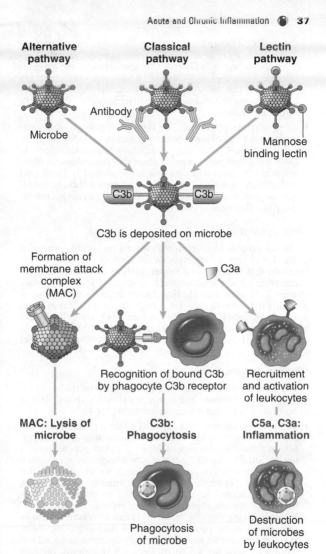

Alternative pathway

Classical pathway

Lectin pathway

Antibody

Microbe

Mannose binding lectin

C3b | C3b

C3b is deposited on microbe

Formation of membrane attack complex (MAC)

C3a

Recognition of bound C3b by phagocyte C3b receptor

Recruitment and activation of leukocytes

MAC: Lysis of microbe

C3b: Phagocytosis

C5a, C3a: Inflammation

Phagocytosis of microbe

Destruction of microbes by leukocytes

FIGURE 2–5 The activation and functions of the complement system. Activation of complement by different pathways leads to cleavage of C3. The functions of the complement system are mediated by breakdown products of C3 and other complement proteins and by the membrane attack complex (MAC). (The steps in the activation and regulation of complement are described in Box 2–2, p. 66).

cleave C5 into C5a and C5b pieces. C5b binds the late components (C6–C9), culminating in the formation of the *membrane attack complex* (*MAC*, composed of multiple C9 molecules).

- The biologic functions of complement fall into two general categories: MAC-induced cell lysis and the complement fragment-induced changes in vascular permeability, chemotaxis, and opsonization.

C3a and C5a (so-called *anaphylatoxins*) stimulate histamine release from mast cells and thereby increase vascular permeability and vasodilation. C5a also activates the arachidonate metabolism causing additional inflammatory mediator release.

C5a is a powerful leukocyte chemoattractant.

C3b is an opsonin.

- Complement activation is tightly regulated by cell-associated (e.g., *decay-accelerating factor*, or DAF) and circulating (e.g., *C1 inhibitor*) regulatory proteins. Defects in DAF will cause *paroxysmal nocturnal hemoglobinuria*, characterized by recurrent complement-mediated red cell lysis and anemia (p. 636). C1 inhibitor deficiency will cause *hereditary angioneurotic edema*, characterized by episodic, potentially life-threatening edema.

Kinin System (p. 65)

Plasma protein *kininogens* are cleaved by specific proteases called *kallikreins* to generate *bradykinin*, a vasoactive nonapeptide that causes blood vessel dilation, increased vascular permeability, and pain. Surface activation of *Hageman factor* (*factor XII*) produces clotting factor XIIa, which converts plasma prekallikrein into kallikrein; the latter cleaves high-molecular-weight kininogen to produce bradykinin. Kallikrein is also a potent activator of Hageman factor (forms an autocatalytic loop), has chemotactic activity, and causes neutrophil aggregation.

Clotting System (p. 65)

The clotting system is divided into two interrelated systems, designated the *intrinsic* and *extrinsic pathways*, that converge to activate a hemostatic mechanism (Chapter 4).

- The *intrinsic pathway* is a series of plasma proenzymes that can be activated by Hageman factor, resulting in the activation of *thrombin*, cleavage of *fibrinogen*, and generation of a fibrin clot. During this process, *fibrinopeptides* are formed that induce vascular permeability and are chemotactic for leukocytes. Thrombin also has inflammatory properties, causing increased leukocyte adhesion to endothelium via binding to specific *protease-activated receptors (PARs)*.
- While inducing clotting, factor XIIa can also activate the *fibrinolytic system*, producing *plasmin* that degrades fibrin, thereby solubilizing the clot. Plasmin contributes to inflammation by cleaving C3 to produce C3 fragments, forming fibrin *split* products that increase vascular permeability and activating Hageman factor.

Arachidonic Acid Metabolites: Prostaglandins, Leukotrienes, and Lipoxins (p. 68)

Cells respond to activating stimuli by generating lipid short-range signaling molecules (*eicosanoids*) from cell membrane–derived arachidonic acid (AA). These are synthesized by two major enzyme classes (Fig. 2–6):

- Cyclooxygenases (inhibited by aspirin) generate *prostaglandins* and *thromboxanes*
- Lipoxygenases produce *leukotrienes* and *lipoxins*

Some of the eicosanoid products and their effects include the following:

- Prostaglandin I$_2$ (*prostacyclin*) and prostaglandin E$_2$ cause vasodilation,
- Prostaglandin E$_2$ increases sensitivity to painful stimuli and can mediate fever.

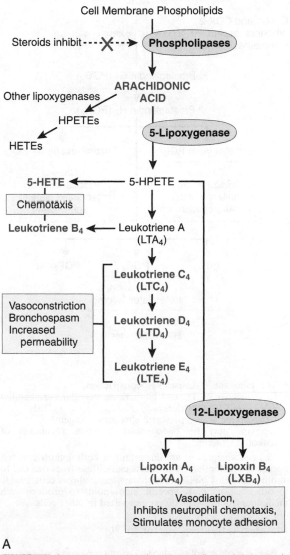

FIGURE 2-6 Generation of arachidonic acid metabolites and their roles in inflammation. The molecular targets of action of some anti-inflammatory drugs are indicated by an X. COX, cyclooxygenase; HETE, hydroxyeicosatetraenoic acid; HPETE, hydroperoxyeicosatetraenoic acid. *Continued*

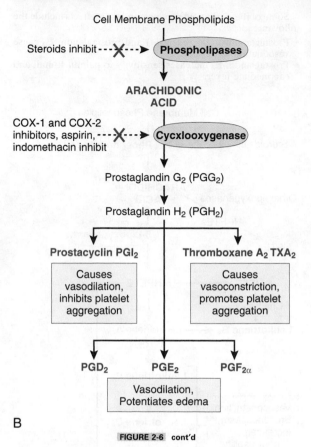

Cell Membrane Phospholipids

Steroids inhibit ---✗---▶ **Phospholipases**

ARACHIDONIC ACID

COX-1 and COX-2 inhibitors, aspirin, ---✗---▶ **Cycxlooxygenase** indomethacin inhibit

Prostaglandin G_2 (PGG$_2$)

Prostaglandin H_2 (PGH$_2$)

Prostacyclin PGI$_2$

Causes vasodilation, inhibits platelet aggregation

Thromboxane A$_2$ TXA$_2$

Causes vasoconstriction, promotes platelet aggregation

PGD$_2$ PGE$_2$ PGF$_{2\alpha}$

Vasodilation, Potentiates edema

B

FIGURE 2-6 cont'd

- Thromboxane A_2 causes vasoconstriction.
- Leukotrienes C_4, D_4, and E_4 increase vascular permeability and cause vasoconstriction.
- Leukotriene B_4 is a powerful chemotactic agent.
- Lipoxins may be endogenous negative regulators of leukotriene action.

Cell-cell interactions are important in both leukotriene and lipoxin biosynthesis. AA products can diffuse from one cell to another and this *transcellular biosynthesis* allows cells unable to otherwise generate specific eicosanoids to produce such mediators from intermediates generated in other cells.

Platelet-Activating Factor (p. 70)

PAF is a phospholipid-derived mediator produced by mast cells and other leukocytes after various stimuli, including IgE-mediated reactions. PAF causes platelet aggregation and release, bronchoconstriction, vasodilation, increased vascular permeability, increased leukocyte adhesion, and leukocyte chemotaxis. Thus, PAF can elicit most of the cardinal features of inflammation.

Cytokines and Chemokines
(p. 70 and Chapter 6)

Cytokines are proteins produced principally by activated lymphocytes and macrophages (but also endothelium, epithelium, and connective tissue cells) that modulate the function of other cell types. *Chemokines* are cytokines that also stimulate leukocyte movement (chemotaxis).

Tumor Necrosis Factor and Interleukin 1 (p. 71)

These are the major cytokines mediating inflammation; they are produced primarily by activated macrophages. Their most important actions in inflammation include effects on endothelium, leukocytes, and induction of the systemic acute-phase reactions (Fig. 2–7).

- Secretion is stimulated by endotoxin, immune complexes, toxins, physical injury, and a variety of inflammatory products.
- TNF and IL1 induce *endothelial activation*, including induction of endothelial adhesion molecules and chemical medi-

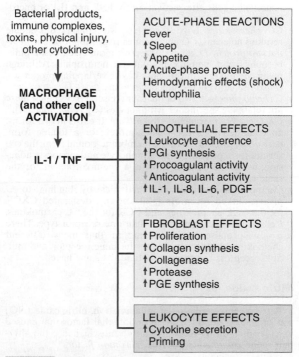

FIGURE 2–7 Major effects of interleukin 1 (IL1) and tumor necrosis factor (TNF) in inflammation.

ators (e.g., other cytokines [IL6], chemokines [IL8], growth factors, eicosanoids [PGI$_2$ and PAF], and nitric oxide), enzymes associated with matrix remodeling, and increases in endothelial thrombogenicity.

- IL1 and TNF induce systemic *acute-phase responses* associated with infection or injury: fever; anorexia; lethargy; neutrophilia; release of corticotropin and corticosteroids; and hemodynamic effects of septic shock—hypotension, decreased vascular resistance, increased heart rate, and acidosis (Chapter 4).
- TNF-α also *regulates body mass* by promoting lipid and protein mobilization and by suppressing appetite. Sustained TNF production contributes to *cachexia*, a pathologic state characterized by weight loss and anorexia that accompanies some infections and neoplasias.

Chemokines (p. 71)

Chemokines are a family (>40 known) of small proteins expressed by a wide range of cell types; they act primarily as chemoattractants and activators for leukocytes. Chemokines are classified into four major classes, according to the arrangement of conserved cysteine (C) residues:

- *CXC chemokines* have one amino acid residue separating the first two conserved cysteine residues. The CXC chemokines act primarily to recruit neutrophils. *IL8* is typical of this group; it is produced by macrophages and endothelial cells after activation by TNF and IL1 or microbial products.
- *CC chemokines* have the first two conserved cysteine residues adjacent. CC chemokines (e.g., *monocyte chemoattractant protein-1*) generally recruit monocytes, eosinophils, basophils, and lymphocytes but not neutrophils. Although many chemokines in this class have overlapping properties, *eotaxin* selectively recruits eosinophils.
- *C chemokines* lack two of the four conserved cysteines; these are relatively specific for lymphocytes (e.g., *lymphotactin*).
- *CX$_3$C chemokines* include *fractalkine*. It exists in two forms: an endothelial surface–bound protein or a soluble form, derived by proteolysis of the membrane-bound form; the cell surface form promotes firm lymphocyte and monocyte adhesion, while the soluble form is a chemoattractant for the same cells.
- Chemokines mediate their activities by binding to G protein–linked receptors (>20 known), designated CXCR for the CXC chemokines, and CCR for the CC chemokines. Cells typically express more than one receptor type. There is also promiscuity in binding in that many different chemokine ligands can bind to the same receptor, and multiple receptors can frequently bind the same ligand.

Nitric Oxide (p. 72)

A pleiotropic mediator of inflammation, nitric oxide (NO) was originally identified as an endothelial factor that caused vascular dilation by relaxing smooth muscle, hence the alternate name *endothelium-derived relaxation factor*.

- Besides vasodilation, NO acts in its local environment to (i) inhibit platelet aggregation and adhesion and (ii) kill certain microbes and tumor cells (via free radical formation).

- NO is synthesized from arginine, molecular oxygen, NADPH, and other cofactors by *nitric oxide synthase* (NOS).
- There are three types of NOS (endothelial [eNOS], neuronal [nNOS], and cytokine inducible [iNOS]) exhibiting two distinct expression patterns: (i) eNOS and nNOS are constitutively expressed but become active only in the setting of increased cytoplasmic calcium; (ii) iNOS is not constitutively expressed but is instead synthesized by macrophages after induction by certain cytokines (e.g., interferon-γ).
- NO plays several important roles during an inflammatory response. eNOS is important in maintaining *vascular tone*, and NO production via iNOS is a compensatory mechanism to reduce leukocyte recruitment. NO production by activated macrophages (via iNOS) is also important in the pathogenesis of *septic shock*.
- NO is involved in responses to infection. NO and reactive oxygen species combine to form antimicrobial metabolites such as peroxynitrite [OONO⁻], S-nitrosothiols, and nitrogen dioxide [$NO_2^{\cdot}$]). These can all kill microbes, but at the risk of causing damage to host cells.

Lysosomal Constituents of Leukocytes
(p. 73)

Release of lysosome granule content by neutrophils and monocytes contributes to the inflammatory response as well as to tissue injury.

- *Neutrophils* have two types of granules; smaller *specific (or secondary) granules* contain lysozyme, collagenase, gelatinase, lactoferrin, plasminogen activator, and histaminase; larger *azurophil (or primary) granules* contain myeloperoxidase, bactericidal factors (lysozyme, defensins), acid hydrolases, and a variety of neutral proteases (elastase, cathepsin G, collagenases).
- Specific and azurophil granules can prematurely empty into phagocytic vacuoles not yet completely surrounding engulfed material; alternatively, the contents can be directly secreted extracellularly, or released after cell death. Acid proteases normally degrade proteins, bacteria, and debris only within the acidic phagolysosome, whereas neutral proteases can degrade extracellular components at neutral pH. Monocytes and macrophages also contain hydrolases (collagenase, elastase, phospholipase, and plasminogen activator) that are particularly important in chronic inflammatory reactions.
- Lysosomal constituents can potentiate vascular permeability and chemotaxis, as well as cause tissue damage. The potentially harmful effects of proteases are normally held in check by multiple serum and tissue *antiproteases* (e.g., α₁-antitrypsin inhibits neutrophil elastase). Inhibitor deficiency may result in sustained leukocyte protease activity and disease (e.g., α₁-antitrypsin deficiency, Chapter 18).

Oxygen-Derived Free Radicals (p. 73)

Oxygen-derived free radicals (including O_2^-, H_2O_2, and hydroxyl radical) are released extracellularly from leukocytes after phagocytosis and after exposure to chemotactic agents or immune complexes. These metabolites can also combine with NO to form other reactive nitrogen intermediates. Effects of these reactive oxygen species (ROS) include:

- Endothelial cell damage causing increased vascular permeability
- Inactivation of antiproteases, resulting in unopposed protease activity
- Injury to multiple cell types (e.g., tumor cells, red cells, parenchymal cells)

Tissues are normally protected from the damaging effects of ROS by multiple pathways (p. 17, Fig. 1–14), including the serum proteins ceruloplasmin and transferrin, and enzymes such as superoxide dismutase, catalase, and glutathione peroxidase. The net effect of ROS on tissues depends on the balance between production and inactivation.

Neuropeptides (p. 74)

Neuropeptides play a role in initiating and propagating inflammatory responses. *Substance P*, for example, is a powerful mediator of vascular permeability, transmits pain signals, regulates blood pressure, and stimulates immune and endocrine cell secretion. Local substance P release leads to plasma influx and amplification of an initial inflammatory stimulus.

Other Mediators (p. 74)

The mediators described above account for inflammatory responses to many types of injury, but do not completely explain the mechanisms underlying inflammation in two common pathologic conditions:

- *Response to hypoxia.* Hypoxia alone can directly induce an inflammatory response; this is largely mediated by the protein *hypoxia-induced factor 1α (HIF-1α)* produced by cells deprived of oxygen.
- *Response to necrotic cells.* Necrosis elicits inflammatory reactions designed to eliminate these cells. The molecular basis of the response is still unknown, although uric acid, a product of DNA breakdown, can crystallize at high concentrations and thereby potentially stimulate inflammation and subsequent immune responses (as in the disease *gout*).

Summary of Chemical Mediators of Acute Inflammation (p. 74)

Although there are a plethora of inflammatory mediators (see Table 2–5, p. 74), a relative few may be most relevant clinically (Table 2–2).

OUTCOMES OF ACUTE INFLAMMATION (p. 75)

Acute inflammation will be altered by the nature and intensity of injury, the tissue affected, and host responsiveness; the process has one of three general outcomes:

TABLE 2–2   **Role of Mediators in Different Reactions of Inflammation**

Reaction	Mediator
Vasodilation	Prostaglandins Nitric oxide Histamine
Increased vascular permeability	Vasoactive amines C3a and C5a (through liberating amines) Bradykinin Leukotrienes C_4, D_4, E_4 PAF Substance P
Chemotaxis, leukocyte recruitment and activation	C5a Leukotriene B_4 Chemokines IL-1, TNF Bacterial products
Fever	IL-1, TNF Prostaglandins
Pain	Prostaglandins Bradykinin
Tissue damage	Neutrophil and macrophage lysosomal enzymes Oxygen metabolites Nitric oxide

- *Complete resolution*, with regeneration of native cells and restoration to normalcy.
- *Healing by connective tissue replacement (fibrosis)* occurs after substantial tissue destruction, when inflammation occurs in nonregenerating tissues, or in the setting of abundant fibrin exudation. In pyogenic infections, intense neutrophil infiltration and tissue liquefaction may result in *abscess formation*; eventually, this will be replaced by fibrosis.
- *Progression to chronic inflammation*, outlined in greater detail below.

MORPHOLOGIC PATTERNS OF ACUTE INFLAMMATION (p. 76)

Although all acute inflammatory reactions are characterized by vascular changes and leukocyte infiltration, there are frequently distinctive morphologic changes that suggest possible causes.

Serous Inflammation (p. 76)

Serous inflammation is reflected by tissue fluid accumulation and indicates a modest increase in vascular permeability. In the peritoneal, pleural, and pericardial cavities, this is called an *effusion*, but it can occur elsewhere (e.g., skin burn blisters).

Fibrinous Inflammation (p. 76)

Fibrinous inflammation is a more marked increase in vascular permeability, with exudates containing large amounts of fibrinogen. The fibrinogen is converted to fibrin through coagulation system activation. Involvement of serosal surfaces (e.g., pericardium or pleura) is referred to as *fibrinous pericarditis* or *pleuritis*.

Suppurative or Purulent Inflammation (p. 77)

This pattern is characterized by production of purulent exudates (*pus*) consisting of leukocytes and necrotic cells. An *abscess* refers to a localized collection of purulent inflammatory tissue accompanied by liquefactive necrosis (e.g., staphylococcal abscess).

Ulcers (p. 77)

Ulcers are local erosions of epithelial surfaces produced by sloughing of inflamed necrotic tissue (e.g., gastric ulcers).

SUMMARY OF ACUTE INFLAMMATION (p. 77)

When encountering an injurious agent (e.g., microbe or dead cells), phagocytes attempt to eliminate these agents and secrete cytokines, eicosanoids, and other mediators. These mediators in turn act on endothelial cells to promote plasma efflux and further leukocyte recruitment. Recruited leukocytes are activated and will phagocytize offending agents. As the injurious agent is eliminated, anti-inflammatory counterregulatory mechanisms quench the process and the host returns to a normal state of health. If the injurious agent cannot be quickly eliminated, the result may be chronic inflammation.

CHRONIC INFLAMMATION (p. 78)

Chronic inflammation is a prolonged process (weeks or months) in which active inflammation, tissue destruction, and attempts at healing may all be proceeding simultaneously. Chronic inflammation can occur:

- Following acute inflammation, either because the inciting stimulus persists or because normal healing is somehow interrupted
- From repeated bouts of acute inflammation
- Most commonly as a low-grade, smoldering response *without* prior acute inflammation, due to:

  Persistent infection by intracellular microbes (e.g., tubercle bacilli, viruses) of low direct toxicity but nevertheless capable of evoking immunologic responses

  Prolonged exposure to potentially toxic exogenous (e.g., silica, causing pulmonary silicosis) or endogenous substances (e.g., lipids, causing atherosclerosis)

  Immune reactions, particularly those against one's own tissues (e.g., autoimmune diseases)

In contrast to acute inflammation—characterized by vascular changes, edema, and neutrophilic infiltration—chronic inflammation is typified by:

- *Infiltration with mononuclear inflammatory cells*, including macrophages, lymphocytes, and plasma cells

- *Tissue destruction*, largely induced by persistent injury and the inflammatory cells
- Attempts at healing by connective tissue replacement, accomplished by vascular proliferation (angiogenesis) and fibrosis

Mononuclear Cell Infiltration (p. 79)

Macrophages are the dominant cellular players in chronic inflammation.

- Macrophages derive from circulating monocytes induced to emigrate across the endothelium by chemokines or other chemoattractants. After reaching the extravascular tissue, monocytes transform into the phagocytic macrophage (Fig. 2–8).
- Macrophages are central figures in chronic inflammation because of the numerous biologically active products they secrete after being activated. Macrophages are activated through cytokines produced by immune-activated T cells (especially interferon-γ [IFN-γ]) or by nonimmune factors (e.g., endotoxin) (see Fig. 2–8).
- Although macrophage products are important for host defense, some mediators induce tissue damage. These include reactive oxygen and nitric oxide metabolites that are toxic to cells, and proteases that degrade extracellular matrix. Other products cause fibroblast proliferation, connective tissue production, and angiogenesis.
- In chronic inflammation, macrophage accumulation persists by continued recruitment of monocytes due to ongoing adhesion molecule and chemotactic factor expression.

Other Cells in Chronic Inflammation (p. 81)

- *Lymphocytes* are mobilized in both antibody- and cell-mediated immune reactions (driven by contact with specific antigen) and are involved even in nonimmune inflammation (e.g., through the effects of endotoxin). Activated T lymphocytes (particularly through IFN-γ production) activate monocytes and macrophages; activated macrophages, in turn, influence T (and B) lymphocyte function. *Plasma cells* are terminally differentiated B cells that produce antibodies directed against either foreign antigen or altered tissue components.
- *Eosinophils* are characteristic of immune reactions mediated by IgE and in parasitic infections. Eosinophil recruitment depends on *eotaxin*, a CC chemokine. Eosinophils have granules containing *major basic protein (MBP)*, a cationic molecule that is toxic to parasites but also lyses mammalian epithelium (Chapter 6).
- *Mast cells* are widely distributed in connective tissues and participate in both acute and chronic inflammation. They express surface receptors that bind the Fc portion of IgE. In acute reactions, binding of specific antigens to these IgE antibodies leads to mast cell degranulation and mediator release (e.g., histamine). This type of response occurs during anaphylactic reactions to foods, insect venom, or drugs (Chapter 6).

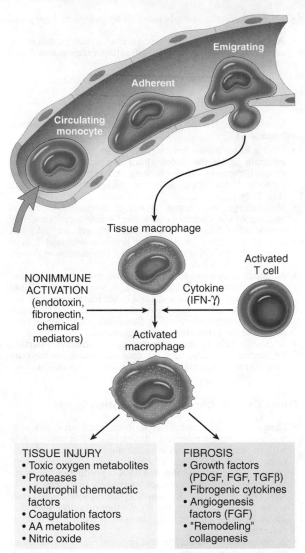

FIGURE 2–8 The roles of activated macrophages in chronic inflammation. Macrophages are activated by cytokines from immune-activated T cells (particularly IFN-γ) or by nonimmune stimuli such as endotoxin. The products made by activated macrophages that cause tissue injury and fibrosis are indicated. AA, arachidonic acid; PDGF, platelet-derived growth factor; FGF, fibroblast growth factor; TGFβ, transforming growth factor β.

Granulomatous Inflammation (p. 82)

This distinctive form of chronic inflammation is characterized by focal accumulations of activated macrophages (*granulomas*); macrophage activation is reflected by the cells becoming enlarged and flattened (so-called *epithelioid* macrophages).

- Nodules of epithelioid macrophages in granulomatous inflammation are surrounded by a collar of lymphocytes elaborating factors necessary to induce macrophage activation. Activated macrophages may fuse to form multinucleate *giant cells*, and central necrosis may be present in some granulomas (particularly from infectious causes).
- *Foreign body granulomas* are incited by relatively inert foreign bodies, while *immune granulomas* are formed by immune T cell–mediated responses to persistent antigens. IFN-γ from activated T cells causes macrophage transformation to epithelioid cells and multinucleate giant cells. The prototypical immune granuloma is caused by the tuberculosis bacillus; in that setting, the granuloma is called a *tubercle* and *classically exhibits central caseous necrosis.*
- *Granulomatous inflammation* is a distinctive inflammatory reaction with relatively few (albeit important) possible causes, either infectious or noninfectious (Table 2–3).

Lymphatics in Inflammation (p. 83)

Lymphatics and lymph nodes filter and "police" extravascular fluids. With the mononuclear phagocyte system, they represent a secondary line of defense whenever a local inflammatory response cannot contain an external agent.

- *Lymphatics* are delicate channels lined by endothelium with loose, overlapping cell junctions, scant basement membrane, and no muscular support except in the larger ducts. In inflammation, lymphatic flow is increased to drain edema fluid, leukocytes, and cell debris from the extravascular space.
- In severe injuries, drainage may also transport the offending agent; lymphatics may become inflamed *(lymphangitis)*, as may the draining lymph nodes *(lymphadenitis)*. In hand infections, for example, red *lymphangitic* streaks may follow the course of lymphatics up the arm, accompanied by painful axillary lymph node enlargement. The nodal enlargement is usually due to lymphoid follicle and sinusoidal phagocyte hyperplasia (termed *reactive lymphadenitis*, Chapter 14).
- Although lymphatics and lymph nodes typically contain infections, severe cases can result in organisms gaining access to the vascular circulation, so-called *bacteremia*. Phagocytes of liver, spleen, and bone marrow then constitute the next line of defense; in massive infections, bacteria may still seed distant tissues of the body (heart valves, meninges, kidneys, and joints are favored sites).

SYSTEMIC EFFECTS OF INFLAMMATION (p. 84)

Systemic changes associated with inflammation are collectively called the *acute phase response,* or—in severe cases—the systemic inflammatory response syndrome (SIRS). These rep-

TABLE 2–3 **Examples of Granulomatous Inflammations**

Disease	Cause	Tissue Reaction
Bacterial		
Tuberculosis	*Mycobacterium tuberculosis*	*Noncaseating tubercle* (*granuloma prototype*): a focus of epithelioid cells, rimmed by fibroblasts, lymphocytes, histiocytes, occasional Langhans' giant cell *Caseating tubercle*: central amorphous granular debris, loss of all cellular detail, acid-fast bacilli
Leprosy (tuberculoid form)	*Mycobacterium leprae*	Acid-fast bacilli in macrophages; granulomas and epithelioid types
syphilis	*Treponema pallidum*	*Gumma*: Microscopic to grossly visible lesion, enclosing wall of histiocytes; plasma cell infiltrate; center cells are necrotic without loss of cellular outline
Cat-scratch disease	Gram-negative bacillius	Rounded or stellate granuloma containing central granular debris and recognizable neutrophils; giant cells uncommon
Parasitic		
Schistosomiasis	*Schistosoma mansoni, S. haematobium, S. japonicum*	Egg emboli; eosinophils
Fungal		
	Cryptococcus neoformans	Organism is yeastlike, sometimes budding; 5–10 mm; large, clear capsule
	Coccidioides immitis	Organism appears as spherical (30–80 mm) cyst containing endospores of 3–5 mm each
Inorganic Metals and Dusts		
Silicosis, berylliosis		Lung involvement; fibrosis
Unknown		
Sarcoidosis		*Noncaseating granuloma*: giant cells (Langhans' and foreign-body types); asteroids in giant cells; occasional Schaumann body (concentric calcific concretion); no organisms

resent responses to cytokines produced either by bacterial products (e.g., endotoxin) or by other inflammatory stimuli. The acute phase response consists of several clinical and pathologic changes:

- *Fever:* temperature elevation (1–4°C) is produced in response to *pyrogens*, substances that stimulate prostaglandin synthesis in the hypothalamus. For example, endotoxin stimulates leukocyte release of IL1 and TNF to increase cyclooxygenase production of prostaglandins. In the hypothalamus, PGE_2 stimulates intracellular second signals (e.g., cyclic AMP) that reset the temperature set point. Thus, aspirin reduces fever by inhibiting cyclooxygenase activity to block prostaglandin synthesis.

- *Acute-phase proteins* are plasma proteins, mostly synthesized in the liver, whose synthesis increases several hundred-fold in response to inflammatory stimuli (e.g., cytokines such as IL6 and TNF). Three of the best-known examples are C-reactive protein (CRP), fibrinogen, and serum amyloid A protein (SAA). CRP and SAA bind to microbial cell walls, and may act as opsonins and fix complement. They may also help clear necrotic cell nuclei and mobilize metabolic stores (see also Chapter 6).
- *Leukocytosis* (increased white cell number in peripheral blood) is a common feature of inflammatory reactions. It occurs by accelerated release of bone marrow cells, typically with increased numbers of immature neutrophils in the blood (*shift to the left*). Prolonged infection also induces proliferation of bone marrow precursors due to increased colony-stimulating factor (CSF) production. The leukocyte count usually climbs to 15,000 to 20,000 cells/μl, but may reach extraordinarily high levels of 40,000 to 100,000 cells/ml (referred to as *leukemoid reactions*). Bacterial infections typically increase neutrophil numbers (*neutrophilia*); viral infections increase lymphocyte numbers (*lymphocytosis*); parasitic infestations and allergic disorders are associated with increased eosinophils (*eosinophilia*).
- *Other manifestations of the acute phase response* include increased pulse and blood pressure; decreased sweating, mainly because of redirection of blood flow from cutaneous to deep vascular beds; rigors (shivering), chills, anorexia, somnolence, and malaise, probably due to systemic effects of cytokines.
- In severe bacterial infections (*sepsis*), the large amounts of organisms and endotoxin in the blood stimulate the production of enormous quantities of several cytokines, notably TNF and IL1. High levels of these cytokines result in a clinical triad of disseminated intravascular coagulation (DIC), hypoglycemia, and cardiovascular failure described as *septic shock* (Chapter 4).

CONSEQUENCES OF DEFECTIVE OR EXCESSIVE INFLAMMATION (p. 85)

- *Defective inflammation* typically results in increased susceptibility to infections and delayed healing of wounds and tissue damage. Delayed repair occurs because inflammation is essential for clearing damaged tissues and debris, and provides the necessary stimulus to get the repair process started.
- *Excessive inflammation* is the basis of many categories of human disease, for example, allergies and autoimmune diseases (Chapter 6). Inflammation also plays a critical role in cancer, atherosclerosis and ischemic heart disease, and some neurodegenerative diseases (e.g., Alzheimer disease). Prolonged inflammation and the accompanying fibrosis also cause pathologic changes in chronic infectious, metabolic, and other diseases.

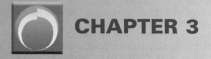

CHAPTER 3

Tissue Renewal and Repair: Regeneration, Healing, and Fibrosis

Repairing injured or dead tissues is critical to survival. Once injury occurs, the host responds to eliminate the offending agent, contain the damage, and prepare surviving cells for replication.

Definitions (p. 89)

Healing Repair involving a combination of regeneration and connective tissue deposition (fibrosis or scar). Scarring occurs when tissues are intrinsically unable to regenerate (e.g., heart, brain), if the underlying connective tissue scaffolding is disrupted, or following extensive exudates.

Regeneration Cell or tissue growth that replaces lost structures; generally involves proliferation of the same cell type, although stem cells may proliferate and differentiate to replace dead cells. Regeneration requires intact connective tissue scaffolding.

CONTROL OF NORMAL CELL PROLIFERATION AND TISSUE GROWTH (p. 89)

Cell populations in adult tissues are regulated by the relative rates of cell proliferation, differentiation, and apoptotic death. General concepts regarding cell proliferation:

- Cell proliferation may involve physiologic (e.g., hormonal) or pathologic stimuli (e.g., injury, mechanical forces, or cell death).

- It is controlled by either soluble or contact-mediated signals.
- Signals may be stimulatory or inhibitory.
- Increased cell proliferation can be accomplished by shortening the cell cycle or—most important—by recruiting quiescent cells into the cell cycle.

Tissue-Proliferative Activity (p. 90)

The cell cycle consists of G_1 (presynthetic), S (DNA synthesis), G_2 (premitotic), and M (mitotic) phases; quiescent cells are in a physiologic state called G_0 (Fig. 3–1). Although most tissues are composed mainly of cells in G_0 (that can periodically enter the cell cycle), various combinations of continuously dividing cells, terminally differentiated cells, and stem cells are also present. Tissues are divided into three groups according to their proliferative capacity:

- *Continuously dividing (labile):* cells proliferate throughout life, replacing those that are destroyed (e.g., surface epithelia and bone marrow hematopoietic cells). Typically, mature cells derive from *stem cells* (see below) with unlimited capacity to regenerate and varying capacity to differentiate.
- *Quiescent (stable):* cells are normally involved in low-level replication but are capable of rapid division in response to

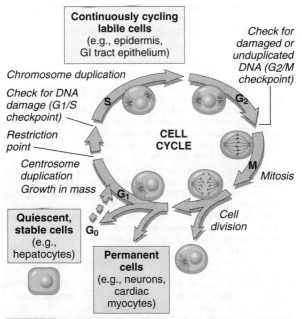

FIGURE 3–1 Cell cycle landmarks. The figure shows the cell cycle phases (G_0, G_1, G_2, S, and M), the location of the G_1 restriction point, and the G_1/S and G_2/M checkpoints. Cells from labile tissues such as the epidermis and the gastrointestinal tract may cycle continuously; stable cells such as hepatocytes are quiescent but can enter the cell cycle; permanent cells such as neurons and cardiac myocytes have lost the capacity to regenerate. (Modified from Pollard TD, Earnshaw WC: Cell Biology. Philadelphia, WB Saunders, 2002.)

stimuli (e.g., liver, kidney, fibroblasts, smooth muscle, and endothelial cells).

- *Nondividing (permanent):* cells cannot undergo division in postnatal life (e.g., neurons, skeletal muscle, and cardiac muscle).

Stem Cells (p. 91)

Stem cells are characterized by prolonged *self-renewal capacity* and by *asymmetric replication* (i.e., with each cell division, one cell retains self-renewing property while the other differentiates to become a mature, nondividing cell).

Embryonic Stem Cells (p. 91)

These pleuripotent stem cells are capable of differentiating into any tissue type. Isolated from normal blastocysts, embryonic stem (ES) cells may be maintained as undifferentiated cell lines or induced to differentiate along a variety of cell lineages. ES cells are:

- Used to identify signals required for normal tissue differentiation
- Central in generating animals congenitally deficient in specific genes (*knockouts*) by inactivating or deleting a gene in an ES cell and then incorporating the modified ES cell into a developing blastocyst
- Potentially of use in repopulating damaged organs

Adult Stem Cells (p. 91)

Small numbers of reservoir cells in normal adult tissues located in *niches* unique to each tissue (e.g., bulge area of hair follicles); compared to ES cells, these cells have a more restricted differentiation capability and tend to be lineage-specific. Nevetheless, adult stem cells with relatively broad differentiation potential occur in bone marrow and in *tissue stem cells* outside the bone marrow.

- Bone marrow contains *hematopoietic stem cells (HSCs)* capable of regenerating all blood cell elements; bone marrow also contains multipotential stromal cells (capable of differentiating, e.g., into bone, cartilage, fat, or muscle).
- HSCs (mesodermal lineage cells) are capable of differentiating into neurons (ectoderm), hepatocytes (endoderm), and other adult cell lineages, so-called *transdifferentiation*.
- Stem cells may also fuse with host cells, transferring genetic material and giving the (false) impression of transdifferentiation.
- Despite impressive *plasticity* (breadth of differentiation potential), HSCs do not contribute significantly to normal tissue homeostasis or to replacement of injured tissues; their role may be in local production of growth factors to promote healing.
- *Multipotent adult progenitor cells (MAPCs)* are also found in bone marrow and in multiple other tissue sites (e.g., brain, skin, and muscle); these cells proliferate in culture without senescence and have broad developmental capacity.

Role of Stem Cells in Tissue Homeostasis
(p. 93)

Tissue stem cells are typically responsible for generating the mature cells of the organ in which they reside, thereby maintaining normal tissue homeostasis; they also have variable potential to differentiate more broadly and to repopulate tissues following injury.

- *Epithelium:* Most epithelial surfaces (e.g., skin, mucous membranes, gastrointestinal tract) are constantly maintained by stem cells with a discrete set of differentiation lineages. Terminally differentiated cells do not divide and are continuously sloughed at the external surface. After injury, stem cells can repopulate the tissue.
- *Liver:* Liver stem cells reside in the canals of Hering (junction of hepatocytes and the bile duct system) and give rise to *oval cells*, with a capacity to form hepatocytes or biliary epithelium; they are typically only active if direct hepatocyte proliferation is not possible (e.g., fulminant hepatic failure).
- *Brain:* Although neurons are the prototype of nondividing, permanent cells, *neural stem cells* exist and can even be integrated into neural circuits. Their functional role is unknown.
- *Striated muscle:* Skeletal and cardiac myocytes cannot proliferate; regeneration of injured skeletal muscle is accomplished by proliferation of *satellite cells*, a stem cell pool in adult muscle. *If* similar cells are present in heart (controversial), they do not contribute to any significant extent to myocardial regeneration (e.g., after infarction).

Growth Factors (p. 95)

A plethora of growth factors are known; some act on multiple cell types, while others have restricted cell targets. Besides stimulating proliferation, they can affect cell movement, contractility, differentiation, and angiogenesis—all important processes in wound healing (see later). Major growth factors in regeneration and wound healing are summarized in Table 3–1:

- *Epidermal growth factor (EGF)* and *transforming growth factor-α (TGF-α)* have extensive homology and exert their effects primarily through binding to the same EGF receptor (EGFR1 or ERB B1), a transmembrane molecule with intrinsic tyrosine kinase activity. They are mitogenic for epithelial cells, hepatocytes, and fibroblasts.
- *Hepatocyte growth factor (HGF)* is produced by fibroblasts, endothelial cells, and hepatocytes; it has mitogenic effects on most epithelial cells, as well as promoting embryonic development. The HGF receptor (product of the *c-MET* proto-oncogene) is overexpressed in many tumors.
- *Vascular endothelial growth factor (VEGF)* is a family of proteins that promotes blood vessel formation in early development (*vasculogenesis*) and plays a central role in new blood vessel growth in adults (*angiogenesis*); it is particularly important in the angiogenesis associated with chronic inflammatory states and in healing wounds. VEGF members act by binding to receptors with intrinsic tyrosine kinase activity (VEGFR1-VEGFR3); VEGFR-2 is expressed by endothelial cells (ECs) and is the main receptor for vasculogenesis/angiogenesis. VEGF-C and -D bind to

TABLE 3–1 Growth Factors and Cytokines Involved in Regeneration and Wound Healing

Cytokine	Symbol	Source	Functions
Epidermal growth factor	EGF	Platelets, macrophages, saliva, urine, milk, plasma	Mitogenic for keratinocytes and fibroblasts; stimulates keratinocyte migration and granulation tissue formation
Transforming growth factor alpha	TGF-α	Macrophages, T lymphocytes, keratinocytes, and many tissues	Similar to EGF; stimulates replication of hepatocytes and certain epithelial cells
Hepatocyte growth factor/scatter factor	HGF	Mesenchymal cells	Enhances proliferation of epithelial and endothelial cells, and of hepatocytes; increases cell motility
Vascular endothelial cell growth factor (isoforms A, B, C, D)	VEGF	Mesenchymal cells	Increases vascular permeability; mitogenic for endothelial cells
Platelet-derived growth factor (isoforms A, B, C, D)	PDGF	Platelets, macrophages, endothelial cells, keratinocytes, smooth muscle cells	Chemotactic for PMNs, macrophages, fibroblasts, and smooth muscle cells; activates PMNs, macrophages, and fibroblasts; mitogenic for fibroblasts, endothelial cells, and smooth muscle cells; stimulates production of MMPs, fibronectin, and HA; stimulates angiogenesis and wound contraction; remodeling; inhibits platelet aggregation; regulates integrin expression
Fibroblast growth factor-1 (acidic), -2 (basic)	FGF	Macrophages, mast cells, T lymphocytes, endothelial cells, fibroblasts, and many tissues	Chemotactic for fibroblasts; mitogenic for fibroblasts and keratinocytes; stimulates keratinocyte migration, angiogenesis, wound contraction, and matrix deposition

Transforming growth factor beta (isoforms 1, 2, 3); other members of the family are BMP and activin	TGF-β	Platelets, T lymphocytes, macrophages, endothelial cells, keratinocytes, smooth muscle cells, fibroblasts	Chemotactic for PMNs, macrophages, lymphocytes, fibroblasts, and smooth muscle cells; stimulates TIMP synthesis, keratinocyte migration, angiogenesis, and fibroplasia; inhibits production of MMPs and keratinocyte proliferation; regulates integrin expression and other cytokines; induces TGF-β production
Keratinocyte growth factor (also called FGF-7)	KGF	Fibroblasts	Stimulates keratinocyte migration, proliferation, and differentiation
Insulin-like growth factor-1	IGF-1	Macrophages, fibroblasts, and other cells	Stimulates synthesis of sulfated proteoglycans, collagen, keratinocyte migration, and fibroblast proliferation; endocrine effects similar to growth hormone
Tumor necrosis factor	TNF	Macrophages, mast cells, T lymphocytes	Activates macrophages; regulates other cytokines; multiple functions
Interleukins	IL1, etc.	Macrophages, mast cells, keratinocytes, lymphocytes, and many tissues	Many functions. Some examples: chemotactic for PMNs (IL1), fibroblasts (IL4), stimulation of MMP-1 synthesis (IL1), angiogenesis (IL8), TIMP synthesis (IL6); regulation of other cytokines
Interferons	IFN-α, etc.	Lymphocytes and fibroblasts	Activates macrophages; inhibits fibroblast proliferation and synthesis of MMPs; regulates other cytokines

BMP, bone morphogenetic proteins; PMNs, polymorphonuclear leukocytes; MMPs, matrix metalloproteinases; HA, hyaluronic acid; TIMP, tissue inhibitor of matrix metalloproteinase.
Modified from Schwartz SI: Principles of Surgery. New York, McGraw-Hill 1999.

VEGFR-3 to induce lymphatic endothelial proliferation (*lymphangiogenesis*).

- *Platelet-derived growth factor (PDGF)* is a protein family found in platelet α-granules, but is also made by ECs, macrophages, and smooth muscle cells. By binding to distinct α- or β-receptors, PDGF causes migration and proliferation of fibroblasts, monocytes, and smooth muscle cells.
- *Fibroblast growth factors (FGFs)* are a growth factor family including acidic and basic forms; they are secreted by a wide variety of cells and bind to extracellular matrix heparan sulfate to form reservoirs of inactive factors. Basic FGF, in particular, has the ability to induce all the steps necessary for angiogenesis (see below), and FGF members are centrally involved in wound repair, tissue development, and hematopoiesis.
- *TGF-β* belongs to a large family of growth factors with wide-ranging functions. Produced by a variety of cell types (especially macrophages), TGF-β is a growth inhibitor for most epithelial cells (via receptor kinases that phosphorylate *Smad* cytoplasmic transcription factors), and has potent anti-inflammatory effects. It also promotes fibrosis by stimulating fibroblast chemotaxis, proliferation, and extracellular matrix synthesis, and by inhibiting collagen degradation.

Cytokines are primarily important as mediators of immune and inflammatory responses (Chapter 6); however, many also have growth-promoting activities.

Signaling Mechanisms in Cell Growth (p. 97)

Growth factor *ligands* bind to specific target cell receptors; receptor ligation transmits intracellular signals to induce gene transcription and promote entry into the cell cycle. General schemes of intercellular signaling are:

- *Autocrine:* Cells respond to signaling substances produced by themselves.
- *Paracrine:* A cell produces substances that affect target cells in close proximity.
- *Endocrine:* Cells synthesize hormones that circulate in the blood to act on distant targets.

Overview of Receptors and Signal Transduction Pathways (p. 98)

The pathways by which ligand and receptor interactions transduce intracellular signals is schematized in Figure 3–2. Receptor-ligand interactions typically induce receptor dimerization or trimerization that then transduces a signal; single receptor molecules can also transduce signals but usually only after recruitment of secondary cytosolic adapter proteins. Simplistically, signaling (conversion of extracellular stimuli to intracellular events) occurs by generating cascades of sequential protein kinases that commit entry into the cell cycle.

- *Receptors with intrinsic kinase activity:* Most growth factor receptors (e.g., PDGFR, EGFR, FGFR) have intrinsic tyrosine kinase activities that are activated following ligand binding. The active kinases then phosphorylate downstream effector molecules leading to *their* activation. Phosphory-

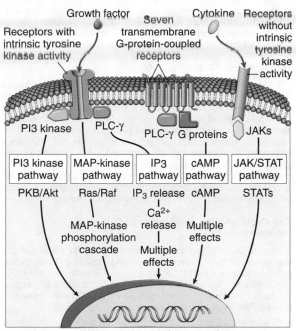

Transcription factor activation

FIGURE 3–2 Examples of signal transduction systems that require cell surface receptors. Shown are receptors with and without intrinsic kinase activity, and seven transmembrane G protein–coupled receptors.

lated receptor tyrosines also permit docking and activation of various cytosolic proteins, including those in the Ras signaling pathway, the phosphoinositide-3 (PI-3)-kinase pathway, phospholipase Cγ (PLCγ) in the protein kinase C pathway, and members of the *Src* family of kinases.

- Activated Ras binds to Raf, which phosphorylates a family of mitogen-activated protein (MAP) kinases.
- The PI 3 pathway activates a series of kinases including Akt, leading eventually to cell survival.
- PLCγ activation leads to inositol 1,4,5-triphosphate (IP_3) production followed by calcium release from endoplasmic reticulum, and diacylglycerol formation with protein kinase C activation (and additional protein phosphorylations).
- *Receptors without intrinsic kinase activity:* These receptors associate with and activate cytosolic protein kinases; for example, cytoplasmic Janus kinases (JAKs) link activated receptors with downstream STATs (signal transduction and activation of transcription) that shuttle into the nucleus and activate gene transcription.
- *G protein–linked receptors:* These receptors (>1500 described to date) all contain seven transmembrane spans; they include the chemokine receptors (Chapter 2) as well as receptors for epinephrine and glucagon. Ligand binding activates a signal transducing G protein complex generating intracellular second messengers including calcium and 3′,5′-cyclic adenosine monophosphate (cAMP).

- *Steroid hormone receptors:* Ligands for these receptors are lipophilic and therefore directly diffuse through plasma membranes; receptors are typically intranuclear transcription factors that are activated by ligand binding.

Transcription Factors (p. 100)

These factors include products of growth-promoting genes (e.g., c-*MYC* and c-*JUN*) and cell cycle–inhibiting genes (e.g., *p53*); they have a modular design with separate domains for DNA binding and transcriptional regulation. The end result of most signal transduction is altered gene transcription driven by changes in transcription factor activity. In general, the rapid responses demanded by cell signaling do not permit new synthesis of transcription factors, but rather rely on post-translational modifications that allow transcription factor migration into the nucleus. Modifications include dimerization, phosphorylation, or release of constitutively bound inhibitors.

Cell Cycle and the Regulation of Cell Proliferation (p. 100)

In general, cell proliferation is stimulated by some combination of soluble growth factors and signaling from extracellular matrix (ECM) components. Details of cell cycle regulation are covered in Chapter 7 in the context of cancer; the broad strokes of the cell cycle (see Fig. 3–3 in *Robbins and Cotran Pathologic Basis of Disease,* 7th ed.) include:

- A cascade of protein phosphorylation pathways involving *cyclins* and *cyclin-dependent kinases (CDKs)*. CDKs are constitutively expressed protein kinases that become active only after forming complexes with specific cyclins. Cyclins are regulatory proteins whose concentrations rise and fall during the cell cycle.
- Different combinations of cyclins and CDKs are associated with each of the important *transitions* in the cell cycle. For example, the G_1/S transition is a critical restriction point since the cell must make a major commitment of cellular resources to replicating its DNA. Cyclin-CDK complexes regulate the cell cycle by phosphorylating various target proteins (e.g., those involved in initiation of DNA replication or mitotic spindle formation). Cyclin-CDK complexes are regulated by catabolism or by binding of *CDK inhibitors*.
- *Checkpoints* provide a *surveillance mechanism* for ensuring that critical transitions in the cell cycle occur in the correct order and that important events are completed with fidelity. For example, the tumor-suppressor gene *p53* is activated in response to DNA damage and inhibits further progression through the cell cycle by increasing expression of a CDK inhibitor (it can even induce apoptosis).

MECHANISMS OF TISSUE REGENERATION
(p. 101)

Amphibians have impressive regenenerative capabilities attributed to the ability of quiescent cells (even cardiac myocytes) to reenter the cell cycle, and an efficient differentiation of stem cells in areas of injury. Mammals (unfortunately) lack this capacity and regeneration in damaged tissues is largely just compensatory growth involving cell hypertrophy and hyperplasia; this will usually restore functional capacity but does not necessarily reconstitute the original anatomy. The inadequacy of true regeneration in mammals is ascribed to a rapid fibroproliferative response and scar formation after wounding. Although some adult human tissues can regenerate to a significant extent (e.g., compensatory liver hyperplasia), other organs (kidney, pancreas, adrenal glands, thyroid, and lungs) have extremely limited regenerative capacity beyond the first few years of life. Thus, because adult kidneys cannot produce new nephrons, growth of the remaining kidney after unilateral nephrectomy involves nephron hypertrophy and limited tubular epithelial replication. Regeneration of pancreatic β cells involves stem cell differentiation or transdifferentiation of pancreatic ductal cells. Liver regeneration after partial hepatectomy involves the replication of mature cells without stem cell participation.

EXTRACELLULAR MATRIX AND CELL-MATRIX INTERACTIONS (p. 103)

ECM markedly influences cell growth and function; it consists of *fibrous structural proteins* (e.g., collagen) and *adhesive glycoproteins* embedded in a gel of *proteoglycans and hyaluronan*. These macromolecules assemble into an *interstitial matrix*, present in the spaces between cells, or into a *basement membrane*, apposed to cell plasma membranes.

Collagen (p. 104)

These connective tissue proteins provide tensile strength. Generically, at least some part of each collagen molecule is composed of a triple helix braid of three polypeptide chains, each having a primary glycine-X-Y repeating sequence (X and Y are any amino acid). There are at least 27 types of collagen (Table 3–2). Types I, II, III, V, and XI are the fibrillar collagens, and are most abundant; the collagen of skin and bone is mostly type I, while cartilage collagen is mostly type II. Type IV forms sheets instead of fibrils and is the major collagen found in basement membrane (BM). Other collagens may form ECM meshworks, or participate in cellular anchorage.

Procollagens are synthesized as individual α chains, followed by enzymatic hydroxylation of prolines and lysines. Three chains then align to form a triple helix and the product is secreted. In the extracellular space, the globular C- and N-terminal fragments are proteolytically cleaved, and lysine oxidase (whose enzymatic activity depends on vitamin C) oxidizes lysines and hydroxylysines to permit interchain cross-linking and stabilize the fibrils.

Elastin, Fibrillin, and Elastic Fibers (p. 104)

Elastin provides ECM with elasticity (stretch and recoil). Elastic fibers consist of an *elastin* central core with an associated scaffolding network of fibrillin, a 350-kD glycoprotein. Inherited defects in fibrillin (e.g., in Marfan syndrome) result in formation of abnormal elastic fibers (Chapter 5).

TABLE 3–2 **Main Types of Collagens, Tissue Distribution, and Genetic Disorders**

Collagen Type	Tissue Distribution	Genetic Disorders
Fibrillar Collagens		
I	Ubiquitous in hard and soft tissues	Osteogenesis imperfecta
		Ehlers-Danlos syndrome— arthrochalasias type
II	Cartilage, intervertebral disc, vitreous	Achondrogenesis type II, spondyloepiphyseal dysplasia syndrome
III	Hollow organs, soft tissues	Vascular Ehlers-Danlos syndrome
V	Soft tissues, blood vessels	Classical Ehlers-Danlos syndrome
XI	Cartilage, vitreous	Stickler syndrome
Basement Membrane Collagens		
IV	Basement membranes	Alport syndrome
Other Collagens		
VI	Ubiquitous in microfibrils	Bethlem myopathy
VII	Anchoring fibrils at dermal-epidermal junctions	Dystrophic epidermolysis bullosa
IX	Cartilage, intervertebral disks	Multiple epiphyseal dysplasias
XVII	Transmembrane collagen in epidermal cells	Benign atrophic generalized epidemolysis bullosa
XV and XVIII	Endostatin-forming collagens, endothelial cells	Knobloch syndrome (type XVIII collagen)

Courtesy of Dr. Peter H. Byers, Department of Pathology, University of Washington, Seattle, WA.

Cell Adhesion Proteins (p. 104)

These proteins are classified into four main families: *immunoglobulin family, cadherins, integrins,* and *selectins.* In cell membranes they act as receptors that bind to similar or different molecules in other cells. Cadherins and integrins are transmembrane proteins that link the cell surface (and thus ECM) with the intracellular cytoskeleton.

- *Cadherins* (>90 types!) mediate calcium-dependent interactions with cadherins on adjacent cells and interact with the cytoskeleton via *catenins;* cadherins bind β-catenins that link to α-catenins that connect to actin. Cell-cell interactions mediated through cadherins and catenins play major roles in cell motility and differentiation; they also account for the "contact inhibition" of cell proliferation that occurs when cells touch. β-Catenin mutations are involved in carcinogenesis (Chapter 7).
- *Integrins* participate in cell-cell adhesion, as well as adhesion to the ECM by binding to fibronectin and laminin.
- *Fibronectin* binds to many molecules (e.g., collagen, fibrin, proteoglycans, and cell surface receptors). Alternate splicing of fibronectin mRNA produces either tissue fibronectin (forming fibrillar aggregates at sites of wound healing) or

plasma fibronectin (forming provisional blood clots in wounds preceding ECM deposition).

- *Laminin* is the most abundant glycoprotein in the BM; it has binding domains for both ECM and cell surface receptors.
- Ligand binding to integrins causes clustering and formation of *focal adhesion* complexes; these function as activated receptors to trigger signal transduction pathways (many of the same ones used by soluble growth factors in Figure 3–2). There is functional overlap between integrin and growth factor receptor signaling; both transmit environmental cues that the cell integrates to regulate proliferation, apoptosis, or differentiation.
- Other significant secreted adhesion molecules are:

  SPARC (secreted protein acidic and rich in cysteine), also known as *osteonectin;* contributes to tissue remodeling after injury, and is an angiogenesis inhibitor.

  Thrombospondins, a family of large multifunctional proteins; some inhibit angiogenesis.

  Osteopontin, which regulates calcification and also mediates leukocyte migration.

  Tenacins, large multimeric proteins involved in morphogenesis and cell adhesion.

Proteoglycans and Hyaluronic Acid (p. 106)

These ECM components have a core protein linked to one or more polysaccharides called *glycosaminoglycans*—long repeating polymers of modified disaccharides (e.g., heparan sulfate). Proteoglycans can also be integral membrane proteins (e.g., the *syndecans*). *Hyaluronan* is a huge molecule with many disaccharide repeats; it serves as a ligand for cell surface receptors and other core proteins. Hyaluronan binds large amounts of water, giving ECM its turgor and ability to resist compression.

REPAIR BY HEALING, SCAR FORMATION, AND FIBROSIS (p. 107)

After injury, tissues may regenerate or heal. Regeneration involves restitution of tissue identical to that lost by injury; healing is a fibroproliferative response that "patches" rather than restores a tissue. Some tissues can be completely reconstituted after injury (e.g., bone after a fracture, or epithelium after a superficial skin wound). For tissues incapable of regeneration, repair is accomplished by ECM deposition, producing a *scar.* If damage is ongoing, inflammation becomes chronic, and tissue damage and repair may occur concurrently; ECM deposition in that setting is called *fibrosis.* Generically, fibrosis applies to *any* abnormal deposition of connective tissue. The sequence of healing involves:

- An inflammatory response to eliminate the initial stimulus, remove injured tissue, and initiate ECM deposition
- Proliferation and migration of parenchymal and connective tissue cells
- Formation of new blood vessels (*angiogenesis*) and *granulation tissue* (see below)
- Synthesis of ECM proteins

TABLE 3-3 **Growth Factors and Cytokines Affecting Various Steps in Wound Healing**

Activity in Wound Healing	Factors Involved
Monocyte chemotaxis	PDGF, FGF, TGF-β
Fibroblast migration	PDGF, EGF, FGF, TGF-β, TNF, IL1
Fibroblast proliferation	PDGF, EGF, FGF, TNF
Angiogenesis	VEGF, Ang, FGF
Collagen synthesis	TGF-β, PDGF
Collagenase secretion	PDGF, FGF, EGF, TNF, TGF-β inhibits

- Tissue remodeling
- Wound contraction and acquisition of wound strength

The principal factors involved in each step are listed in Table 3–3.

Repair begins early in inflammation. As early as 24 hours after injury, fibroblasts and vascular EC begin proliferating to form *granulation tissue,* a hallmark of healing; the term derives from its pink, soft, granular appearance on wound surfaces. Histologically, there are proliferating fibroblasts with numerous new blood vessels in a loose matrix. The interstitium is edematous because new vessels are leaky, allowing protein and erythrocyte passage.

Angiogenesis (p. 107)

Angiogenesis is critical to wound healing, to tumor growth, and to the vascularization of ischemic tissues. During embryonic development, vessels arise by *vasculogenesis*—a primitive vascular network assembled from EC precursor *angioblasts*. In adult tissues, vessel formation is called *angiogenesis* (or *neovascularization*); it occurs by branching of preexisting vessels and by recruitment of endothelial precursor cells (EPCs) from bone marrow.

Angiogenesis from Endothelial Precursor Cells (p. 108)

In embryonic development, a common precursor *hemangioblast* generates both hematopoietic stem cells and angioblasts; the latter proliferate, migrate to peripheral sites, and can differentiate into ECs, pericytes, and vascular smooth muscle cells. Angioblast-like EPCs are also stored in adult bone marrow and can initiate angiogenesis; they participate in replacing lost ECs, in vascular implant endothelization, and in neovascularizing ischemic organs, cutaneous wounds, and tumors.

Angiogenesis from Preexisting Vessels (p. 108)

Angiogenesis from preexisting vessels occurs in stepwise fashion:

- Nitric oxide dilates preexisting vessels.
- VEGF induces increased permeability.
- Metalloproteinases degrade the basement membrane (BM).
- Plasminogen activator disrupts EC cell-cell contact.
- ECs proliferate and migrate toward the angiogenic stimulus.
- EC maturation occurs, including growth inhibition and remodeling into capillary tubes.

- Periendothelial cells (pericytes for small capillaries and vascular smooth muscle cells for larger vessels) are recruited.

Growth Factors and Receptors Involved in Angiogenesis (p. 109)

VEGF and the *angiopoietins* (Ang) are the most important factors; the VEGFR-2 tyrosine kinase receptor (largely restricted to ECs and EC precursors) is the most important receptor for angiogenesis (although FGF-2 can also enhance EC proliferation, differentiation, and migration). VEGF/VEGFR-2 interactions:

- Mobilize EPC from bone marrow and enhance their proliferation and differentiation at sites of angiogenesis
- Stimulate proliferation and motility of existing ECs, promoting capillary sprouting

Stabilization of new fragile vessels requires the recruitment of pericytes and smooth muscle cells and the deposition of ECM proteins; *angiopoietins 1 and 2,* PDGF, and TGF-β participate in this process.

- Angiopoietin 1 interacts with the EC receptor *Tie2* to recruit periendothelial cells. The interaction also mediates vessel maturation from simple tubes into more elaborate vascular structures and helps maintain EC quiescence. Angiopoietin 2-Tie2 interactions have the opposite effect; ECs become more responsive to VEGF stimulation.
- PDGF recruits smooth muscle cells.
- TGF-β stabilizes newly formed vessels by enhancing ECM production.

ECM Proteins as Regulators of Angiogenesis (p. 109)

The directed migration of ECs in angiogenesis is controlled by

- *Integrins,* especially $\alpha_v\beta_3$ (critical for forming and maintaining newly formed vessels).
- *Matricellular proteins,* including thrombospondin 1, SPARC, and tenascin C (see above).
- *Proteases* (e.g., plasminogen activators and metalloproteinases) that remodel tissue during EC invasion. They release matrix-bound VEGF and FGF-2 to stimulate angiogenesis, as well as inhibitors of angiogenesis (e.g., *endostatin,* a small fragment of collagen XVIII).

Scar Formation (p. 110)

Scar deposition occurs within the initial granulation tissue framework. Three general steps occur.

Fibroblast Migration and Proliferation (p. 110)

Increased vascular permeability causes plasma protein deposition (e.g., fibronectin and fibrinogen), providing a provisional matrix for fibroblast ingrowth. PDGF, EGF, FGF, and TGF-β and the cytokines IL1 and TNF regulate fibroblast migration and proliferation.

ECM Deposition and Scar Formation (p. 110)

As repair progresses, the numbers of proliferating ECs and fibroblasts decrease; fibroblasts become more synthetic and deposit more collagen and other ECM components. ECM synthesis is stimulated by growth factors (e.g., PDGF, FGF, TGF-β) and cytokines (e.g., IL1) secreted by fibroblasts and leukocytes in healing wounds. ECM degradation is also diminished (see below). Eventually, the granulation tissue scaffolding is converted into a scar composed of fibroblasts and collagen.

Tissue Remodeling (p. 110)

The replacement of granulation tissue with a scar ultimately involves changes in ECM composition. Besides driving ECM synthesis, the various growth factors also modulate the synthesis and activation of *matrix metalloproteinases* (MMPs), a family of more than 20 enzymes that degrade ECM; MMP production is inhibited by TGF-β. MMPs are secreted as proenzymes and activated extracellularly; they require zinc for their activity.

- *Interstitial collagenases* cleave fibrillar collagen types I, II, and III.
- *Gelatinases* degrade amorphous collagen as well as fibronectin.
- *Stromelysins* act on a variety of ECM components, including proteoglycans, laminin, fibronectin, and amorphous collagens.
- *ADAMs* (*disintegrin and metalloproteinase-domain*) are membrane-bound MMPs that release extracellular domains of cell surface proteins (e.g., precursor forms of TNF and TGF-α).

Activated MMPs are rapidly inhibited by various *tissue inhibitors of metalloproteinases (TIMPs)*. The net effect of ECM *synthesis* versus *degradation* results in debridement of injured sites and *remodeling* of the connective tissues framework.

CUTANEOUS WOUND HEALING (p. 111)

Wound healing in the skin is illustrative of repair principles for most tissues. In very superficial wounds, the epithelium is reconstituted and there may be little scar formation. With more extensive injury, the end product may not be functionally perfect; epidermal appendages (hair, sweat glands) do not regenerate, and connective tissue scar replaces the mechanically efficient collagen meshwork in the native dermis.

Wound healing progresses in an orderly fashion through overlapping phases of the processes described above (Fig. 3–3):

- Induction of inflammation by the initial injury
- Granulation tissue formation and reepithelialization
- ECM deposition and remodeling with wound contraction

Skin wounds are classically described as healing by *primary* or *secondary intention*. The healing process is essentially the same in both; the distinction is due more to the nature (extent) of the wounds (see Fig. 3–21, in *Robbins and Cotran Pathologic Basis of Disease*, 7th ed., p. 112).

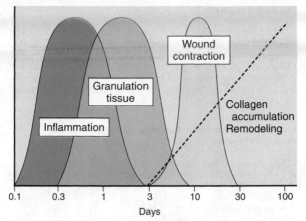

FIGURE 3–3 Phases of wound healing. (From Physiology, Biochemistry, and Molecular Biology of the Skin, 2 volumes, second edition, edited by Lowell A. Goldsmith, copyright 1991 by Oxford University Press, Inc.)

Healing by First Intention (Wounds with Opposed Edges) (p. 111)

A clean surgical approximated incision causes minimal cell death and minimal BM disruption. The healing process involves several steps:

- *0 hours:* The incision is filled with clotted blood.
- *3 to 24 hours:* Neutrophils infiltrate the clot.
- *24 to 48 hours:* Epithelial cells migrate from the edges of the wound depositing BM; proliferation is minimal.
- *Day 3:* Neutrophils are replaced by macrophages. Granulation tissue begins to appear.
- *Day 5:* The incision space is filled with granulation tissue, neovascularization and epithelial proliferation is maximal; collagen fibrils begin to appear.
- *Week 2:* Inflammation, edema, and increased vascularity have waned; fibroblast proliferation accompanies continued collagen accumulation.
- *Month 2:* Scar now consists of connective tissue devoid of inflammation covered by intact epidermis. Tensile strength of the wound will continue to accrue.

Healing by Second Intention (Wounds with Separated Edges) (p. 113)

This occurs when there is more extensive tissue loss. The resulting inflammatory response is greater, and much more abundant granulation tissue will ensue; there will be substantial scar deposition and the overlying epidermis will be thinned. Most significantly, secondary healing is characterized by *wound contraction* in which the defect is markedly reduced from its original size, largely through the contractile activity of *myofibroblasts*.

Wound Strength (p. 113)

Wound strength is initially largely dependent on suturing; when the sutures are removed (typically at 1 week), wound strength is only about 10% of normal. Tensile strength eventually plateaus at 70% to 80% of normal within 3 months; this is associated with increased collagen synthesis exceeding collagen degradation, followed by cross-linking and increased collagen fiber size.

Local and Systemic Factors That Influence Wound Healing (p. 114)

- Size, location, and type of the wound influence healing.
- *Local factors that delay healing* include infections, mechanical forces (e.g., motion or wound tension), and foreign bodies.
- Systemic factors:

  Nutritional status of the host (e.g., protein nutrition and vitamin C intake)

  Metabolic status (diabetes mellitus delays healing)

  Circulatory status or vascular adequacy

  Hormones (e.g., glucocorticoids) (can impede the inflammatory-reparative process)

Complications in Cutaneous Wound Healing (p. 114)

- *Deficient scar formation:* Inadequate granulation tissue or collagen deposition and remodeling can lead to either *wound dehiscence or ulceration.*
- *Excessive repair:* Excessive granulation tissue (*exuberant granulation* or *proud flesh*) can protrude above the surrounding skin and block reepithelialization. Excessive collagen accumulation forms a raised *hypertrophic scar;* progression beyond the original area of injury without subsequent regression is termed a *keloid.*
- *Formation of contractures:* Although wound contraction is a normal part of healing, an exaggerated process is designated a *contracture.* It will cause wound deformity (e.g., producing hand *claw* deformities, or limit joint mobility).

FIBROSIS (p. 115)

The cell proliferation, cell-cell and cell–matrix interactions, and ECM deposition involved in wound healing also underlie the fibrosis associated with chronic inflammatory diseases such as rheumatoid arthritis and cirrhosis. The chronic inflammatory diseases are marked by persistence of the initial injury (e.g., ongoing toxic exposure) or persistence of the inflammatory response (e.g., radiation injury or autoimmunity). In most cases, lymphocyte–macrophage interactions sustain the synthesis and secretion of growth factors and fibrogenic cytokines, proteases, and other biologically active molecules; consequently, the ongoing inflammation drives progressive tissue injury and fibrosis.

CHAPTER 4

Hemodynamic Disorders, Thromboembolic Disease, and Shock

Normal fluid homeostasis involves maintaining vessel wall integrity, intravascular pressure, and osmolarity within physiologic ranges; failure to do so results in interstitial water accumulation (*edema*). Normal fluid homeostasis also involves maintaining blood as a liquid until such time as injury necessitates clot formation. Clotting at inappropriate sites (*thrombosis*) or migration of clots (*embolism*) will obstruct blood flow to tissues and lead to cell death (*infarction*). Conversely, inability to clot after vascular injury results in *hemorrhage;* local bleeding can compromise regional tissue perfusion, while more extensive hemorrhage can result in hypotension (*shock*) and death. Overall, disturbances in normal blood flow are major sources of human morbidity and death.

EDEMA (p. 120)

Edema is increased fluid in interstitial tissue spaces or body cavities (e.g., *hydrothorax, hydropericardium; hydroperitoneum* is also called *ascites*). Edema may be localized (e.g., secondary to isolated venous or lymphatic obstruction) or systemic (as in heart failure); severe systemic edema is called *anasarca*. Table 4–1 lists the pathophysiologic categories of edema; these can be broadly grouped into *noninflammatory* (yields protein-poor *transudates*) and *inflammatory* (yields protein-rich *exudates,* see Chapter 2).

Noninflammatory causes of edema:

• *Increased hydrostatic pressure* forces fluid out of the vessels. *Congestive heart failure* (CHF) (Chapter 12) falls in this

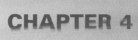

TABLE 4–1   **Pathophysiologic Categories of Edema**

Increased Hydrostatic Pressure
Impaired venous return
   Congestive heart failure
   Constrictive pericarditis
   Ascites (liver cirrhosis)
   Venous obstruction or compression
      Thrombosis
      External pressure (e.g., mass)
      Lower extremity inactivity with prolonged dependency
Arteriolar dilation
   Heat
   Neurohumoral dysregulation

Reduced Plasma Osmotic Pressure (Hypoproteinemia)
Protein-losing glomerulopathies (nephrotic syndrome)
Liver cirrhosis (ascites)
Malnutrition
Protein-losing gastroenteropathy

Lymphatic Obstruction
Inflammatory
Neoplastic
Postsurgical
Postirradiation

Sodium Retention
Excessive salt intake with renal insufficiency
Increased tubular reabsorption of sodium
   Renal hypoperfusion
   Increased renin-angiotensin-aldosterone secretion

Inflammation
Acute inflammation
Chronic inflammation
Angiogenesis

Modified from Leaf A, Cotran RS: Renal Pathophysiology, 3rd ed. New York, Oxford University Press, 1985, p. 146. Used by permission of Oxford Press, Inc.

category and *is the most common cause of systemic edema.*
Edema in CHF is caused mainly by increased venous hydrostatic pressure, although reduced cardiac output (with renal hypoperfusion and resulting sodium and water retention) contributes.

• *Decreased osmotic pressure* reduces movement of fluid into vessels. This occurs with albumin loss (most important cause is proteinuria in *nephrotic syndrome*, Chapter 20) or reduced albumin synthesis (e.g., with cirrhosis [Chapter 18] or as a consequence of protein malnutrition). Reduced osmotic pressure leads to a net fluid movement into the interstitium with plasma volume contraction. As with CHF, edema due to *hypoproteinemia* is exacerbated by secondary salt and fluid retention.

• *Lymphatic obstruction* blocks removal of interstitial fluid. Obstruction is usually localized and related to inflammation or neoplastic processes.

• *Primary sodium retention,* with obligatory associated water retention, causes *both* increased hydrostatic pressure and reduced osmotic pressure. Sodium retention can occur with any renal dysfunction (e.g., acute renal failure or poststreptococcal glomerulonephritis, Chapter 20).

Morphology (p. 122)

Edema is most easily appreciated grossly; microscopically, edema manifests only as subtle cell swelling and separation of the extracellular matrix.

- *Subcutaneous edema* may be diffuse or occur where hydrostatic pressures are greatest (e.g., influenced by gravity, so-called *dependent edema* [legs when standing, sacrum when recumbent]). Dependent edema is typical of CHF. Edema resulting from hypoproteinemia is generally more severe and diffuse; it is most evident in loose connective tissue (e.g., eyelids, causing *periorbital edema*).
- *Edema of solid organs* results in increased size and weight; histologically, there is only separation of parenchymal elements.
- *Pulmonary edema* (Chapter 15) is typical in left ventricular failure but is also seen with renal failure, adult respiratory distress syndrome, infections, and hypersensitivity reactions. The lungs are two to three times their normal weight; sectioning reveals a frothy, blood-tinged mixture of air, edema fluid, and erythrocytes.
- *Brain edema* may be localized to sites of injury (e.g., abscess or neoplasm) or may be generalized (e.g., encephalitis, hypertensive crises, or obstruction to venous outflow). When generalized, the brain is grossly swollen with narrowed sulci and distended gyri flattened against the skull.

HYPEREMIA AND CONGESTION (p. 122)

Both terms mean increased volume of blood in a particular site.

- *Hyperemia* is an *active process* due to augmented blood inflow from arteriolar dilation (e.g., skeletal muscle during exercise or at sites of inflammation). Tissues are redder owing to engorgement with oxygenated blood.
- *Congestion* is a *passive process* caused by impaired outflow from a tissue. Isolated venous obstruction may cause local congestion; systemic venous obstruction occurs in CHF (Chapter 12). Tissues are blue-red (*cyanosis*), particularly as worsening congestion leads to accumulated deoxyhemoglobin. Long-standing stasis of deoxygenated blood can result in hypoxia severe enough to cause cell death.

Morphology (p. 122)

In *acute congestion,* vessels are distended, and organs are grossly hyperemic; capillary bed congestion is also commonly associated with interstitial edema. In *chronic congestion,* capillary rupture may cause focal hemorrhage; subsequent erythrocyte breakdown results in hemosiderin-laden macrophages. Parenchymal cell atrophy or death (with fibrosis) may also be present. Grossly, tissues appear brown, contracted, and fibrotic. Lungs and liver are commonly affected.

- The *lungs* are typically involved in left ventricular failure of any cause. Acutely, there is capillary engorgement, with interstitial edema and airspace transudates. Chronically, hemosiderin-laden macrophages *(heart failure cells)* are seen, with edematous to fibrotic septa *(brown induration)*.

- The *liver* is involved when there is right-sided heart failure, or rarely with hepatic vein or inferior vena cava obstruction. Acutely, there is central vein and sinusoidal distention; central hepatocyte degeneration may also be present. Chronically, the central regions of the hepatic lobules are grossly red-brown and slightly depressed (loss of cells) relative to the surrounding uncongested tan liver (so-called *nutmeg liver*). Microscopically, there is *centrilobular necrosis* with hepatocyte dropout and hemorrhage including hemosiderin-laden macrophages. In severe, long-standing congestion, there may even be hepatic fibrosis *(cardiac cirrhosis)*. Because the central portion of the hepatic lobule is the last to receive blood, centrilobular necrosis can occur whenever hepatic perfusion is reduced; previous hepatic congestion is not necessary.

HEMORRHAGE (p. 123)

Hemorrhage refers to blood extravasation following vessel rupture. Rupture of a large artery or vein is usually due to vascular injury (e.g., trauma, atherosclerosis, or inflammatory or neoplastic erosion of the vessel). Capillary bleeding can occur with chronic congestion. A tendency to hemorrhage from insignificant injury is seen in a variety of disorders called *hemorrhagic diatheses* (Chapter 13). Hemorrhage may be external or enclosed within a tissue; the latter is called a *hematoma*. Hematomas may be trivial (e.g., a bruise) or may accumulate sufficient blood to cause death (e.g., retroperitoneal hematoma resulting from an aortic aneurysm rupture). Hemorrhage is categorized according to size:

- *Petechiae:* Minute, 1- to 2-mm hemorrhages in skin, mucous membranes, or serosal surfaces; these occur with increased intravascular pressure, low platelet counts *(thrombocytopenia)*, defective platelet function, or clotting factor deficits.
- *Purpura:* Larger (≥3 mm) hemorrhages; these occur for the same reasons as petechiae, as well as with trauma, local vascular inflammation *(vasculitis)*, or increased vascular fragility (e.g., amyloidosis).
- *Ecchymoses:* Larger (>1–2 cm) subcutaneous hematomas (commonly called *bruises*). Ecchymoses typically follow trauma but are exacerbated by any of the above conditions.
- Large accumulations of blood in body cavities are called *hemothorax*, *hemopericardium*, *hemoperitoneum*, or *hemarthrosis*, depending on the location.

Erythrocytes in hemorrhages are degraded by macrophages. The hemoglobin (red-blue color) is converted to bilirubin and biliverdin (blue-green color) and eventually to hemosiderin (golden brown), accounting for the characteristic color changes in a bruise. Patients with extensive hemorrhages occasionally develop jaundice from massive erythrocyte breakdown and systemic bilirubin release.

The clinical significance of hemorrhage depends on the volume and rate of blood loss. Rapid loss of less than 20%, or slow losses of even larger amounts, may have little impact; greater losses result in *hemorrhagic (hypovolemic) shock*. Location is also important: bleeding that would be inconsequential in subcutaneous tissues may cause death in the brain.

HEMOSTASIS AND THROMBOSIS (p. 124)

Hemostasis and thrombosis are closely related processes dependent on three components: *endothelium, platelets,* and *coagulation cascade. Hemostasis is a normal physiologic process* maintaining blood in a fluid, clot-free state in normal vessels, while inducing a rapid, localized hemostatic plug at sites of vascular injury. *Thrombosis represents a pathologic state*; it is inappropriate activation of hemostatic mechanisms in uninjured vasculature or thrombotic occlusion after relatively minor injury.

Normal Hemostasis (p. 124)

After injury, there is a characteristic hemostatic response (Fig. 4–1):

- *Reflex neurogenic arteriolar vasoconstriction* is augmented by *endothelin* (potent endothelium-derived vasoconstrictor).
- *Platelet adhesion and activation* (shape change and secretory granule release) are promoted by exposed subendothelial extracellular matrix (ECM). Secreted products recruit other platelets to form a *temporary hemostatic plug.*
- *Activation of the coagulation cascade* is driven by *tissue factor,* a membrane-bound lipoprotein procoagulant factor synthesized by endothelium and exposed after injury. Activation of coagulation culminates in *thrombin* generation and conversion of circulating fibrinogen to insoluble *fibrin* (see below). Thrombin also induces platelet recruitment and granule release. Polymerized fibrin and platelet aggregates form a solid, *permanent plug.*
- *Activation of counter-regulatory mechanisms* (e.g., tissue plasminogen activator [t-PA]) restricts the hemostatic plug to the site of injury.

Endothelium (p. 124)

Endothelial cells (ECs) modulate several, frequently opposing aspects of hemostasis. ECs normally exhibit antiplatelet, anticoagulant, and fibrinolytic properties. However, after injury or activation, ECs exhibit *procoagulant function* (Fig. 4–2). The balance between EC anti- and prothrombotic activities determines whether thrombus formation, propagation, or dissolution occurs.

Platelets (p. 126)

Platelets are crucial for normal hemostasis and thrombosis. After vascular injury, platelets encounter ECM constituents (collagen, proteoglycans, fibronectin, and other adhesive glycoproteins) normally sequestered beneath an intact endothelium. Platelets then undergo *activation* involving adhesion and shape change, secretion (release reaction), and aggregation.

- *Platelet-ECM adhesion* is mediated through von Willebrand factor (vWF), acting as a bridge between platelet receptors (mostly glycoprotein Ib) and exposed collagen. Genetic deficiencies of vWF (von Willebrand disease) or glycoprotein-Ib (Bernard-Soulier syndrome) result in bleeding disorders.
- *Platelet granule secretion (release reaction)* occurs shortly after adhesion. *Alpha granules* express P-selectin adhesion

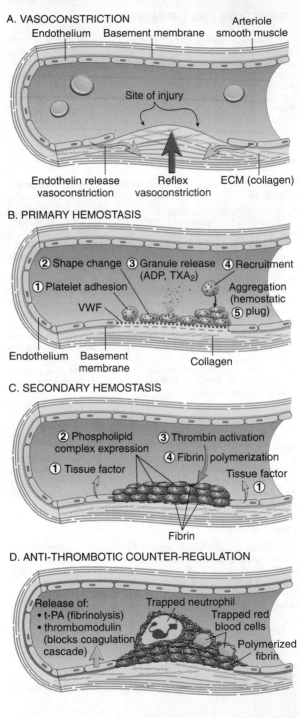

A. VASOCONSTRICTION

Endothelium   Basement membrane   Arteriole smooth muscle

Site of injury

Endothelin release vasoconstriction   Reflex vasoconstriction   ECM (collagen)

B. PRIMARY HEMOSTASIS

② Shape change ③ Granule release (ADP, TXA₂) ④ Recruitment

① Platelet adhesion   Aggregation (hemostatic ⑤ plug)

VWF

Endothelium   Basement membrane   Collagen

C. SECONDARY HEMOSTASIS

② Phospholipid complex expression   ③ Thrombin activation

① Tissue factor   ④ Fibrin polymerization   Tissue factor ①

Fibrin

D. ANTI-THROMBOTIC COUNTER-REGULATION

Release of:
• t-PA (fibrinolysis)
• thrombomodulin (blocks coagulation cascade)

Trapped neutrophil   Trapped red blood cells

Polymerized fibrin

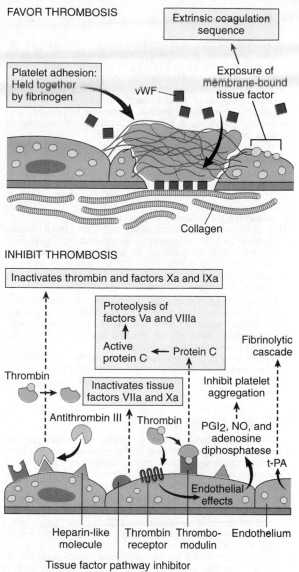

FAVOR THROMBOSIS

Extrinsic coagulation sequence

Platelet adhesion: Held together by fibrinogen

vWF

Exposure of membrane-bound tissue factor

Collagen

INHIBIT THROMBOSIS

Inactivates thrombin and factors Xa and IXa

Proteolysis of factors Va and VIIIa

Active protein C ← Protein C

Fibrinolytic cascade

Thrombin

Inactivates tissue factors VIIa and Xa

Inhibit platelet aggregation

Antithrombin III   Thrombin

PGI₂, NO, and adenosine diphosphatese

t-PA

Endothelial effects

Heparin-like molecule   Thrombin receptor   Thrombo-modulin   Endothelium

Tissue factor pathway inhibitor

FIGURE 4–2 Schematic illustration of some of the pro- and anticoagulant activities of endothelial cells. Not shown are the pro- and antifibrinolytic properties. vWF, von Willebrand factor; PGI$_2$, prostacyclin; NO, nitric oxide; t-PA, tissue plasminogen activator.

FIGURE 4–1 Diagrammatic representation of the normal hemostatic process. *A,* After vascular injury, local neurohumoral factors induce a transient vasoconstriction. *B,* Platelets adhere to exposed extracellular matrix (ECM) via von Willebrand factor (vWF) and are activated, undergoing a shape change and granule release; released adenosine diphosphate (ADP) and thromboxane A$_2$ (TxA$_2$) lead to further platelet aggregation to form the primary hemostatic plug. *C,* Local activation of the coagulation cascade (involving tissue factor and platelet phospholipids) results in fibrin polymerization, "cementing" the platelets into a definitive secondary hemostatic plug. *D,* Counter-regulatory mechanisms, such as release of tissue type plasminogen activator (t-PA) (fibrinolytic) and thrombomodulin (interfering with the coagulation cascade), limit the hemostatic process to the site of injury.

molecules and contain coagulation and growth factors; *dense bodies* or *delta granules* contain adenosine nucleotides (adenosine diphosphate [ADP] and adenosine triphosphate [ATP]), calcium, and vasoactive amines (e.g., histamine). ADP is a potent mediator of *platelet aggregation,* and calcium is important for the coagulation cascade. The release reaction also results in surface expression of *phospholipid complex,* providing a locus for calcium and coagulation factor interactions in the *clotting cascade.*

- *Platelet aggregation* (platelets adhering to other platelets) is promoted by ADP and thromboxane A_2.

    ADP activation changes the conformation of platelet GpIIb-IIIa receptors to allow binding to fibrinogen; fibrinogen then acts to connect multiple platelets together to form large aggregates (GpIIb-IIIa deficiencies result in *Glanzmann thrombasthenia* bleeding disorder).

    Platelet-derived thromboxane A_2 activates platelet aggregation and is a potent vasoconstrictor; EC-derived prostaglandin I_2 (Chapter 2) inhibits platelet aggregation and is a potent vasodilator. Interplay between prostaglandin I_2 and thromboxane A_2 can finely modulate platelet function.

- Platelet aggregation creates the *primary hemostatic plug,* which is reversible. Activation of the coagulation cascade (see below) generates *thrombin* and *fibrin* to form an irreversibly fused mass of platelets and fibrin constituting the definitive *secondary hemostatic plug.*
- Erythrocytes and leukocytes also aggregate in hemostatic plugs; leukocytes adhere to platelets via P-selectin and contribute to the inflammatory response accompanying thrombosis.

Coagulation Cascade (p. 127)

A sequence of conversions of inactive proenzymes into activated enzymes, culminating in the generation of insoluble *fibrin* from the soluble plasma protein *fibrinogen.* Traditionally, coagulation has been divided into *extrinsic* and *intrinsic* pathways, converging where factor X is activated (Fig. 4–3).

- The intrinsic cascade is classically initiated by activation of Hageman factor (factor XII); the extrinsic cascade is activated by *tissue factor* (see above). There is a rather broad overlap between the two pathways and the division is largely an artifact of *in vitro* testing.
- Each reaction in the various pathways results from assembly of a complex held together by *calcium ions* on a *phospholipid complex* and composed of

    Enzyme (activated coagulation factor)
    Substrate (proenzyme form of coagulation factor)
    Cofactor (reaction accelerator)

    Thus, clotting tends to remain localized to sites where assembly can occur (e.g., surfaces of activated platelets or endothelium).

- Besides catalyzing the cleavage of fibrinogen to fibrin, thrombin also exerts numerous effects on local vessel wall and inflammatory cells; it even *limits* the extent of hemostasis (see below). Most such effects are mediated through *protease-activated receptors (PARs),* seven-transmembrane

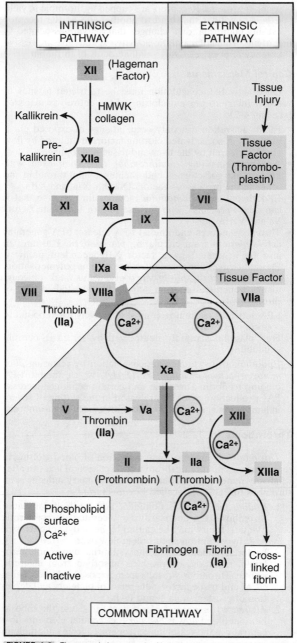

FIGURE 4–3 The coagulation cascade. Note the common link between the intrinsic and extrinsic pathways at the level of factor IX activation. Activated factors are indicated with a lowercase "a." PL, phospholipid surface; HMWK, high-molecular-weight kininogen. Not shown are the anticoagulant inhibitory pathways (see Fig. 4–2).

spanner proteins. Receptors are clipped by thrombin to yield *tethered* peptides that bind to another site on the receptor causing conformational changes that activate associated G proteins. This autocatalytic activity explains the impressive potency of even relatively small amounts of thrombin.

Control Mechanisms

Once activated, coagulation must be restricted to sites of vascular injury to prevent clotting of the entire vascular tree (see Fig. 4–2):

- Factor activation can only occur at sites of exposed phospholipids. Also, activated clotting factors are diluted by flow and are cleared by the liver and tissue macrophages.
- Antithrombins (e.g., *antithrombin III*), complexed with heparin-like cofactors on endothelium, inhibit thrombin and other serine proteases—factors IXa, Xa, XIa, and XIIa.
- Endothelial *thrombomodulin* modifies thrombin so that it can cleave *proteins C and S;* these, in turn, inactivate factors Va and VIIIa.
- Thrombin induces endothelial t-PA release; t-PA generates active *plasmin* from circulating *plasminogen.* Plasmin can also be generated by a factor XII–dependent pathway. Plasmin cleaves fibrin and interferes with its polymerization; the resulting *fibrin split products* also act as weak anticoagulants. Functional plasmin activity is restricted to sites of thrombosis:

   t-PA activates plasminogen most effectively when bound to fibrin meshwork.

   Free plasmin is rapidly neutralized by serum α_2-plasmin inhibitor.

- Endothelium modulates anticoagulation by releasing *plasminogen activator inhibitors (PAIs),* which inhibit t-PA binding to fibrin. Thrombin and certain cytokines increase PAI production; cytokines released in the setting of severe inflammation can therefore cause intravascular thrombosis.

Thrombosis (p. 130)

Thrombosis is inappropriate activation of blood clotting in uninjured vasculature or thrombotic occlusion of a vessel after relatively minor injury. There are three primary influences on thrombus formation, so-called *Virchow's triad:*

1. *Endothelial injury* is dominant and by itself can cause thrombosis (e.g., endocarditis or ulcerated atherosclerotic plaque). Injury may be caused by hemodynamic stresses (e.g., hypertension or turbulent flow over scarred valves), bacterial endotoxins, homocystinuria, hypercholesterolemia, radiation, or products absorbed from cigarette smoke. Thrombosis results from exposed subendothelial ECM and tissue factor, adherence of platelets, and depletion of prostaglandin I_2 and PAIs.

2. *Alterations in normal blood flow* can cause thrombosis. Normal blood flow is *laminar* (i.e., cellular elements flow centrally in the vessel lumen, separated from endothelium by a plasma clear zone). Stasis and turbulence (the latter forms eddy currents with local pockets of stasis):

   Disrupt laminar flow and bring platelets into contact with the endothelium.

Prevent dilution of activated clotting factors by flowing blood.

Retard the inflow of clotting inhibitors and permit thrombus accumulation.

Promote endothelial cell activation.

Stasis causes thrombosis in the venous circulation, cardiac chambers, and arterial aneurysms; turbulence in the arterial circulation also directly causes endothelial injury and dysfunction. Hyperviscosity syndromes (e.g., polycythemia) or deformed erythrocytes (e.g., sickle cell anemia) result in small vessel stasis and also predispose to thrombosis.

3. *Hypercoagulability* contributes less frequently to thrombotic states but is important in certain states; it is loosely defined as any alteration of the coagulation pathways that predisposes to thrombosis (Table 4–2).

Heritable hypercoagulable states: factor V gene mutations are the most common; 2% to 15% of caucasians (60% of patients with recurrent deep vein thrombosis) carry the so-called *Leiden mutation* that renders their factor V resistant to inactivation by protein C. Others with inherited anticoagulants deficiencies (e.g., antithrombin III, protein C or S) also typically present with venous thrombosis and recurrent thromboembolism.

Acquired thrombotic diatheses have diverse causes:

Oral contraceptives or the hyperestrogenic state of pregnancy may cause hypercoagulability by increasing hepatic synthesis of coagulation factors and reduced synthesis of antithrombin III.

TABLE 4–2 **Hypercoagulable States**

Primary (Genetic)
Common
Mutation in factor V gene (factor V_{Leiden})
Mutation in prothrombin gene
Mutation in methyltetrahydrofolate gene
Rare
Antithrombin III deficiency
Protein C deficiency
Protein S deficiency
Very rare
Fibrinolysis defects
Secondary (Acquired)
High risk for thrombosis
Prolonged bed rest or immobilization
Myocardial infarction
Atrial fibrillation
Tissue damage (surgery, fracture, burns)
Cancer
Prosthetic cardiac valves
Disseminated intravascular coagulation
Heparin-induced thrombocytopenia
Antiphospholipid antibody syndrome (lupus anticoagulant syndrome)
Lower risk for thrombosis
Cardiomyopathy
Nephrotic syndrome
Hyperestrogenic states (pregnancy)
Oral contraceptive use
Sickle cell anemia
Smoking

Certain malignancies can release procoagulant tumor products.

Heparin-induced thrombocytopenia syndrome occurs when unfractionated heparin induces circulating antibodies that activate platelets and injure ECs.

Antiphospholipid antibody syndrome occurs in patients with antibodies against anionic phospholipids that can putatively activate platelets or interfere with protein C activity. Patients may have a well-defined autoimmune disease, e.g., systemic lupus erythematosus (i.e., *lupus anticoagulant syndrome*), or may exhibit only a hypercoagulable state.

Morphology of Thrombi (p. 132)

Thrombi may form anywhere in the cardiovascular system. Aortic or cardiac thrombi are typically *nonocclusive (mural)* as a result of rapid and high-volume flow; smaller arterial thrombi may be *occlusive.* All these thrombi usually begin at sites of endothelial injury (e.g., atherosclerotic plaque) or turbulence (vessel bifurcation). Venous thrombi characteristically occur in sites of stasis and are *occlusive.*

At sites of origin, thrombi are generally firmly attached. Arterial thrombi tend to extend retrograde from the attachment point, whereas venous thrombi extend in the direction of blood flow. The propagating tail may not be well attached and may fragment to create an *embolus.*

- *Cardiac and arterial thrombi* are gray-red and have gross and microscopic laminations (*lines of Zahn*) produced by pale layers of platelets and fibrin alternating with darker erythrocyte-rich layers. Major sites include the left ventricle overlying an infarct, ruptured atherosclerotic plaques, and aneurysmal sacs.
- *Venous thrombosis (phlebothrombosis)* often creates a long red-blue cast of the vein lumen because it occurs in a relatively static environment; the thrombus contains more enmeshed erythrocytes among sparse fibrin strands (*red or stasis thrombi*). Fibrin and vessel wall attachment distinguish stasis thrombi from postmortem clots. Phlebothrombosis most commonly affects the veins of the lower extremities (>90% of cases).
- *Thrombi may also form on heart valves.* In *infective endocarditis,* organisms form large infected thrombotic masses (*vegetations*), causing underlying valve damage and systemic infection. Sterile vegetations *(nonbacterial thrombotic endocarditis)* also develop on noninfected valves in hypercoagulable states, particularly in those with malignancies. Rarely, noninfective, *verrucous (Libman-Sacks) endocarditis* occurs in patients with systemic lupus erythematosus (owing to circulating immune complexes).

Fate of the Thrombus (p. 133)

If a patient survives the immediate (generally ischemic or venous obstructive) effects of a thrombus, some combination of the following occurs:

- *Propagation,* causing complete vessel obstruction
- *Embolization* to other sites in the vasculature is especially common with lower extremity venous thrombi embolizing to the lung

- *Dissolution* by fibrinolytic activity
- *Organization and recanalization,* reestablishing flow by ingrowth of endothelial cells, smooth muscle cells, and fibroblasts to create vascular channels, or by incorporating the thrombus as a subendothelial swelling of the vessel wall

Rarely, when microbial seeding of a thrombus occurs, a *mycotic aneurysm* may result.

Clinical Correlations (p. 134)

Thrombi are significant because they (1) *cause obstruction of arteries and veins,* and (2) *are possible sources of emboli.* In each instance, the relevance depends on the site of thrombosis. Thus, although venous thrombi may cause congestion and edema in distal vascular beds, a more dire consequence is their propensity to embolize (e.g., from deep leg vein to lung). Conversely, although arterial thrombi can embolize, their role in local vascular obstruction (e.g., causing myocardial or cerebral infarctions) is much more important.

Venous Thrombosis (Phlebothrombosis)

Venous thrombosis occurs in most instances in the superficial or deep leg veins.

- Superficial thrombi usually occur in varicose saphenous veins, causing local congestion and pain but rarely embolizing. Local edema and impaired venous drainage predispose to skin infections and *varicose ulcers.*
- *Deep thrombi* in larger leg veins above the knee (e.g., popliteal, femoral, and iliac veins) more readily embolize. Although they may cause pain and edema, venous obstruction is usually offset by collateral flow. Thus, deep vein thromboses are entirely asymptomatic in *approximately 50% of patients* and are recognized only after embolization. Deep venous thrombosis occurs in multiple clinical settings:

  Advanced age, bed rest, or immobilization, diminishing the milking action of muscles in the lower leg and slowing venous return.

  Congestive heart failure (CHF).

  Trauma, surgery, and burns result in reduced physical activity, injury to vessels, release of procoagulant substances from tissues, and reduced tPA.

  The puerperal and postpartum states are associated with amniotic fluid embolization (see below) and hypercoagulability.

  Tumor-associated procoagulant release, causing the thrombosis seen with malignancies (*migratory thrombophlebitis* or *Trousseau syndrome*); this may affect multiple sites simultaneously or sequentially.

Arterial Thrombosis

Besides the obstructive consequences of arterial thrombi, cardiac and aortic mural thrombi can also embolize peripherally; the brain, kidneys, and spleen are prime targets. *Myocardial infarction* with dyskinesis and endocardial damage may result in mural thrombi. *Rheumatic valvular disease* can cause mitral valve stenosis, followed by left atrial dilation and thrombus formation within the atrium or auricular appendages; concurrent atrial fibrillation augments atrial blood stasis.

Atherosclerosis is a major cause of arterial thrombi, related to abnormal vascular flow and loss of endothelial integrity.

Disseminated Intravascular Coagulation
(p. 135)

Disseminated intravascular coagulation (DIC) refers to widespread fibrin microthrombi in the microcirculation. This is caused by disorders ranging from obstetric complications to advanced malignancy. DIC is not a primary disease but rather a complication of any diffuse thrombin activation. The microthrombi can cause diffuse circulatory insufficiency, particularly in the brain, lungs, heart, and kidneys; there is also concurrent consumption of platelets and coagulation factors (*consumption coagulopathy*) with fibrinolytic pathway activation, leading to uncontrollable bleeding. DIC is discussed in greater detail in Chapter 13.

EMBOLISM (p. 135)

Embolism refers to any intravascular solid, liquid, or gaseous mass carried by blood flow to a site distant from its origin. Most (99%) arise from thrombi, hence the term *thromboembolism;* unless otherwise specified, embolism is considered thrombotic in origin. Other forms include droplets of fat, gas bubbles, atherosclerotic debris (*atheroemboli*), tumor fragments, bone marrow, or foreign bodies such as bullets. Emboli lodge in vessels too small to permit further passage, resulting in partial or complete vascular occlusion and ischemic necrosis of distal tissue (*infarction*).

Pulmonary Thromboembolism
(p. 136; Chapter 15)

Pulmonary thromboembolism has an incidence of 20 to 25 per 100,000 hospitalized patients and causes about 200,000 deaths annually in the United States. Greater than 95% of pulmonary emboli originate from deep leg vein thrombi; depending on the size, a pulmonary embolus (PE) may occlude the main pulmonary artery, impact across the bifurcation (*saddle embolus*), or pass into smaller arterioles. Multiple emboli may occur, either sequentially or as a shower of small emboli from a single large mass; in general, *one PE puts a patient at risk for more*. Rarely, emboli pass through atrial or ventricular defects into the systemic circulation (*paradoxic embolism*).

- Most PEs (60%–80%) are small and clinically silent. They eventually organize and get incorporated into the vessel wall or leave a delicate, bridging fibrous *web*. Embolic obstruction of small end-arteriolar branches may cause infarction.
- Embolic obstruction of medium-sized arteries may result in pulmonary hemorrhage but usually does not cause pulmonary infarction because of collateral bronchial artery flow. However, with left-sided cardiac failure (and diminished bronchial circulation), infarcts can result.
- Sudden death, right-sided heart failure (*cor pulmonale*), or cardiovascular collapse occurs when 60% or more of the pulmonary circulation is obstructed with emboli. Multiple emboli over time may cause pulmonary hypertension.

Systemic Thromboembolism (p. 136)

Systemic thromboembolism refers to emboli in the arterial circulation. Approximately 80% arise from intracardiac mural thrombi; two thirds are secondary to myocardial infarcts, and 25% arise within dilated left atria (e.g., owing to rheumatic valvular disease). The remainder of systemic emboli originate from aortic aneurysms, thrombi on ulcerated atherosclerotic plaques, or valvular vegetations, and only rarely from paradoxic emboli. Roughly 10% are of unknown origin. Major sites for arteriolar embolization are the lower extremities (75%), brain (10%), viscera (10%), and upper extremities (5%). Consequences of systemic emboli depend on collateral vascular supplies, tissue vulnerability to ischemia, and vessel caliber; usually, arterial emboli cause distal infarction.

Fat Embolism (p. 136)

Fat embolism is the second most common form of embolism (after thromboembolism). It results from release of microscopic fat globules after fractures of long bones or, rarely, after burns or soft tissue trauma. Fat embolism occurs in 90% of severe skeletal injuries; fewer than 10% have any clinical findings.

Fat embolism syndrome, fatal in approximately 10% of cases, is heralded by sudden pulmonary insufficiency 1 to 3 days after injury; 20% to 50% of patients have a diffuse petechial rash and may have neurologic symptoms (irritability and restlessness) that progress to delirium or coma. Thrombocytopenia and anemia can also occur.

- *Pathogenesis* involves mechanical obstruction by microemboli of neutral fat, followed by local platelet and erythrocyte aggregation. Subsequent fatty acid release causes toxic injury to endothelium; platelet activation and granulocyte recruitment contribute free radicals, proteases, and eicosanoids.
- *Diagnosis* depends on identifying microvascular fat globules. Because routine histologic solvents dissolve lipids out of tissues, documentation requires special fat stains performed on frozen sections. Edema and hemorrhage (and pulmonary hyaline membranes) may also be seen microscopically.

Air Embolism (p. 137)

Air embolism refers to gas bubbles within the circulation obstructing vascular flow and causing ischemia. Air may enter the circulation during obstetric procedures or following chest wall injury; generally, more than 100 cc are required to have a clinical effect.

Decompression sickness is a special form of air embolism caused by sudden changes in atmospheric pressure; deep-sea divers and individuals in unpressurized aircraft in rapid ascent are at risk. Air breathed at high pressure (e.g., during a deepsea dive) causes increasing amounts of gas (particularly nitrogen) to be dissolved in blood and tissues. Subsequent rapid ascent (depressurization) allows the dissolved gases to expand and bubble out of solution to form gas emboli.

- Formation of gas bubbles in skeletal muscles and joints causes painful *bends*. In lungs, edema, hemorrhage, and focal emphysema lead to respiratory distress, or *chokes*. Gas emboli may also cause focal ischemia in a number of tissues, including brain and heart. Treatment consists of repressurization to force gas bubbles back into solution, followed by subsequent slow decompression.
- A more chronic form of decompression sickness is *caisson disease;* persistent gas emboli in poorly vascularized portions of the skeleton (heads of the femurs, tibia, and humeri) lead to ischemic necrosis.

Amniotic Fluid Embolism (p. 137)

Amniotic fluid embolism is a serious (mortality rate > 80%) but uncommon (1 in 50,000 deliveries) complication of labor and postpartum period caused by amniotic fluid infusion into the maternal circulation. Classic findings include fetal squamous cells, mucin, lanugo hair, and vernix caseosa fat in the maternal pulmonary microcirculation. The syndrome is characterized by sudden severe dyspnea, cyanosis, and hypotensive shock, followed by seizures and coma. Pulmonary edema, *diffuse alveolar damage,* and DIC ensue from release of toxic (fatty acid) and thrombogenic substances in amniotic fluid.

INFARCTION (p. 137)

Infarction is an area of ischemic necrosis caused by occlusion of either the arterial supply (97% of cases) or venous drainage in a particular tissue. Almost all infarcts result from thrombotic or embolic events; other causes include vasospasm; extrinsic compression of a vessel by tumor, edema, or entrapment in a hernia sac; and twisting of vessels, such as testicular torsion or bowel volvulus; traumatic vessel rupture is a rare cause. Occluded venous drainage (e.g., venous thrombosis) most often induces congestion only; usually, bypass channels rapidly open providing outflow. Infarcts resulting from venous thrombosis are more likely in organs with a single venous outflow, such as testis or ovary.

Morphology (p. 138)

Infarcts may be either *red (hemorrhagic)* or *white (pale, anemic)* and may be either *septic* or *bland.*

- Red infarcts occur in

  Venous occlusions (e.g., ovarian torsion)
  Loose tissues (such as lung)
  Tissues with dual circulations (e.g., lung and small intestine)
  Tissues previously congested because of sluggish venous outflow
  Sites of previous occlusion and necrosis when flow is reestablished

- *White infarcts* occur in solid organs (such as heart, spleen, and kidney) with end-arterial circulations (i.e., few collaterals).
- All infarcts tend to be wedge-shaped; the occluded vessel marks the apex, and the organ periphery forms the base.

Lateral margins may be irregular, reflecting the pattern of adjacent vascular supply.

- The dominant histologic characteristic of infarction is *ischemic coagulative necrosis*. An initial inflammatory response (lasting hours to days) is followed by a reparative response (lasting days to weeks) beginning in the preserved margins (Chapter 3). In stable or labile tissues, some parenchymal regeneration may occur where the underlying stromal architecture is spared; most infarcts are ultimately replaced by scar tissue.
- The brain is an exception; ischemic injury results in *liquefactive necrosis* (Chapter 1).
- Septic infarctions occur when infected heart valve vegetations embolize or when microbes seed an area of necrosis; the infarct becomes an *abscess*.

Clinical Correlations: Factors That Influence Development of an Infarct (p. 139)

The effects of vascular occlusion range from nothing to death of a tissue or even the individual. Major determinants of outcome:

- *Anatomic pattern of vascular supply* (i.e., availability of alternative supply): Dual circulations (lung, liver) or anastomosing circulations (radial and ulnar arteries, circle of Willis, small intestine) protect against infarction. Obstruction of end-arterial vessels generally causes infarction (spleen, kidneys).
- *Rate of development of occlusion:* Slowly developing occlusions less often cause infarction by providing time to develop alternate perfusion pathways (e.g., collateral coronary circulation).
- *Vulnerability to hypoxia:* Neurons undergo irreversible damage after 3 to 4 minutes of ischemia; myocardial cells die after only 20 to 30 minutes. In contrast, fibroblasts within ischemic myocardium are viable even after many hours.
- *Oxygen content of blood:* Anemia, cyanosis, or CHF (with hypoxia) can cause infarction in an otherwise inconsequential blockage.

SHOCK (p. 139)

Shock is systemic hypoperfusion resulting from reduction in either cardiac output or the effective circulating blood volume; the result is hypotension, followed by impaired tissue perfusion and cellular hypoxia. Shock is the final common pathway for many lethal events, including severe hemorrhage, extensive trauma, large myocardial infarction, massive pulmonary embolism, and sepsis.

Shock is grouped into three major categories (Table 4–3). The basic mechanism underlying *cardiogenic* and *hypovolemic shock* is *low cardiac output. Septic shock* is caused by systemic microbial infection and has a more complicated pathogenesis (see below). Rarer causes of shock are *neurogenic,* with loss of vascular tone and peripheral pooling (anesthetic accident or spinal cord injury), and *anaphylactic,* with systemic vasodilation and increased vascular permeability (IgE-mediated hypersensitivity, Chapter 6).

TABLE 4–3 **Three Major Types of Shock**

Type of Shock	Clinical Examples	Principal Mechanisms
Cardiogenic		
	Myocardial infarction Ventricular rupture Arrhythmia Cardiac tamponade Pulmonary embolism	Failure of myocardial pump owing to intrinsic myocardial damage, extrinsic pressure, or obstruction to outflow
Hypovolemic		
	Hemorrhage Fluid loss, e.g., vomiting, diarrhea, burns, or trauma	Inadequate blood or plasma volume
Septic		
	Overwhelming microbial infections Endotoxic shock Gram-positive septicemia Fungal sepsis Superantigens	Peripheral vasodilation and pooling of blood; endothelial activation/injury; leukocyte-induced damage; disseminated intravascular coagulation; activation of cytokine cascades

Pathogenesis of Septic Shock (p. 139)

With a 25% to 50% mortality rate and 200,000 deaths annually in the United States, septic shock ranks first among the causes of death in intensive care units. The incidence is increasing as a result of improved life support for high-risk patients, increasing use of invasive procedures, and more immunocompromised hosts.

- Septic shock results from spread of an initially localized infection (e.g., abscess, pneumonia) into the bloodstream.
- Most cases (70%) are caused by gram-negative bacilli expressing endotoxin (*endotoxic shock*). Endotoxins are bacterial lipopolysaccharides (LPS) released when cell walls are degraded. LPS consists of a toxic fatty acid (*lipid A*) core and a complex polysaccharide (including O antigens). Analogous molecules on fungi and gram-positive bacteria can also elicit septic shock.
- All the effects of septic shock are reproduced by LPS alone. LPS binds (as a complex with a normal serum protein) to CD14 molecules on leukocytes (especially monocytes and macrophages), endothelial cells, and other cell types; the LPS molecule then interacts with membrane toll-like receptor 4 (TLR-4) that transduces an intracellular signal.
- TLR-4 engagement profoundly activates cytokine and chemokine production; depending on LPS dosage and the numbers of macrophages activated, there are different outcomes:

At *low doses,* LPS mainly activates complement and monocyte/macrophages, leading to enhanced bacterial eradication. Mononuclear phagocytes produce tumor necrosis factor (TNF), interleukin 1 (IL1), and chemokines. IL1 and TNF act on ECs to increase adhesion molecule expression and production of additional cytokines and chemokines (Chapter 2). The net effect is an enhanced local inflammatory response and improved clearance of infections.

At *moderate doses,* cytokine-induced secondary effectors (e.g., nitric oxide, Chapter 2) become significant. Also, systemic effects of TNF and IL1 are seen (e.g., fever and synthesis of acute-phase reactants). Higher-dose LPS also directly down-regulates EC anticoagulation mechanisms (e.g., reduced thrombomodulin), tipping the coagulation cascade toward thrombosis.

At *high doses,* septic shock supervenes with high-level cytokines and secondary mediators resulting in:

• Systemic vasodilation (hypotension)
• Diminished myocardial contractility
• Widespread endothelial injury and activation, with systemic leukocyte adhesion and pulmonary alveolar capillary damage (*adult respiratory distress syndrome,* Chapter 15)
• Activation of the coagulation system, culminating in DIC

The resulting hypoperfusion causes *multiorgan system failure* affecting the liver, kidneys, and central nervous system. Unless the underlying infection (and LPS overload) is brought under control, the patient usually dies.

Morphology (p. 141)

Shock of any form causes nonspecific cell and tissue changes largely reflecting hypoxic injury; brain, heart, lungs, kidneys, adrenals, and gastrointestinal tract are particularly affected. Outside of neuron and myocyte loss, virtually all tissues may recover if the patient survives.

• The *brain* shows hypoxic encephalopathy (Chapter 28).
• The *heart* shows coagulation necrosis and *contraction band necrosis* (Chapter 12)
• The *kidneys* develop extensive tubular ischemic injury (*acute tubular necrosis,* Chapter 20), causing oliguria, anuria, and electrolyte disturbances.
• The *lungs* are seldom affected in pure hypovolemic shock; however, diffuse alveolar damage (*shock lung,* Chapter 15) may occur in septic or traumatic shock.

Clinical Course (p. 142)

The clinical manifestations depend on the precipitating insult.

• In hypovolemic and cardiogenic shock, the patient presents with hypotension; a weak, rapid pulse; tachypnea; and cool, clammy, cyanotic skin. In septic shock, the skin may initially be warm and flushed owing to peripheral vasodilation.
• Beyond the catastrophe that precipitated the shock state (e.g., myocardial infarct, hemorrhage, or sepsis), cardiac, cerebral, and pulmonary changes secondary to the shock state worsen the situation.
• Patients surviving the initial complications enter *a second phase dominated by renal insufficiency* and marked by a progressive fall in urine output, as well as severe fluid and electrolyte imbalances.

- The prognosis varies with the origin and duration of shock. Thus, 80% to 90% of young, otherwise healthy patients with hypovolemic shock survive with appropriate management, whereas cardiogenic shock associated with extensive myocardial infarction or septic shock carry mortality rates near 75%.

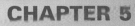

CHAPTER 5

Genetic Disorders

Genetic disorders (p. 146) are extremely common with a lifetime frequency estimated at 670 per 1000; the number includes not only "classic" genetic disorders with mendelian inheritance, but also cancer and cardiovascular diseases that increasingly are appreciated to have prominent (albeit complex and multifactorial) genetic components. Genetic disorders can be classified as follows:

- Mendelian disorders
- Multifactorial disorders
- Single-gene disorders with nonclassic inheritance
- Chromosomal (cytogenetic) disorders

Moreover, the genetic diseases encountered in clinical practice are very much only the tip of the iceberg, since the vast majority of genetic disorders do not result in viable conceptuses. Nevertheless, approximately 1% of all newborns have a gross chromosomal abnormality, and 5% of individuals younger than age 25 have a serious disease with a significant genetic component.

Sequencing of the human genome has provided some startling insights regarding the genetic basis of disease. Greater than 50% of the genome represents blocks of repetitive nucleotides of uncertain significance, and *only* less than 2% of the genome actually codes for proteins; remarkably, there is coding for only roughly 30,000 genes (although with alternative splicing, >100,000 proteins can be synthesized). With completion of the draft sequence of the human genome, *genomics* now putatively permits the study of all the relevant genes in a particular pathologic entity, as well as their interactions. Although genomic microarray analysis of tumors is already being applied (Chapter 7), genomics will more importantly permit the unraveling of complex multifactorial diseases.

On average, any two individuals share 99.9% of their DNA sequences, so that the remarkable diversity of humanity (and the basis of genetic disease) rests in less than 0.1% of the DNA (or roughly 3 million base pairs). The most common form of variation is the single nucleotide polymorphism (SNP); interestingly, only less than 1% of these SNPs occur in coding regions. Clearly, these may have significance in causing disease states; however, most SNPs simply represent a marker coin-herited with the *real* genetic disease locus.

MUTATIONS (p. 147)

A mutation is a permanent change in the DNA; mutations in germ cells are transmitted to progeny (and cause heritable disease) while mutations in somatic cells are not transmissible but may contribute to change (e.g., malignant transformation). There are three categories of mutations:

- *Genome mutations:* involving loss or gain of whole chromosomes (e.g., monosomy or trisomy)
- *Chromosome mutations:* rearranged genetic material giving rise to visible changes in chromosome structure
- *Gene mutations:* submicroscopic genetic changes including:

  Point mutations: due to single nucleotide substitutions
  Frameshift mutations (changes in the reading frame of the DNA): due to insertion or deletion of nucleotides

Gene mutations may involve changes in coding or noncoding regions of the genome.

Mutations in the Coding Region (Exons)

- *Missense mutations: Point mutations in the coding sequences* can potentially change the triplet base code and therefore substitute a different amino acid in the final translated protein product (*missense mutation*). If the substituted amino acid is not significantly different from the original, the result is a *conservative missense mutation* and minimal (if any) consequences occur; if the amino acid is quite different (size, charge, etc.), the result is a *nonconservative missense mutation*, which can potentially lead to loss of function, misfolding and degradation of the protein, or gain of function.
- *Nonsense mutations: Point mutations in the coding sequences* can potentially result in the formation of an inappropriate "stop" codon (*nonsense mutation*). In that case, the resulting protein may be truncated with loss of normal activity.
- *Frameshift mutations:* insertions or deletions of multiples of three nucleotides may have no effect other than adding or deleting a new amino acid; frameshifts of other numbers of nucleotides rapidly lead to defective protein products (missense or nonsense).

Mutations Within Noncoding Regions (Introns)

- Point mutations or deletions in enhancer or promoter regions can significantly affect the regulation or level of gene transcription.
- Point mutations can lead to defective splicing and thus failure to form mature mRNA species.

Trinucleotide Repeat Mutations

This is a special category of mutations, since these are characterized by amplification of three nucleotide sequences.

Trinucleotide repeats are a common feature of many normal genetic sequences; what makes the trinucleotide mutations unusual is the 10-fold to 200-fold amplification that happens in certain disease states (e.g., fragile X syndrome or Huntington disease), frequently leading to abnormal gene expression. This type of mutation is also dynamic, with the length of the trinucleotide repeat sequences frequently expanding during gametogenesis.

MENDELIAN DISORDERS (p. 149)

Mendelian disorders result from mutations in single genes of large effect. Whether a particular mutation will have an adverse outcome is also influenced by additional factors (e.g., compensatory genes and environmental factors that can influence whether a particular mutation is manifested as a discernible phenotype).

Definitions (p. 150)

Codominance   refers to full expression of both alleles of a gene pair in a heterozygote.

Genetic heterogeneity   means production of a given trait by different mutations at multiple loci.

Penetrance   is the percentage of individuals carrying an autosomal dominant gene and expressing the trait.

Pleiotropism   refers to multiple end effects of a single mutant gene.

Polymorphism   means multiple allelic forms of a single gene.

Variable expressivity   refers to a variable expression of autosomal dominant trait in affected individuals.

Transmission Patterns of Single-Gene Disorders (p. 150)

Autosomal Dominant Disorders (p. 150)

Autosomal dominant disorders have the following general features:

- Mutations affect structural (e.g., collagen) or regulatory (e.g., receptor) proteins. In some instances (e.g., collagen), the product of the mutant allele interferes with the function of the normal protein. Such mutant alleles, called *dominant negative*, can produce severe protein deficiency, as in osteogenesis imperfecta (Chapter 26).
- There is reduced penetrance and variable expressivity.
- Onset of clinical features may be later than in autosomal recessive disorders.

Autosomal Recessive Disorders (p. 151)

Autosomal recessive disorders include most inborn errors of metabolism. In contrast to autosomal dominant disorders, the following features generally apply:

- Age of onset is frequently in early life.
- Clinical features tend to be more uniform.
- In many patients, enzyme proteins, rather than structural proteins, are affected.

X-Linked Disorders (p. 152)

All sex-linked disorders are X-linked, and almost all X-linked disorders are recessive. They are fully expressed in males because mutant genes on the X chromosome do not have a Y chromosome counterpart. In contrast, heterozygous females usually partially express the disease because the paired normal allele is randomly inactivated in some, but not all, cells (e.g., glucose-6-phosphate dehydrogenase [G6PD] deficiency).

Biochemical and Molecular Basis of Single-Gene (Mendelian) Disorders (p. 152)

Virtually any type of protein may be affected in these disorders. Some examples are provided in Table 5–1.

Enzyme Defects and Their Consequences (p. 152)

Mutations can result in the synthesis of a defective enzyme (reduced activity), or reduced synthesis of a normal enzyme. In either event, the result is a metabolic block with:

- Accumulation of substrate (which may be directly toxic, e.g., phenylalanine in *phenylketonuria*)
- Decreased amount of end product (which may be necessary for normal function, e.g., melanin in *albinism*)
- Absence of an important regulatory component (necessary to control inflammatory states, e.g., α_1-antitrypsin)

Defects in Receptors and Transport Systems (p. 154)

These defects can affect the intracellular accumulation of an important precursor (e.g., low-density lipoprotein in *familial hypercholesterolemia*) or export of a metabolite necessary for normal tissue homeostasis (e.g., chloride in *cystic fibrosis*).

Alterations in Structure, Function, or Quantity of Nonenzyme Proteins (p. 154)

The hemoglobinopathies (e.g., sickle cell disease) are good examples of diseases in which insufficient or abnormal hemoglobins can have profound consequences.

Genetically Determined Adverse Reactions to Drugs (p. 154)

These otherwise clinically silent mutations are "unmasked" when specific compounds/substrates are administered that cannot be appropriately catabolized or that lead to toxic intermediates.

Disorders Associated with Defects in Structural Proteins (p. 154)

Marfan Syndrome (p. 154)

Marfan syndrome results from mutations in the *fibrillin-1* gene (mapped to 15q21.1). Fibrillin, a glycoprotein secreted by fibroblasts, is a component of microfibrils that provides a scaffolding for the deposition of elastin; abnormal fibrillin disrupts assembly of microfibrils by a dominant-negative effect. There

TABLE 5–1 Biochemical and Molecular Basis of Some Mendelian Disorders

Protein Type/Function	Example	Molecular Lesion	Disease
Enzyme	Phenylalanine hydroxylase	Splice site mutation: reduced amount	Phenylketonuria
	Hexosaminidase	Splice site mutation or frameshift mutation with stop codon: reduced amount	Tay-Sachs disease
	Adenosine deaminase	Point mutations: abnormal protein with reduced activity	Severe combined immunodeficiency
Enzyme Inhibitor	α_1-Antitrypsin	Missense mutations: impaired secretion from liver to serum	Emphysema and liver disease
Receptor	Low-density lipoprotein receptor	Deletions, point mutations: reduction of synthesis, transport to cell surface, or binding to low-density lipoprotein	Familial hypercholesterolemia
Transport			
Oxygen	Vitamin D receptor	Point mutations: failure of normal signaling	Vitamin D–resistant rickets
	Hemoglobin	Deletions: reduced amount	α-Thalassemia
		Defective mRNA processing: reduced amount	β-Thalassemia
		Point mutations: abnormal structure	Sickle cell anemia
Ions	Cystic fibrosis transmembrane conductance regulator	Deletions and other mutations	Cystic fibrosis
Structural			
Extracellular	Collagen	Deletions or point mutations cause reduced amount of normal collagen or normal amounts of mutant collagen	Osteogenesis imperfecta; Ehlers-Danlos syndromes
	Fibrillin	Missense mutations	Marfan syndrome
Cell membrane	Dystrophin	Deletion with reduced synthesis	Duchenne/Becker muscular dystrophy
	Spectrin, ankyrin, or protein 4.1	Heterogeneous	Hereditary spherocytosis
Hemostasis	Factor VIII	Deletions, insertions, nonsense mutations, and others: reduced synthesis or abnormal factor VIII	Hemophilia A
Growth Regulation	Rb protein	Deletions	Hereditary retinoblastoma
	Neurofibromin	Heterogeneous	Neurofibromatosis type 1

is secondary weakness of the connective tissue, particularly in the aorta, mitral valve, and ciliary zonules. The end result is a disorder of connective tissues affecting predominantly the *skeletal, ocular,* and *cardiovascular systems,* with most patients ultimately dying due to rupture of a dissecting aneurysm or from heart failure.

Skeletal changes

- Tall stature with exceptionally long extremities
- Long, tapering fingers and toes (arachnodactyly)
- Laxity of joint ligaments, producing hyperextensibility
- Spinal deformities (e.g., kyphosis and scoliosis)

Ocular changes

- Bilateral dislocation of lenses (ectopia lentis)
- Increased axial length of the globe, giving rise to retinal detachments

Cardiovascular lesions

- Mitral valve prolapse is most common, although not life-threatening; affected valves are floppy, associated with mitral regurgitation.
- Cystic medial degeneration of the aorta is less common than mitral valve lesions but clinically more important. Histologically, the media exhibits elastin fragmentation with excess glycosaminoglycan deposition, causing aortic ring dilation and valvular incompetence. More important, the cystic medial degeneration predisposes to medial dissections (a dissecting aneurysm); cleavage of the aortic wall may extend proximally or distally, often resulting in aortic rupture.

Ehlers-Danlos Syndromes (p. 155)

Ehlers-Danlos syndromes (EDS) are a clinically and genetically heterogeneous group of disorders that result from *defects in collagen synthesis;* the major manifestations involve the following systems:

- *Skin:* Skin is hyperextensible, extremely fragile, and vulnerable to trauma; surgical repair of wounds is markedly impaired owing to defective collagen synthesis.
- *Joints:* Joints are hypermobile and prone to dislocation.
- *Internal complications:* Manifestations include rupture of the colon and large arteries; ocular fragility with corneal rupture and retinal detachment; and diaphragmatic hernias.

EDS is divided into six variants on the basis of predominant clinical manifestations and patterns of inheritance (Table 5–2). Some of the better characterized defects are as follows:

- Reduced activity of lysyl-hydroxylase, an enzyme essential for collagen cross-linking.
- Abnormalities of type III collagen, due to distinct structural gene mutations. Because a structural rather than an enzyme protein is affected, the pattern of inheritance is autosomal dominant.
- Defective conversion of type I procollagen to mature collagen due to mutant procollagen chains that resist cleavage of N-terminal peptides, essential for the formation of normal collagen. Even if only one of the two alleles is mutant, the abnormal products interfere with the formation of normal

TABLE 5–2 Classification of Ehlers-Danlos Syndromes (EDS)

EDS Type*	Clinical Findings	Inheritance	Gene Defects
Classical (I/II)	Skin and joint hypermobility, atrophic scars, easy bruising	Autosomal dominant	COL5A1, COL5A2
Hypermobility (III)	Joint hypermobility, pain, dislocations	Autosomal dominant	Unknown
Vascular (IV)	Thin skin, arterial or uterine rupture, bruising, small joint hyperextensibility	Autosomal dominant	COL3A1
Kyphoscoliosis (VI)	Hypotonia, joint laxity, congenital scoliosis, ocular fragility	Autosomal recessive	Lysyl-hydroxylase
Arthrochalasia (VIIa,b)	Severe joint hypermobility, skin changes mild, scoliosis, bruising	Autosomal dominant	COL1A1, COL1A2
Dermatosparaxis (VIIc)	Severe skin fragility, cutis laxa, bruising	Autosomal recessive	Procollagen N-peptidase

*EDS were previously classified by Roman numerals. Parentheses show previous numerical equivalents.

collagen helices, and hence heterozygotes have severe disease (a *dominant-negative* effect).

- Defective copper metabolism secondarily reduces the activity of the enzyme lysyl oxidase, essential for collagen and elastin cross-linking. It is inherited as an X-linked recessive trait.

Disorders Associated with Defects in Receptor Proteins (p. 156)

Familial Hypercholesterolemia (p. 156)

Familial hypercholesterolemia results from a mutation in the gene encoding the receptor for low-density lipoprotein (LDL). At least 900 mutations have been identified affecting different aspects of LDL uptake, metabolism, and regulation.

Normal Cholesterol Transport and Metabolism

Figure 5–1 illustrates LDL metabolism. Only a few salient features are emphasized:

- LDL is the major transport form of cholesterol in plasma.
- Although many cells in the body possess high-affinity receptors that recognize apoprotein B-100 of the LDL molecule, about 70% of plasma LDL is cleared by the liver. The remaining 30% is transported into other cells, especially mononuclear phagocytes, by binding to distinct *scavenger* receptors for chemically altered (e.g., acetylated) LDL.
- The transport of and metabolism of LDL into the liver occurs through several steps:

  Binding to specific surface receptors
  Internalization, followed by transport to and fusion with lysosomes

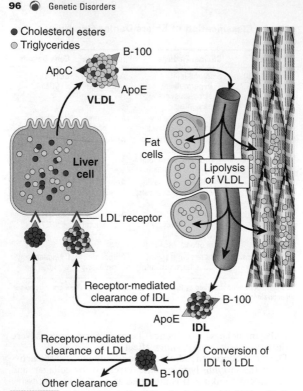

● Cholesterol esters
○ Triglycerides

FIGURE 5–1 Schematic illustration of low-density lipoprotein (LDL) metabolism and the role of the liver in its synthesis and clearance. Lipolysis of very-low-density lipoprotein (VLDL) by lipoprotein lipase in the capillaries releases triglycerides that are then stored in fat cells and used as a source of energy in skeletal muscles. IDI, intermediate density lipoprotein; ApoE, Apoprotein E.

Lysosomal processing, leading to release of free cholesterol into cytoplasm

Free cholesterol affects three processes:

1. Suppresses cholesterol synthesis by inhibiting the rate-limiting enzyme hydroxymethylglutaryl coenzyme A reductase
2. Activates enzymes that esterify cholesterol
3. Suppresses LDL receptor synthesis, thereby limiting further cholesterol transport

Mutations in Familial Hypercholesterolemia

Based on the normal metabolic pathways in LDL uptake and metabolism, the various mutations can be clustered into five general classes.

- *Class I* mutations impair transcription, resulting in defective LDL receptor protein synthesis.
- *Class II* mutations prevent transport of newly sythesized LDL receptors from the endoplasmic reticulum to the Golgi complex for export to the cell surface.
- *Class III* mutations are associated with production of an LDL receptor protein that has reduced binding capacity.

- *Class IV* mutations give rise to proteins that can bind LDL but cannot internalize it.
- *Class V* mutations result in LDL receptor proteins that are expressed and internalized but cannot be recycled.

Clinical Features

Familial hyercholesterolemia is an extremely common disorder with a gene frequency of 1 in 500. Heterozygotes have the following features:

- Cells possess 50% of the normal number of high-affinity LDL receptors. Plasma LDL cholesterol level is two to three times higher than normal, resulting from both impaired clearance of plasma LDL and increased synthesis.
- Hypercholesterolemia leads to premature atherosclerosis and accumulation of cholesterol in soft tissues and skin, producing xanthomas.

Homozygotes have much greater elevations of plasma LDL cholesterol and are at much greater risk of developing widespread atherosclerosis; ischemic heart disease often develops before age 20. Xanthomas of the skin are also more prominent.

Disorders Associated with Defects in Enzymes (p. 158)

Lysosomal Storage Diseases (p. 158)

The synthesis, transport, and functions of lysosomal enzymes should be reviewed (see Fig. 5–11 in *Robbins and Cotran Pathologic Basis of Disease*, 7th ed.). Lysosomal storage disorders result from an inherited lack of functional lysosomal enzymes or other proteins essential for their function. In the absence of normal lysosomal processing, catabolism of complex substrates is impaired, leading to accumulation of partially degraded insoluble metabolites within lysosomes. The lysosomes, packed with undigested macromolecules, are enlarged and interfere with normal cell function.

Lysosomal storage diseases are classified on the basis of the biochemical nature of the accumulated metabolite (Table 5–3). Distribution of the stored material and resultant clinical features depend on:

- The site where most of the material to be degraded is normally found
- The site where most of the degradation normally occurs

Because cells of the mononuclear phagocytic system are particularly rich in lysosomes and are responsible for degradation of several substrates, organs rich in phagocytic cells (e.g., liver and spleen) are often affected.

Tay-Sachs Disease (GM$_2$-Gangliosidosis) (p. 160)

Tay-Sachs disease results from mutations that affect the α-subunit of the hexosaminidase enzyme complex; the resultant hexosaminidase A deficiency prevents GM$_2$-ganglioside degradation. It is most common in Jews of Eastern European origin.

The clinical features derive primarily from accumulation of GM$_2$-ganglioside in neurons of the central and autonomic nervous systems and retina:

- Motor and mental deterioration commencing at about 6 months of age

TABLE 5-3 **Lysosomal Storage Diseases**

Disease	Enzyme Deficiency	Major Accumulating Metabolites
Glycogenosis		
Type 2—Pompe disease	α-1,4-Glucosidase (lysosomal glucosidase)	Glycogen
Sphingolipidoses		
GM$_1$ gangliosidosis	GM$_1$ ganglioside β-galactosidase	GM$_1$ ganglioside, galactose-containing oligosaccharides
Type 1—infantile, generalized		
Type 2—juvenile		
GM$_2$ gangliosidosis		
Tay-Sachs disease	Hexosaminidase-α subunit	GM$_2$ ganglioside
Sandhoff disease	Hexosaminidase-β subunit	GM$_2$ ganglioside, globoside
GM$_2$ gangliosidosis, variant AB	Ganglioside activator protein	GM$_2$ ganglioside
Sulfatidoses		
Metachromatic leukodystrophy	Arylsulfatase A	Sulfatide
Multiple sulfatase deficiency	Arylsulfatases A, B, C; steroid sulfatase; iduronate sulfatase; heparan N-sulfatase	Sulfatide, steroid sulfate, heparan sulfate, dermatan sulfate
Krabbe disease	Galactosylceramidase	Galactocerebroside
Fabry disease	α-Galactosidase A	Ceramide trihexoside

Gaucher disease	Glucocerebrosidase	Glucocerebroside
Niemann-Pick disease: types A and B	Sphingomyelinase	Sphingomyelin
Mucopolysaccharidoses (MPS)		
MPS I H (Hurler)	α-L-Iduronidase	Dermatan sulfate, heparan sulfate
MPS II (Hunter)	L-Iduronosulfate sulfatase	
Mucolipidoses (ML)		
I-cell disease (ML II) and pseudo-Hurler polydystrophy	Deficiency of phosphorylating enzymes essential for the formation of mannose-6-phosphate recognition marker; acid hydrolases lacking the recognition marker cannot be targeted to the lysosomes but are secreted extracellularly	Mucopolysaccharide, glycolipid
Other Diseases of Complex Carbohydrates		
Fucosidosis	α-Fucosidase	Fucose-containing sphingolipids and glycoprotein fragments
Mannosidosis	α-Mannosidase	Mannose-containing oligosaccharides
Aspartylglycosaminuria	Aspartylglycosamine amide hydrolase	Aspartyl-2-deoxy-2-acetamido-glycosylamine
Other Lysosomal Storage Diseases		
Wolman disease	Acid lipase	Cholesterol esters, triglycerides
Acid phosphate deficiency	Lysosomal acid phosphatase	Phosphate esters

- Blindness
- A cherry-red spot in the retina
- Death by age 2 or 3 years

Antenatal diagnosis and carrier detection are possible by DNA probe analysis and enzyme assays on cells obtained from amniocentesis.

Morphology

- Ballooning of neurons with cytoplasmic vacuoles staining positive for lipids
- Whorled configurations in the cytoplasmic vacuoles, revealed by electron microscopy
- Progressive destruction of neurons with proliferation of microglia
- Accumulation of lipids in retinal ganglion cells, rendering them pale in color, thus accentuating the normal red color of the macular choroid (cherry-red spot)

Niemann-Pick Diseases Types A and B (p. 163)

Niemann-Pick diseases types A and B are two related disorders associated with sphingomyelinase deficiency and consequent accumulation of sphingomyelin in mononuclear phagocytes and other cell types.

Sphingomyelinase-deficient type A variant is the most common form:

- Diffuse neuronal involvement, leading eventually to cell death and shrinkage of the brain; there is a retinal cherry-red spot similar to that seen in Tay-Sachs disease.
- Extreme accumulation of lipids in mononuclear phagocytes, giving rise to massive splenomegaly, enlargement of liver and lymph nodes, and infiltration of bone marrow.
- Visceral involvement affecting the gastrointestinal tract and lungs.

Affected cells everywhere are enlarged and filled with numerous small vacuoles that impart cytoplasmic foaminess. Clinical manifestations appear soon after birth and consist of hepatosplenomegaly, failure to thrive, and deterioration of psychomotor functions. Survival is limited to 1 or 2 years.

Gaucher Disease (p. 163)

Gaucher disease refers to a cluster of autosomal recessive disorders in which mutations affecting the glucocerebrosidase locus reduce the levels of this enzyme. Consequently, cleavage of ceramide (derived from cell membranes of senescent leukocytes and red blood cells as well as from turnover of brain gangliosides) is impaired. Glucocerebroside accumulation occurs in mononuclear phagocytes and (in some forms) in the central nervous system. Two important variants of Gaucher disease are identified:

- *Type I,* the most common form, occurs in adults. This chronic, non-neuronopathic form is associated with glucocerebroside storage in mononuclear phagocytes; there is no brain involvement but massive splenomegaly; involvement of bone marrow produces small or large areas of bone erosions that can cause pathologic fractures; pancytopenia or thrombocytopenia results from hypersplenism; life span is not affected.
- *Type II,* also known as the *acute neuronopathic form,* is associated with hepatosplenomegaly as well as central nervous

system involvement; symptoms such as convulsions and mental deterioration dominate the clinical picture, and death occurs at a young age.

Morphology

Histologically, affected cells (Gaucher cells) are distended with periodic acid–Schiff (PAS)–positive material that has a fibrillary appearance resembling crumpled tissue paper.

Clinical Features

These patterns, resulting from different allelic mutations in the structural gene for the enzyme, run within families. Prenatal diagnosis is possible by enzyme assay of amniotic fluid or by DNA probe analysis.

Mucopolysaccharidoses (p. 165)

Mucopolysaccharidoses (MPS) are a group of disorders resulting from inherited deficiencies of enzymes involved in the degradation of mucopolysaccharides. The mucopolysaccharides that accumulate in the cells include heparan sulfate, dermatan sulfate, keratan sulfate, and chondroitin sulfate.

Several clinical variants of MPS have been described, each resulting from the deficiency of one specific enzyme. Some better known examples are autosomal recessive Hurler disease (MPS I) and X-linked recessive Hunter disease (MPS II). In general, all forms are progressive, and are characterized by

- Coarse facial features
- Hepatosplenomegaly
- Corneal clouding
- Lesions of cardiac valves
- Narrowing of coronary arteries
- Joint stiffness
- Mental retardation

Morphology

Histologically, affected cells are distended with clear cytoplasm (balloon cells) that contains PAS-positive material. Accumulated mucopolysaccharides are found in many cell types, including mononuclear phagocytes (giving rise to hepatosplenomegaly), fibroblasts throughout the body, endothelial cells and intimal smooth muscle cells (giving rise to narrowing of coronary arteries), and neurons.

Glycogen Storage Disorders (Glycogenoses) (p. 165)

Glycogen storage disorders are a group of autosomal recessive disorders resulting from defects in the synthesis or catabolism of glycogen. On the basis of specific enzyme deficiencies and resultant clinical pictures, glycogen storage diseases have been divided into three major groups (Table 5–4):

Hepatic forms

The prototype is von Gierke disease (type I glycogenosis). This results from deficiency of the hepatic enzyme glucose-6-phosphatase, essential for converting glucose 6-phosphate to glucose. The major effects of this enzyme deficiency are:

TABLE 5-4 Principal Subgroups of Glycogenoses

Clinicopathologic Category	Specific Type	Enzyme Deficiency	Morphologic Changes	Clinical Features
Hepatic Type	Hepatorenal—von Gierke disease (type I)	Glucose-6-phosphatase	Hepatomegaly—intracytoplasmic accumulations of glycogen and small amounts of lipid; intranuclear glycogen Renomegaly—intracytoplasmic accumulations of glycogen in cortical tubular epithelial cells	In untreated patients: failure to thrive, stunted growth, hepatomegaly, and renomegaly. Hypoglycemia due to failure of glucose mobilization, often leading to convulsions. Hyperlipidemia and hyperuricemia resulting from deranged glucose metabolism; many patients develop gout and skin xanthomas. Bleeding tendency due to platelet dysfunction. With treatment most survive and develop late complications, e.g., hepatic adenomas.
Myopathic Type	McArdle syndrome (type V)	Muscle phosphorylase	Skeletal muscle only—accumulations of glycogen predominant in subsarcolemmal location	Painful cramps associated with strenuous exercise. Myoglobinuria occurs in 50% of cases. Onset in adulthood (>20 years). Muscular exercise fails to raise lactate level in venous blood. Serum creatine kinase always elevated. Compatible with normal longevity.
Miscellaneous Types	Generalized glycogenosis—Pompe disease (type II)	Lysosomal glucosidase (acid maltase)	Mild hepatomegaly—ballooning of lysosomes with glycogen, creating lacy cytoplasmic pattern Cardiomegaly—glycogen within sarcoplasm as well as membrane-bound Skeletal muscle—similar to changes in heart	Massive cardiomegaly, muscle hypotonia, and cardiorespiratory failure within 2 years. A milder adult form with only skeletal muscle involvement, presenting with chronic myopathy.

- Accumulation of glycogen because it cannot be broken down to free glucose
- Low blood glucose (hypoglycemia)

Myopathic forms

These disorders result from deficiencies of enzymes that fuel glycolysis in striated muscles. McArdle disease (type V glycogenosis) is caused by lack of muscle phosphorylase. Deficiency of this enzyme leads to

- Storage of glycogen in skeletal muscles
- Muscle weakness
- Muscle cramps after exercise
- Absence of exercise-induced rise in blood lactate

Miscellaneous forms

There are several of these forms, the most important being type II glycogenosis, or Pompe disease, resulting from deficiency of the lysosomal enzyme acid maltase (α-glucosidase). As in other lysosomal storage diseases, many organs are involved, but storage of glycogen is most prominent in the heart. Affected neonates have massive cardiomegaly, and death results from cardiac failure by age 2.

Alkaptonuria (Ochronosis) (p. 167)

Lack of homogentisic oxidase blocks the metabolism of phenylalanine and leads to accumulation of homogentisic acid. Excessive homogentisic acid is associated with the following:

- Excretion in urine, imparting to it a black color if allowed to stand.
- Ochronosis, a blue-black pigmentation of the ears, nose, and cheeks resulting from binding of homogentisic acid to connective tissue and cartilage.
- Arthropathy associated with articular cartilage deposition: The pigmented cartilage loses resilience and is readily eroded; the vertebral column, knee, shoulders, and hips are usually affected.

Disorders Associated with Defects in Proteins That Regulate Cell Growth (p. 168)

Neurofibromatosis: Types 1 and 2 (p. 168)

Neurofibromatosis types 1 and 2 (NF-1 and -2) are two genetically distinct autosomal dominant disorders, both characterized by the presence of tumors of the nerves.

Neurofibromatosis type 1

Previously called *von Recklinghausen disease,* this type is characterized by three main features:

- *Multiple neural tumors* involve nerve trunks in skin as well as internal organs. Three types of lesions are found: cutaneous, subcutaneous, and plexiform. The last-mentioned are subcutaneous tumors that contain numerous tortuous thickened nerves. They sometimes cause massive enlargement of a limb or other body parts. Histologically, neurofibromas reveal proliferation of neurites, Schwann cells, and fibroblasts, all embedded in loose myxoid stroma.

- *Cutaneous pigmentations,* present in more than 90% of patients, taking the form of light brown macules located over nerve trunks (*café au lait* spots).
- *Lisch nodules* or pigmented iris hamartomas are present in almost all cases.

There are also several associated abnormalities:

- There are skeletal lesions (bone cysts, scoliosis, and erosion of the bone surface) in 30% to 50% of patients.
- There is an increased risk of the development of other tumors, especially meningiomas, optic gliomas, and pheochromocytomas.
- There is a tendency toward reduced intelligence.

Neurofibromatosis type 2

Previously called *acoustic neurofibromatosis*, this type is characterized by

- Bilateral acoustic nerve tumors in all cases
- Gliomas, particularly ependymomas
- Café au lait spots
- Absence of Lisch nodules

Pathogenesis

- The *NF-1* gene locus on chromosome 17 encodes *neurofibromin*, a protein that down-regulates the function of the $p21^{Ras}$ oncoprotein. *NF-1* is therefore formally a tumor-suppressor gene, and when it is not adequately expressed, the various tissue overgrowths of neurofibromatosis type 1 occur.
- The *NF-2* locus is on chromosome 22 and also encodes a tumor-suppressor gene encoding the protein *merlin;* merlin shares homology with the ezrin, radixin, and moesin (ERM) family of cytoskeletal proteins. *Merlin* is thought to regulate contact inhibition and Schwann cell proliferation.

DISORDERS WITH MULTIFACTORIAL INHERITANCE (p. 169)

Disorders with multifactorial inheritance are the consequence of the interplay of two or more mutant genes combined with environmental factors. Multifactorial inheritance underlies many congenital malformations and common disorders, such as diabetes mellitus, gout, hypertension, and coronary heart disease. Disorders with multifactorial inheritance exhibit these characteristics:

- Although the risk of expression is conditioned by the number of mutant genes inherited, environmental influences significantly modify the risk of expression; hence the concordance rate—even in identical twins—is only 20% to 40%.
- The risk of recurrence of the disorder in first-degree relatives is 2% to 7%.
- If two children in a family have the disorder, the risk of recurrence in subsequent offspring rises to 9%.

CYTOGENETIC DISORDERS (p. 173)

Cytogenetic disorders may be due to alterations in the *number* or in the *structure* of chromosomes.

Numerical Disorders

Common types of numerical disorders include

- *Monosomy,* associated with one less normal chromosome (2n – 1)
- *Trisomy,* associated with one extra chromosome (2n + 1)
- *Mosaicism,* associated with one or more populations of cells, some with normal chromosomal complement, others with extra or missing chromosomes

Numerical disorders of chromosomes result from errors during cell division. Monosomy and trisomy usually result from chromosomal nondisjunction during gametogenesis (the first meiotic division), whereas mosaics are produced when mitotic errors occur in the zygote. Monosomy or trisomy of autosomes usually results in early fetal death and spontaneous abortion, whereas similar imbalances in sex chromosomes are typically better tolerated.

Structural Aberrations

Structural aberrations of chromosomes include (Fig. 5–2):

- *Deletion:* Loss of a terminal or interstitial (midpiece) segment of a chromosome.
- *Translocation:* Involves transfer of a segment of one chromosome to another:

    Balanced reciprocal, involving exchange of chromosomal material between two chromosomes with no net gain or loss of genetic material.

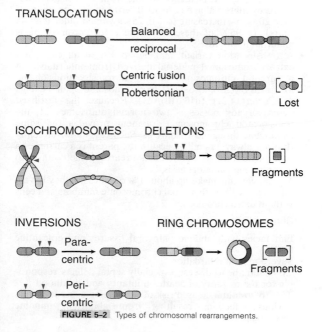

FIGURE 5–2 Types of chromosomal rearrangements.

Robertsonian (centric) fusion, or reciprocal translocation between two acrocentric chromosomes involving the short arm of one and the long arm of the other; transfer of segments leads to formation of one abnormally large chromosome and one extremely small one. The latter is usually lost. This translocation predisposes to the formation of abnormal (unbalanced) gametes.

- *Isochromosome:* Formed when one arm (short or long) is lost and the remaining arm is duplicated, resulting in a chromosome of two short arms only or of two long arms. In live births, the most common isochromosome is designated i(Xq), that is, duplication of long arm and deletion of short arm of the X chromosome.

- *Inversion:* Rearrangement associated with two breaks in a chromosome, followed by inversion and reincorporation of the broken segment.

- *Ring chromosome:* Deletion affecting both ends, followed by fusion of the damaged ends.

Cytogenetic Disorders Involving Autosomes
(p. 175)

Trisomy 21 (Down Syndrome) (p. 170)

Down syndrome is the most common chromosomal disorder (1 in 700 births).

Pathogenesis

Karyotypic features are as follows:

- About 95% have a complete extra chromosome 21 (47,XY,+21). The incidence of this form is strongly influenced by maternal age (1 in 1550 births in women younger than 20 years, increasing to 1 in 25 in women older than 45 years). In 95% of these cases, the extra chromosome is maternal in origin.

- A translocation variant, making up 4% of all cases, has extra chromosomal material derived from inheritance of a parental chromosome bearing a translocation of the long arm of chromosome 21 to chromosome 22 or 14 (e.g., 46,XX,der(14;21) (q10;q10),+21). Because the fertilized ovum already possesses two normal autosomes 21, the translocated chromosomal fragment provides the same triple-gene dosage as trisomy 21. Such cases are frequently (but not always) familial because the parent is a carrier of a robertsonian translocation. Such a rearrangement may also occur during gametogenesis.

- Mosaic variants make up about 1% of all cases; they have a mixture of cells with normal chromosome numbers and cells with an extra chromosome 21.

Clinical Features (Fig. 5–3)

- Flat facies with oblique palpebral fissures and epicanthic folds
- Severe mental retardation
- Congenital heart disease, especially septal defects, responsible for the majority of deaths in infancy and childhood
- Ten- to 20-fold increased risk of developing acute leukemia
- Serious infections resulting from abnormal immune responses

- Premature Alzheimer disease in those who survive after 35 years of age

Other Trisomies (p. 176)

Trisomy 18 (*Edwards syndrome*) and trisomy 13 (*Patau syndrome*) occur much less commonly than trisomy 21; affected infants have severe malformations and usually die within the first year of life (see Fig. 5–3).

Chromosome 22q11.2 Deletion Syndrome (p. 176)

In chromosome 22q11.2 deletion syndrome, there is a small deletion of band 11.2 on the long arm of chromosome 22; it is best visualized by fluorescence *in situ* hybridization.

Clinical Features

- Congenital heart defects
- Abnormalities of palate
- Facial dysmorphism
- Developmental delay
- Variable T-cell deficiency
- Hypoparathyroidism

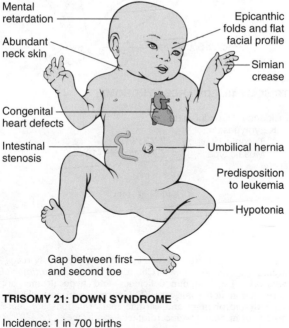

TRISOMY 21: DOWN SYNDROME

Incidence: 1 in 700 births
Karyotypes:

Trisomy 21 type:	47,XX, +21
Translocation type:	46,XX,der(14;21)(q10;q10),+21
Mosaic type:	46,XX/47,XX, +21

A

FIGURE 5–3 Clinical features and karyotypes of selected autosomal trisomies.

Continued

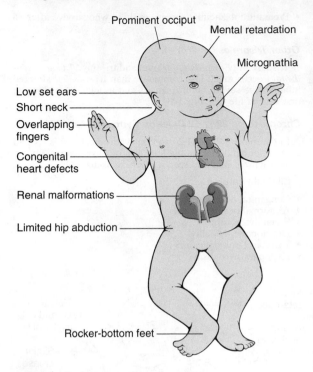

Prominent occiput

Mental retardation

Micrognathia

Low set ears

Short neck

Overlapping fingers

Congenital heart defects

Renal malformations

Limited hip abduction

Rocker-bottom feet

TRISOMY 18: EDWARDS SYNDROME

Incidence: 1 in 8000 births
  Karyotypes:
    Trisomy 18 type: 47,XX, +18
    Mosaic type: 46,XX/47,XX, +18

B

FIGURE 5–3 cont'd

These clinical features are shared by the previously recognized *DiGeorge syndrome* (Chapter 6) and *velocardiofacial syndrome*. T-cell immunodeficiency and hypocalcemia are more prominent in some cases (DiGeorge syndrome), whereas facial dysmorphology and cardiac malformations are more prominent in others (velocardiofacial syndrome).

Cytogenetic Disorders Involving Sex Chromosomes (p. 178)

Imbalances of sex chromosomes are better tolerated than similar imbalances of autosomes, and hence sex chromosome disorders are more common than autosomal disorders. The

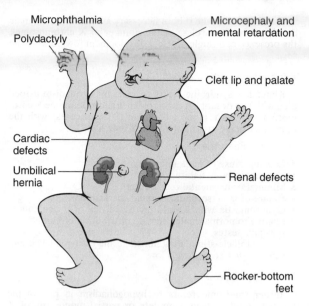

Microphthalmia

Polydactyly

Microcephaly and mental retardation

Cleft lip and palate

Cardiac defects

Umbilical hernia

Renal defects

Rocker-bottom feet

TRISOMY 13: PATAU SYNDROME

Incidence: 1 in 15,000 births
   Karyotypes:
   Trisomy 13 type: 47,XX, +13
   Translocation type: 46,XX,+13,der(13;14)(q10;q10)
   Mosaic type: 46,XX/47,XX, +13

C

FIGURE 5–3 cont'd

milder nature of X chromosome–associated aberrations is, in part, related to the fact that there is normally random inactivation of one X chromosome (Lyon hypothesis):

- All but one X chromosome is genetically inactive (although several genes—up to 20% on the short arm of any "inactivated" X chromosome—escape being "shut off").
- Random inactivation of either paternal or maternal X chromosome occurs early in embryogenesis and leads to the formation of a Barr body.
- Normal females are functional mosaics with two cell populations, one with an inactivated paternal X chromosome and the other with an inactivated maternal X chromosome.

Because numerical aberrations of X chromosomes (extra or missing) are associated with somatic and gonadal abnormalities, the Lyon hypothesis has to be modified as follows:

- Both X chromosomes are required for normal gametogenesis; the inactivated X is selectively reactivated in germ cells during gamete formation.
- X inactivation spares certain regions of the chromosome necessary for normal growth and development.

The Y chromosome is both necessary and sufficient for male development. Regardless of the number of X chromosomes, the presence of a single Y drives development toward the male sex.

Klinefelter Syndrome (p. 179)

Klinefelter syndrome refers to male hypogonadism associated with two or more X chromosomes and at least one Y chromosome; 47,XXY is most common (80% of cases) with the remainder being mosaics (e.g., 46,XY/47,XXY).

Clinical Features

- Leading cause of male infertility
- Eunuchoid body habitus
- Minimal or no mental retardation
- Failure of male secondary sexual characteristics
- Gynecomastia with 20-fold increased risk of breast cancer relative to normal males; female distribution of hair
- Atrophic testes
- Plasma follicle-stimulating hormone and estrogen levels elevated; testosterone levels low

Turner Syndrome (p. 179)

Turner syndrome refers to hypogonadism in phenotypic females resulting from complete or partial monosomy of X chromosome. Traditional cytogenetics reveals that 45,X occurs in some 57% of cases, although mosaics (e.g., 45,X/46,XX) also frequently occur; by using more sensitive techniques, mosaicism is revealed in up to 75% of cases, and the majority of Turner syndrome patients are actually probably mosaics. 46,X,i(Xq) (isochromosome of the long arm with deletion of the short arm) also yields a Turner phenotype.

Clinical Features

There are wide-ranging degrees of abnormalities that occur, presumably depending on the exact karyotype; 45,X is most severely affected. Typical features include

- Lymphedema of neck, hands, and feet
- Webbing of neck
- Short stature
- Broad chest and widely spaced nipples
- Primary amenorrhea
- Failure of breast development
- Infantile external genitalia
- Ovaries severely atrophic and fibrous (streak ovaries)
- Congenital heart disease, particularly aortic coarctation

Hermaphroditism and Pseudohermaphroditism (p. 181)

True hermaphrodites are extremely rare. These individuals have both ovaries and testes, either combined as an ovotestis or with one gonad on each side. Fifty percent have 46,XX karyotype; of the remaining, approximately equal numbers have 46,XY and 45,X/46,XY karyotypes.

Pseudohermaphrodites have disparate gonadal and phenotypic sexual characteristics.

- *Female pseudohermaphrodites* have a 46,XX karyotype. Ovaries and internal genitalia are normal, but external genitalia are ambiguous or virilized. The most common cause is inappropriate exposure to androgenic steroids during gestation. The condition may occur in congenital adrenal hyperplasia or in the presence of androgen-secreting maternal tumors.

● *Male pseudohermaphrodites* have Y chromosomes; the gonads are therefore exclusively testes, but external genitalia are either ambiguous or completely female. The condition results from defective virilization of the male embryo because of reduced androgen synthesis or resistance to action of androgens. The most common form is *complete testicular feminization* associated with mutation in the structural gene for the androgen receptor located on Xq11-Xq12.

SINGLE-GENE DISORDERS WITH NONCLASSIC INHERITANCE (p. 181)

These disorders are classified into four categories:

* Triplet repeat mutations (e.g., fragile X syndrome)
* Mutations in mitochondrial genes (e.g., Leber hereditary optic neuropathy)
* Defective genomic imprinting (e.g., Prader-Willi and Angelman syndromes)
* Gonadal mosaicism

Triplet Repeat Mutations—Fragile X Syndrome (p. 181)

Several disorders, such as Huntington disease, myotonic dystrophy, and fragile X syndrome, are characterized by triplet repeat mutations. In these mutations, there is a long repeated sequence of three nucleotides, and most affected sequences share the nucleotides guanine (G) and cytosine (C). Approximately 10 known disorders have been associated with a similar type of mutation; in virtually all cases, neurodegenerative changes dominate the clinical picture (Table 5–5).

Fragile X syndrome is the prototypic disorder in this category and is a common cause of familial mental retardation. It is characterized cytogenetically by a fragile site on Xq27.3, which is visualized as a discontinuity of chromosomal staining. At this site, there are multiple tandem repeats of the nucleotide sequence CGG in the 5′-untranslated region of the *FMR-1* gene. In normal individuals, the average number of repeats is 29 (range of 10–55), whereas affected individuals have 200 to 4000 repeats; patients with *premutations* are characterized by 55 to 200 CGG repeats. In carrier females, the premutations undergo amplification during oogenesis, resulting in full mutations that are then passed on to progeny.

Because the mutations are carried on the X chromosome, this is an X-linked recessive disorder. However, because premutations are silent and are amplified only during oogenesis in carrier females, the transmission pattern differs from classic X-linked disorders. Consequently, carrier males with premutations do not have any symptoms; approximately 50% of carrier females are affected. The molecular basis of fragile X syndrome is not clear. Presence of greater than 230 CGG repeats causes transcriptional suppression of the *FMR-1* gene.

TABLE 5-5 **Summary of Trinucleotide Repeat Disorders**

Disease	Gene	Locus	Protein	Repeat	Number of Repeats Normal	Number of Repeats Disease
Expansions Affecting Noncoding Regions						
Fragile X syndrome	*FMR1/FRAXA*	Xq27.3	FMR-1 protein (FMRP)	CGG	6–53	60–200 (pre) >230 (full)
Friedreich ataxia	*X25*	9q13–21.1	Frataxin	GAA	7–34	34–80 (pre) >100 (full)
Myotonic dystrophy	*DMPK*	19q13	Myotonic dystrophy protein kinase (DMPK)	CTG	5–37	50–thousands
Expansions Affecting Coding Regions						
Spinobulbar muscular atrophy (Kennedy disease)	*AR*	Xq13–21	Androgen receptor (AR)	CAG	9–36	38–62
Huntington disease	*HD*	4p16.3	Huntingtin	CAG	6–35	36–121
Dentatorubral-pallidoluysian atrophy (Haw River syndrome)	*DRPLA*	12p13.31	Atrophin-1	CAG	6–35	49–88
Spinocerebellar ataxia type 1	*SCA1*	6p23	Ataxin-1	CAG	6–44	39–82
Spinocerebellar ataxia type 2	*SCA2*	12q24.1	Ataxin-2	CAG	15–31	36–63
Spinocerebellar ataxia type 3 (Machado–Joseph disease)	*SCA3 (MJD1)*	14q32.1	Ataxin-3	CAG	12–40	55–84
Spinocerebellar ataxia type 6	*SCA6*	19p13	α_{1A}-Voltage-dependent calcium channel subunit	CAG	4–18	21–33
Spinocerebellar ataxia type 7	*SCA7*	3p12–13	Ataxin-7	CAG	4–35	37–306

Clinical Features

Affected males have severe mental retardation, and 80% have an enlarged testis. Other physical features, such as an elongated face and large mandible, are inconsistent. The clinical features of fragile X syndrome worsen with each successive generation because of amplification of nucleotide repeats during oogenesis. This phenomenon is called *anticipation*.

Mutations in Mitochondrial Genes—Leber Hereditary Optic Neuropathy (p. 185)

Ova contain multiple mitochondria, whereas spermatozoa contain few; hence the mitochondrial content of zygotes is derived almost entirely from the ovum (sperm mitochondria also tend to be selectively degraded after formation of the fertilized zygote). Thus, mitochondrial DNA is transmitted entirely by females, and diseases resulting from mutations in mitochondrial genes are *maternally inherited*.

Affected females transmit the disease to all their offspring—male and female; however, daughters and not sons pass the disease further to their progeny. When a cell carrying normal and mutant mitochondrial DNA divides, the proportion of normal and mutant DNA in the daughter cells is random and quite variable. Hence, expression of disorders resulting from mutations in mitochondrial genes is unpredictable.

Genes contained in the mitochondria encode enzymes involved in oxidative phosphorylation. Consequently, diseases in this category predominantly affect organs heavily dependent on mitochondrial energy metabolism. These include the neuromuscular system, liver, heart, and kidney. As an example, Leber hereditary optic neuropathy causes blindness, neurologic dysfunction, and cardiac conduction defects.

Defective Genomic Imprinting

Genomic imprinting (p. 185) is an epigenetic process that results in differential inactivation of either the maternal or the paternal alleles of certain genes. The process involves differential DNA methylation or histone H4 deacetylation, leading to selective gene inactivation. *Maternal imprinting* refers to transcriptional silencing of the maternal allele, whereas *paternal imprinting* refers to inactivation of the paternal allele. Two syndromes resulting from genomic imprinting are described below.

Prader-Willi Syndrome and Angelman Syndrome (p. 186)

- *Prader-Willi syndrome* is characterized by mental retardation, short stature, hypotonia, obesity, and hypogonadism; it results from the deletion of genes located at 15q12 in the paternally derived chromosome 15. In some cases, an entire paternal chromosome 15 is absent, replaced instead by two maternally derived chromosomes 15 (uniparental disomy). In the latter case, the patients do not exhibit any structural or numerical cytogenetic abnormality.
- *Angelman syndrome* patients are born with deletion of the same chromosomal region derived from their mothers, or uniparental disomy of paternal chromosome 15. These

patients, in addition to mental retardation, have ataxia, seizures, and inappropriate laughter.

The molecular mechanisms underlying these syndromes are only slowly coming to light. In Angelman syndrome, the affected gene is *UBE3A*, coding for a ubiquitin protein-ligase with a role in directing proteasomal degradation of a variety of intracellular proteins. The converse gene(s) in Prader-Willi syndrome are not yet known.

Gonadal Mosaicism (p. 187)

Gonadal mosaicism results from mutations that selectively affect cells destined to form gonads during early embryogenesis. Because all somatic cells are normal, the affected individual is phenotypically normal. However, because germ cells are affected, one or more offspring can manifest disease.

DIAGNOSIS OF GENETIC DISEASES (p. 187)

Diagnosis of genetic diseases involves cytogenetic and molecular analyses. Such evaluations are indicated for a number of clinical reasons:

- Prenatal evaluation, performed on fetal cells obtained by amniocentesis or chorionic villus biopsy because of:

  Advanced maternal age (>34 years)
  A parent with a structural chromosomal abnormality (e.g., Robertsonian translocation)
  Previous child with chromosomal abnormality
  A parent who is carrier of an X-linked disease (to determine fetal sex)

- Postnatal evaluation, performed on peripheral blood lymphocytes because of:

  Multiple congenital anomalies
  Unexplained mental retardation
  Suspected chromosomal abnormalities
  Suspected fragile X syndrome
  Infertility, to rule out sex chromosomal abnormality
  Recurrent abortion (both parents must be evaluated to rule out carriers of balanced translocation)

Two different approaches are applied to the diagnosis of genetic diseases by recombinant DNA technology:

- *Direct gene diagnosis,* involving detection of the mutant gene
- *Indirect gene diagnosis,* involving detection of linkage of the disease gene with a harmless *marker gene*

Direct Gene Diagnosis (p. 188)

Direct gene diagnosis is based on the identification of a qualitative difference between DNA sequences in normal *versus* abnormal genes. Three methods are used:

- Some mutations alter or destroy normal DNA restriction sites. For example, the normal factor V gene has two restriction sites for the enzyme Mn11, one of which is lost if there is a factor V mutation. This results in the production of different-sized products when DNA from normal or affected individuals is amplified by polymerase chain reaction (PCR) and then cut with Mnl1. The different products are visualized on gel electrophoresis.

- Oligonucleotide probe analysis is used when point mutations produce an abnormal gene that does not alter any known restriction site. Two oligonucleotides 18 to 20 bases long are synthesized, having at their centers the single base by which the normal and mutant genes differ. Each oligonucleotide hybridizes strongly to the corresponding (normal) gene but weakly to the gene that does not share the exact sequence. Thus, after PCR amplification of target DNA, the normal and mutant genes can be distinguished on the basis of the *strength* of hybridization with the two oligonucleotide probes.

- Mutations that affect the length of DNA (e.g., deletions or expansions) can also be detected by PCR analysis. For example, in the fragile X syndrome, amplifications of the DNA by primers that flank the region affected by trinucleotide repeats generate products of different sizes when DNAs from normal carrier males and affected individuals are compared.

Indirect DNA Diagnosis: Linkage Analysis
(p. 189)

In many genetic diseases, the mutant gene and its normal counterpart have not yet been identified or sequenced, and thus direct gene diagnosis cannot be used. It is therefore necessary to employ *linkage analysis,* which determines whether a given family member or fetus inherited the same relevant chromosomal region(s) as a previously affected family member. This technique requires that chromosomes carrying the normal and mutant genes in heterozygotes be distinguishable.

To accomplish this, advantage is taken of naturally occurring variations in DNA sequences in the vicinity of (and linked to) the mutant gene. Such variations may result from differences in specific nucleotides (site polymorphisms) or differences in the number of nucleotide repeats (length polymorphisms). Site polymorphisms, also called *restriction fragment length polymorphisms,* result from DNA polymorphisms that give rise to fragments of different lengths by Southern blot analysis. Length polymorphisms result from differences between the number of repeats of short sequences of noncoding DNA. These can be detected by PCR analysis of the DNA because the product size depends on the number of nucleotide repeats. Single nucleotide polymorphisms (SNPs) are also a form of site polymorphism that are being increasingly used to identify linkages with certain disease entities.

Linkage analysis has proved useful in antenatal detection of several genetic disorders, such as cystic fibrosis, Huntington disease, polycystic kidney disease, fragile X syndrome, and Duchenne muscular dystrophy. It has certain limitations:

- For prenatal diagnosis, several affected and unaffected family members must be available for testing.
- Key family members (e.g., parents, siblings) must be heterozygous for the polymorphism (i.e., the normal chromosome and that carrying the mutant gene must be

distinguishable). Because length polymorphisms have multiple alleles, there are much greater chances of heterozygosity. These, therefore, are more useful than restriction site polymorphisms.

- Recombination between homologous chromosomes during gametogenesis may lead to loss of linkage between any given DNA polymorphism and the mutant gene.

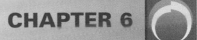

CHAPTER 6

Diseases of Immunity

The immune system evolved primarily to defend against microbial invasion; it accomplishes this by distinguishing self from nonself (exogenous or foreign) molecules and marshaling a plethora of effector mechanisms to either eliminate or neutralize the perceived invader. The pathways to recognition and elimination involve both *innate* (nonspecific) and *adaptive* (antigen-specific) components and are well reviewed in pages 194 to 205 of *Robbins and Cotran Pathologic Basis of Disease*, 7th ed. Although the pathways of the immune system are exquisitely tuned and generally well regulated, overly exuberant responses to foreign invaders can lead to pathologic consequences. Moreover, the immune system occasionally loses tolerance for self components and can thereby incite effector responses to a variety of normal tissue components—the basis of autoimmune disease.

DISORDERS OF THE IMMUNE SYSTEM (p. 205)

Pathology related to the immune system falls into four broad general categories:

- *Hypersensitivity* reactions (e.g., anaphylaxis)
- *Autoimmunity* (i.e., immune responses to self)
- *Deficiency* states, congenital or acquired
- *Amyloidosis*, a disorder of extracellular protein accumulation, frequently with an underlying immunologic association

Mechanisms of Hypersensitivity Reactions (p. 205)

Hypersensitivity reactions are divided into four general categories based on the underlying mechanisms of immune injury (Table 6–1).

TABLE 6-1 **Mechanisms of Immunologically Mediated Diseases**

Type	Prototype Disorder	Immune Mechanisms	Patholgic Lesions
Immediate (type I) hypersensitivity	Anaphylaxis; allergies; bronchial asthma (atopic forms)	Production of IgE antibody → immediate release of vasoactive amines and other mediators from mast cells; recruitment of inflammatory cells (late-phase reaction)	Vascular dilation, edema, smooth muscle contraction, mucus production, inflammation
Antibody-mediated (type II) hypersensitivity	Autoimmune hemolytic anemia; Goodpasture syndrome	Production of IgG, IgM → binds to antigen on target cell or tissue → phagocytosis or lysis of target cell by activated complement or cells bearing Fc receptors; recruitment of leukocytes	Cell lysis; inflammation
Immune complex–mediated (type III) hypersensitivity	Systemic lupus erythematosus; some forms of glomerulonephritis; serum sickness; Arthus reaction	Deposition of antigen-antibody complexes → complement activation → recruitment of leukocytes by complement products and Fc receptors → release of enzymes and other toxic molecules	Necrotizing vasculitis (fibrinoid necrosis); inflammation
Cell-mediated (type IV) hypersensitivity	Contact dermatitis; multiple sclerosis; type I diabetes; transplant rejection; tuberculosis	Activated T lymphocytes → (i) release of cytokines and macrophage activation; (ii) T cell–mediated cytotoxicity	Perivascular cellular infiltrates; edema; cell destruction; granuloma formation

Immediate (Type I) Hypersensitivity (p. 206)

Immediate (type I) hypersensitivity is mediated by immunoglobulin E (IgE) antibodies directed against specific antigens (allergens). Synthesis of IgE antibody requires the induction of CD4+ helper T cells of the T_H2 type; these T_H2-type cells produce multiple cytokines that contribute to various aspects of type I hypersensitivity responses. In particular, interleukin 4 (IL4) produced by T_H2 cells is essential for IgE synthesis; IL3, IL5, and granulocyte-macrophage colony-stimulating factor (GM-CSF) promote production and survival of *eosinophils*—important effector cells in type I hypersensitivity responses. IgE antibodies synthesized in response to prior exposure to allergens are normally bound to mast cells and basophils via specific surface Fc receptors. On re-exposure, allergen binds to and cross-links the IgE on mast cells and results in (Fig. 6–1):

- Release *(degranulation)* of preformed vesicles containing *primary mediators*
- De novo synthesis and release of *secondary mediators*

Mast cell and basophil degranulation can also be triggered by a variety of other physical and chemical stimuli (yielding responses similar to those elicited by allergens):

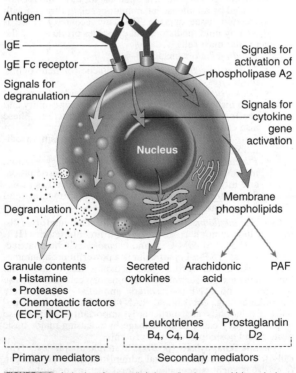

FIGURE 6–1 Activation of mast cells in immediate hypersensitivity and release of their mediators. ECF, eosinophil chemotactic protein; NCF, neutrophil chemotactic protein; PAF, platelet-activating factor.

- Complement fragments C3a and C5a *(anaphylatoxins)*
- Certain drugs (codeine, morphine, adenosine)
- Mellitin (in bee venom)
- Sunlight
- Trauma
- Heat or cold

In type I hypersensitivity, *two phases* characteristically occur (see Fig. 6–1):

1. *An initial (rapid) response*, evident within 5 to 30 minutes of allergen exposure, with resolution within 30 minutes. Primary mast cell mediators that induce the initial rapid response include:

   Biogenic amines (e.g., histamine), which cause bronchial smooth muscle contraction, increased vascular permeability and dilation, and increased mucous gland secretions

   Chemotactic mediators (e.g., eosinophil chemotactic factors and neutrophil chemotactic factors)

   Enzymes contained in granule matrix (e.g., chymase, tryptase) that generate kinins and activated complement by acting on their precursor proteins

   Proteoglycans (e.g., heparin)

2. *A second (delayed) phase,* with onset 2 to 24 hours after initial allergen exposure; this can last for days, and is characterized by an intense inflammatory cell infiltration with associated tissue damage. This late secondary phase is driven by lipid mediators and cytokines produced by the activated mast cells.

   Lipid mediators include:

   - *Leukotriene B_4* is highly chemotactic for neutrophils, monocytes, and eosinophils.
   - *Leukotrienes C_4, D_4*, and E_4 are 1000-fold more potent than histamine in increasing vascular permeability and causing bronchial smooth muscle contraction. These also cause marked mucous gland secretion.
   - *Prostaglandin D_2* causes intense bronchospasm, vasodilation, and mucous secretion.
   - *Platelet-activating factor* causes platelet aggregation, histamine release, bronchoconstriction, vasodilation, and increased vascular permeability. It also has proinflammatory effects, such as chemoattraction and degranulation of neutrophils.

Cytokine mediators recruit and activate inflammatory cells; these include tumor necrosis factor (TNF)-α, interleukins (IL1, IL3, IL4, IL5, IL6), GM-CSF, and *chemokines* (chemoattractant proteins). TNF-α in particular is a powerful proinflammatory cytokine that recruits and activates many additional inflammatory cells. Recruited inflammatory cells also release cytokines, and TNF-α–activated epithelial cells secrete chemokines (e.g., eotaxin and RANTES) that recruit eosinophils. Eosinophils are particularly important in late-phase responses; they cause tissue damage by releasing major basic protein and eosinophil cationic protein.

Systemic Anaphylaxis (p. 209). Systemic anaphylaxis typically follows parenteral or oral administration of an allergen (e.g., drugs such as penicillin, or food such as peanuts). The severity reflects the level of sensitization, and even minuscule doses may induce anaphylactic shock in an appropriate host.

Pruritus, urticaria, and erythema occur minutes after exposure, followed by bronchoconstriction and laryngeal edema; this can escalate into laryngeal obstruction, hypotensive shock, and death within minutes to hours.

Local Immediate Hypersensitivity Reactions (p. 210). These reactions are exemplified by *atopic allergies*. There is an hereditary predisposition affecting 10% of the population (mapping to 5q31, where many genes for T_H2-type cytokines are located); affected individuals tend to develop local type I responses to common inhaled or ingested allergens. Symptoms include urticaria, angioedema, rhinitis, and asthma.

Antibody-Mediated (Type II) Hypersensitivity (p. 210)

Antibody-mediated (type II) hypersensitivity is mediated by antibodies against intrinsic antigens or extrinsic antigens adsorbed on cell surfaces or extracellular matrix. Subsequent pathology occurs secondary to three major pathways (Fig. 6–2):

- *Opsonization and complement- and Fc receptor–mediated phagocytosis*: Cells can be directly lysed via the C5–C9 complement membrane attack complex (MAC) or they can be *opsonized* (enhanced phagocytosis) as a result of fixation of antibody or C3b fragments. Low concentrations of bound antibody (IgG or IgE) can also cause cell lysis (without phagocytosis) by nonsensitized cells bearing Fc receptors (e.g., natural killer [NK] cells), so-called *antibody-dependent cell-mediated cytotoxicity (ADCC)*.

- *Complement- and Fc receptor–mediated inflammation:* The deposition of antibodies (with subsequent complement activation) in the extracellular matrix leads to the recruitment and activation of nonspecific inflammatory cells (neutrophils and macrophages). These activated cells can release injurious proteases and reactive oxygen species that lead to tissue pathology.

- *Antibody-mediated cellular dysfunction*: Without causing tissue damage per se, certain antibodies can inappropriately activate or block normal cellular or hormonal function.

Examples of antibody-mediated type II hypersensitivity diseases are given in Table 6–2.

Immune Complex–Mediated (Type III) Hypersensitivity (p. 210)

Immune complex–mediated (type III) hypersensitivity is mediated by antigen-antibody complexes—immune complexes—forming either in the circulation or at sites of antigen deposition. Antigens can be exogenous (e.g., infectious agents) or endogenous. and immune complex–mediated disease can be either systemic or local. Examples of immune complex–mediated diseases are given in Table 6–3.

Systemic Immune Complex Disease (p. 212). Systemic immune complex disease is characterized by circulating immune complexes that are systemically deposited. *Acute serum sickness* is the prototypical systemic immune complex disease. It is caused by administration of large amounts of a foreign protein; after inoculation, newly synthesized antibodies complex with the foreign antigen to form circulating immune complexes. Small immune complexes (antigen excess)

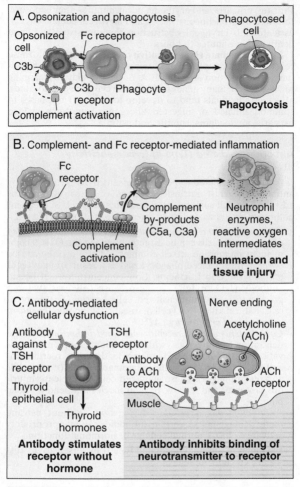

A. Opsonization and phagocytosis

Opsonized cell

Fc receptor

C3b

C3b receptor

Complement activation

Phagocyte

Phagocytosed cell

Phagocytosis

B. Complement- and Fc receptor-mediated inflammation

Fc receptor

Complement activation

Complement by-products (C5a, C3a)

Neutrophil enzymes, reactive oxygen intermediates

Inflammation and tissue injury

C. Antibody-mediated cellular dysfunction

Antibody against TSH receptor

TSH receptor

Thyroid epithelial cell

Thyroid hormones

Antibody stimulates receptor without hormone

Nerve ending

Acetylcholine (ACh)

Antibody to ACh receptor

ACh receptor

Muscle

Antibody inhibits binding of neurotransmitter to receptor

FIGURE 6–2 Schematic illustration of the three major mechanisms of antibody-mediated injury. *A,* Opsonization of cells by antibodies and complement components and ingestion by phagocytes. *B,* Inflammation induced by antibody binding to leukocyte Fc receptors and by activated complement fragments. *C,* Antireceptor antibodies disturb receptor function (e.g., anti–thyroid-stimulating hormone [TSH] receptor antibodies activate thyroid epithelial cells in Graves disease, or antiacetylcholine [ACh] receptor antibodies impair neuromuscular synaptic transmission in myasthenia gravis).

circulate for long periods because they bind with low avidity to mononuclear phagocytes and are ineffectively cleared; these complexes are prone to deposit within a capillary or arteriolar walls, causing *vasculitis*. Immune complex deposition is enhanced by increased vascular permeability resulting from inflammatory cell activation by immune complex binding to Fc or C3b receptors. The activated inflammatory cells release vasoactive mediators, including cytokines. Affected tissues include renal glomeruli (causing glomerulonephritis),

TABLE 6-2 Examples of Antibody-Mediated Diseases (Type II Hypersensitivity)

Disease	Target Antigen	Mechanisms of Disease	Clinicopathologic Manifestations
Autoimmune hemolytic anemia	Erythrocyte membrane proteins (Rh blood group antigens, blood group antigen)	Opsonization and phagocytosis of erythrocytes	Hemolysis, anemia
Autoimmune thrombocytopenic purpura	Platelet membrane proteins (GpIIb:IIIa or GpIb/IX)	Opsonization and phagocytosis of platelets	Bleeding
Pemphigus vulgaris	Proteins in intercellular junctions of epidermal cells (cadherin)	Antibody-mediated activation of proteases, disruption of intercellular adhesions	Skin vesicles (bullae)
Vasculitis caused by ANCA	Neutrophil granule proteins, presumably released from activated neutrophils	Neutrophil degranulation and inflammation	Vasculitis
Goodpasture syndrome	Noncollagenous protein in basement membranes of kidney glomeruli and lung alveoli	Complement- and Fc receptor–mediated inflammation	Nephritis, lung hemorrhage
Acute rheumatic fever	Streptococcal cell wall antigen; antibody cross-reacts with myocardial antigen	Inflammation, macrophage activation	Myocarditis, arthritis
Myasthenia gravis	Acetylcholine receptor	Antibody inhibits acetylcholine binding, down-modulates receptors	Muscle weakness, paralysis
Graves disease (hyperthyroidism)	TSH receptor	Antibody-mediated stimulation of TSH receptors	Hyperthyroidism
Insulin-resistant diabetes	Insulin receptor	Antibody inhibits binding of insulin	Hyperglycemia, ketoacidosis
Pernicious anemia	Intrinsic factor of gastric parietal cells	Neutralization of intrinsic factor, decreased absorption of vitamin B_{12}	Abnormal erythropoies, anemia

ANCA, antineutrophil cytoplasmic antibodies; TSH, thyroid-stimulating hormone.
From Abbas AK, Lichtman H: Cellular and Molecular Immunology, 5th ed. WB Saunders, Philadelphia, 2003.

TABLE 6–3 **Examples of Immune Complex–Mediated Diseases**

Disease	Antigen Involved	Clinicopathologic Manifestations
Systemic lupus erythematosus	DNA, nucleoproteins, others	Nephritis, arthritis, vasculitis
Polyarteritis nodosa	Hepatitis B virus surface antigen (in some cases)	Vasculitis
Poststreptococcal glomerulonephritis	Streptococcal cell wall antigen(s); may be "planted" in glomerular basement membrane	Nephritis
Acute glomerulonephritis	Bacterial antigens (*Treponema*); parasite antigens (malaria, schistosomes); tumor antigens	Nephritis
Reactive arthritis	Bacterial antigens (*Yersinia*)	Acute arthritis
Arthus reaction	Various foreign proteins	Cutaneous vasculitis
Serum sickness	Various proteins, e.g., foreign serum (anti-thymocyte globulin)	Arthritis, vasculitis, nephritis

joints (arthritis), skin, heart, and serosal surfaces. With continued antibody production, large immune complexes eventually form (antibody excess); these are cleared by phagocytes, ending the disease process.

Deposition of immune complexes activates the complement cascade and subsequent tissue injury derives largely from complement–mediated inflammation and cells bearing Fc receptors.

- C3b enhances opsonization.
- C5a (chemotactic factor) release promotes neutrophil and monocyte recruitment with subsequent protease and reactive oxygen species elaboration.
- C3a and C5a release increases vascular permeability and causes smooth muscle contraction.
- Cytolysis mediated by the MAC.
- Immune complexes also *aggregate platelets* (with subsequent degranulation) and *activate factor XII* (Hageman factor). The coagulation cascade and kinin systems are thus involved as well.

Morphology

There is fibrinoid deposition within vessel walls with neutrophil infiltration and surrounding hemorrhage and edema—*acute necrotizing vasculitis (fibrinoid necrosis)*. Superimposed thrombosis and downstream tissue necrosis may also be present. Immune complexes and complement can be visualized by immunofluorescence or by electron microscopy (electron-dense deposits). With time and clearance (catabolism) of the inciting antigen and immune complex, the lesions resolve. In *chronic serum sickness*—resulting from recurrent or prolonged antigen exposures and ongoing immune complex deposition (e.g., systemic lupus erythematosus, SLE)—there is intimal thickening and vascular and/or parenchymal scarring.

Local Immune Complex Disease (Arthus Reaction) (p. 215). This reaction is characterized by a localized tissue vasculitis and necrosis. This occurs (rather than systemic immune complex disease) because:

- Formation or deposition of immune complexes is extremely localized (e.g., *intracutaneous* antigen injection in previously sensitized hosts carrying the appropriate circulating antibody).
- Relevant antigen is *planted* (deposited) only within a particular tissue (e.g., the renal glomerulus) with subsequent *in situ* immune complex formation.

Cell-Mediated (Type IV) Hypersensitivity (p. 215)

Cell-mediated (type IV) hypersensitivity is initiated by specifically sensitized T lymphocytes and includes delayed-type hypersensitivity and T cell–mediated cytotoxicity (Fig. 6–3).

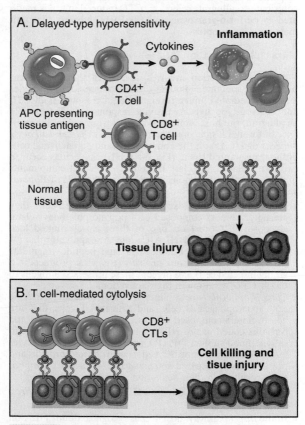

FIGURE 6–3 Mechanisms of T cell–mediated (type IV) hypersensitivity reactions. *A,* In delayed-type hypersensitivity reactions, CD4+ T cells (and sometimes CD8+ T cells) respond to local antigens by secreting cytokines that stimulate inflammation and activate phagocytes leading to tissue injury. *B,* In some diseases, CD8+ cytolytic T lymphocytes (CTLs) directly kill tissue cells. APC, antigen-presenting cell.

Delayed-Type Hypersensitivity (p. 216). Delayed-type hypersensitivity is the principal pattern of response to *Mycobacterium tuberculosis*, fungi, protozoa, and parasites, as well as contact skin sensitivity and allograft rejection. This response is largely mediated by CD4+ (T_H1) cells that secrete specific cytokines after encounter with processed antigen expressed by antigen presenting cells (APCs). The T_H1 response is driven by IL12 secreted by activated macrophages. T_H1 cytokines include interferon (IFN)-γ, IL2, and TNF-α; these cytokines mediate injury by recruiting and activating antigen-nonspecific monocytes and macrophages (Chapter 2). With persistent or nondegradable antigens, an initial infiltrate of T cells and macrophages can be eventually replaced by a nodule of activated ("epithelioid") macrophages, forming a *granuloma*.

T Cell–Mediated Cytotoxicity (p. 217). Generation of CD8+ cytotoxic T lymphocytes (CTLs) is the principal pattern of response to many viral infections and to tumor cells; CTLs also contribute to allograft rejection. CTL-induced injury is mediated by perforin-granzyme and Fas-FasL pathways that ultimately induce apoptosis.

Transplant Rejection (p. 218)

Transplant rejection involves several of the mechanisms of immune-mediated injury discussed previously; besides antibody-mediated injury, foreign allografts induce both CTL and delayed-type hypersensitivity responses. In the case of an allograft, the host immune system is triggered by the presence of foreign *histocompatibility molecules* (*human leukocyte antigens* or *HLAs*) on the endothelium and parenchymal cells of the transplanted tissue (Fig. 6–4). HLA molecules occur in two forms, class I and class II, that drive distinct components of the host immune response (see also pp. 203–205 of *Robbins and Cotran Pathologic Basis of Disease,* 7th ed.).

- *Class I molecules* are expressed on all nucleated cells; they are heterodimers composed of a polymorphic heavy-chain glycoprotein (coded on one of three closely linked loci: HLA-A, HLA-B, and HLA-C) and a nonpolymorphic $β_2$-microglobulin. Class I molecules bind peptide fragments derived from *endogenous proteins* (e.g., viral products in a virally infected cell) and present these processed antigens to *CD8+ CTL*, resulting in their activation.

- *Class II molecules* are confined to *APCs*, including dendritic cells, macrophages, B cells, and activated T cells; they are heterodimers composed of noncovalently associated α and β chains coded in the HLA-D region (with three serologically defined subloci DP, DQ, and DR). Class II molecules bind peptide fragments derived from *exogenous proteins* and present these processed antigens to *CD4+ helper T lymphocytes*, resulting in their activation.

Host T cells recognize allograft HLA by two pathways, *direct* and *indirect*:

- In the *direct pathway*, host T cells recognize donor HLA on APCs derived from the donor; the most important cells in this process are donor *dendritic cells*. Host CD8+ T cells recognize donor class I HLA molecules and mature into CTL; host CD4+ T cells recognize donor class II HLA molecules;

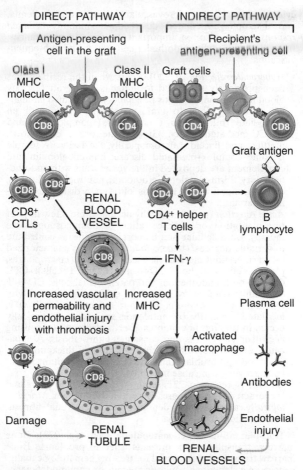

DIRECT PATHWAY | INDIRECT PATHWAY

FIGURE 6–4 Schematic representation of the events that lead to the destruction of histoincompatible grafts. In the direct pathway, class I and class II antigens on donor antigen-presenting cells are recognized by host CD8+ cytotoxic T cells and CD4+ helper T cells, respectively. CD4+ cells proliferate and produce cytokines that induce tissue damage by a local delayed hypersensitivity reaction, and stimulate B cells and CD8+ T cells. CD8+ T cells responding to graft antigens differentiate into cytotoxic T lymphocytes that kill graft cells. In the indirect pathway, graft antigens are displayed by host APCs and activate CD4+ T cells, which damage the graft by a local delayed hypersensitivity reaction. The example shown is for a kidney allograft.

they proliferate and differentiate to form a T_H1 effector cell population.
- In the *indirect pathway*, host T cells recognize donor HLA after they have been processed and presented on the *host APC* (analogous to any other exogenous processed antigen). The principal response is therefore a delayed-type hypersensitivity response mediated by CD4+ T lymphocytes.

Consequences of Allograft Recognition (see Fig. 6–4). These consequences include direct CTL-mediated cytolysis as well as microvascular injury, tissue ischemia, and macrophage-mediated destruction. *Antibody-mediated responses* may also be important in some circumstances; these tend to induce endothelial cell injury and subsequent vasculitis.

- *Hyperacute rejection* (p. 220) occurs when the recipient has been previously sensitized to antigens in a graft (e.g., by blood transfusion, previous pregnancy). Preformed circulating antibody binds to graft endothelial HLA with an immediate (minutes to 1 or 2 days) complement- and ADCC-mediated injury. Grossly, the organ is cyanotic, mottled, and flaccid. Microscopically, the lesions resemble immune complex–mediated disease; immunoglobulin and complement are deposited in the vessel walls with endothelial injury, fibrin-platelet microthrombi, neutrophil infiltrates, and arteriolar fibrinoid necrosis followed by distal parenchymal infarction.

- *Acute rejection* (p. 220) typically occurs within a few days of transplantation or after cessation of immunosuppressive therapy. Both cellular and humoral mechanisms contribute to variable degrees. *Acute cellular rejection* is characterized by an interstitial mononuclear cell infiltrate (macrophages, plasma cells, and both CD4+ and CD8+ T cells). CTL damage both endothelium and parenchymal cells; CD4+ T cells inflict damage by inducing a delayed hypersensitivity reaction. *Acute humoral rejection (rejection vasculitis)* is mediated primarily by antidonor antibodies. It typically occurs in the first few months after transplantation causing necrotizing vasculitis and consequent thrombosis. A subacute vasculitis may also occur, with intimal thickening (by proliferating fibroblasts and macrophages); resultant vascular narrowing can cause infarction.

- *Chronic rejection* (p. 221) occurs over months to years and is characterized by progressive organ dysfunction. *Morphologically*, arteries show dense obliterative intimal fibrosis, causing allograft ischemia.

Transplantation of Hematopoietic Cells (p. 222). Bone marrow transplantation presents special problems. Bone marrow transplantation is used for treating hematologic malignancies (e.g., leukemia), aplastic anemia, or immunodeficiency states. The recipient receives lethal levels of irradiation (or chemotherapy) to eradicate malignant cells, create a satisfactory graft bed, and minimize host rejection of the grafted marrow. Recipient NK cells or radiation-resistant T cells, however, may mediate significant transplant rejection.

The unique problem with marrow transplantation is *graft-versus-host disease (GVHD)*, in which donor immunocompetent cells or precursors are introduced into an immunocompromised HLA-nonidentical host. Consequently, the host cells are recognized by the transplanted immunocompetent T cells as being foreign with ensuing CD8+ and CD4+ T cell–mediated injury. Biliary epithelium, skin, and gastrointestinal mucosa are most typically affected. There is also profound immunosuppression and reactivation of cytomegalovirus infection, particularly in the lung. Chronic GVHD produces skin changes similar to those seen in systemic sclerosis (discussed later).

GVHD and complications (e.g., infections) are often lethal; to minimize its severity, close HLA matching and selective donor marrow T-cell depletion (and/or immunosuppression) are attempted to reduce the severity of GVHD. Unfortunately, T cell–depleted marrow engrafts poorly, and in leukemic patients the relapse rate of leukemia is increased when T cell–depleted marrow is used (donor T cells exert a potent graft-versus-leukemia effect).

Autoimmune Diseases (p. 223)

Autoimmune diseases result from breakdown in *self-tolerance*, the normal state of nonresponsiveness to one's own antigens.

Immunologic Tolerance (p. 223)

Tolerance can be central or peripheral:

- *Central tolerance* (p. 223): Many self-antigens are expressed in the thymus and presented by thymic APCs in association with HLA molecules. T-cell clones with high-affinity T-cell receptors for self-antigens are deleted in the thymus during development. A similar negative selection also occurs during B-cell development. Clonal deletion is not perfect, however, and numerous normal B cells can be found with surface immunoglobulin against self-antigens (e.g., DNA, myelin, collagen, and thyroglobulin).
- *Peripheral tolerance*: Autoreactive T cells that escape thymic deletion can be removed or inactivated in the periphery via one of the following mechanisms:

  Anergy: Irreversible functional inactivation of T cells may occur when they recognize self-antigen in the absence of necessary costimulatory signals from normal parenchymal cells.

  Suppression by regulatory T cells: Regulatory T cells (largely identified by constitutive expression of CD4 and the α chain of the IL2 receptor [CD25]) may inhibit lymphocyte activation and effector functions by secreting cytokines such as IL10 and transforming growth factor (TGF)-β.

  Clonal deletion by activation-induced cell death: Those self-antigens that are abundant in the peripheral tissue may cause persistent activation of self-reactive T cells, leading to expression of FasL on these cells. Such cells undergo apoptosis by engaging Fas co-expressed on these cells.

  Antigen sequestration: Immune-privileged sites such as testis, eye, and brain may sequester tissue antigens across a relatively impermeant blood-tissue barrier.

Mechanisms of Autoimmune Diseases (p. 226)

Because helper T cells control both cellular and humoral immunity, T-helper cell tolerance is considered critical for prevention of autoimmune diseases. Multiple pathways allow tolerance to be bypassed, all involving some combination of susceptibility genes and environmental triggers (especially infections).

- *Role of susceptibility genes.* Although multiple autoimmune diseases are strongly associated with specific HLA alleles, the expression of particular HLA molecules is not—by itself—the cause of autoimmunity. Defects in pathways that would normally regulate either peripheral or central tolerance have also been implicated; thus, defects in the Fas-FasL pathway or other molecules involved in activation-induced death may prevent apoptosis of autoreactive T cells. Defective T regulatory cell development or defective expression of self-antigens by thymic epithelium are also pathways by which tolerance may be bypassed. *Most human autoimmune disorders have complex, multigenic patterns of susceptibility and are not attributable to single gene mutations.*

• *Role of infections.* The onset of many autoimmune diseases is temporally associated with infections. This may occur because infections up-regulate costimulator molecule expression on APCs and overcome that pathway of peripheral tolerance. Infections might also break tolerance by *molecular mimicry* whereby some infectious agents share epitopes with self-antigens; hence, immune responses against such epitopes could damage normal tissues. Tissue injury occurring in the course of response to infection could structurally alter self-antigens, or release normal self-antigens; these molecules could activate T cells that are not tolerant to the altered, or previously cryptic antigens.

Once induced, autoimmune diseases tend to be progressive (albeit with occasional relapses and remissions). An important mechanism for the persistence and evolution of autoimmunity is the phenomenon of *epitope spreading.* The molecular structure of certain self-antigens normally prevents exposure of some self-epitopes to developing T cells; hence, T cells are not tolerized to such *cryptic* epitopes. However, if such epitopes become recognizable in postnatal life as a result of molecular alteration of self-antigens, T cells reactive to such epitopes can cause persistent autoimmunity. The phenomenon is called *epitope spreading* because the immune response "spreads" to determinants that were not initially recognized.

Systemic Lupus Erythematosus (p. 227)

SLE is the prototypical systemic autoimmune disorder, characterized by numerous autoantibodies, especially *antinuclear antibodies (ANAs).* Incidence approaches 1 in 2500 in some general populations; the female-male ratio is 9:1. ANAs are commonly detected by indirect immunofluorescence. The patterns of immunofluorescence (e.g., homogeneous, peripheral, speckled, nucleolar), although nonspecific, can suggest the type of circulating autoantibody. ANAs can also occur in other autoimmune disorders (and in up to 10% of normal individuals) (Table 6–4), but *anti–double-stranded DNA and anti-Smith antigen antibodies strongly suggest SLE.*

In addition to ANAs, SLE patients produce many other autoantibodies, some directed against blood elements (red blood cells, platelets, leukocytes). Moreover, 40% to 50% of SLE patients have antibodies to phospholipid-associated proteins (*antiphospholipid antibodies*). Some bind to cardiolipin antigen, giving rise to false-positive Venereal Disease Research Laboratory (VDRL) tests. Others interfere with (prolong) in vitro coagulation assays. These so-called *lupus anticoagulants* actually exert a *pro*coagulant effect *in vivo*, causing recurrent vascular thromboses, miscarriages, and cerebral ischemia (*secondary antiphospholipid antibody syndrome*).

TABLE 6-4 **Antinuclear Antibodies in Various Autoimmune Diseases**

Nature of Antigen	Antibody System	Disease, % Positive					
		SLE	Durg-Induced LE	Systemic Sclerosis—Diffuse	Limited Scleroderma—CREST	Sjögren Syndrome	Inflammatory Myopathies
Many nuclear antigens (DNA, RNA, proteins)	Generic ANA (indirect IF)	>95	>95	70–90	70–90	50–80	40–60
Native DNA	Anti-double-stranded DNA	40–60	<5	<5	<5	<5	<5
Histones	Antihistone	50–70	>95	<5	<5	<5	<5
Core proteins of small nuclear ribonucleoprotein particles (Smith antigen)	Anti-Sm	20–30	<5	<5	<5	<5	<5
Ribonucleoprotein (U1RNP)	Nuclear RNP	30–40	<5	15	10	<5	<5
RNP	SS-A(Ro)	30–50	<5	<5	<5	70–95	10
RNP	SS-B(La)	10–15	<5	<5	<5	60–90	<5
DNA topoisomerase I	Scl-70	<5	<5	28–70	10–18	<5	<5
Centromeric proteins	Anticentromere	<5	<5	22–36	90	<5	<5
Histidyl-t-RNA synthetase	Jo-1	<5	<5	<5	<5	<5	25

Boxed entries indicate high correlation.
SLE, systemic lupus erythematosus; LE, lupus erythematosus; ANA, antinuclear antibodies; RNP, ribonucleoprotein.

Pathogenesis

Monozygotic twin concordance (>20%) and familial and HLA clustering suggest a *genetic predisposition*. In addition, *exogenous factors*, such as drug exposure (see later discussion), ultraviolet irradiation, and estrogens, are also involved. Although the cause is unknown, the pathogenesis is thought to involve some basic defect in the maintenance of B-cell peripheral self-tolerance. This may occur secondary to some combination of:

- Heritable defects in the regulation of B-cell proliferation.
- Helper T-cell hyperactivity; a primary defect in CD4+ helper T cells may drive self-antigen–specific B cells to produce autoantibodies.

Tissue damage occurs by formation of immune complexes (type III hypersensitivity) or by antibody-mediated injury to blood cells (type II hypersensitivity). Although ANAs cannot penetrate cells, these circulating autoantibodies may nevertheless form immune complexes with intracellular contents released from otherwise damaged cells.

Morphology

Typical in all tissues is a type III hypersensitivity response with an acute necrotizing vasculitis and fibrinoid deposits, involving small arteries and arterioles. Immunoglobulin, dsDNA, and C3 may be found within vessel walls. Skin and muscle are most commonly involved. A perivascular lymphocytic infiltrate is frequently present. In chronic cases, vessels show a fibrous thickening and luminal narrowing.

Kidney. Kidney is involved in virtually all cases of SLE; the principal mechanism of injury is immune complex deposition. Five patterns of *lupus nephritis* are regonized:

Class I: Normal by light, electron, and fluorescence microscopy; rare (<5%).

Class II: Mesangial lupus glomerulonephritis (GN); present in 10% to 25% of patients, associated with minimal hematuria or proteinuria. Slight increase in mesangial matrix and cells with granular mesangial immunoglobulin and complement deposits.

Class III: Focal proliferative GN; in 20% to 35% of patients. Associated with recurrent hematuria, moderate proteinuria, and occasional mild renal insufficiency. Focal and segmental glomerular swelling with endothelial and mesangial proliferation, neutrophil infiltration, and sometimes fibrinoid deposits and capillary thrombi.

Class IV: Diffuse proliferative GN; in 35% to 60% of patients, many of whom are overtly symptomatic, with microscopic to gross hematuria, proteinuria (sometimes nephrotic range), hypertension, and diminished glomerular filtration rate. Most glomeruli show endothelial, mesangial, and occasionally epithelial proliferation. Immune complex deposits are typically *subendothelial* and when extensive form *wire loops*. Frequently, there are also tubular changes with granular immune complex deposits in basement membranes and interstitial changes. Most severe form of lupus nephritis; carries the worst prognosis.

Class V: Membranous GN; in 10% to 15% of patients. Associated with severe proteinuria (nephrotic syndrome).

Diffusely thickened capillary walls similar to idiopathic membranous GN and characterized by *subepithelial* immune complex deposits.

Skin. Classically, there is malar erythema, including bridge of nose *(butterfly rash)*. Also, variable cutaneous lesions ranging from erythema to bullae occur elsewhere. Sunlight exacerbates the lesions. Microscopically, there is basal layer degeneration with dermal-epidermal junction immunoglobulin and complement deposits. The dermis shows variable fibrosis, perivascular mononuclear cell infiltrates, and vascular fibrinoid change.

Joints. In the joints, SLE is characterized by a *nonspecific, nonerosive synovitis*. There is minimal joint deformity in contrast to rheumatoid arthritis.

Central Nervous System. Neuropsychiatric manifestations are probably secondary to endothelial injury and occlusion (antiphospholipid antibodies) or impaired neuronal function as a result of autoantibodies to a synaptic membrane antigen.

Pericarditis and Other Serosal Cavity Involvement. Serositis is initially fibrinous with focal vasculitis, fibrinoid necrosis, and edema; progress to adhesions, possibly obliterating serosal cavities (i.e., the pericardial sac).

Cardiovascular System. Principal involvement is pericarditis; myocarditis is much less common. Characteristic *nonbacterial verrucous (Libman-Sacks) endocarditis* occurs much less frequently with the current clinical use of steroids. Typically, numerous small, warty vegetations (1 to 3 mm) occur on the inflow or outflow surfaces (or both) of the mitral and tricuspid valves. Subtle or overt valvular abnormalities readily detected by echocardiography are common. They affect mitral and aortic valves and may cause stenosis or regurgitation. An increasing number of younger patients, especially those treated with corticosteroids, have clinical evidence of coronary artery disease; exacerbation of traditional risk factors (e.g., hypertension, hypercholesterolemia) and immune complex– and antiphospholipid antibody-mediated injury may also contribute

Spleen. Moderate splenomegaly occurs with capsular thickening and follicular hyperplasia. Marked perivascular fibrosis around penicilliary arteries (containing immunoglobulin, C3, and dsDNA) is characteristic, producing an *onion-skin* appearance.

Lungs. Pleuritis occurs with pleural effusions in 50% of patients; there is also interstitial pneumonitis, and diffuse fibrosing alveolitis, all probably related to immune complex deposition.

Clinical Features

The clinical manifestations of SLE are protean. It typically presents insidiously as a systemic, chronic, recurrent, febrile illness with symptoms referable to virtually any tissue but especially joints, skin, kidneys, and serosal membranes. Autoantibodies to hematologic components may induce thrombocytopenia, leukopenia, and anemia. The course of the disease is highly variable; rarely, it is fulminant with death in weeks to months.

- Occasionally may cause minimal symptoms (hematuria, rash) and remit even without treatment.

- More often, the disease is characterized by recurrent flares and remissions over many years and is held in check by immunosuppressive regimens.
- Ten-year survival is approximately 80%; death is most commonly caused by renal failure or intercurrent infections.

Chronic Discoid Lupus Erythematosus (p. 235). This disease is limited to cutaneous lesions that grossly and microscopically mimic SLE. Only 35% of patients have a positive ANA. As in SLE, there is deposition of immunoglobulin and C3 at the dermal-epidermal junction. After many years, 5% to 10% of affected individuals develop systemic manifestations.

Drug-Induced Lupus Erythematosus (p. 235). Drugs such as hydralazine, procainamide, isoniazid, and D-penicillamine frequently induce a positive ANA and less often a lupus erythematosus–like syndrome. With the latter, although there is multiorgan involvement, renal and central nervous system disease is uncommon. Anti-dsDNA antibodies are rare, but antihistone antibodies are common. There is linkage with HLA-DR4. Drug-related lupus erythematosus usually remits after removal of the offending agent.

Rheumatoid Arthritis (see Chapter 26)

Sjögren Syndrome (p. 235)

Sjögren syndrome is characterized by dry eyes *(keratoconjunctivitis sicca)* and dry mouth *(xerostomia)*, resulting from immune-mediated lacrimal and salivary gland destruction. About 40% of cases occur in isolation (the primary form or *sicca syndrome*), and the remaining 60% occur in association with other autoimmune diseases, such as rheumatoid arthritis (most common), SLE, or scleroderma; 90% of patients are women between ages 35 and 45.

- Most patients have rheumatoid factor in the absence of rheumatoid arthritis; ANAs against ribonucleoproteins SS-A (Ro) and SS-B (La) are especially common (see Table 6–4).
- Injury is probably a consequence of both cellular and humoral mechanisms; it is most likely initiated by activation of CD4+ T cells reacting to an unknown self-antigen. There is some association with Epstein-Barr virus and hepatitis C, as well as human T-cell lymphotropic virus (HTLV)-1 infection; patients with human immunodeficiency virus (HIV)-1 infection can develop similar lesions.

Morphology

The lacrimal and salivary glands (other exocrine glands may also be involved) initially show a periductal lymphocytic infiltrate (predominantly CD4+ T cells with some B cells) with ductal epithelial hyperplasia and luminal obstruction. This is followed by acinar atrophy, fibrosis, and eventual fatty replacement. Secondary changes include corneal inflammation, erosion, and ulceration, and atrophy of oral mucosa with inflammatory fissuring and ulceration; the latter changes result in difficulty in swallowing food.

Clinical Features. Patients frequently develop nasal drying and crusting, with ulceration and, rarely, septal perforation. Laryngitis, bronchitis, or pneumonitis can result from respiratory involvement.

To distinguish lacrimal and salivary gland enlargement caused by Sjögren syndrome (*Mikulicz syndrome*) from other causes (e.g., sarcoidosis, leukemia, lymphoma), lip biopsy (to examine minor salivary glands) is helpful.

Some cases of Sjögren syndrome have extraglandular involvement:

- Commonly a tubulointerstitial nephritis with tubular atrophy occurs; this causes renal tubular acidosis with excess urate and phosphate excretion. Glomerular involvement is rare.
- Adenopathy may occur with pleomorphic lymph node infiltrates. There is a 40-fold increased risk of developing a B-cell lymphoma in involved glands.

Systemic Sclerosis (Scleroderma) (p. 237)

Scleroderma involves excessive systemic fibrosis, most commonly in the skin (where it may be confined for years); the fibrosis eventually involves the gastrointestinal tract, kidneys, heart, muscles, and lung. The female-male ratio is 3:1, with peak incidence in the 50- to 60-year age group. The disease initially presents with symmetric edema and thickening skin of hands and fingers or with *Raynaud phenomenon* (paroxysmal pallor or cyanosis of tips of fingers or toes). This initial presentation is followed by:

- Articular symptoms that mimic rheumatoid arthritis
- Dysphagia from esophageal fibrosis (up to 50% of patients)
- Gastrointestinal involvement leading to malabsorption, intestinal pain, or obstruction
- Pulmonary fibrosis, causing respiratory or right-sided heart failure
- Direct cardiac involvement, which can induce arrhythmias or heart failure secondary to microvascular infarction
- Development of malignant hypertension, potentially culminating in fatal renal failure

Systemic sclerosis is subclassified as:

- *Diffuse scleroderma*: Widespread cutaneous and early visceral involvement with rapid progression. Associated with DNA topoisomerase I ANA (see Table 6–4).
- Localized scleroderma *(CREST syndrome)*: CREST is an acronym for *c*alcinosis, *R*aynaud phenomenon, *e*sophageal dysmotility, *s*clerodactyly, and *t*elangiectasia. There is minimal cutaneous involvement (typically fingers and face) with late visceral involvement and a relatively benign course. This type is associated with anticentromere antibodies (see Table 6–4).

Pathogenesis

Although the cause is unknown (and may be multifactorial), the final common pathway of systemic sclerosis involves vascular injury due to abnormal immune responses; this results in the local accumulation of growth factors that drive fibroblast proliferation and stimulate collagen synthesis. Etiologic possibilities include:

- Activation of CD4+ T cells by an unidentified antigen with cytokine production (TNF-α, IL1, IL4, platelet-derived growth factor, or TGF-β) that promotes collagen synthesis
- Recurrent endothelial injury (owing to toxic mediators released by activated T cells or environmental triggers) causing platelet aggregation and subsequent release of

activating factors that alter vascular permeability and stimulate fibroblasts

Although a host of autoantibodies—refelecting deranged humoral immunity—is also present, there is no evidence that these antibodies cause injury. The autoantibodies include (see Table 6–4):

- Antibodies to DNA topoisomerase I (anti-Scl 70); this ANA is highly specific for diffuse scleroderma
- Anticentromere antibody, characteristic of the CREST syndrome

Morphology

Skin. Grossly, there is diffuse sclerosis with atrophy. Initially, affected areas are edematous with a doughy consistency. Eventually, fibrotic fingers become tapered and claw-like with diminished mobility, and the face becomes a drawn mask. Focal obliteration of the vascular supply causes ulceration. Occasionally, fingertips undergo autoamputation.

Microscopically, there are perivascular lymphocytic infiltrates with early capillary and arteriolar injury and partial occlusion; edema and collagen fiber degeneration are followed by progressive dermal fibrosis and vascular hyaline thickening.

Alimentary Tract. Progressive atrophy and collagenization of muscularis occurs, mostly in the esophagus; the lower two thirds may develop rubber-hose inflexibility. Throughout the alimentary tract, mucosa may be thinned and ulcerated with mural collagenization; vascular changes are as described for skin.

Musculoskeletal System. Typically, an inflammatory synovitis progressing to fibrosis is present; joint destruction is uncommon. Muscle involvement begins proximally with edema and mononuclear perivascular infiltrates, progressing to interstitial fibrosis with myofiber degeneration; vessels show basement membrane thickening.

Kidneys. Kidneys are affected in two thirds of patients; *renal failure accounts for 50% of deaths in systemic sclerosis.* The most prominent changes are in vessel walls (especially interlobular arteries) with intimal proliferation and deposition of mucinous or collagenous material. Hypertension is present in 30% of cases, 10% of which have a malignant course. Hypertension further accentuates the vascular changes, often resulting in fibrinoid necrosis with thrombosis and necrosis.

Lungs. Lungs show variable fibrosis of small pulmonary vessels with diffuse interstitial and alveolar fibrosis progressing in some cases to honeycombing.

Heart. Perivascular infiltrates with interstitial fibrosis occasionally evolve into a restrictive cardiomyopathy. There may also be conduction system involvement with resultant arrhythmias.

Inflammatory Myopathies (see Chapter 27)

Mixed Connective Tissue Disease (p. 239)

It is controversial whether mixed connective tissue disease represents a heterogeneous subgroup of other autoimmune disorders or is a separate clinical entity. It is characterized by:

- Features suggestive of SLE, polymyositis, and systemic sclerosis (e.g., Raynaud phenomenon, esophageal dysmotility, myositis, leukopenia-anemia, fever, lymphadenopathy, and hypergammaglobulinemia)

- High ANA titers to ribonucleoproteins (and in contrast to SLE *no* antibodies to native DNA or Smith antigens) (see Table 6-4)
- Infrequency of renal disease
- Excellent response to steroids

Polyarteritis Nodosa and Other Vasculitides
(see Chapter 11)

Immunologic Deficiency Syndromes (p. 240)

Immunologic deficiency syndromes can be subdivided into primary and secondary forms:

- *Primary immunodeficiency disorders* are usually hereditary, typically manifesting between 6 months and 2 years of life as maternal antibody protection is lost.
- *Secondary immunodeficiencies* result from altered immune function due to infections, malnutrition, aging, immunosuppression, irradiation, chemotherapy, or autoimmunity.

Primary Immunodeficiencies (p. 240)

X-Linked Agammaglobulinemia of Bruton (p. 240). This is one of the most common primary immunodeficiency syndromes. This X-linked disorder presents as *recurrent bacterial infections* (e.g., *Staphylococcus, Haemophilus influenzae, Streptococcus pneumoniae*) beginning after 6 months of age. There is virtually no serum immunoglobulin, but cell-mediated immune function is normal; consequently, most viral and fungal infections are handled appropriately. Exceptions include enterovirus, echovirus (causing a fatal encephalitis), and vaccine-associated poliovirus (causing paralysis) because these viruses are normally neutralized by circulating antibodies. *Giardia lamblia*, an intestinal parasite that is normally neutralized by secreted IgA, can also cause persistent infections.

- The basic defect is lack of *mature* B cells due to mutations in the B-cell tyrosine kinase gene (*BTK*); *BTK* is normally expressed in early B cells and is critical for transduction of signals from the antigen receptor complex that drive B-cell maturation. Pre-B cells are present in normal numbers in marrow, but lymph nodes and spleen lack germinal centers, and plasma cells are absent from all tissues.
- T-cell numbers and function are entirely normal.
- For unknown reasons, these patients have an increased frequency (up to 20%) of autoimmune connective tissue diseases, including a rheumatoid-like arthritis that responds to gammaglobulin therapy.

Common Variable Immunodeficiency (p. 242). Common variable immunodeficiency comprises a heterogeneous group of disorders, congenital and acquired, sporadic and familial. The common feature is hypogammaglobulinemia, generally affecting all immunoglobulin classes but occasionally only IgG.

The pathogenesis of antibody deficiency is not clear and may differ among patients. There may be intrinsic B-cell defects or, more commonly, defective B-cell maturation as a result of defects in T cells. Some patients show linkage with the complement genes within HLA complex, as do certain patients with selective IgA deficiency, suggesting some genetically determined defect in B-cell differentiation. Clinical features resemble X-linked agammaglobulinemia (i.e., recurrent sinopulmonary infections, serious enterovirus infections, and persistent *G. lamblia* infections). In contrast to X-linked agammaglobulinemia, symptoms start in childhood or adolescence. These patients are also prone to autoimmune diseases and lymphoid malignancies.

Isolated IgA Deficiency (p. 242). This is a common immunodeficiency (1 in 600 people) with *virtual absence of serum and secretory IgA and occasionally of IgG₂ and IgG₄ subclasses.* This immunodeficiency may be familial or acquired after toxoplasmosis, measles, or other viral infection.

* Although usually asymptomatic, patients can have recurrent sinopulmonary and gastrointestinal infections and are prone to respiratory tract allergies and autoimmune diseases (SLE, rheumatoid arthritis).
* The basic defect is failure of maturation of IgA-positive B cells. Immature forms are present in normal numbers.
* About 40% of patients have antibodies to IgA. Transfusion of IgA-containing blood products may induce anaphylaxis.

Hyper-IgM Syndrome (p. 242). This syndrome is characterized by the production of IgM but failure to produce IgG, IgA, and IgE antibodies. It results from failure of T cells to cause B-cell switching to form immunoglobulins other than IgM. Such isotype switching depends on interaction of CD40L on T cells with CD40 on B cells. In 70% of patients, there is mutation of *CD40L* gene encoded on X chromosome (Xq26); hence the disease is X-linked. In the other patients, there are mutations in CD40 or in an enzyme called *activation-induced deaminase*; the latter is a DNA-editing enzyme required for isotype switching.

Clinically, lack of opsonizing IgG leads to recurrent bacterial infections; in addition, because T-cell/macrophage interactions in cell-mediated immune responses also involve CD40-CD40L ligations, there is susceptibility to *Pneumocystis jiroveci (carinii)*.

DiGeorge Syndrome (Thymic Hypoplasia) (p. 243). This multiorgan congenital disorder results from failure of development of the third and fourth pharyngeal pouches before the eighth week of gestation. Characteristics are as follows:

* *Thymic hypoplasia or aplasia*: T-cell deficiency with lack of cell-mediated responses (especially to fungi and viruses); B cells and immunoglobulin levels are usually normal.
* *Parathyroid hypoplasia*: Abnormal calcium regulation with hypocalcemic tetany.
* Congenital defects of heart and great vessels.
* Dysmorphic facies.

DiGeorge syndrome results from the deletion of a gene mapping to 22q11; this chromosomal abnormality is seen in 90% of cases. Patients may be treated with fetal thymus or thymic epithelium transplants. If children survive into their fifth year, T-cell function tends to normalize even with thymic aplasia.

Severe Combined Immunodeficiency Disease (p. 243). Severe combined immunodeficiency disease (SCID) refers to a heterogeneous group of autosomal or X-linked recessive disorders *characterized by lymphopenia and defects* *in T-cell and B-cell function.* Pathogenetic mechanisms fall into two general categories:

- In 50% to 60% of cases, SCID is an X-linked disorder resulting from a mutation in the common γ chain (γc) subunit of several cytokine receptors. Because of the defective receptor subunit, lymphoid progenitors fail to be stimulated by IL2, IL4, IL7, IL9, IL11, and IL15; in particular, the defect in IL7 stimulatory pathways is most profound because IL7 is required for the proliferation of lymphoid progenitors. Consequently, there is a severe defect in T-cell development with a lesser B-cell developmental defect.
- The remaining cases of SCID are inherited as autosomal recessive disorders; in this group, the most common cause is deficiency of the enzyme adenosine deaminase. This deficiency leads to an accumulation of lymphocyte-toxic metabolites, such as deoxy–adenosine triphosphate (deoxy-ATP).

Because T-cell defects lead to secondary B-cell defects, patients with SCID have impairment of both cellular and humoral immunity, manifested as recurrent bacterial, viral, and fungal infections. Their lymphoid tissues (thymus, lymph nodes) are hypoplastic. Bone marrow transplantation is the current mainstay of therapy, although X-linked SCID is the first human disease in which gene therapy has been successful; the normal γc gene was expressed in patient bone marrow stem cells using retroviral vectors, and the cells were transplanted back. Unfortunately, a cohort of these patients developed leukemia—apparently due to retroviral genome integration into an area of the host genome expressing a tumor suppressor gene—so that this gene therapy approach is on hold.

Immunodeficiency with Thrombocytopenia and Eczema (Wiskott-Aldrich Syndrome) (p. 244). This X-linked recessive disease is characterized by thrombocytopenia, eczema, and recurrent infections with a predilection for lymphoma development.

- The thymus is morphologically normal, but there is peripheral T-cell depletion in lymphoid tissues with an associated defect in cellular immunity.
- Antibody responses are variable but are characteristically poor to polysaccharide antigens.
- The defect maps to Xp11.23, the location for the gene for Wiskott-Aldrich syndrome protein (WASP); WASP links cell surface receptors and intracellular cytoskeleton and is therefore important for cytoskeletal integrity and signal transduction.
- Bone marrow transplantation is the only current therapy.

Genetic Deficiencies of the Complement System (p. 244). Deficiencies have been described for virtually all complement components and for two inhibitors. A deficiency of C2 is the most common, but it is not associated with serious infections, presumably because the alternative complement pathway is unaffected. Deficiency of C3 impairs both complement pathways and hence leads to increased susceptibility to bacterial infections. Inherited deficiencies of C1q and C4 impair clearance of immune complexes and hence increase the risk of immune complex–mediated diseases (e.g., SLE). An absence of C1 esterase inhibitor is associated with *hereditary angioedema*, resulting from uncontrolled generation of vasoactive kinins. Defects in later-acting complement components (C5–C8) result in recurrent neisserial infections.

Acquired Immunodeficiency Syndrome (AIDS) (p. 245)

AIDS is an infectious secondary form of immunodeficiency caused by HIV-1. It is characterized by profound suppression of T cell–mediated immunity, opportunistic infections, secondary neoplasms, and neurologic disease.

Epidemiology (p. 245)

Transmission of HIV occurs through:

- Sexual contact
- Parenteral inoculation
- Vertical transmission from infected mothers to fetuses or newborns

In the United States, there are five major risk groups:

1. *Homosexual/bisexual men*: Over 50% of reported cases of AIDS (in homosexual men the virus enters via lymphocytes in semen through traumatized rectal mucosa). This mode of transmission is in decline; only 42% of new AIDS cases can be attributed to male homosexual contacts.
2. *Intravenous drug users* (without a history of homosexual contact): Approximately 25% of all patients. The virus is tranmitted through sharing of contaminated needles and drug paraphernalia.
3. *Hemophiliacs*: Approximately 0.5% of cases. Especially those receiving large amounts of pooled factor VIII concentrate before 1985.
4. *Blood/component recipients (excluding hemophiliacs)*: Approximately 1% of all patients. Transmission by this route has been virtually eliminated in the United States.
5. *Other high-risk groups*: About 10% of patients acquire the disease through heterosexual contacts with members of other high-risk groups. Roughly a third of new cases are attributable to heterosexual contact.

In approximately 6% of cases, no risk factors can be identified. Ninety percent of children with AIDS have an HIV-infected mother and have had transplacental or perinatal transmission. Ten percent of pediatric AIDS patients received blood or blood products before 1985.

Some other aspects of transmission are as follows:

- Risk of seroconversion after an accidental needle-stick with infected blood is approximately 0.3%.
- HIV is *not* transmitted by casual (nonsexual) contact.
- Outside the United States and Europe, male-to-female transmission (most through vaginal intercourse) is the most common mode of spread.
- Increased heterosexual transmission is beginning to outpace other modes in the United States.
- Although HIV has been found in vaginal and cervical secretions, monocytes, and endothelium, female-to-male transmission is still uncommon in the United States (20-fold less common than male-to-female heterosexual transmission).
- All forms of sexual transmission are facilitated by co-existence of sexually transmitted diseases with genital ulcerations.

Etiology: The Properties of HIV (p. 246)

HIV-1 is a human type C retrovirus in the same family as the animal lentivirus family. It is also closely related to HIV-2, which causes a similar disease, primarily in West Africa.

- HIV is a *nontransforming cytopathic retrovirus* inducing immunodeficiency by destruction of target T cells.
- The HIV-1 lipid envelope, derived from the infected host membrane during budding, is studded with two viral glycoproteins, gp120 and gp41, which are critical for HIV infection of cells.
- The virus core contains major capsid protein p24, nucleocapsid protein, genomic RNA, and three viral enzymes: protease, integrase, and reverse transcriptase. Antiviral therapy is directed against the reverse transcriptase and protease.
- HIV has several genes not present in the other retroviruses. These genes include *TAT, VPU, VIF, NEF,* and *REV.* Many, such as *TAT* and *REV,* regulate HIV transcription and hence may be targeted for therapy.

Pathogenesis of HIV Infection and AIDS (p. 248)

CD4+ helper T-cell depletion is the central pathogenic pathway of AIDS. The CD4 antigen (also present at lower levels on monocytes and macrophages) is the high-affinity receptor for the gp120 protein on HIV-1. In addition to CD4, gp120 must also bind to coreceptors on target cells in order to affect cell entry. The major coreceptors are the chemokine receptors CCR5 and CXCR4; individuals who have mutations in the CCR5 chemokine receptor are resistant to HIV infection.

- After binding gp120 to CD4 and subsequently to one of the chemokine coreceptors, the noncovalently linked gp41 protein undergoes a conformational change that allows the virus to be internalized.
- The genome undergoes reverse transcription, and the proviral DNA is then integrated into the host genome.
- Transcription/translation and viral propagation may subsequently occur only with T-cell activation (e.g., antigenic stimulation). In the absence of T-cell activation, the infection enters a latent phase.
- Early in the course of the disease, HIV colonizes the lymphoid organs including infecting monocytes and macrophages that are refractory to HIV cytopathic effects; these infected monocyte/macrophages can act as HIV reservoirs (perhaps transferring virus to T cells during antigen presentation), as well as vehicles for viral transport, especially to the central nervous system.
- In addition to macrophages, the follicular dendritic cells in the germinal center of lymph nodes are also important reservoirs of HIV. Viral particles coated with anti-HIV antibodies attach to the Fc receptor on follicular dendritic cells. These HIV virions continually infect T cells as they come in close contact with the follicular dendritic cells during passage through lymph nodes.
- T-cell depletion ensues. The majority of the cell loss is due to intracellular viral replication with subsequent cell lysis. Approximately 1 billion to 2 billion CD4+ T cells are lysed daily; however, early in the disease this loss is largely replenished by regeneration, and T-cell loss appears deceptively small.

- T-cell loss also occurs by:

  Progressive destruction of the architecture and cellular composition of the lymphoid organs, including cells important for maintaining a cytokine environment conducive to CD4+ maturation

  Chronic activation of uninfected cells (responding to HIV or opportunistic infections), leading eventually to *activation-induced cell death*

  Fusion of infected and noninfected cells via gp120 leading to cell death

  Binding of soluble gp120 to noninfected CD4+ T cells leading to activation of apoptotic pathways or to CTL-mediated killing

- The consequences of HIV infection on immune function are listed in Table 6–5. In addition to T-cell depletion, there are also qualitative defects in T-cell function, with a selective loss of T-cell memory early in the course of disease. There is also paradoxic polyclonal B-cell activation; nevertheless, patients with AIDS are unable to mount appreciable antibody responses to new antigens, probably owing to CD4+ T-cell depletion, intrinsic B-cell defects, or both.

Pathogenesis of Central Nervous System Involvement (p. 253)

The central nervous system is a major target in HIV infection. This occurs predominantly, if not exclusively, via infected monocytes that circulate to the brain and are either activated to release toxic cytokines directly or to recruit other neuron-damaging inflammatory cells.

TABLE 6–5 **Major Abnormalities of Immune Function in AIDS**

Lymphopenia
Predominantly due to selective loss of the CD4+ helper-inducer T-cell subset; inversion of CD4: CD8 ratio

Decreased T-Cell Function *In Vivo*
Preferential loss of memory T cells
Susceptibility to opportunistic infections
Susceptibility to neoplasms
Decreased delayed-type hypersensitivity

Altered T-Cell Function *In Vitro*
Decreased proliferative response to mitogens, alloantigens, and soluble antigens
Decreased specific cytotoxicity
Decreased helper function for pokeweed mitogen-induced B-cell immunoglobulin production
Decreased IL2 and TNF-α production

Polyclonal B-Cell Activation
Hypergammaglobulinemia and circulating immune complexes
Inability to mount *de novo* antibody responses to a new antigen or vaccine
Refractoriness to the normal signals for B-cell activation *in vitro*

Altered Monocyte or Macrophage Functions
Decreased chemotaxis and phagocytosis
Decreased HLA class II expression
Diminished capacity to present antigen to T cells
Increased spontaneous secretion of IL1, TNF, IL6

IL, interleukin; TNF, tumor necrocis factor.

Natural History of HIV Infection (p. 253)

On the basis of interactions of HIV with the host immune system, HIV infection can be divided into three phases (Fig. 6–5). In each of the three phases of HIV infection, viral replication continues, and hence HIV infection lacks a phase of true microbiologic latency.

- *Early, acute phase* is characterized by transient viremia, widespread seeding of lymphoid tissue, a temporary fall in

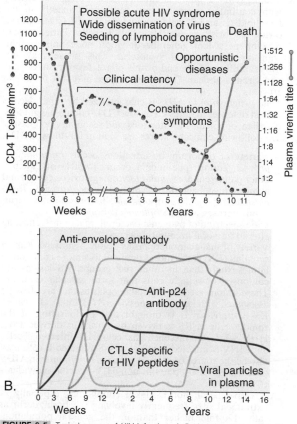

FIGURE 6–5 Typical course of HIV infection. *A,* During the early period after primary infection, there is widespread dissemination of virus and a sharp decrease in the number of CD4+ T cells in peripheral blood. An immune response to HIV ensues, with a decrease in viremia followed by a prolonged period of clinical latency. During this period, viral replication continues. The CD4+ T-cell count gradually decreases during the following years, until it reaches a critical level below which there is a substantial risk of opportunistic diseases. (Redrawn from Fauci AS, Lane HC: Human immunodeficiency virus disease: AIDS and related conditions. In Fauci AS, et al. (eds): Harrison's Principles of Internal Medicine, 14th ed. New York, McGraw-Hill, 1997, p 1791.) *B,* Immune response to HIV infection. A cytolytic T lymphocyte (CTL) response to HIV is detectable 2 to 3 weeks after the initial infection and peaks by 9 to 12 weeks. Marked expansion of virus-specific CD8+ T-cell clones occurs during this time, and up to 10% of a patient's CTLs may be HIV specific at 12 weeks. The humoral immune response to HIV peaks at about 12 weeks.

CD4+ T cells, followed by seroconversion and control of viral replication by generation of CD8+ antiviral T cells. Clinically, a self-limited acute illness with sore throat, nonspecific myalgias, and aseptic meningitis may develop. Clinical recovery and near-normal CD4+ T-cell counts occur within 6 to 12 weeks. The viral load at the end of the acute phase reflects the balance between HIV production and host defenses. This viral set-point is an important predictor of the rate of progression of HIV disease. Those with high viral loads at the end of the acute phase progress to AIDS more rapidly.

- *Middle, chronic phase* is characterized by clinical latency with continued vigorous viral replication mainly in the lymphoid tissue but only gradual decline of CD4+ counts owing to brisk regeneration of T cells. Patients may develop persistent generalized lymph node enlargement, with no constitutional symptoms. This phase may last for years. Toward the end of this phase, fever, rash, fatigue, and viremia appear. The chronic phase may last from 7 to 10 years.
- *Final progression to AIDS* is characterized by rapid decline in host defenses manifested by low CD4+ counts, weight loss, diarrhea, opportunistic infections, and secondary neoplasms. The following clinical features are seen in full-blown AIDS:

A variety of opportunistic infections occur. *Pneumocystis jiroveci (carinii)* pneumonia occurs in 50% of patients; other pathogens are *Candida*, cytomegalovirus, typical and atypical mycobacteria, *Cryptococcus neoformans, Toxoplasma gondii, Cryptosporidium*, herpes simplex virus, papovaviruses, and *Histoplasma capsulatum.*

A wide spectrum of pyogenic bacterial infections (reflecting altered humoral immunity) occurs.

A variety of malignant neoplasms occur. Aggressive *Kaposi sarcoma* (KS) is the most common; it is more common in homosexuals than in other risk groups. KS lesions are composed of spindle cells that form vascular channels. These lesions are monoclonal neoplasms that are strongly associated with human herpesvirus-8 (HHV-8), also called *KS herpesvirus*. It is thought that proliferation of the spindle cells in KS is driven by cytokines derived from HHV-8–infected mesenchymal cells, HIV-infected T cells, and HHV-8–infected B cells; HHV-8–infected B cells may also be the source of *primary effusion lymphomas* in AIDS patients. KS also occurs in non–HIV-infected individuals (Chapter 11).

Aggressive B-cell non-Hodgkin lymphomas, especially at extranodal sites, frequently involving the brain, occur at rates 120-fold higher than in the general population. Epstein-Barr virus is important in the pathogenesis of AIDS-associated lymphomas. Fifty percent of systemic lymphomas and 100% of central nervous system lymphomas carry the Epstein-Barr virus genome. Patients with AIDS also have increased incidence of squamous cell carcinoma of the uterine cervix most likely caused by greater susceptibility to human papillomavirus infection.

Clinical neurologic involvement occurs in 40% to 60% of patients, manifesting as:

Acute aseptic meningitis
Vacuolar myelopathy
Peripheral neuropathy

Most commonly, a progressive encephalopathy, designated AIDS-dementia complex

Although great therapeutic strides have been made in combined antiretroviral therapies, treated patients still carry viral DNA in their lymphoid tissues and can develop active infection if treatment is stopped.

Morphology

With the exception of the central nervous system, the tissue changes in AIDS are neither specific nor diagnostic; the pathologic features are those of the various opportunistic infections and neoplasms. The opportunistic infections and AIDS-associated neuropathy are discussed elsewhere in the organ-specific chapters.

Lymph Nodes. Adenopathy in early HIV infection reflects the initial polyclonal B-cell proliferation and hypergammaglobulinemia, showing nonspecific, predominantly follicular hyperplasia with mantle zone attenuation and intense medullary plasmacytosis. HIV particles can be demonstrated in germinal centers by *in situ* hybridization, localized mainly on the surface of follicular dendritic cells.

With progression to full-blown AIDS, the lymphoid follicles become involuted *(burned out)*, with general lymphocyte depletion and disruption of the organized follicular dendritic cell network. Inflammatory responses to infections may be sparse or atypical, and infectious organisms may not be apparent without special stains. Similar lymphoid depletion occurs in the spleen and thymus.

Patients frequently develop diffuse high-grade malignant B-cell lymphomas (the second most common malignancy, after KS), perhaps because of prolonged B-cell proliferation in the face of deteriorating regulatory controls.

Amyloidosis (p. 258)

Amyloid is a heterogeneous group of pathogenetic fibrillar proteins that accumulate within tissues and organs, either because of excess synthesis or because of resistance to catabolism. *All these proteins share the ability to aggregate into an insoluble, cross-beta-pleated sheet tertiary conformation*; all are deposited extracellularly in a variety of tissues and in a large array of clinical settings. As amyloid accumulates, it produces pressure atrophy of adjacent parenchyma. Depending on tissue distribution and degree of involvement, amyloid may be asymptomatic and found only as an unsuspected anatomic change or may be life threatening.

Physical and Chemical Nature of Amyloid (p. 259). By electron microscopy, amyloid is composed predominantly (95%) of nonbranching fibrils of indeterminate length and 7.5 to 10 nm diameter. These fibrils are associated with a minor (5%) *P component*, consisting of stacks of pentagonal, doughnut-shaped structures with homology to C-reactive protein.

Of the 15 biochemically distinct forms of amyloid thus far identified, three are most common (Table 6–6):

- *Amyloid light-chain protein* (AL): Immunoglobulin light chains (or amino-terminal fragments thereof) derived from plasma cells; amyloid due to lambda light chains occurs much more often than amyloid due to kappa light chains. *Frequently associated with B-cell dyscrasias (e.g., multiple myeloma).*

TABLE 6–6   **Classification of Amyloidosis**

Clinicopathologic Category	Associated Diseases	Major Fibril Protein	Chemically Related Precursor Protein
Systemic (Generalized) Amyloidosis			
Immunocyte dyscrasias with amyloidosis (primary amyloidosis)	Multiple myeloma and other monoclonal B-cell proliferations	AL	Immunoglobulin light chains, chiefly λ light chain
Reactive systemic amyloidosis (secondary amyloidosis)	Chronic inflammatory conditions	AA	SAA
Hemodialysis-associated amyloidosis	Chronic renal failure	Aβ₂m	β₂-microglobulin
Hereditary amyloidosis			
Familial Mediterranean fever	—	AA	SAA
Familial amyloidotic neuropathies (several types)	—	ATTR	Transthyretin
Systemic senile amyloidosis		ATTR	Transthyretin
Localized Amyloidosis			
Senile cerebral	Alzheimer disease	Aβ	APP
Endocrine			
Medullary carcinoma of thyroid	—	A Cal	Calcitonin
Islet of Langerhans	Type II diabetes	AIAPP	Islet amyloid peptide
Isolated atrial amyloidosis	—	AANF	Atrial natriuretic factor
Prion diseases	Various prion diseases of the central nervous system	Misfolded prion protein (PrPˢᶜ)	Normal prion protein PrP

- *Amyloid-associated protein* (AA): An 8500-dalton nonimmunoglobulin protein derived from a 12,000-dalton serum precursor called *SAA* (serum amyloid-associated) protein that is synthesized in liver; SAA is elevated in inflammatory states.
- β_2-*Amyloid protein* ($A\beta_2$): A peptide found in Alzheimer disease; it forms the core of cerebral plaques and deposits within cerebral vessel walls. It derives from a transmembrane glycoprotein precursor (APP) (Chapter 28).

Some less common forms of amyloid are seen in particular clinical settings:

- *Transthyretin (TTR)*: A normal serum protein that binds and transports thyroxine and retinol. A mutant form is deposited as amyloid in a group of hereditary diseases called *familial amyloid polyneuropathy*.

- *β₂-Microglobulin*: The smaller nonpolymorphic peptide component of class I HLA molecules and a normal serum protein; it is deposited in the form of amyloidosis that complicates long-term hemodialysis.

Classification of Amyloidosis (p. 260)

Amyloidosis is subdivided into *systemic* (generalized) and *localized* (tissue-specific) forms and is further classified on the basis of predisposing conditions (see Table 6–6).

Systemic amyloidosis is associated with the following conditions:

- *B-cell dyscrasias (also called primary amyloidosis)*: The most common form in the United States. Composed of AL-type amyloid. AL-type systemic amyloidosis occurs in 5% to 15% of patients with multiple myeloma. Tumorous plasma cells synthesize abnormal quantities of a single immunoglobulin (*M spike* on serum protein electrophoresis) or immunoglobulin light chain (*Bence Jones* protein). By virtue of their smaller size, Bence Jones proteins are frequently excreted in the urine. The vast majority of cases of AL-type systemic amyloidosis are *not* associated with *overt* B-cell neoplasms. Nevertheless, they have elevated monoclonal immunoglobulins, light chains, or both. Typically (but not always), AL-type amyloid involves the heart, gastrointestinal tract, peripheral nerves, skin, and tongue more than other organs.
- *Secondary or reactive amyloidosis*: Marked by AA-type amyloid. Secondary amyloidosis is associated with chronic inflammatory states (infectious and noninfectious) (e.g., rheumatoid arthritis, scleroderma, dermatomyositis, bronchiectasis, chronic osteomyelitis). Typically, kidneys, liver, spleen, lymph nodes, adrenals, and thyroid are involved.
- *Hemodialysis-related amyloidosis*: Affects 60% to 80% of patients on chronic hemodialysis. This form is due to deposition (in joints, synovium, and tendon sheaths) of β₂-microglobulin not filtered by normal dialysis membranes.
- *Hereditary forms*: Include many rare entities, often confined to specific geographic locations. Most common and best characterized form is *familial Mediterranean fever*, a recurrent, febrile illness typically in Sephardic Jews, Armenians, and Arabs, characterized by bouts of serosal inflammation. The systemic amyloid is of AA type, suggesting that chronic inflammation plays a pivotal role. *Familial amyloidotic polyneuropathies* have autosomal dominant transmission and show deposition of mutant transthyretins principally in peripheral and autonomic nerves.

Localized amyloidosis is confined to amyloid in a single organ or tissue. The following conditions are associated:

- *Nodular (tumor-forming) deposits*: Often AL protein with associated plasma cell infiltrates. These deposits occur most frequently in lung, larynx, skin, bladder, tongue, and periorbitally. This may represent localized forms of B-cell dyscrasias.
- *Endocrine amyloid*: Deposition in a variety of tumors associated with catabolism of polypeptide hormones or prohormones (e.g., thyroid medullary carcinoma [procalcitonin]).
- *Amyloidosis of aging* occurs typically in the eighth and ninth decades and is most commonly due to deposition of nonmutant transthyretin. Although amyloid distribution is systemic, the dominant involvement is of the heart, and it

presents with a restrictive cardiomyopathy or arrhythmias. In addition to the sporadic senile systemic amyloidosis, there is another form, affecting predominantly the heart, in which mutant transthyretin is deposited. This condition is more common in blacks.

Morphology (p. 263)

Macroscopically, affected tissues are stained blue-violet with iodine and dilute sulfuric acid. Microscopically, routine stains reveal only amorphous, acellular, hyaline, eosinophilic extracellular material. With special stains (e.g., Congo red), amyloid is salmon-pink, and characteristic yellow-green birefringence may be seen using polarized light.

Kidneys. Kidneys are classically enlarged, pale gray, waxy, and firm. In advanced disease, chronic vascular occlusion (owing to amyloid deposits) may result in a shrunken, contracted organ. Amyloid deposits in several areas:

- *Glomeruli*, initially mesangial and subendothelial: With continued accumulation, there is hyalinization of glomeruli.
- *Peritubular regions:* Deposits begin in the tubular basement membrane and gradually extend into the interstitium.
- *Blood vessels*: Hyaline thickening of arterial and arteriolar walls with narrowing lumen eventually causes ischemia with tubular atrophy and interstitial fibrosis.

Spleen. The spleen may be enlarged (up to 800 gm). Amyloid deposits begin between cells. With time, one of two patterns emerges:

- *Sago spleen*: Deposits are limited to the splenic follicles, giving rise to *tapioca-like* granules on gross inspection.
- *Lardaceous spleen*: Amyloid largely spares the follicles and is deposited in the red pulp. Fusion of deposits forms large geographic areas of amyloid.

Liver. Amyloid induces hepatomegaly with a pale, waxy gray, firm appearance. Microscopically, amyloid first deposits in the space of Disse, gradually encroaching on parenchyma and sinusoids to produce pressure atrophy with massive hepatic replacement.

Heart. Distinctive (although not always present) are minute, typically atrial, pink-gray subendocardial droplets representing focal amyloid accumulations. Vascular and subepicardial deposits may also occur. Microscopically, there are interstitial and perimyocyte deposits, progressively leading to pressure atrophy.

Clinical Features (p. 264)

Diagnosis is made on the basis of biopsy and characteristic Congo red stain. Favored biopsy sites are the kidney (when renal manifestations are present) and the rectum or gingiva (in systemic disease).

- Abdominal fat pad aspirates may also yield diagnostic tissue.
- In amyloidosis associated with B-cell dyscrasias, serum and urine electrophoresis and bone marrow biopsy (for plasmacytosis) are indicated.
- In systemic amyloidosis, the prognosis is poor. Median survival after diagnosis in the setting of B-cell dyscrasias is about 24 months. Reactive amyloidosis may have a slightly better outlook, depending on the ability to control the underlying condition.

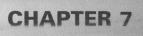

CHAPTER 7

Neoplasia

A tumor is an abnormal mass of tissue, the growth of which is virtually autonomous and exceeds that of normal tissues. In contrast to non-neoplastic proliferations (Chapter 3), the growth of tumors persists after cessation of the stimuli that initiated the change. Tumors are classified into two broad categories: benign and malignant; the type of neoplasm is based on the characteristics of its parenchyma.

NOMENCLATURE (p. 270)

Tumor nomenclature is summarized in Table 7–1. All tumors have two basic components:

- The *transformed* neoplastic cells
- The supporting stroma composed of nontransformed elements, such as connective tissues and blood vessels

Benign Tumors (p. 270)

The names of these tumors typically (but not uniformly) end with the suffix *-oma*. For example, benign mesenchymal tumors include lipoma, fibroma, angioma, osteoma, and leiomyoma. The nomenclature of benign epithelial tumors is somewhat complex and is based on both histogenesis and architecture, for example:

- *Adenomas*: Benign epithelial tumors arising in glands or forming glandular patterns
- *Cystadenomas*: Adenomas producing large cystic masses, seen typically in the ovary
- *Papillomas*: Epithelial tumors forming microscopic or macroscopic finger-like projections
- *Polyp*: A tumor projecting from the mucosa into the lumen of a hollow viscus (e.g., stomach or colon)

Malignant Tumors (p. 271)

Malignant tumors are called *cancers* and are divided into two general categories:

TABLE 7-1 **Nomenclature of Tumors**

Tissue of Origin	Benign	Malignant
Composed of One Parenchymal Cell Type		
Tumors of mesenchymal origin		
Connective tissue and derivatives	Fibroma	Fibrosarcoma
	Lipoma	Liposarcoma
	Chondroma	Chondrosarcoma
	Osteoma	Osteogenic sarcoma
Endothelial and related tissues		
Blood vessels	Hemangioma	Angiosarcoma
Lymph vessels	Lymphangioma	Lymphangiosarcoma
Synovium		Synovial sarcoma
Mesothelium		Mesothelioma
Brain coverings	Meningioma	Invasive meningioma
Blood cells and related cells		
Hematopoietic cells		Leukemias
Lymphoid tissue		Lymphomas
Muscle		
Smooth	Leiomyoma	Leiomyosarcoma
Striated	Rhabdomyoma	Rhabdomyosarcoma
Tumors of epithelial origin		
Stratified squamous	Squamous cell papilloma	Squamous cell or epidermoid carcinoma
Basal cells of skin or adnexa		Basal cell carcinoma
Epithelial lining of glands or ducts	Adenoma	Adenocarcinoma
	Papilloma	Papillary carcinomas
	Cystadenoma	Cystadenocarcinoma
Respiratory passages	Bronchial adenoma	Bronchogenic carcinoma
Renal epithelium	Renal tubular adenoma	Renal cell carcinoma
Liver cells	Liver cell adenoma	Hepatocellular carcinoma
Urinary tract epithelium (transitional)	Transitional cell papilloma	Transitional cell carcinoma
Placental epithelium	Hydatidiform mole	Choriocarcinoma
Testicular epithelium (germ cells)		Seminoma
		Embryonal carcinoma
Tumors of melanocytes	Nevus	Malignant melanoma
More Than One Neoplastic Cell Type—Mixed Tumors, Usually Derived from One Germ Cell Layer		
Salivary glands	Pleomorphic adenoma (mixed tumor of salivary origin)	Malignant mixed tumor of salivary gland origin
Renal anlage		Wilms tumor
More Than One Neoplastic Cell Type Derived from More Than One Germ Cell Layer—Teratogenous		
Totipotential cells in gonads or in embryonic rests	Mature teratoma, dermoid cyst	Immature teratoma, teratocarcinoma

- *Carcinomas,* arising from epithelial cells
- *Sarcomas,* arising from mesenchymal tissues

The nomenclature of specific types of carcinomas or sarcomas is based on their appearance and presumed histogenetic origin (Table 7–1). Thus, malignant epithelial tumors with glandular growth patterns are referred to as *adenocarcinomas,* whereas sarcomas arising from or resembling smooth muscle cells are called *leiomyosarcomas.*

Some tumors appear to have more than one parenchymal cell type. Two important members of this category:

- *Mixed tumors* are derived from one germ cell layer that differentiates into more than one parenchymal cell type. For example, mixed salivary gland tumor contains epithelial cells as well as myxoid stroma and cartilage-like tissue. All elements arise from altered differentiation of ductal epithelial cells.
- *Teratomas* are made up of a variety of parenchymal cell types representative of more than one germ cell layer, usually all three. They arise from totipotential cells that retain the ability to form endodermal, ectodermal, and mesenchymal tissues. Such tumors are found principally in the testis and ovary.

There are two *non-neoplastic* lesions that grossly resemble tumors; moreover, their names are deceptively similar to tumors and sound ominous:

- *Choristomas:* Ectopic rests of nontransformed tissues (e.g., pancreatic cells under the small bowel mucosa).
- *Hamartomas:* Masses of disorganized tissue indigenous to a particular site (i.e., a hamartomatous nodule in the lung may contain islands of cartilage, bronchi, and blood vessels).

BIOLOGY OF TUMOR GROWTH: BENIGN AND MALIGNANT NEOPLASMS (p. 272)

The distinction between benign and malignant tumors is based on appearance (morphology) and ultimately on behavior (clinical course), using four criteria:

- Malignant change (transformation) of the target cell (i.e., differentiation versus anaplasia)
- Rate of growth
- Local invasion
- Metastases

Differentiation and Anaplasia (p. 272)

Differentiation is the extent to which tumor cells resemble comparable normal cells. Cells within most benign tumors closely mimic corresponding normal cells. Thus, thyroid adenomas are composed of normal-looking thyroid acini, and the cells in lipomas look like those in normal adipose tissue. Although malignant neoplasms are in general less well differentiated than their benign counterparts, they nevertheless can range from well differentiated to very poorly differentiated.

Lack of differentiation is called *anaplasia,* and is a hallmark of malignant cells. The following cytologic features are used to characterize anaplasia:

- *Nuclear and cellular pleomorphism:* Variation in the shape and size of cells and nuclei.
- *Hyperchromasia:* Darkly stained nuclei that frequently contain prominent nucleoli.
- *Nuclear-cytoplasmic ratio:* Approaches 1:1 instead of 1:4 or 1:6, reflecting nuclear enlargement.
- *Abundant mitoses:* Reflect proliferative activity. Mitotic figures may be abnormal (e.g., tripolar).
- *Loss of polarity:* Anaplastic cells show disturbed orientation, and tend to form anarchic, disorganized masses.
- *Tumor giant cells:* Containing a single large polyploid nucleus or multiple nuclei.

Poorly differentiated, anaplastic tumors also demonstrate a total disarray of tissue architecture. Thus, in an anaplastic uterine cervical malignancy, the normal orientation of squamous epithelial cells relative to each other is lost. Well-differentiated tumors, whether benign or malignant, tend to retain the functional characteristics of their normal counterparts. Thus, there may be hormone production by endocrine tumors or keratin production by squamous epithelial tumors.

Dysplasia refers to disorderly but non-neoplastic growth; it is usually encountered in epithelia (e.g., the uterine cervix). Pleomorphism, hyperchromasia, and loss of normal orientation may occur, without sufficient changes to merit the designation of malignancy. Mild degrees of dysplasia do not always result in cancer and are often reversible when the inciting cause (e.g., chronic irritation) is removed. Nevertheless, when dysplastic changes are marked and *involve the entire thickness of the epithelium*, the lesion is considered a preinvasive neoplasm and is referred to as *carcinoma in situ*. This lesion is a forerunner, in many cases, of invasive carcinoma.

Rates of Growth (p. 276)

Most malignant tumors grow more rapidly than benign tumors. Nevertheless, some cancers grow slowly for years, and only then enter a phase of rapid growth; others expand rapidly from the outset. Growth of cancers arising from hormone-sensitive tissues (e.g., the breast) may be affected by hormonal variations associated with pregnancy and menopause. Ultimately, the progression of tumors and their growth rates are determined by an excess of cell production over cell loss.

- Fast-growing tumors can have a high cell *turnover,* that is, rates of proliferation and apoptosis are both high.
- The proportion of cells in a tumor population that are actively proliferating is called the *growth fraction.* The growth fraction of tumor cells has a profound impact on susceptibility to therapeutic intervention, because most anti-cancer treatments act only on cells that are in cycle.
- Malignant tumors grow more rapidly than do benign lesions. In general (but not always), the growth rate of tumors correlates with the level of differentiation.

Cancer Stem Cells and Cancer Cell Lineages (p. 278)

A clinically detectable tumor (typically containing 10^9 cells) is a heterogeneous population of cells originating from the clonal growth of the progeny of a single cell. Tumor stem cells have the capacity to initiate and ultimately sustain tumor growth; however, these cells constitute a small fraction of the total population (0.1%–2%) and have an extremely low rate of replication. This concept is important because therapies that efficiently kill the rapidly replicating progeny may very well leave in place the stem cells that are wholly capable of regenerating the entire tumor.

Local Invasion (p. 278)

In benign *versus* malignant lesions, local invasion is characterized as follows:

- *Benign tumors:* Most benign tumors grow as cohesive expansile masses that develop a rim of condensed connective tissue, or *capsule*, at the periphery. These tumors do not penetrate the capsule or the surrounding normal tissues, and the plane of cleavage between the capsule and the surrounding tissues facilitates surgical enucleation.
- *Malignant neoplasms* are invasive and infiltrative, and destroy normal tissues surrounding them. They lack a well-defined capsule and plane of cleavage, making enucleation difficult or impossible. Consequently, surgical treatment of such tumors requires removal of a considerable margin of healthy and apparently uninvolved tissue.

Metastasis (p. 279)

The process of metastasis involves invasion of lymphatics, blood vessels, or body cavities by tumor, followed by transport and growth of secondary tumor cell masses that are discontinuous with the primary tumor. *This is the single most important feature distinguishing benign from malignant tumors.* With the notable exception of tumors in the brain and basal cell carcinomas of the skin, almost all malignant tumors have the capacity to metastasize.

Pathways of Spread (p. 279)

Metastasis occurs by three routes:

- *Spread into body cavities:* This occurs by seeding surfaces of the peritoneal, pleural, pericardial, or subarachnoid spaces. Carcinoma of the ovary, for example, spreads transperitoneally to the surface of the liver or other abdominal viscera.
- *Invasion of lymphatics:* This is followed by transport of tumor cells to regional nodes and, ultimately, other parts of the body; it is common in the initial spread of carcinomas. Although tumors do not contain functional lymphatics, lymphatic vessels at tumor margins are apparently sufficient to facilitate lymphatic spread. Lymph nodes in the lymphatic drainage of tumors are frequently enlarged; in some cases, this results from the growth of metastatic tumor cells, but in other cases can result from nodal reactive hyperplasia to tumor antigens.
- *Hematogenous spread:* This is typical of all sarcomas but also is the favored route for certain carcinomas (e.g., those originating in the kidney). Because of their thinner walls, veins are more frequently invaded than arteries, and metastasis

follows the pattern of venous flow; understandably, lung and liver are the most common sites of hematogenous metastases. Other major sites of hematogenous spread include brain and bones.

EPIDEMIOLOGY (p. 281)

A variety of factors predispose an individual or a population to the development of cancer. Cancers of the prostate, lung, and colon are the most common cancers in men; breast, lung, and colon cancers are the most common in women. In the United States, cancer is responsible for approximately 23% of all deaths annually, although the age-adjusted cancer death rate declined by roughly 1% between 1990 and 2000.

Geographic and Environmental Factors (p. 283)

Environmental factors significantly influence the occurrence of specific forms of cancer in different parts of the world. In Japan, for example, the death rate from gastric cancer is about seven times that in the United States. Conversely, carcinoma of the colon is much less common as a cause of death in Japan. In Japanese immigrants to the United States, the death rates for stomach and colon cancer are intermediate between those of natives of Japan and the United States, pointing to environmental and cultural influences. Other examples of environmental factors in carcinogenesis:

- Increased risk of certain cancers with exposure to asbestos, vinyl chloride, and 2-naphthylamine
- Association of carcinomas of the oropharynx, larynx, and lung with cigarette smoking

Age (p. 284)

Cancer is more common in those older than 55 years of age, and is the main cause of death in women aged 40 to 79 and in men aged 60 to 79. Nevertheless, certain cancers are particularly common in children younger than 15 years of age:

- Tumors of the hematopoietic system (leukemias and lymphomas)
- Neuroblastomas
- Wilms tumors
- Retinoblastomas
- Sarcomas of bone and skeletal muscle

Genetic Predisposition to Cancer (p. 284)

Heredity plays a role in the development of cancer even in the presence of clearly defined environmental factors. Nevertheless, less than 10% of cancer patients have inherited mutations that predispose to malignancy; the frequency is even lower (0.1%) for certain cancers. Despite the low frequency, understanding the hereditary aspects of cancer has had a major impact on understanding neoplastic pathogenesis; moreover, heritable genes frequently also play a role in the more common

TABLE 7–2 **Inherited Predisposition to Cancer**

Gene	Inherited Predisposition
Inherited Cancer Syndromes (Autosomal Dominant)	
RB	Retinoblastoma
p53	Li-Fraumeni syndrome (various tumors)
p16INK4A	Melanoma
APC	Familial adenomatous polyposis/colon cancer
NF1, NF2	Neurofibromatosis 1 and 2
BRCA1, BRCA2	Breast and ovarian tumors
MEN1, RET	Multiple endocrine neoplasia 1 and 2
MSH2, MLH1, MSH6	Hereditary nonpolyposis colon cancer
PATCH	Nevoid basal cell carcinoma syndrome
Familial Cancers	
Familial clustering of cases, but role of inherited predisposition not clear for each individual	
Breast cancer	
Ovarian cancer	
Pancreatic cancer	
Inherited Autosomal Recessive Syndromes of Defective DNA Repair	
Xeroderma pigmentosum	
Ataxia-telangiectasia	
Bloom syndrome	
Fanconi anemia	

sporadic tumors. Genetic predisposition to cancer can be divided into three categories (Table 7–2):

1. Autosomal dominant inherited cancer syndromes (p. 284) are characterized by inheritance of single mutant genes that greatly increase the risk of developing a certain type of tumor. The inherited mutation is usually a point mutation occurring in a single allele of a tumor suppressor gene; the defect in the second allele occurs in somatic cells, typically as a consequence of chromosome deletion or recombination. Retinoblastoma and familial adenomatous polyposis are prominent examples. Inherited cancer syndromes have some characteristic features:

   There is tumor involvement in only specific sites or tissues (e.g., multiple endocrine neoplasia, type II due to mutations of the *RET* oncogene only affects thyroid, parathyroid, and adrenal glands); there is no increased predilection to cancers in general.

   Tumors usually have an associated *marker phenotype* (e.g., multiple benign tumors in familial polyposis of colon).

   As in other autosomal dominant conditions, incomplete penetrance and variable expression are seen.

2. *Defective DNA repair syndromes* (p. 286) are characterized by chromosome or DNA instability that greatly increases the predisposition to environmental carcinogens (e.g., hereditary nonpolyposis colon cancer [HNPCC] due to inactivation of a DNA mismatch repair gene).

3. *Familial cancers* (p. 287) are characterized by familial clustering of specific forms of cancer, but the transmission pattern is not clear in an individual case; familial forms of common cancers (e.g., breast, colon, brain, and ovary) are

included in this category. These familial cancers have several features in common:

Early age at onset is usual, occasionally with multiple or bilateral tumors.

There is no marker phenotype (e.g., familial colon cancers do not arise in preexisting polyps).

The predisposition to familial tumors is usually autosomal dominant, but multifactorial inheritance cannot be excluded, and susceptibility may be due to multiple low-penetrance alleles.

Nonhereditary Predisposing Conditions
(p. 287).

Certain clinical conditions are associated with an increased risk of developing cancers (e.g., liver cirrhosis and hepatocellular carcinoma, or ulcerative colitis and colon cancer).

Chronic Inflammation and Cancer (p. 287)

Although the precise mechanisms linking chronic inflammation and carcinogenesis are not known, chronic inflammatory reactions can cause ongoing local production of cytokines that can stimulate the growth of transformed cells or can directly promote genomic instability by the production of reactive oxygen species. Inflammation can also increase the local pool of stem cells that can be subject to the effects of mutagens.

Precancerous Conditions (p. 287)

Although in the great majority of such lesions no malignant transformation occurs, certain non-neoplastic disorders (e.g., leukoplakia of the oral mucosa) have a well-defined association with cancer. Certain benign tumors are also associated with the subsequent development of cancer. Although the development of cancers in benign tumors is uncommon, there are a few exceptions (e.g., villous adenomas of the colon often develop into cancer). Most malignant tumors, however, arise *de novo*.

MOLECULAR BASIS OF CANCER (p. 288)

A simplified scheme of the molecular pathogenesis of cancer is provided in Figure 7–1:

- Cancer is a genetic disease. *Nonlethal genetic damage lies at the heart of carcinogenesis*. The genetic injury may be acquired in somatic cells by environmental agents or inherited in the germ line.
- Tumors develop as clonal progeny of a single genetically damaged progenitor cell; such monoclonality of tumors can be verified by study of X-linked markers.
- Four classes of normal regulatory genes are the targets of genetic damage:

Growth-promoting proto-oncogenes
Growth-inhibiting tumor-suppressor genes
Genes that regulate apoptosis
Genes that regulate DNA repair

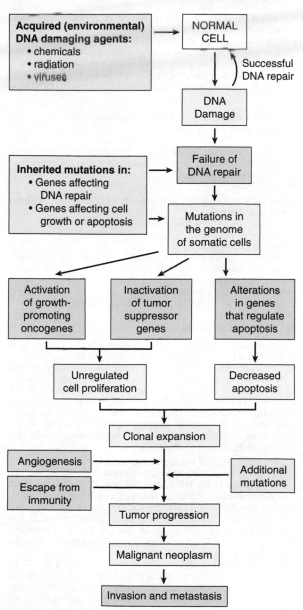

FIGURE 7–1 Flow chart depicting a simplified scheme of the molecular basis of cancer.

- Defects in DNA repair predispose to genomic mutations (*mutator phenotype*) and thus to neoplastic transformation.
- Carcinogenesis is a multistep process. The attributes of malignancy (e.g., invasiveness, excessive growth, escape from the immune system) are acquired in a stepwise fashion, a process called *tumor progression*. At the genetic level, progression results from accumulation of successive mutations.

Essential Alterations for Malignant Transformation (p. 289)

Certain fundamental changes in cell physiology contribute to the development of a malignant phenotype; the genes that contribute to malignant transformation act on one or more of these pathways:

- Self-sufficiency in growth signals (proliferation without external stimuli)
- Insensitivity to growth-inhibitory signals
- Evasion of apoptosis
- Defects in DNA repair
- Limitless replicative potential (related to telomere maintenance)
- Sustained angiogenesis
- Ability to invade and metastasize
- Ability to escape immune recognition and regulation

The Normal Cell Cycle (p. 289)

The orderly progression of cells through the cell cycle is orchestrated by cyclins and cyclin-dependent kinases (CDKs), and by their inhibitors. CDKs are expressed constitutively and drive the cell cycle by phosphorylating certain target proteins; CDK activity is regulated by the binding of cyclins that are selectively synthesized and degraded throughout the cell cycle. Following cyclin-CDK activation, the relevant cyclin is degraded and the activity declines rapidly. The details of the process are elaborated in Chapter 3, but important highlights are summarized here (Table 7–3):

- The cyclin D-CDK4 complex has a critical role in cell cycle regulation by phosphorylating the retinoblastoma susceptibility protein (RB). RB is a central "on-off" switch for DNA replication and modulates the G_1/S restriction point; in its hypophosphorylated "off" state, it binds to elongation factor 2 (E2F) and prevents DNA transcription. When RB is hyperphosphorylated by cyclin D-CDK4, E2F is released, thus permitting DNA transcription and progression into the cell cycle S phase.
- The next major decision point in the cell cycle is the G_2/M transition. Cyclin A-CDK2 and cyclin B-CDK1 complexes decrease microtubule stability, induce centrosome separation, and drive chromosome condensation, steps critical for entering mitosis.
- CDK inhibitors are important regulators of cyclin-CDK activity. The two main classes are *Cip/Kip family* (includes p21, p27, and p57) and the *INK4/ARF family* (includes p16INK4a and p14ARF). Transcriptional activation of p21 is controlled by p53; the role of p53 in the cell cycle is surveillance, triggering checkpoint controls that slow or stop cell cycle progression of damaged cells.

TABLE 7–3 Main Cell-Cycle Components and Their Inhibitors

Cell-Cycle Component	Main Function
Cyclin-Dependent Kinases	
• CDK4	Forms a complex with cyclin D. The complex phosphorylates RB, allowing the cell to progress through the G_1 restriction point.
• CDK2	Forms a complex with cyclin E in late G_1, which is involved in the G_1/S transition. Forms a complex with cyclin A at the S phase that facilitates the G_2/M transition.
• CDK1	Forms a complex with cyclin B, which acts at the G_2/M transition.
Inhibitors	
• Cip/Kip family: p21, p27	Block the cell cycle by binding to cyclin–CDK complexes. p21 is induced by the tumor suppressor p53. p27 responds to growth suppressors such as transforming growth factor-β.
• 1NK4/ARF family: p16INK4A, p14ARF	p16INK4a binds to cyclin D–CDK4 and promotes the inhibitory effects of RB. p14ARF increases p53 levels by inhibiting MDM2 activity.
Checkpoint Components	
• p53	Tumor suppressor altered in the majority of cancers; causes cell-cycle arrest and apoptosis. Acts mainly through p21 to cause cell-cycle arrest. Causes apoptosis by inducing the transcription of pro-apoptotic genes such as *BAX*. Levels of p53 are negatively regulated by MDM2 through a feedback loop. p53 is required for the G_1/S checkpoint and is a main component of the G_2/M checkpoint.
• Ataxia-telangiectasia mutated (*ATM*)	Activated by mechanisms that sense double-stranded DNA breaks. Transmits signals to arrest the cell cycle after DNA damage. Acts through p53 in the G_1/S checkpoint. At the G_2/M checkpoint, it acts both through p53-dependent mechanisms and through the inactivation of CDC25 phosphatase, which disrupts the cyclin B–CDK1 complex. Component of a network of genes that include *BRCA1* and *BRCA2*, which link DNA damage with cell-cycle arrest and apoptosis.

- In the G_1/S checkpoint, cell cycle arrest is mostly mediated through p53, via production of p21. The G_2/M checkpoint involves both p53-dependent and p53-independent pathways.

Self-Sufficiency in Growth Signals (p. 292)

Tumor growth autonomy occurs when the normal steps of cell proliferation occur in the absence of growth-promoting signals. Normal cell proliferation involves the following steps that can potentially be subverted by oncogenes:

- Growth factor binding to cell surface receptor
- Transient and limited activation of the growth factor receptor with activation of signal-transduction proteins on the cytoplasmic side of the plasma membrane
- Transmission—via second messengers or signal transduction molecules—of signal to the nucleus

- Induction and activation of nuclear regulatory factors that initiate DNA transcription
- Entry and progression of the cell through the cell cycle

Protooncogenes, Oncogenes, and Oncoproteins
(p. 293)

- *Oncogenes* are genes that promote autonomous cell growth in cancer cells.
- *Protooncogenes* are normal cellular genes that affect growth and differentiation.
- *Oncoproteins* are the protein products of oncogenes; they resemble the normal products of protooncogenes except that they are devoid of normal regulatory elements.
- Protooncogenes can be converted into oncogenes by:

  Transduction into retroviruses (viral oncogene or v-*onc*).
  Changes in situ that affect protooncogene expression, function, or both, thereby converting them into c-*onc* (cellular oncogenes). Constitutive expression of normal protooncogenes results in oncoproteins that endow cells with growth self-sufficiency.

- Protooncogenes may be converted to oncogenes by one of three mechanisms:

  Point mutations
  Chromosomal rearrangements
  Gene amplification

Most human tumors are not caused by v-*oncs*, but rather by c-*oncs*. The presence of c-*onc* is detected by transfection of tumor-derived DNA into mouse fibroblast cell lines. If the tumor DNA contains transforming sequences (c-*onc*), the transfected fibroblasts acquire the growth characteristics of neoplastic cells: loss of contact inhibition, growth in soft agar, and tumor formation in immunosuppressed mice. The products of protooncogenes are organized in the following list and in Table 7–4 on the basis of their role in signal transduction.

- *Growth factors* (p. 293): Some protooncogenes code for growth factors, such as platelet-derived growth factor (PDGF) (by the *SIS* protooncogene). Many tumors that produce growth factors are also responsive to the growth-promoting effects of the secreted growth factors and hence subject to autocrine stimulation.
- *Growth factor receptors* (p. 294): Several oncogenes encode growth factor receptors. Both structural alterations (mutations) and overexpression of the receptor genes have been found in association with malignant transformation. Mutations in several tyrosine-kinase types of growth factor receptors lead to their constitutive activation without binding to their ligands. As an example, mutations and rearrangements of the *RET* gene occur in MEN2A, MEN2B, and papillary carcinoma of the thyroid.

  Overexpression commonly involves members of the epidermal growth factor receptor family (e.g., c-*erb* B1 is overexpressed in the majority of squamous cell carcinomas of lung; c-*erb* B2 [also called c-*neu*] is amplified in adenocarcinomas of the breast, ovary, lung, stomach, and so on). In breast cancers that have amplified c-*erb* B2, the prognosis is poor, presumably because their cells are sensitive to smaller quantities of growth factors.

TABLE 7-4 Selected Oncogenes, Their Mode of Activation, and Associated Human Tumors

Category	Protooncogene	Mode of Activation	Associated Human Tumor
Growth Factors			
PDGF-β chain	SIS	Overexpression	Astrocytoma
			Osteosarcoma
Fibroblast growth factors	HST-1	Overexpression	Stomach cancer
	INT-2	Amplification	Bladder cancer
			Breast cancer
			Melanoma
TGFα	TGFα	Overexpression	Astrocytomas
			Hepatocellular carcinomas
HGF	HGF	Overexpression	Thyroid cancer
Growth Factor Receptors			
EGF-receptor family	ERB-B1 (ECFR)	Overexpression	Squamous cell carcinomas of lung, gliomas
	ERB-B2	Amplification	Breast and ovarian cancers
CSF-1 receptor	FMS	Point mutation	Leukemia
Receptor for neurotrophic factors	RET	Point mutation	Multiple endocrine neoplasia 2A and B, familial medullary thyroid carcinomas
PDGF receptor	PDGF-R	Overexpression	Gliomas
Receptor for stem cell (steel) factor	KIT	Point mutation	Gastrointestinal stromal tumors and other soft tissue tumors

Continued

TABLE 7-4 Selected Oncogenes, Their Mode of Activation, and Associated Human Tumors—cont'd

Category	Protooncogene	Mode of Activation	Associated Human Tumor
Proteins Involved in Signal Transduction			
GTP-binding	K-RAS	Point mutation	Colon, lung, and pancreatic tumors
	H-RAS	Point mutation	Bladder and kidney tumors
	N-RAS	Point mutation	Melanomas, hematologic malignancies
Nonreceptor tyrosine kinase	ABL	Translocation	Chronic myeloid leukemia
			Acute lymphoblastic leukemia
RAS signal transduction	BRAF	Point mutation	Melanomas
WNT signal transduction	β-catenin	Point mutation	Hepatoblastomas, hepatocellular carcinoma
		Overexpression	
Nuclear Regulatory Proteins			
Transcriptional activators	C-MYC	Translocation	Burkitt lymphoma
	N-MYC	Amplification	Neuroblastoma, small cell carcinoma of lung
	L-MYC	Amplification	Small cell carcinoma of lung
Cell-Cycle Regulators			
Cyclins	CYCLIN D	Translocation	Mantle cell lymphoma
		Amplification	Breast and esophageal cancers
	CYCLIN E	Overexpression	Breast cancer
Cyclin-dependent kinase	CDK4	Amplification or point mutation	Glioblastoma, melanoma, sarcoma

- *Signal-transducing proteins* (p. 296): These proteins are biochemically heterogeneous; the best-studied is the RAS family of guanine triphosphate (GTP)-binding proteins (G proteins).

The *RAS* Oncogene (p. 296)

Approximately 15% to 20% of all human tumors carry mutant RAS proteins; the vast majority of the RAS proteins differ from their normal protooncogene counterparts by point mutations. Normal RAS proteins flip back and forth between an activated (GTP-bound) signal-transmitting form and an inactive (guanosine diphosphate [GDP]-bound) quiescent form. The conversion of active RAS to inactive RAS is mediated by its intrinsic GTPase activity, and is augmented by a family of GTPase-activating proteins (GAPs). Mutant RAS proteins bind GAPs, but still lack GTPase activity, and hence remain trapped in the signal-transmitting GTP-bound form; in this state, the active RAS turns on the MAP kinase pathway and promotes mitogenesis.

- *Alterations in nonreceptor tyrosine kinases* (p. 297): An example in this category is the c-*ABL* gene, which in its normal form exerts a regulated tyrosine-kinase activity. In chronic myeloid leukemia, translocation of c-*ABL* with fusion to the *BCR* gene produce a hybrid protein with potent, unregulated tyrosine-kinase activity.
- *Transcription factors* (p. 297): The products of *MYC, JUN, FOS,* and *MYB* oncogenes are nuclear proteins. They are expressed in a highly regulated fashion during proliferation of normal cells, and regulate transcription of growth-related genes. Their oncogenic versions are typically associated with overexpression. Dysregulation of MYC expression (e.g., due to gene duplication, rearrangements with gene translocation, or changes in posttranslational regulation) occurs in Burkitt lymphoma, neuroblastomas, and small cell cancer of the lung.
- *Cyclins and CDKs* (p. 298): Overexpression of cyclin D and CDK4 is common in many types of cancer, with loss of the checkpoint in the G_1/S transition.

Insensitivity to Growth Inhibitory Signals: Tumor-Suppressor Genes (p. 298)

Cancer may arise not only by activation of growth-promoting oncogenes, but also by inactivation of genes that normally suppress cell proliferation (tumor-suppressor genes). The *RB* gene located on chromosome 13q14 is the prototypic tumor-suppressor gene (others include von Hippel–Lindau [*VHL*] and Wilms tumor [*WT-1*] genes) (see Table 7–5 for selected tumor-suppressor genes involved in human neoplasms). It is relevant to the pathogenesis of the childhood tumor retinoblastoma; 40% of retinoblastomas are familial, and the rest are sporadic. To account for the familial and sporadic occurrence, a *two-hit* hypothesis has been proposed:

- Both normal alleles of the *Rb* locus must be inactivated (two hits) for the development of retinoblastoma.
- In familial cases, children inherit one defective copy of the *RB* gene in the germ line; the other copy is normal. Retinoblastoma develops when the normal *RB* gene is lost in retinoblasts as a result of somatic mutation.

TABLE 7-5 Selected Tumor Suppressor Genes Involved in Human Neoplasms

Subcellular Location	Gene	Function	Tumors Associated with Somatic Mutations	Tumors Associated with Inherited Mutations
Cell surface	TGF-β receptor	Growth inhibition	Carcinomas of colon	Unknown
	E-cadherin	Cell adhesion	Carcinoma of stomach	Familial gastric cancer
Inner aspect of plasma membrane	NF-1	Inhibition of RAS signal transduction and of p21 cell-cycle inhibitor	Neuroblastomas	Neurofibromatosis type 1 and sarcomas
Cytoskeleton	NF-2	Cytoskeletal stability	Schwannomas and meningiomas	Neurofibromatosis type 2, acoustic schwannomas and meningiomas
Cytosol	APC/β-catenin	Inhibition of signal transduction	Carcinomas of stomach, colon, pancreas; melanoma	Familial adenomatous polyposis coli/colon cancer
	PTEN	PI-3 kinase signal transduction	Endometrial and prostate cancers	Unknown
	SMAD 2 and SMAD 4	TGF-β signal transduction	Colon, pancreas tumors	Unknown
Nucleus	RB	Regulation of cell cycle	Retinoblastoma; osteosarcoma carcinomas of breast, colon, lung	Retinoblastomas, osteosarcoma
	p53	Cell-cycle arrest and apoptosis in response to DNA damage	Most human cancers	Li-Fraumeni syndrome; multiple carcinomas and sarcomas
	WT-1	Nuclear transcription	Wilms tumor	Wilms tumor
	p16 (INK4a)	Regulation of cell cycle by inhibition of cyclin-dependent kinases	Pancreatic, breast, and esophageal cancers	Malignant melanoma
	BRCA-1 and BRCA-2	DNA repair	Unknown	Carcinomas of female breast and ovary; carcinomas of male breast
	KLF6	Transcription factor	Prostate	Unknown

- In sporadic cases, both normal *RB* alleles are lost by somatic mutation in one of the retinoblasts.
- Cancer develops when the cells become homozygous for the mutant tumor-suppressor genes. Because heterozygous cells are normal, these genes are also called *recessive cancer genes*.
- The *RB* locus may be involved in the pathogenesis of several cancers because patients with familial retinoblastoma are at greatly increased risk of developing osteosarcomas and soft tissue sarcomas.

Tumor-Suppressor Genes

The functions of tumor-suppressor genes (and the human tumors related to them) are summarized in Table 7–5. The following paragraphs offer a sampling of different genes and their gene products and tumorigenic mechanisms:

RB **Gene** (p. 299). The *RB* gene product regulates the advancement of cells from the G_1 to S phase of the cell cycle (see earlier discussion). With *RB* mutations, E2F transcription factor regulation is lost, and cells continue to cycle in the absence of a growth stimulus. Several oncogenic DNA viruses (e.g., human papillomavirus [HPV]) synthesize proteins that bind to pRb and displace the E2F transcription factors, thereby contributing to persistent cell cycling. Transforming growth factor-β (TGF-β) is a growth-inhibiting cytokine that up-regulates CDK inhibitors (e.g., p27), thus preventing RB hyperphosphorylation.

p53 **Gene** (p. 302). The function of the normal *p53* gene (located on 17p13.1) is to prevent the propagation of genetically damaged cells. When DNA is damaged by ultraviolet light, chemicals, or irradiation, the normal *p53* transcription is up-regulated, subsequently resulting in transcription of several genes that cause cell cycle arrest and DNA repair. The cell cycle arrest in G_1 is mediated by p53-dependent transcription of the CDK inhibitor *p21*. If during the pause in cell cycle the DNA can be repaired, the cell is allowed to continue to S phase; however, if DNA damage cannot be repaired, p53 induces apoptosis by increasing transcription of the pro-apoptic gene *BAX*. The *p53* tumor-suppressor gene is mutated in greater than 50% of all human cancers. Those who inherit a mutant copy of the *p53* gene (e.g., *Li-Fraumeni syndrome*) are at a high risk of developing a malignant tumor by inactivation of the second normal allele in somatic cells. Patients with the Li-Fraumeni syndrome develop many different types of tumors, including leukemias, sarcomas, breast cancer, and brain tumors. With homozygous loss of *p53*, DNA damage goes unrepaired, and cells carrying mutant genes continue to divide and eventually give rise to cancer. Similar to the *RB* gene, *p53* can also be functionally inactivated by products of DNA oncogenic viruses.

APC **Gene/β-Catenin Pathway** (p. 304). Those born with one mutant allele of this gene develop thousands of adenomatous polyps in the colon, of which one or more develop into colonic cancers (Chapter 17). *APC* mutations with homozygous loss are also found in 70% to 80% of sporadic colon cancers. Normal APC protein binds to and regulates the degradation of β-catenin in the cytoplasm; in the absence of the APC protein, β-catenin levels increase, and it translocates to the nucleus where it up-regulates cellular proliferation by increasing the transcription of c-*MYC, cyclin D1,* and other genes. Thus, APC is a negative regulator of β-catenin.

TGF-β Pathway (p. 304). This pathway up-regulates growth inhibitory genes, including CDK inhibitors, by binding to TGF-β receptors. The gene encoding the type II TGF-β receptor is inactivated in more than 70% of colon cancers that develop in HNPCC patients, in sporadic colon cancer with microsatellite instability, and in gastric cancers in HNPCC patients. The mutated TGF-β receptors prevent the growth-restraining effects of TGF-β. In addition, downstream mediators of the TGF-β signaling cascade (e.g., SMAD 2 and SMAD 4) are also mutated or inactivated in pancreatic and colorectal tumors.

NF-1 Gene (p. 305). This tumor-suppressor gene regulates signal transduction by the RAS pathway. Homozygous loss of *NF-1* impairs the conversion of active (GTP-bound) RAS to inactive (GDP-bound) RAS; cells are continuously stimulated to divide. As with *APC*, germ line inheritance of one mutant allele of *NF-1* predisposes to the development of numerous benign neurofibromas when the second NF-1 gene is lost or mutated (Chapter 5); some of these tumors progress to malignancy.

WT-1 Gene (p. 306). Mutational inactivation of *WT-1* (located on chromosome 11p13), either in the germ line or in the somatic cells, is associated with the development of Wilms tumors. The WT-1 protein is a transcriptional activator of genes involved in renal and gonadal differentiation; although not precisely known, the tumorigenic function of WT-1 deficiency is connected to its role in the differentiation of genitourinary tissues.

Evasion of Apoptosis (p. 306)

The accumulation of neoplastic cells requires not only the activation of oncogenes or inactivation of tumor suppressor genes, but also mutations in the genes that regulate apoptosis. The prototypic gene in this group, *BCL2*, prevents programmed cell death, (apoptosis) via the mitochondrial pathway (protein products of *BCL2* and related genes control apoptosis by regulating cytochrome *c* exit from the mitochondria; cytochrome *c* activates the proteolytic enzyme caspase 9 [Chapter 1]). Overexpression of *BCL2* presumably extends cell survival, and if cells are genetically damaged, they continue to suffer additional mutations in oncogenes and tumor suppressor genes. The most dramatic example of *BCL2* overexpression is seen in follicular B-cell lymphomas. Approximately 85% of these tumors exhibit a t(14;18) translocation juxtaposing *BCL2* with a transcriptionally active immunoglobulin heavy chain locus; the result is *BCL2* overexpression. Other genes of the *BCL2* family (e.g., *BAX*) can be pro-apoptotic, and genes not directly related to the *BCL2* family can also regulate apoptosis; *p53* was already mentioned, although it is noteworthy that lack of p53 activity actually reduces apoptosis by decreasing *BAX* transcription. In addition, if *MYC*-driven cells do not have sufficient growth factors in their environs, they undergo apoptosis, which effect can be prevented by *BCL2* overexpression.

DNA Repair and Genomic Instability in Cancer Cells (p. 307)

DNA repair genes do not contribute directly to cell growth or proliferation. They act indirectly by correcting errors in DNA that occur spontaneously during cell division or those that follow exposure to mutagenic chemicals or irradiation. Patients born with inherited mutations of DNA repair proteins are at greatly increased risk of developing cancer (*genomic instability syndromes*). In addition, defects in DNA repair pathways are also present in sporadic human cancers. *DNA repair genes are not directly oncogenic*; however, defective proteins permit mutations to occur in other genes during normal cell division. Defects can occur in three types of DNA repair systems:

- Mismatch repair
- Nucleotide excision repair
- Recombination repair

Hereditary Nonpolyposis Colon Cancer Syndrome (p. 306)

Patients are born with one defective copy of one of several DNA repair genes involved in *mismatch repair* (e.g., *MSH2* and *MLH1*). They develop carcinomas of the cecum or proximal colon without an adenomatous polyp pre-neoplastic stage. Loss of the normal "spell checker" function of the mismatch repair enzymes leads to gradual accumulation of errors in multiple genes including protooncogenes and tumor suppressor genes. Mismatch repair mutations can be readily documented by examining *microsatellite repeats* (tandem repeats of 1–6 nucleotides that are fixed in normal tissues); variation of microsatellites (so-called *microsatellite instability*) is a hallmark of mismatch repair defects.

Xeroderma Pigmentosum (p. 307)

Patients develop skin cancers as a result of the mutagenic effects of ultraviolet (UV) light. These patients have mutated *nucleotide excision repair* genes required for correcting UV light-induced pyrimidine dimer formation.

Inherited Diseases with Defects in DNA Repair by Homologous Recombination (p. 307)

This group of autosomal recessive disorders (including Bloom syndrome, Fanconi anemia, and ataxia-telangiectasia) is characterized by hypersensitivity to other DNA-damaging agents (e.g., ionizing radiation or chemical cross-linking agents). In ataxia-telangiectasia, for example, *ATM* gene mutations result in a protein kinase that can no longer sense DNA double-stranded breaks. Normally the ATM protein would phosphorylate p53 leading to cell cycle arrest or apoptosis; with defective ATM activity, DNA-damaged cells continue to proliferate and are prone to transformation.

BRCA-1 and BRCA-2 (p. 308)

About 5% to 10% of breast cancers are familial, and mutations in *BRCA-1* or *BRCA-2* can account for 80% of such cases. Individuals who inherit defective copies of *BRCA-1* are also at an increased risk of developing ovarian cancers, and those with germ line mutations of *BRCA-2* have an increased risk of ovarian cancer, male breast cancer, melanoma, and pancreatic carcinoma. Mutations in either gene are associated with 60% to 85% lifetime risk of breast cancer and 15% to 40% lifetime risk of ovarian cancer. Such mutations are found in less than 3% of all breast cancers (reflecting the fact that they are not common mutations in sporadic breast cancers). Both genes are involved in the repair of double-stranded DNA breaks by homologous recombination.

Limitless Replicative Potential: Telomerase
(p. 309)

The enzyme telomerase is not active in most somatic cells; as a consequence, the cellular telomeres progressively shorten with each cycle of proliferation until the cell can no longer replicate its DNA and subsequently arrests in a terminally non-dividing state called *replicative senescence* (Chapter 1). Cancer cells overcome this limitation by reactivating telomerase (normally only active in germ cells); more than 90% of human tumors show telomerase activity.

Development of Sustained Angiogenesis (p. 309)

Even with genetic abnormalities that dysregulate cell growth and survival, tumors cannot enlarge beyond 1 to 2 mm in diameter without inducing host blood vessel growth (*angiogenesis*) to provide nutrients and remove wastes. New vessel ingrowth can also stimulate tumor proliferation via the endothelial production of proteins such as insulin-like growth factor and PDGF. Tumors induce angiogenesis by elaborating endothelial growth proteins such as *vascular endothelium growth factor (VEGF)* and *basic fibroblast growth factor (bFGF)* (Chapter 3). However, the new tumor vessels differ from normal vasculature by being tortuous, irregularly shaped, and highly leaky. The switch to an angiogenic phenotype in tumors (thus markedly increased growth potential) may be associated with the loss of angiogenesis inhibitors (e.g., *thrombospondin-1,* which is normally induced by p53). In addition to angiogenic factors, tumor cells also produce antiangiogenic factors (e.g., angiostatin and endostatin). Tumor growth is controlled by the balance between angiogenic and antiangiogenic factors. The latter is under study therapeutically to retard tumor growth.

Invasion and Metastasis (p. 311)

The sequential steps involved in invasion and metastasis are depicted in Figure 7–2. This sequence may be interrupted at any stage by host factors. Experimental studies in animals indicate that cells within a primary tumor are heterogeneous with respect to metastatic abilities. Only certain subclones can complete all the steps outlined in Figure 7–2 and are able to form secondary tumors at distant sites.

Invasion of Extracellular Matrix (p. 312)

Tumor cells must attach to, degrade, and penetrate the extracellular matrix at several steps of the metastatic cascade. Invasion of extracellular matrix can be resolved into four steps:

- *Detachment of tumor cells from each other*: Tumor cells remain attached to each other by several adhesion molecules, including a family of glycoproteins called *cadherins*. In several carcinomas, there is down-regulation of epithelial (E) cadherins, presumably reducing tumor cell cohesion.
- *Attachment to matrix components*: Tumor cells bind to laminin and fibronectin via cell surface receptors. Receptor-mediated binding is an important step in invasion.
- *Degradation of extracellular matrix*: After attachment, tumor cells secrete proteolytic enzymes that degrade the matrix components and create passageways for migration. In experimental systems, the ability of tumor cell variants to degrade extracellular matrix can be correlated with their metastatic

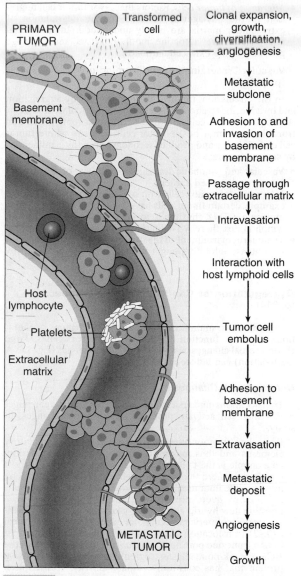

FIGURE 7–2 The metastatic cascade. The sequential steps involved in the hematogenous spread of a tumor are illustrated.

ability. Enzymes that are important in this respect are type IV collagenases (cleave basement membrane collagen), cathepsin D (a cysteine proteinase), and urokinase-type plasminogen activator. These enzymes act on a large variety of substrates, including laminin, fibronectin, and proteoglycan cores.

- *Migration of tumor cells*: Factors that favor tumor cell migration in the passageways created by the degradation of extracellular matrix are poorly understood. Implicated in this process are autocrine motility factors and cleavage products of the extracellular matrix.

Vascular Dissemination and Homing of Tumor Cells (p. 313)

In the circulation, tumor cells form emboli by aggregation and by adhering to circulating leukocytes, particularly platelets. Aggregated tumor cells are thereby afforded some protection from the antitumor host effector cells. The site where tumor cell emboli lodge and produce secondary growths is influenced by several factors:

- Vascular and lymphatic drainage from the site of the primary tumor, as discussed earlier.
- Interaction of tumor cells with organ-specific receptors. For example, certain tumor cells have high levels of an adhesion molecule, CD44, that binds to high endothelial venules in lymph nodes, thereby facilitating nodal metastases.
- The microenvironment of the organ or site (e.g., a tissue rich in protease inhibitors might be resistant to penetration by tumor cells).

Dysregulation of Cancer-Associated Genes (p. 314)

In addition to mutational activation of oncogenes or mutational loss of function of tumor suppressor genes, large chromosomal changes as well as epigenetic changes (e.g., DNA methylation) can induce malignancy.

Chromosomal Changes (p. 314)

Translocations and inversions are chromosome rearrangements that can activate protooncogenes. These changes do so by:

- Removing protooncogenes from their normal regulatory elements and thus making them prone to overexpression; an example is the t (8:14)(q24:q32) translocation in Burkitt lymphoma where the normally tightly regulated c-*myc* gene moves to the immunoglobulin heavy chain gene locus resulting in c-*myc* overexpression.
- Forming new hybrid genes that fortuitously encode growth-promoting chimeric molecules; an example is the reciprocal t (9:22) translocation of the Philadelphia chromosome that joins a truncated portion of the c-*abl* protooncogene with the *BCR* (break-point cluster region) gene to form a fusion protein that has constitutive kinase activity. Transcription factors are often the partners in gene fusions occurring in cancer cells.

Gene Amplification (p. 315)

Reduplication and amplification of DNA sequences may underlie the protooncogene activation associated with overexpression. Examples include N-*myc* overexpression in 25% to 30% of neuroblastomas and *ERB-B2* overexpression in 20% of breast cancers.

Epigenetic Changes: Silencing of Tumor Suppressor Genes by DNA Methylation (p. 315)

Methylation of promoter sequences without any changes in primary DNA base sequences can cause the inactivation of tumor suppressor genes (e.g., *p14ARF* in gastrointestinal cancers and *p16INK4a* in various malignancies). Therapeutic strategies to demethylate selected DNA sequences may be efficacious in these cases.

Molecular Profiles of Cancer Cells (p. 315)

Determination of mRNA levels by microarray analysis now permits obtaining *gene expression signatures* or *molecular profiles* for tumors. Applying the technique to breast cancers and acute lymphoblastic leukemias has identified subtypes with molecular profiles that predict the clinical course.

MOLECULAR BASIS OF MULTISTEP CARCINOGENESIS (p. 315)

No single genetic alteration is sufficient to induce cancers *in vivo*. Multiple controls exerted by multiple categories of genes—oncogenes, tumor suppressor genes, and apoptosis-regulating genes—must be lost for the emergence of cancer cells. This situation is exemplified by the colon adenoma-to-carcinoma sequence (Fig. 7–3); the evolution of benign adenomas to carcinomas is marked by increasing and additive effects of mutations, affecting *RAS*, *APC*, *p53*, and *SMAD 2* and

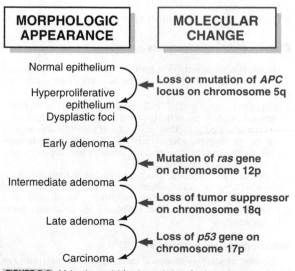

FIGURE 7–3 Molecular model for the evolution of colorectal cancers through the adenoma-carcinoma sequence. Although *APC* mutation is an early event and loss of *p53* occurs late in tumorigenesis, the timing for other changes may be quite variable. Note also that individual tumors may not have all the changes listed. (Adapted from Vogelstein B, Kinzler KW: Colorectal tumors. In Vogelstein B, Kinzler KW: The Genetic Basis of Human Cancer. New York, McGraw-Hill, 2002, p. 583.)

SMAD 4 genes on 18q. The accumulation of mutations, resulting perhaps from genetic instability of cancer cells, may be promoted by loss of *p53*, DNA repair genes, or both. Genes that regulate cellular proliferation in a more or less tissue-specific manner, such as *APC, NF-1*, and *RB*, are called *gatekeeper* genes, whereas those that regulate genomic stability (DNA repair genes) are called *caretaker* genes. These latter genes regulate the likelihood of a particular cell developing a mutator phenotype (cells unusually susceptible to addition mutations) resulting in mutations in the gatekeeper genes.

Tumor Progression and Heterogeneity
(p. 319)

Over time tumors can become more aggressive and acquire greater malignant potential; accelerated growth, invasiveness, angiogenesis, and the ability to form distant metastases are all attributes that are typically acquired in an incremental fashion by acquisition of new mutations. This is manifested as a sequential appearance of cell subpopulations; thus, despite the fact that tumors are initially *monoclonal in origin, by the time they become clinically evident, they are extremely heterogeneous.*

CARCINOGENIC AGENTS AND THEIR CELLULAR INTERACTIONS (p. 319)

Agents that cause genetic damage and induce neoplastic transformation include:

• Chemical carcinogens
• Radiant energy
• Oncogenic viruses and other microbes

Chemical Carcinogenesis (p. 319)

Neoplastic transformation brought about by chemicals is a dynamic multistep process. It can be broadly divided into two stages:

• *Initiation* refers to the induction of certain irreversible changes (mutations) in the genome of cells. Initiated cells are not transformed cells; they do not have growth autonomy or unique phenotypic characteristics. In contrast to normal cells, however, they give rise to tumors when appropriately stimulated by promoting agents.
• *Promotion* refers to the process of tumor induction in previously initiated cells by chemicals referred to as *promoters*. The effect of promoters is relatively short-lived and reversible; they do not affect DNA and are nontumorigenic by themselves.

Initiation of Carcinogenesis (p. 320)

The vast majority of chemical carcinogens are referred to as *procarcinogens* because they require metabolic activation *in vivo* to produce the ultimate carcinogens. Only a few alkylating and acylating agents are direct-acting carcinogens. The activation of procarcinogens in most cases depends on microsomal cytochrome P-450 oxygenases. Individuals who inherit highly inducible forms of these enzymes incur a higher risk of smoking-related lung cancers, for example. Several factors, such as age, sex, and hormones, also modulate the activity of microsomal enzymes and hence the potency of procarcinogens.

Molecular Targets of Chemical Carcinogens (p. 321)

All direct-acting carcinogens and procarcinogens are highly reactive electrophilic compounds that can react with nucleophilic sites in the cell. DNA is the primary and most important target of chemical carcinogens; thus, chemical carcinogens are mutagens that induce mutations in protooncogenes, tumor suppressor genes, and genes that regulate apoptosis. Thus, the *RAS* oncogene is frequently mutated in chemically induced tumors in rodents. Because specific sequences are targeted by different chemicals, an analysis of the mutations found in human tumors may allow linkage to specific carcinogens. Carcinogen-induced changes in DNA, however, do not necessarily lead to the initiation of carcinogenesis because the DNA damage can be repaired. However, if the DNA repair ability is impaired (e.g., xeroderma pigmentosum), the cancer risk significantly increases. Because chemical carcinogens are mutagenic, a simple *in vitro* test for carcinogenicity is the *Ames test*, using the ability of potential carcinogens to induce mutations in selected strains of the bacterium *Salmonella typhimurium*.

Initiated Cell (p. 321)

Unrepaired DNA alterations are essential first steps in initiating tumors; however, the damaged DNA template must also be replicated to make the changes permanent. Thus, many chemicals become metabolically activated in the liver but will not induce tumors unless liver cells proliferate within 3 to 4 days of DNA adduct formation. Quiescent cells may never be affected by chemical carcinogens unless a mitotic stimulus is also provided.

Promotion of Carcinogenesis (p. 321)

The initial mutagenic event in most instances requires subsequent exposure to promoters, including various hormones, drugs, phenols, and phorbol esters. Phorbol esters are the most widely used promoters in experimental systems; they are not mutagenic and seem to exert their effects by epigenetic mechanisms. Tetradecanoyl phorbol acetate (TPA), a commonly used promoter, is a powerful activator of protein kinase C, an enzyme that is a key element in the signal transduction pathways. Activation of protein kinase C leads to a series of phosphorylation reactions that ultimately affect cell proliferation and differentiation. Thus, promoters appear to be involved in the clonal expansion and aberrant differentiation of initiated cells.

Carcinogenic Chemicals (p. 322)

- *Alkylating agents:* These include direct-acting agents, such as cyclophosphamide and busulfan, used in the treatment of cancer as well as immunosuppressants. Patients receiving such therapy are at increased risk of developing another cancer.
- *Polycyclic aromatic hydrocarbons:* These are present in cigarette smoke and may therefore be relevant to the pathogenesis of lung cancer.

- *Aromatic amine and azo dyes*: β-Naphthylamine, an aniline dye used in the rubber industries, was in the past responsible for bladder cancers in exposed workers.
- *Naturally occurring carcinogens*: Aflatoxin B_1, produced by the fungus *Aspergillus flavus*, is a potent hepatocarcinogen in animals and is believed to be a factor in the high incidence of liver cancer in Africa. The fungus grows on moldy grains and peanuts, and the toxin is ingested with contaminated foods.
- *Nitrosamines and amides*: These can be synthesized in the gastrointestinal tract from ingested nitrites or derived from digested proteins and may contribute to the induction of gastric cancer.
- *Miscellaneous agents*: Asbestos, vinyl chloride, and metals such as nickel are carcinogenic. They predispose exposed individuals to the development of cancer. Hormones such as estrogens may play a role in the causation of endometrial cancer.

Radiation Carcinogenesis (p. 323)

Radiant energy in the form of UV rays and ionizing radiations can cause cancer.

Ultraviolet Rays (p. 323)

Natural UV radiation, especially UVB, derived from the sun can cause skin cancer. At greatest risk are fair-skinned people who live in locales that receive a great deal of sunlight; carcinomas and melanomas of exposed skin are particularly common in Australia and New Zealand. Two mechanisms may be involved in UV induction of cancer:

- Damage to DNA by the formation of pyrimidine dimers
- Immunosuppression (but thus far demonstrated only in animal models)

Ionizing Radiation (p. 323)

Electromagnetic and particulate radiations are carcinogenic. The ability of ionizing radiations to cause cancer lies in their ability to induce mutations. Such mutations may result from a direct effect of the radiant energy or an indirect effect mediated by the generation of free radicals from water or oxygen. Particulate radiations (such as α particles and neutrons) are more carcinogenic than electromagnetic radiation (x-rays, gamma rays).

Evidence for the carcinogenicity of ionizing radiation comes from several sources:

- Miners of radioactive ores have an increased risk of lung cancer.
- The incidence of certain forms of leukemia is greatly increased in survivors of atomic bombs in Japan.
- Therapeutic radiation to the neck in children has been associated with the later development of thyroid cancer.

In humans, there is a hierarchy of cellular vulnerability to radiation-induced neoplasms:

- Most common are myeloid leukemias, followed by thyroid cancer in children.
- Cancers of the breast and lung are less commonly radiation induced.

- Skin, bone, and gut are the least susceptible to radiation carcinogenesis.

Viral and Microbial Carcinogenesis (p. 324)

A variety of DNA and RNA viruses are known to cause cancer in animals, and some are implicated in human cancer:

- Human papillomavirus (HPV)
- Epstein-Barr virus (EBV)
- Hepatitis B virus (HBV)
- Kaposi sarcoma herpesvirus (KSHV)

Oncogenic DNA Viruses (p. 324)

The genomes of oncogenic DNA viruses integrate into and form a stable association with the host cell genome. The virus cannot complete its replicative cycle because essential viral genes are interrupted during viral DNA integration; consequently, the virus may remain latent for years. Viral genes that are transcribed early in the viral life cycle are typically important for cellular transformation.

Human Papillomavirus (p. 324)

Approximately 70 genetically distinct types of HPV have been identified. Some types (e.g., 1, 2, 4, and 7) definitely cause benign squamous papillomas (warts) in humans. Evidence supporting the role of HPV in human cancers is as follows:

- Squamous cell cancers of the uterine cervix contain HPV types 16 or 18 in over 90% of cases. These viruses are also contained in presumed precursors (e.g., *carcinoma in situ*) of the invasive cancer.
- Genital warts with low malignant potential are caused by distinct HPV types (*low-risk* types, e.g., HPV-6 and HPV-11).
- Molecular analysis of HPV-associated cervical carcinomas reveals clonal integration of the viral genomes in the host cell DNA. During integration, the viral DNA is interrupted in a manner that leads to overexpression of the E6 and E7 viral proteins. These proteins have the potential to transform cells by binding to and inhibiting the functions of Rb and p53 tumor suppressor gene products.

Epstein-Barr Virus (p. 325)

This member of the herpesvirus family is associated with four human cancers:

- *Burkitt lymphoma* (p. 326) is a tumor of B lymphocytes that is consistently associated with a t(8;14) translocation. In certain parts of Africa, Burkitt lymphoma is endemic, and virtually all patients' tumor cells carry the EBV genome. It is unlikely, however, that EBV alone can cause Burkitt lymphoma. In normal individuals, EBV-driven B-cell proliferation is self-limited and controlled. In patients with subtle or overt immune dysregulation, EBV causes sustained B-cell proliferation because EBV genes dysregulate growth-controlling pathways of B cells. Such B cells acquire additional mutations and sometimes the translocation t(8;14), and eventually become autonomous.
- *Nasopharyngeal carcinoma* (p. 327) is endemic in southern China and some other locales, and the EBV genome is found

in all such tumors. As in Burkitt lymphoma, EBV probably acts in concert with other factors.

- *B-cell lymphomas in immunosuppressed patients*, especially in those with acquired immunodeficiency syndrome (AIDS), may be associated with EBV. The role of normal immune responses in control of EBV-induced B-cell proliferation is illustrated by the occurrence of B-cell lymphomas in patients with AIDS and recipients of immunosuppressive drugs. These patients have polyclonal B-cell proliferations that transform into monoclonal lymphomas. In transplant recipients, withdrawal of immunosuppressive drugs can cause regression of such EBV-induced proliferations.
- Some forms of *Hodgkin lymphoma* have been associated with EBV.

Hepatitis B Virus (p. 327)

There is a close association between HBV infection and liver cancer in many parts of the world. In Taiwan, the risk of developing hepatic cancer is increased 200-fold in those infected with HBV. Cofactors other than HBV are also believed to play roles in the genesis of liver cancer. The mechanism by which HBV causes cancer is probably multifactorial:

- By causing hepatocellular injury and resulting regenerative hyperplasia, the pool of mitotically active cells subject to mutational damage by environmental agents such as aflatoxins is increased.
- HBV encodes a regulatory element called *HBx* that causes transcriptional activation of several protooncogenes.
- HBx protein also binds to p53 and may thus inactivate it.

Hepatitis C virus is also associated with liver cancer. This is believed to be due to the ability of HCV to cause liver injury and subsequent regeneration, as discussed previously.

Oncogenic RNA Viruses (p. 327)

Only one human retrovirus, human T-cell lymphotropic virus type 1 (HTLV-1), has been firmly implicated in carcinogenesis:

- This virus has a strong tropism for CD4+ T cells and causes a T-cell leukemia in 3% to 5% of infected individuals with a 40- to 60-year latent period.
- HTLV-1–associated leukemia/lymphoma is endemic in parts of Japan and the Caribbean basin. It is sporadic elsewhere, including the United States.
- HTLV-1 proviral DNA is detected in DNA of leukemic T cells. The integration shows a clonal pattern.
- The mechanism of HTLV-1–induced transformation is not clear; HTLV-1 does not contain an oncogene, and it is not found integrated near a protooncogene.
- The HTLV-1 genome contains a unique segment referred to as the tax region. The proteins encoded by the *TAX* gene activate the transcription of the T-cell growth factor interleukin-2 (IL-2) as well as its receptor, thus setting up an autocrine stimulatory loop. The resulting polyclonal expansion of T cells is at increased risk of developing additional mutations that can eventually give rise to a monoclonal T-cell tumor.

Helicobacter pylori (p. 328) causes no clinical consequences in the great majority of infected individuals; however, in 20% to 30% of cases, infection leads to peptic ulcer (Chapter 17), gastric lymphoma, and carcinoma. Chronic infection with *H. pylori* is thought to induce *H. pylori*–reactive T cells that cause proliferation of polyclonal B-cell populations via cytokine secretion. These T cell–dependent B cells eventually become monoclonal and T cell independent by accumulating mutations (e.g., t[11:18] translocations). The resultant tumor is called *marginal zone lymphoma* or, sometimes, *MALToma* (for *m*ucosa-*a*ssociated *l*ymphoid *t*issue lymphomas). Before becoming T cell independent, such B-cell proliferations respond to antibiotic treatment.

HOST DEFENSE AGAINST TUMORS—TUMOR IMMUNITY (p. 328)

Tumors are not entirely "self" and may be potentially recognized by the immune system (called *immune surveillance*). This concept is supported by the observations that immune elements accumulate in and around tumors, that certain malignancies show an increased incidence in immunocompromised hosts, and that cancers frequently elicit tumor-specific T cells and antibodies. The fact that tumors also occur in immunocompetent hosts suggests that immune surveillance may be imperfect, and that immune surveillance leads to *cancer immunoediting* that modulates the immunogenicity of neoplasms.

Tumor Antigens (p. 328)

These antigens can be classified into two groups: tumor-specific antigens, present only on tumor cells, and tumor-associated antigens, present on tumor cells as well as some normal cells.

Tumor-specific antigens are readily demonstrated in chemically induced tumors in rodents and some human tumors. Tumor-specific antigens are composed of tumor-derived peptides that are presented on the cell surface by major histocompatibility complex class I molecules and recognized by CD8+ T cells. Several types of proteins can result in tumor-specific antigens not previously encountered by the host immune system:

- Products of mutated oncogenes and tumor suppressor genes (e.g., mutated RAS, p53, and BCR-ABL).
- Products of other mutated genes resulting from intrinsic genetic instability and a mutator phenotype.
- Overexpressed or aberrantly expressed cellular proteins. Frequently, these represent proteins that are expressed at low levels in normal tissues but are markedly overexpressed in tumors (e.g., tyrosinase, expressed in normal melanocytes but overexpressed in melanomas where it induces an immune response).
- Tumor antigens produced by oncogenic viruses.
- Oncofetal antigens that may be normally expressed developmentally but are not normally seen on adult tissues; during malignant transformation, these proteins may elicit immune responses.
- Altered cell surface glycolipids and glycoproteins. Tumors frequently have dysregulated expression of the enzymes responsible for lipid and protein glycosylation, and can lead

to the appearance of tumor-specific epitopes on carbohydrate side chains, or on an aberrantly exposed polypeptide cores.

Tumor-associated antigens include oncofetal antigens (e.g., carcinoembryonic antigen [CEA]) and lineage-specific antigens (e.g., CD10 on B cells). They do not typically evoke immune responses but are useful for tumor diagnosis, and may be targets for immunotherapy.

Antitumor Effector Mechanisms (p. 331)

Cell-mediated and humoral immunity both participate, but CD8+ cytotoxic T lymphocyte (CTL)-mediated killing is the principal mechanism of antitumor immunity; natural killer (NK) cells and activated macrophages may also contribute.

Immune Surveillance (p. 331)

Evidence for the presence of physiologically relevant immune surveillance includes:
- Increased frequency of cancers in patients with congenital or acquired (drug-induced, AIDS) immunodeficiency
- Increased susceptibility to EBV infections and EBV-associated lymphoma in boys with X-linked immunodeficiency

Tumors may escape immunosurveillance by:
- Selective outgrowth of antigen-negative variants.
- Loss or reduced expression of histocompatibility antigens, thus becoming less susceptible to cytotoxic T-cell lysis (although NK cells might be expected to have increased activity in that setting).
- Tumor-induced immunosuppression.
- Failure of sensitization because tumor cells do not express necessary costimulatory molecules.
- Apoptosis of cytotoxic T cells because tumor cells express Fas; the FasL-expressing T cells undergo death when engaged by tumor-associated Fas.

A potential caveat to the hypothesis that failure of immune surveillance contributes to malignancy: Tumors that develop in immunodeficient patients are mainly lymphomas; these could be the consequence of an abnormal immune system rather than failure of immune surveillance.

CLINICAL FEATURES OF TUMORS (p. 332)

Effects of Tumor on Host (p. 333)

Local and Hormonal Effects (p. 333)

- *Related to location*: Intracranial tumors (e.g., pituitary adenoma) can expand and destroy the remaining pituitary gland, giving rise to an endocrine disorder; tumors of the gastrointestinal tract may cause obstruction of the bowel or may ulcerate and cause bleeding.
- *Hormone production*: Tumors of endocrine glands may elaborate hormones; this is more common in benign than in malignant tumors.

Cancer Cachexia (p. 333)

Loss of body fat, wasting, and profound weakness are referred to as *cancer cachexia*. The basis of cachexia is multifactorial:

* Loss of appetite
* Poorly understood metabolic changes that lead to reduced synthesis and storage of fat and increased mobilization of fatty acids from adipocytes
* Production of tumor necrosis factor (previously called *cachectin*) by activated macrophages
* Production of other humoral factors, such as proteolysis-inducing factor (PIF), which can increase the catabolism of muscle and adipose tissue

Paraneoplastic Syndromes (p. 333)

Symptoms of these syndromes are not directly related to the spread of the tumor or elaboration of hormones indigenous to the tissue from which the tumor arose. Paraneoplastic syndromes may be the earliest clinical manifestations of a neoplasm and may mimic distant spread. The most common syndromes include:

* *Endocrinopathies*: Some nonendocrine cancers produce hormones or hormone-like factors (ectopic hormone production); for example, certain cancers of the lung (small cell type) produce *Cushing syndrome* by elaborating corticotropin or related peptides.
* *Hypercalcemia*: Hypercalcemia may occur owing to resorption of bone resulting from the elaboration of parathyroid hormone (PTH)-like peptides or, in some cases, of TGF-α by certain tumors (e.g., squamous cell cancer of the lung, T-cell leukemias/lymphomas). Cancer-associated hypercalcemia can also result from osteolysis induced by bony metastases (a process that is *not* considered a paraneoplastic syndrome).
* *Acanthosis nigricans*: The acquired (nongenetic) form of this verrucous pigmented lesion of the skin is frequently associated with visceral malignancy.
* *Clubbing of fingers and hypertrophic osteoarthropathy*: These conditions are associated with lung cancers and other thoracic lesions.
* *Thrombotic diatheses*: Thrombotic diatheses resulting from production of thromboplastic substance by tumor cells may manifest as disseminated intravascular coagulation, migratory thrombophlebitis (Trousseau syndrome), or vegetations on heart valves (nonbacterial thrombotic endocarditis).

Grading and Staging of Tumors (p. 335)

This assessment provides a semiquantitative estimate of the clinical gravity of a tumor. Both histologic grading and clinical staging are valuable for prognostication and for planning therapy, although staging has proved to be of greater clinical value.

Grading

Grading is based on the degree of differentiation and the number of mitoses within the tumor. Cancers are classified as grades I to IV with increasing anaplasia. In general, higher-grade tumors are more aggressive than lower-grade tumors. Grading is imperfect because:

- Different parts of the same tumor may display different degrees of differentiation.
- The grade of tumor may change as the tumor grows.

Staging

Staging is based on the anatomic extent of the tumor. Relevant to staging are the size of the primary tumor and the extent of local and distant spread. Two methods of staging are in current use: the TNM (*t*umor, *n*ode, *m*etastases) and the AJC (*A*merican *J*oint *C*ommittee) systems. Both systems assign higher stages to tumors that are larger, locally invasive, and metastatic.

Laboratory Diagnosis of Cancer (p. 335)

Histologic and Cytologic Methods (p. 336)

Histologic examination is the most important method of diagnosis. In addition to the usual fromalin-fixed and paraffin-embedded sections, quick-frozen sections are employed to obtain a rapid diagnosis while the patient is still under anesthesia. Proper histologic diagnosis is greatly aided by:

- Availability of all relevant clinical data
- Adequate preservation and sampling of the specimen
- In some cases, examination of the frozen specimen to detect cell surface receptors

Fine-needle aspiration for cytologic evaluation involves aspiration of cells and fluids from tumors or masses that occur in readily palpable sites (e.g., breast, thyroid, lymph nodes). The aspirated cells are smeared, stained, and examined.

Cytologic or Papanicolaou smears involve examination of cancer cells that are readily shed. Exfoliative cytologic examination is used most commonly in the diagnosis of dysplasia, *carcinoma in situ*, and invasive cancer of the uterine cervix and tumors of the stomach, bronchus, and urinary bladder.

Cytologic interpretation is based chiefly on changes in the appearance of individual cells. In the hands of experts, false-positive results are uncommon, but false-negative results do occur because of sampling errors. When possible, cytologic diagnosis must be confirmed by biopsy before therapeutic intervention.

Immunohistochemistry (p. 336)

This technique involves detection of cell products or surface markers by antibodies. The binding of antibodies can be revealed by fluorescent labels or chemical reactions that result in the generation of a colored product. Immunohistochemistry is useful in the following settings:

- Diagnosis of undifferentiated tumors by the detection of tissue-specific intermediate filaments
- Categorization of leukemias and lymphomas by using monoclonal antibodies specific for various lymphohematopoietic cells

- Determination of the site of origin of metastases by using reagents that identify specific cell types (e.g., prostate-specific antigen for prostate cancer)
- Detection of molecules that have prognostic or therapeutic significance (e.g., immunochemical detection of hormone receptors and products of protooncogenes, such as *ERB-B2*, on breast cancers)

Molecular Diagnosis (p. 337)

- DNA probe analysis involves polymerase chain reaction or fluorescence *in situ* hybridization (FISH) analysis. These techniques are currently used most extensively in the diagnosis of lymphoid neoplasms because such tumors are associated with clonal rearrangements of T-cell or B-cell antigen receptor genes.
- Detection of oncogenes such as N-*MYC* is also valuable in assessing the prognosis of certain tumors.
- Diagnosis of chronic myeloid leukemia can be made by detection of the *BCR-ABL* fusion gene product, even in the absence of the Philadelphia chromosome.
- Specific translocations detected by polymerase chain reaction can distinguish between similar-appearing tumors (e.g., small round blue cell tumors in children).
- Hereditary predisposition to certain tumors (e.g., breast cancer and endocrine neoplasms) can be detected by mutational analysis of *BRCA-1*, *BRCA-2*, and *RET* genes.
- *Spectral karyotyping* is a technique used to analyze all chromosomes from a single cell using a pallet of fluorochromes; it can readily detect even small translocations or insertions and can determine the origin of unidentified chromosomes.
- DNA microarray analysis and proteomics are increasingly being used to identify gene expression signatures; these analyses have relevance for identifying tumor subtypes with potential prognostic or therapeutic significance.

Flow Cytometry (p. 338)

Measurement of the DNA content of tumor cells by flow cytometry is useful because with several tumors there is a relationship between abnormal DNA content and prognosis. Flow cytometric detection of cell surface antigens is of value in the diagnosis of leukemias and lymphomas.

Tumor Markers (p. 338)

Tumor-derived or tumor-associated molecules can be detected in blood or other body fluids. They are not primary methods of diagnosis but rather diagnostic adjuncts. They may also be of value in determining the response to therapy or recurrence of tumor after treatment. Two examples of tumor markers are described here:

- *Carcinoembryonic antigen (CEA)*, normally produced by fetal gut, liver, and pancreas, can be elaborated by cancers of the colon, pancreas, stomach, and breast. Less consistently, the levels are elevated in non-neoplastic conditions (e.g., alcoholic cirrhosis, hepatitis, and ulcerative colitis). This antigen is of value in estimating tumor burden in colorectal cancer and in detecting recurrences after surgery.

- α-*Fetoprotein (AFP)* is normally produced by fetal yolk sac and liver. Markedly elevated levels are noted in cancers of the liver and testicular germ cells and can be used to assess recurrences or response to therapy. Non-neoplastic conditions, such as cirrhosis and hepatitis, are also associated with less marked elevations of α-fetoprotein.

CHAPTER 8

Infectious Diseases

In the United States, serious infections affect otherwise healthy people, as well as those immunosuppressed by acquired immunodeficiency syndrome (AIDS), chronic disease, transplantation, or anticancer drugs. Infectious diseases kill more than 10 million persons each year in developing countries, many dying because of the initial failure to prevent infection, or to lack of treatment.

To understand the mechanisms of infectious disease, one must consider:

- The type and virulence properties of the organism
- The host response to the infectious agent

The list of disease-causing microorganisms is constantly expanding:

- *Helicobacter* gastritis, hepatitis B virus (HBV) and hepatitis C virus (HCV) infections, rotavirus diarrhea, human metapneumovirus respiratory disease, and Legionnaires' pneumonia are all diseases with relatively newly recognized pathogens (difficulty in culturing was responsible for the late discoveries).
- Some infectious agents are genuinely new to humans, such as human immunodeficiency virus (HIV, causing AIDS), *Borrelia burgdorferi* (causing Lyme disease), and the coronavirus that causes severe acute respiratory syndrome (SARS).
- Some infections have become more common as a result of AIDS-induced immunosuppression; these pathogens include cytomegalovirus (CMV), human herpesvirus type 8, *Mycobacterium avium-intracellulare, Pneumocystis jiroveci (carinii),* and *Cryptosporidium parvum.*
- Risk of bioterrorism has increased interest in pathogens that pose the greatest danger because of their efficient disease transmission, relative ease of production and distribution, difficulty in defending against, or the ability to provoke alarm and fear in the general public (see Table 8–2 in *Robbins and Cotran Pathologic Basis of Disease,* 7th ed., p. 346).

CATEGORIES OF INFECTIOUS AGENTS
(p. 346) (Table 8–1)

Prions (p. 346)

- Prions are not viruses; they lack RNA and DNA.
- They are composed only of a modified host protein, termed *prion protein* (PrP).
- They cause spongiform encephalopathies (kuru, Creutzfeldt-Jakob disease, "mad-cow disease").
- Prions are associated with neurodegenerative diseases, including fatal familial insomnia.

Viruses (see Table 8–4 in *Robbins and Cotran Pathologic Basis of Disease*, 7th ed., p. 347)

- Viruses are obligate intracellular organisms, requiring host cell metabolism for replication.
- Viruses contain DNA or RNA (but not both) within a protein coat *(capsid)* that may be surrounded by a lipid bilayer *(envelope)*.
- They cause transient acute illness (colds, influenza), chronic disease (HBV, HIV), or lifelong latent infection with potential for long-term reactivation (herpesviruses).

Bacteriophages, Plasmids, Transposons (p. 348)

These agents are mobile genetic elements that indirectly cause human diseases by encoding bacterial virulence factors (adhesins, toxins, or antibiotic resistance).

Bacteria (p. 348; see also Table 8–5 in *Robbins and Cotran Pathologic Basis of Disease*, 7th ed., p. 349)

- Bacteria lack nuclei and other membrane-bound organelles, but have cell walls sandwiched between two phospholipid bilayers (gram-negative bacteria) or outside a single bilayer (gram-positive bacteria). They can grow extracellularly (e.g., *Pneumococcus*) or intracellularly (e.g., *Mycobacterium tuberculosis*).
- Bacteria are major causes of severe infectious diseases.
- Normal persons carry 10^{12} bacteria on the skin (mostly *Staphylococcus epidermidis* and *Propionibacterium acnes*), and 10^{14} bacteria in the gastrointestinal tract (99.9% of which are anaerobic).

Chlamydiae, Rickettsiae, and Mycoplasmas (p. 349)

These infectious agents are similar to bacteria but lack certain structures (mycoplasmas lack cell walls) or metabolic capabilities (chlamydiae cannot synthesize adenosine triphosphate [ATP]). Chlamydiae and rickettsiae are obligate intracellular microbes; mycoplasmas are the smallest of the free-living microbes.

TABLE 8-1 Classes of Human Pathogens and Their Habitats

Taxonomic Category	Size	Site of Propagation	Sample Species	Disease
Viruses	20–300 nm	Obligate intracellular	Poliovirus	Poliomyelitis
Chlamydiae	200–1000 nm	Obligate intracellular	Chlamydia trachomatis	Trachoma, urethritis
Rickettsiae	300–1200 nm	Obligate intracellular	Rickettsia prowazekii	Typhus fever
Mycoplasmas	125–350 nm	Extracellular	Mycoplasma pneumoniae	Atypical pneumonia
Bacteria	0.8–15 µm	Cutaneous	Staphylococcus aureus	Wound
		Mucosal	Vibrio cholerae	Cholera
		Extracellular	Streptococcus pneumoniae	Pneumonia
		Facultative intracellular	Mycobacterium tuberculosis	Tuberculosis
Fungi	2–200 µm	Cutaneous	Trichophyton sp.	Tinea pedis (athlete's foot)
		Mucosal	Candida albicans	Thrush
		Extracellular	Sporothrix schenckii	Sporotrichosis
		Facultative intracellular	Histoplasma capsulatum	Histoplasmosis
Protozoa	1–50 µm	Mucosal	Giardia lamblia	Giardiasis
		Extracellular	Trypanosoma gambiense	Sleeping sickness
		Facultative intracellular	Trypanosoma cruzi	Chagas disease
		Obligate intracellular	Leishmania donovani	Kala-azar
Helminths	3 mm–10 m	Mucosal	Enterobius vermicularis	Enterobiasis
		Extracellular	Wuchereria bancrofti	Filariasis
		Intracellular	Trichinella spiralis	Trichinosis

- Chlamydiae cause urogenital infections, conjunctivitis, trachoma, and respiratory infections.
- Rickettsiae are transmitted by insect vectors, including lice (epidemic typhus), ticks (Rocky Mountain spotted fever [RMSF]), and mites (scrub typhus), and cause hemorrhagic vasculitis or encephalitis (RMSF).
- Mycoplasmas cause atypical pneumonia or nongonococcal urethritis.

Fungi (p. 351)

Fungi are eukaryotes with thick, chitin-containing cell walls; they grow in humans as budding yeast cells and slender tubes (hyphae).

- In otherwise healthy persons, fungi produce superficial infections (e.g., athlete's foot caused by tinea), abscesses (sporotrichosis), or granulomas *(Coccidioides, Histoplasma,* and *Blastomyces)*
- In immunocompromised hosts, opportunistic fungi *(Candida, Aspergillus,* and *Mucor)* cause systemic infections with tissue necrosis, hemorrhage, and vascular occlusion.
- In AIDS patients, the opportunistic fungus *Pneumocystis jiroveci (carinii)* causes pneumonia.

Protozoa (p. 351; see also Table 8–6 in *Robbins and Cotran Pathologic Basis of Disease,* 7th ed., p. 351)

Protozoa are motile, single-celled eukaryotes; they can replicate intracellularly *(Plasmodium* in erythrocytes, *Leishmania* in macrophages) or extracellularly in the urogenital system, intestine, or blood.

- *Trichomonas vaginalis* is transmitted sexually.
- Intestinal protozoa *(Entamoeba histolytica* and *Giardia lamblia)* infect when swallowed.
- Blood-borne protozoa *(Plasmodium* and *Leishmania* species) are transmitted by blood-sucking insects.

Helminths (p. 351)

Roundworms *(nematodes)* infect the intestines *(Ascaris,* hookworms, and *Strongyloides)* or tissues (filariae and *Trichinella).* Flatworms *(cestodes)* are segmented tapeworms living within the intestinal lumen or within tissue cysts (cysticerci and hydatids). The most important fluke *(trematode)* is the blood-dwelling *Schistosoma* (causing schistosomiasis).

- Helminths are highly differentiated parasites with complex life cycles.
- The severity of disease is proportional to the number of infecting organisms.

Ectoparasites (p. 352)

Ectoparasites are arthropods (lice, ticks, bedbugs, fleas) that attach to and live on the skin. They may be vectors for other pathogens (i.e., ticks transmit Lyme disease spirochetes).

TRANSMISSION AND DISSEMINATION OF MICROBES (p. 352)

Host Barriers to Infection (p. 352)

Barriers that prevent microbes from entering the body include intact skin and mucosal surfaces and their secretory products (lysozyme in tears, acid in stomach).

- Skin defenses include keratinized outer layer, fatty acids, and low pH.
- Gastrointestinal defenses include gastric acid, pancreatic bile lytic enzymes, mucous layer, defensins, and secreted IgA.
- Respiratory defenses include ciliary activity, mucous layer, defensins, and secreted IgA.
- Most skin infections are caused by less virulent microbes entering through damaged sites (moist skin, cuts, burns, or insect bites).
- Respiratory, gastrointestinal, and urogenital infections are caused by virulent organisms penetrating intact mucosal barriers.

Spread and Dissemination of Microbes (p. 354)

- Microbes can be transmitted person-to-person via respiratory, fecal-oral, sexual, or transplacental routes. Animal-to-human transmission can occur through direct contact or ingestion *(zoonotic infections);* alternatively, invertebrate vectors may passively spread infection or serve as required hosts for pathogen replication and development.
- Some microbes proliferate locally; others penetrate the epithelial barrier and spread distally via lymphatics, blood, or nerves, so disease manifestations occur at sites distant from microbial entry.

HOW MICROORGANISMS CAUSE DISEASE (p. 356)

Infectious agents damage tissues by:

- Entering cells and directly causing cell death
- Releasing toxins that kill cells at a distance
- Releasing enzymes that degrade tissue components or damage blood vessels
- Inducing host inflammatory cell responses that may directly contribute to tissue damage, including suppuration, scarring, and hypersensitivity reactions

Mechanisms of Viral Injury (p. 356)

Viruses directly damage host cells by entering and replicating within them.

- Viruses have a predilection to infect certain cell types *(tissue tropism)* determined by:

  Binding to specific cell surface proteins (HIV binds to CD4 and the CXCR4 chemokine receptor on T cells)

  Cell type-specific transcription factors (JC virus can only proliferate in oligodendroglia)

Physical barriers, local temperature, and pH (enteroviruses resist gut acid and enzymes)

- Viral infection can be transient (e.g., mumps), chronic latent (varicella-zoster virus [VZV]), or chronic productive (HBV), or can promote cellular transformation and malignancy (human papillomavirus [HPV]).
- Viruses kill host cells by

Inhibiting host DNA, RNA, or protein synthesis (poliovirus)
Damaging the plasma membrane (HIV)
Lysing cells (rhinoviruses and influenzaviruses)
Inducing a host immune response to virus-infected cells (HBV)

Mechanisms of Bacterial Injury (p. 358)

Bacterial damage depends on the ability of the bacteria to adhere to host cells, invade cells and tissues, or deliver toxins.

- Bacterial protein *adhesins* (fimbriae or pili) bind to specific host cells, thereby determining tissue tropisms.
- Intracellular bacteria can kill host cells by rapid replication and lysis *(Shigella* and *Escherichia coli),* or may permit host cell viability while evading intracellular defenses and proliferating within endosomes *(M. tuberculosis)* or cytoplasm *(Listeria monocytogenes).*
- Endotoxin (lipopolysaccharide, LPS) is a cell wall component of gram-negative bacteria; it causes septic shock by inducing high levels of tumor necrosis factor (TNF), interleukin 1 (IL1), and interleukin 12 (IL12).
- Exotoxins are proteins released by bacteria that damage host tissues by several mechanisms:

Extracellular enzymes destroy tissue integrity by digesting structural proteins *(Staphylococcus aureus* exfoliative toxin).
Exotoxins can have a binding (B) component that delivers a toxic active (A) component into the cell cytoplasm, where it alters signaling pathways to cause cell death *(Bacillus anthracis* toxins).
The components of neurotoxins block neurotransmitter release, causing paralysis *(Clostridium* species).

- Superantigens stimulate large numbers of T cells by binding between class II MHC (major histocompatibility complex) molecules and T-cell receptors, resulting in massive T-cell proliferation and cytokine release (e.g., toxic shock syndrome due to *S. aureus).*

Injurious Effects of Host Immunity (p. 359)

Host immune responses to microbes sometimes causes tissue injury:

- Granulomatous responses to certain microbes (e.g., *M. tuberculosis)* function to sequester the pathogen, but can cause tissue damage and fibrosis.
- Liver damage following HBV infection is due to the immune response against infected liver cells (see Chapter 18).
- Post-streptococcal glomerulonephritis occurs when anti-streptococcal antibodies form complexes with streptococcal antigens and deposit in renal glomeruli and produce nephritis (see Chapter 20).

Immune Evasion by Microbes (p. 359)

The success of immune evasion is an important determinant of microbial virulence. Mechanisms include:

- Replication in sites inaccessible to host immune response (*Clostridium difficile* replicates in the small bowel lumen), or rapid invasion of host cells before immune responses become effective (malaria sporozoites entering hepatocytes)
- Constantly changing surface antigens (*N. gonorrhoeae* and African trypanosomes)
- Escaping phagocytosis or complement-mediated lysis (the carbohydrate capsule of *Streptococcus pneumoniae* prevents phagocytsosis)
- Inhibiting innate immune mechanisms (viruses produce cytokine homologues that function as antagonists)
- Decreased recognition of infected cells by T cells (herpesviruses alter MHC expression and impair antigen presentation) or compromising lymphocyte function (HIV)

Infections in Immunosuppressed Hosts
(p. 360)

The nature of such infections depends on which effector mechanisms are impaired.

- Genetic immunodeficiencies:

  B cells (X-linked agammaglobulinemia is associated with *S. pneumoniae, Haemophilus influenzae, S. aureus,* rotavirus, and enterovirus infections)
  Complement proteins (*S. pneumoniae, H. influenzae,* and *Neisseria meningitidis* infections)
  Neutrophil function (*S. aureus* infections)

- Acquired immunodeficiencies: HIV infection kills T-helper cells, and is associated with viral (herpes simplex and varicella-zoster), bacterial (many), and parasitic infections (cryptococcus).

- Immunosuppression in organ transplantation or during bone marrow engraftment renders patients susceptible to virtually all organisms, including common environmental microbes (*Aspergillus* and *Pseudomonas*).

SPECIAL TECHNIQUES FOR DIAGNOSING INFECTIOUS AGENTS (p. 361)

Some infectious agents can be directly observed in hematoxylin and eosin–stained sections (e.g., CMV inclusion bodies; *Candida* and *Mucor;* most protozoans; all helminths). Most microbes are best visualized after special stains that take advantage of particular cell wall characteristics (Table 8–2). In addition, cultures of lesional tissues may be performed to speciate organisms and to determine drug sensitivity. Nucleic acid tests are used to diagnose *M. tuberculosis, N. gonnorrhoeae,* and *Chlamydia trachomatis,* and to quantify HIV, HBV, and HCV to monitor response to treatment.

TABLE 8–2 Special Techniques for Diagnosing Infectious Agents

Technique	Organisms
Gram stain	Most bacteria
Acid-fast stain	Mycobacteria, nocardiae (modified)
Silver stains	Fungi, legionellae, pneumocystis
Periodic acid–Schiff stain	Fungi, amebae
Mucicarmine stain	Cryptococci
Giemsa stain	Campylobacteria, leishmaniae, malaria, parasites
Antibody probes	Viruses, rickettsiae
Culture	All classes
DNA probes	Viruses, bacteria, protozoa

SPECTRUM OF INFLAMMATORY RESPONSES TO INFECTION (p. 361)

Although microbes have impressive molecular diversity, tissue responses to them follow five histologic patterns. Notably, similar patterns can be seen in response to physical or chemical agents or in inflammatory diseases of unknown etiology.

Suppurative (Polymorphonuclear) Inflammation (p. 361)

- Inflammation is usually caused by pyogenic bacteria, mostly extracellular gram-positive cocci and gram-negative rods.
- Inflammation results from increased vascular permeability and neutrophil recruitment by bacterial chemoattractants.
- Lesions vary from tiny microabscesses to diffuse involvement of entire lung lobes *(S. pneumoniae);* these may resolve without sequelae (pneumococcal pneumonia) or scar *(Klebsiella pneumoniae).*

Mononuclear and Granulomatous Inflammation (p. 362)

- Usually is induced by viruses, intracellular bacteria, spirochetes, intracellular parasites, and helminths.
- The cell type that predominates depends upon the nature of the host immune response: plasma cells in chancres of primary syphilis, lymphocytes in viral infections of the brain, or macrophages in *M. avium-intracellulare* infections of AIDS patients.
- Granulomatous inflammation, characterized by accumulation of activated macrophages, is usually evoked by slowly dividing pathogens *(M. tuberculosis).*

Cytopathic-Cytoproliferative Inflammation (p. 362)

- Usually induced by viral infections, it is characterized by cell proliferation and necrosis with sparse inflammation
- May show inclusion bodies (CMV), polykaryons (measles viruses), blisters (herpesviruses), or warty excrescences (papillomaviruses).

Necrotizing Inflammation (p. 362)

- Caused by rampant viral infection (fulminant HBV infection), secreted bacterial toxins *(Clostridium perfringens)*, or direct protozoan cytolysis of host cells *(E. histolytica)*
- Results in severe tissue necrosis in the absence of inflammation

Chronic Inflammation and Scarring (p. 363)

- Outcomes range from complete healing to scarring; excessive scarring may cause dysfunction (schistosomiasis).
- Inflammation may be severe despite a paucity of organisms *(M. tuberculosis)*.

The patterns of inflammation may be mixed because of multiple simultaneous infections; the same microbe may also cause different patterns in different patients due to host idiosyncratic responses (e.g., mostly lymphocytes in patients exhibiting *tuberculoid leprosy* and mostly macrophages in patients exhibiting *lepromatous leprosy*). Patterns should be consistent with the organisms cultured or identified by microscopy.

VIRAL INFECTIONS (p. 363)

Transient Infections

Viruses that cause transient infections are structurally heterogenous, but each elicits an immune response that effectively eliminates the virus.

Measles (Rubeola) (p. 363)

- An RNA paramyxovirus, it is a leading cause of vaccine-preventable death and illness worldwide.
- Most hosts develop T cell–mediated immunity that controls the viral infection; the characteristic measles rash is due to hypersensitivity to viral antigens in the skin.
- Subacute sclerosing panencephalitis and inclusion body encephalitis (in immunocompromised individuals) are rare late complications.
- Ulcerated mucosal lesions in the oral cavity near the opening of Stensen ducts (pathognomonic *Koplik spots*) show necrosis, neutrophils, and neovascularization.
- Lymphoid organs exhibit marked follicular hyperplasia, large germinal centers, and pathognomonic multinucleated giant cells with eosinophilic nuclear and cytoplasmic inclusion bodies, called *Warthin-Finkeldey cells* (also seen in lungs and sputum).

Mumps (p. 364)

- This paramyxovirus is related to measles virus, respiratory syncytial virus (major cause of infantile lower respiratory infections), and parainfluenzavirus (common cause of croup).
- It causes transient inflammation and enlargement of the parotid glands; less often mumps spreads to other sites including the testes, pancreas, and central nervous system.

- Lesions show interstitial edema and diffuse macrophage, lymphocyte, and plasma cell infiltrates.

Poliovirus (p. 364)

- Poliovirus is a spherical, unencapsulated RNA enterovirus. Other members of the enterovirus family cause rashes (coxsackievirus A), conjunctivitis (enterovirus 70), meningitis (coxsackievirus and echovirus), myopericarditis (coxsackievirus B), and jaundice (hepatitis A).
- Although usually asymptomatic, poliovirus invades the central nervous system in 1 of 100 infected persons, replicating in motor neurons of the spinal cord (causing muscular paralysis) or brain stem (*bulbar poliomyelitis* potentially causing respiratory paralysis).
- Poliovirus is the target of a worldwide vaccination campaign. Each of the three major strains of the virus is included in the Salk formalin-fixed (killed) and the Sabin oral, attenuated (live) vaccines.

West Nile Virus (p. 364)

- West Nile virus is an arthropod-borne virus *(arbovirus)* of the flavivirus group; the group also includes viruses causing dengue fever, Eastern encephalitis, and yellow fever.
- The virus is normally transmitted by mosquitoes to birds (the major viral reservoir) and mammals; humans are usually only incidental hosts.
- CNS complications (meningitis, encephalitis, meningoencephalitis) develop in roughly 1 of 150 clinically apparent infections, with acute flaccid paralysis clinically indistinguishable from polio. Rarely, patients can develop hepatitis, myocarditis, or pancreatitis.
- Immunosuppressed and elderly individuals are at greatest risk. Development of meningoencephalitis carries a 10% mortality rate; survivors may exhibit long-term cognitive and neurologic impairment.

Viral Hemorrhagic Fevers (p. 365)

- These systemic infections are characterized by fever and hemorrhage, and caused by enveloped RNA viruses from four different families (arenaviruses, filoviruses, bunyaviruses, and flaviviruses).
- Viral hemorrhagic fever (VHF) viruses are transmitted to humans by infected insects or animals; the spectrum of illness ranges from mild acute disease (fever, headache, rash, myalgia, neutropenia, and thrombocytopenia) to severe life-threatening hemodynamic deterioration and shock.
- Most VHF viruses infect endothelial cells; hemorrhagic manifestations are due to endothelial or platelet dysfunction or to thrombocytopenia.

Chronic Latent Infections (Herpesvirus Infections) (p. 365)

These large, encapsulated double-stranded DNA viruses cause acute infection followed by latent infection in which the virus persists in a noninfectious form, with periodic reactivation and shedding of infectious virus.

Herpes Simplex Virus (p. 365)

- Herpes simplex virus (HSV) lesions range from self-limited cold sores and gingivostomatitis (HSV-1), to genital sores (mainly HSV-2) and corneal blindness (HSV-1 is the major infectious cause of corneal blindness in the United States), to life-threatening disseminated visceral infections and encephalitis.
- In primary infections, HSV replicates in skin and mucous membranes (at the site of viral entry) causing vesicular lesions.
- During reactivation, HSV, residing latent in neurons, spreads from regional ganglia back to skin or mucous membranes.
- HSV lesions show large, pink-purple, virion-containing intranuclear inclusions, compressing host chromatin against the nuclear membrane *(Cowdry-type A inclusions)*.
- HSV also produces characteristic inclusion-bearing multi-nucleated syncytia; these may be visualized from smears of fluid from intraepithelial blisters *(Tzanck preparation)*.
- HSV corneal lesions include:

    Herpes stromal keratitis with mononuclear cell infiltrates around keratinocytes and endothelial cells; neovascularization, scarring, opacification of the cornea, and blindness may result.

    Herpes epithelial keratitis with viral-induced epithelial cytolysis.

Cytomegalovirus (p. 366)

- CMV infection is nearly always asymptomatic in healthy children and adults, but may manifest as a mononucleosis-like syndrome. In neonates and immunosuppressed patients, CMV causes esophagitis, colitis, hepatitis, pneumonitis, renal tubulitis, chorioretinitis, and meningoencephalitis.
- Infection is spread by intrauterine or perinatal transmission, in mother's milk, respiratory droplets, saliva, semen and vaginal fluid, and iatrogenically in blood transfusions or by transplanting infected grafts.
- Although 95% of congenitally infected infants are asymptomatic, CMV can produce cytomegalic inclusion disease (CID) in infants, especially if the initial maternal infection occurs during pregnancy. CID manifestations include hemolytic anemia, jaundice, hepatosplenomegaly (due to extramedullary hematopoiesis), pneumonitis, deafness, chorioretinitis, brain damage, and thrombocytopenia.
- CMV is the most common opportunistic pathogen in AIDS.
- Disseminated CMV in immunocompromised hosts is life-threatening; lungs, gastrointestinal tract, and retina are primarily affected, with associated focal necrosis and minimal inflammation.
- CMV infection causes marked cellular enlargement, with characteristic large purple intranuclear inclusions surrounded by a clear halo, as well as smaller basophilic cytoplasmic inclusions.

Varicella-Zoster Virus (p. 368)

- Acute VZV infection causes *chickenpox;* reactivation of latent VZV causes *shingles* (or *herpes zoster*).
- VZV infects mucous membranes, skin, and neurons, establishing a latent infection in sensory ganglia.

- VZV is transmitted by aerosols, disseminates hematogenously, and causes vesicular skin lesions (chickenpox) initially on the trunk with progression to head and extremities.
- Each skin lesion evolves rapidly from a macule to a vesicle, classically resembling "a dew drop on a rose petal."
- Histologically, vesicles contain epithelial cell intranuclear inclusions and blisters identical to HSV.
- Shingles occurs when latent VZV in dorsal root ganglia reactivates, infecting sensory nerves that carry viruses to the skin, and causing painful vesicular lesions, typically in a dermatomal distribution.

Chronic Productive Infections (p. 368)

In some infections, the immune system cannot eliminate the virus, resulting in persistent viremia. High mutation rates (e.g., in HIV and HBV) may be a mechanism to evade the immune system.

Hepatitis B Virus (p. 369) (see also Chapter 18)

- DNA virus member of the hepadnavirus family and the etiologic agent of "serum hepatitis," HBV is a significant cause of acute and chronic liver disease.
- HBV can be transmitted percutaneously, perinatally, and sexually.
- The DNA genome is synthesized by reverse transcription of an RNA template; lack of a proofreading function in the reverse transcriptase leads to the characteristically high mutation rate.
- HBV infects hepatocytes; cellular injury occurs mainly due to immune responses to infected liver cells and *not* cytopathic effects of the virus.
- The effectiveness of the cytotoxic T-cell immune response largely determines whether a person clears the virus or becomes a chronic *carrier*.
- Chronic hepatitis is associated with lymphocytic inflammation, apoptotic hepatocytes, and progressive destruction of the liver parenchyma; liver cirrhosis and increased risk for hepatocellular carcinoma may result.

Transforming Infections (p. 369)

Viruses implicated in causing human cancer include Epstein-Barr virus (EBV), human papillomavirus (HPV), and human T-cell lymphotropic virus 1 (HTLV-1).

Epstein-Barr Virus (p. 369)

- EBV causes *infectious mononucleosis,* a benign, self-limited lymphoproliferative disease characterized by fever, sore throat, generalized lymphadenopathy, splenomegaly, and increased white blood cell count in the blood (as high as 18,000 cells/µL, 95% of which are activated "atypical" cytototoxic T lymphocytes).
- EBV infection begins in nasopharyngeal and oropharyngeal epithelial cells, followed by infection of B cells in underlying lymphoid tissues. B cells become the eventual reservoir of latent infection. T-cell counts increase as a response to clear the EBV-infected B cells.

- The lymph nodes in the posterior cervical, axillary, and groin regions are enlarged, show increased numbers of T cells in their paracortical zones, and contain large binucleate cells, Reed-Sternberg–like cells.
- In immunocompromised individuals, EBV is associated with B-cell lymphoma (see Chapter 14).
- In EBV-associated *Burkitt's lymphoma,* there is a characteristic 8:14 translocation of the c-*myc* oncogene into the immunoglobulin heavy chain region.

Human Papillomavirus (p. 371)

- Nonenveloped DNA papovaviruses, HPVs are transmitted mainly by skin or genital contact.
- HPVs cause benign tumors of squamous cells of the skin (warts). Some HPV serotypes are associated with cervical or anogenital squamous cell carcinoma.
- HPVs cause characteristic perinuclear vacuolization of epithelial cells *(koilocytosis).*
- HPV proteins promote cell growth; HPV E6 and E7 gene products dysregulate the cell cycle and may thereby promote malignancy.

BACTERIAL INFECTIONS (p. 371)

Gram-Positive Bacterial Infections (p. 371)

Staphylococci and streptococci are commensal *cocci* (round); *Corynebacterium diphtheriae, L. monocytogenes,* and *B. anthracis* are *bacilli* (rod-shaped).

Staphylococcal Infections (p. 371)

These cocci grow in clusters.

- *S. aureus* causes skin infections, osteomyelitis, pneumonia, endocarditis, food poisoning, and toxic shock syndrome; the organism causes pyogenic inflammation that is distinctive for its local destructiveness.
- Virulence factors include:
  Surface proteins that allow host cell adherence
  Enzymes that degrade host proteins, promoting invasion and tissue destruction
  Toxins that damage host cell membranes (hemolysins), or induce skin sloughing (exfoliative toxins), vomiting (enterotoxins), or shock (via superantigens)
- Less virulent staphylococci infect catheterized patients, patients with prosthetic heart valves, or intravenous drug abusers *(S. epidermidis),* or cause urinary tract infections *(Staphylococcus saprophyticus).*

Streptococcal Infections (p. 373)

These facultative or obligate anaerobic gram-positive cocci grow in pairs or chains. The bacteria are classified by the pattern of hemolysis on blood agar: β (complete or clear hemolysis), α (partial or green hemolysis), and γ (no hemolysis, rarely pathogenic).

- β-Hemolytic streptococci are grouped by their carbohydrate (Lancefield) antigens and include the following:

Streptococcus pyogenes (group A) causes pharyngitis, scarlet fever, erysipelas, impetigo, rheumatic fever, toxic shock syndrome, necrotizing fasciitis, and glomerulonephritis.

Streptococcus agalactiae (group B) colonizes the female genital tract and causes chorioamnionitis in pregnancy, as well as neonatal sepsis and meningitis.

- α-Hemolytic streptococci include:

S. pneumoniae, a common cause of adult community-acquired pneumonia and meningitis

Viridans-group streptococci, a normal component of the oral flora, which cause dental caries *(Streptococcus mutans)* and endocarditis

- *Enterococci* (previously classified as streptococci but now a separate genus) cause endocarditis and urinary tract infections.

- *Streptococcus* carries several virulence factors:

Capsules resist phagocytosis *(S. pyogenes* and *S. pneumoniae)*.

M-proteins inhibit the alternate pathway of complement activation *(S. pyogenes)*.

Pneumolysin destroys host-cell membranes and damages tissue *(S. pneumoniae)*.

- Streptococcal infections are characterized by diffuse interstitial neutrophilic infiltrates with minimal host tissue destruction.

Diphtheria (p. 374)

C. diphtheriae is a slender gram-positive rod with clubbed ends.

- Diphtheria is a life-threatening disease characterized by a durable membrane at the site of *C. diphtheriae* growth in the oropharynx, and exotoxin-mediated damage to the heart, nerves, and other organs.
- Diphtheria toxin is a phage-encoded two-component toxin; an A subunit blocks protein synthesis by ADP ribosylation of elongation factor-2 (leading to inactivation); the B fragment binds to the cell surface and facilitates entry of the A subunit.
- Release of toxin in the pharynx causes epithelial necrosis with a fibrinosuppurative exudate.

Listeriosis (p. 375)

L. monocytogenes is a gram-positive, facultative intracellular bacillus.

- *Listeria* causes food-acquired sepsis and meningitis in elderly and immunosuppressed people, and placental infections in pregnant women with consequent neonatal infections *(granulomatosis infantiseptica)*.
- *L. monocytogenes* enters epithelial cells by binding E-cadherin and stimulating phagocytosis; the bacillus then uses listeriolysin O and two phospholipases to degrade the phagolysosome membrane to escape into the cytoplasm.
- In the cytoplasm, a bacterial protein (ActA) induces actin polymerization to propel the bacteria into adjacent cells.
- *L. monocytogenes* evokes exudative inflammation with numerous neutrophils.

Anthrax (p. 375)

B. anthracis is a spore-forming gram-positive bacillus common in animals having contact with spore-contaminated soil.

- Humans contract anthrax through exposure to contaminated animal products or powdered spores (a biologic weapon).
- Three major anthrax syndromes are:

  Cutaneous: painless, pruritic papules developing into edematous vesicles followed by a black eschar

  Inhalational: rapidly leads to sepsis, shock, and frequently death

  Gastrointestinal: contracted by eating contaminated meat; causes severe, bloody diarrhea and often death

- Anthrax toxin comprises a B subunit (protective factor) and one of two A subunits (edema factor or lethal factor) that act in host cell cytoplasm:

  Edema factor converts ATP to cyclic adenosine monophosphate (cAMP) leading to cellular water efflux.

  Lethal factor is a protease that causes cell death by destroying mitogen-activated protein kinase kinases.

- Anthrax lesions exhibit necrosis with neutrophilic and macrophage infiltration, and large, rectangular gram-positive extracellular bacteria in chains.

Nocardia (p. 376)

Nocardia asteroides is an aerobic gram-positive bacterium growing in branched chains.

- *N. asteroides* causes opportunistic, indolent respiratory infections frequently with CNS dissemination.
- Nocardiosis elicits a suppurative response, surrounded by granulation tissue and fibrosis. Irregularly stained gram-positive organisms in branching filaments will also stain with modified acid-fast protocols (Fite-Faraco stain).

Gram-Negative Bacterial Infections (p. 377)

Some gram-negative pathogens are discussed in the appropriate chapters of organ systems. Anaerobic gram-negative organisms are considered later in this chapter.

Neisserial Infections (p. 377)

Neisseria are aerobic, gram-negative diplococci.

- *N. meningitidis* causes suppurative, bacterial meningitis in individuals typically 5 to 19 years old.

  Bacteria colonize the oropharynx and spread by the respiratory route.

  Meningitis occurs when people living in crowded quarters (college dormitories) acquire serotypes to which they are not immune.

  Meningitis risk is higher with C5 to C9 complement deficiencies.

- *N. gonorrhoeae* is the second most common sexually transmitted bacterial infection in the United States.

In males it causes symptomatic urethritis.

In women it is often asymptomatic and, if untreated, can lead to pelvic inflammatory disease, infertility, and ectopic pregnancy.

In adults, rare disseminated infections cause septic arthritis and hemorrhagic rash.

Neonatal infections cause blindness and, rarely, sepsis.

Organisms elicit acute purulent responses; if untreated, granulation tissue and scarring result.

- *Neisseria* organisms use antigenic variation to evade immune responses. These arise by expression of alternative genes for adhesive pili and OPA proteins (so-called because they make cultured bacterial colonies opaque).

Whooping Cough (p. 378)

Bordetella pertussis is a gram-negative coccobacillus.

- Whooping cough is a communicable illness characterized by paroxysms of violent coughing.
- Coordinated expression of virulence factors is regulated by the *Bordetella* virulence gene locus (*bvg*).
- Pertussis toxin ADP ribosylates and inactivates guanine nucleotide-binding proteins; as a result, G proteins cannot transduce plasma membrane receptor signals.
- Infection causes laryngotracheobronchitis with mucosal erosion, and mucopurulent exudate associated with peripheral lymphocytosis.

Pseudomonas Infection (p. 378)

Pseudomonas aeruginosa is an opportunistic aerobic gram-negative bacillus.

- This pathogen is frequently seen in patients with cystic fibrosis, burns, or neutropenia.
- This organism has co-regulated pili and adherence proteins (bind to epithelial cells and lung mucin), endotoxin, and exotoxin A (inhibits protein synthesis by the same mechanism as diphtheria toxin).
- In patients with cystic fibrosis, *P. aeruginosa* in the lungs secretes an exopolysaccharide (alginate) that forms a slimy biofilm that protects bacteria from antibodies, complement, phagocytes, and antibiotics.
- In neutropenic individuals, *Pseudomonas* pneumonia can cause extensive tissue necrosis by vascular invasion with subsequent thrombosis.

Plague (p. 379)

Yersinia is a gram-negative intracellular bacterium with three clinically important species.

- *Yersinia pestis* causes plague; it is transmitted from rodents to humans by flea bites or aerosols.
- *Yersinia enterocolitica* and *Yersinia pseudotuberculosis* cause fecal-oral transmitted ileitis and mesenteric lymphadenitis.
- *Yersinia* toxins (called *Yops*) are injected by bacteria into host phagocytes by a syringe-like mechanism; the toxins block phagocytosis and cytokine production.
- Plague causes lymph node enlargement *(buboes)*, pneumonia, or sepsis, with massive bacterial proliferation, tissue necrosis, and neutrophilic infiltrates.

Chancroid (Soft Chancre) (p. 380)

Chancroid is an acute, ulcerative genital infection caused by *Hemophilus ducreyi,* most common in Africa and Southeast Asia. The ulcer contains neutrophils and fibrin, with an underlying zone of granulation tissue, necrosis, and thrombosis and a lymphoplasmacytic infiltrate.

Granuloma Inguinale (p. 380)

Granuloma inguinale is a sexually transmitted disease caused by *Calymmatobacterium donovani,* a minute, encapsulated coccobacillus.

- Infection begins as a papule on the genitalia or extragenital sites (oral mucosa or pharynx) that ulcerates and granulates to form a soft, painless mass.
- Left untreated, the lesion may scar and cause urethral, vulvar, or anal strictures.
- Histologic examination reveals epithelial hyperplasia at the borders of the ulcer with underlying neutrophils and mononuclear inflammatory cells.

Mycobacteria (p. 381)

Mycobacteria are aerobic bacilli that grow in chains and have a waxy cell wall composed of mycolic acid; the cell wall retains certain dyes after acid treatment (hence the name *acid-fast bacilli*).

Tuberculosis (p. 381)

M. tuberculosis causes tuberculosis, the second leading infectious cause of death in the world, after HIV. Tuberculosis affects 1.7 billion people worldwide and kills 1.7 million people each year. Over 50 million people worldwide are coinfected with HIV and *M. tuberculosis*, leading to particularly severe tuberculosis. There are about 16,000 new cases of tuberculosis in the United States annually, most among immigrant, economically disadvantaged, jailed, or HIV-infected individuals.

- Outcomes related to *M. tuberculosis* infections depend upon host immunity; immune responses can both control infections as well as contribute to the pathologic manifestations of disease:

  Macrophages phagocytize inhaled *M. tuberculosis* after binding bacterial wall lipoarabinomannan, as well as complement that has opsonized the bacteria.

  Within macrophages, *M. tuberculosis* blocks phagosome-lysosome fusion, allowing unchecked bacterial proliferation in the phagosome.

  Within 2 to 4 weeks of infection, T lymphocytes specific for *M. tuberculosis* proliferate and produce IFN-γ (interferon-γ).

  IFN-γ activates macrophages to kill bacteria via inducible nitric oxide synthase producing bactericidal nitric oxide (see Chapter 2).

- After the T-cell delayed-type hypersensitivity to the bacterium develops, intradermal injection of purified protein derivative (PPD) of the bacteria will result in local induration and permit diagnosis of current (or previous) infection.

- *Primary tuberculosis* occurs in previously unexposed (unsensitized) people:

  95% of people have asymptomatic infections with a persistent, latent lung infection focus.

  5% have symptomatic infections with lobar consolidation, hilar adenopathy, and pleural effusion.

  Rare lymphohematogenous spread can lead to tuberculous meningitis and *miliary tuberculosis*.

- *Secondary tuberculosis* occurs in a previously exposed (sensitized) host:

  Infection usually occurs from reactivation of latent infection when immune resistance is weakened.

  Typically, infection causes cavitation in apex of upper lung lobes, with associated low-grade fever, night sweats, and weight loss.

- Manifestations of tuberculosis in HIV depends on the extent of immunosuppression:

  More than 300 CD4 cells/mm^3: similar to secondary tuberculosis.

  Fewer than 200 CD4 cells/mm^3: similar to progressive primary tuberculosis.

  Extrapulmonary involvement is more common with advanced HIV.

- Diagnosis of tuberculosis may be made by:

  Identifying acid-fast bacilli in sputum or tissue

  Culture of *M. tuberculosis* from sputum or tissue (allows drug sensitivity testing)

  Polymerase chain reaction is highly sensitive

- The pathologic appearance of tuberculosis depends on disease stage, infection site, and immune status.

  Caseating granulomas are characteristic of tuberculosis; central necrotic tissue is surrounded by lymphocytes and activated macrophages (see Chapter 2).

  In primary tuberculosis, there are lung and draining lymph node granulomas, known as the *Ghon complex*.

  In secondary tuberculosis, the initial lesion is a circumscribed focus of caseation, usually involving the apical pleura.

  Secondary pulmonary tuberculosis may heal with fibrosis (spontaneously or after therapy). Alternatively, it may progress to rupture into blood vessels, causing hematogenous spread, or into airways, releasing bacteria during coughing.

Mycobacterium avium-intracellulare *Complex*
(p. 386)

These common environmental bacteria cause widely disseminated infections (characterized by abundant acid-fast organisms) in immunocompromised hosts (e.g., advanced HIV).

Leprosy (p. 387)

Leprosy (Hansen disease) is a slowly progressive infection caused by *Mycobacterium leprae;* it affects skin and peripheral nerves with resultant disabling deformities.

- Inhaled *M. leprae* are phagocytized by monocytes and pulmonary macrophages, with subsequent spread through the blood; however, they grow primarily only in cooler tissues of the periphery.

- Leprosy has two patterns of disease (depending on the host immune response):

  Tuberculoid leprosy: insidious, dry, scaly skin lesions lacking sensation, with asymmetric peripheral nerve involvement.

  Lepromatous (anergic) leprosy: disfiguring cutaneous thickening and nodules, with nervous system damage due to mycobacterial invasion into perineural macrophages and Schwann cells.

  Tuberculoid leprosy is associated with a T-helper type 1 response (IFN-γ), and lepromatous leprosy is associated with an ineffective T-helper type 2 response (see Chapter 6).

Spirochetes (p. 388)

Spirochetes are gram-negative, slender corkscrew-shaped bacteria with axial periplasmic flagella. An outer sheath membrane can mask bacterial antigens from host immune responses.

Syphilis (p. 388)

Treponema pallidum causes syphilis, a sexually or transplacentally transmitted infection.

- *Primary syphilis* occurs about 3 weeks after sexual contact with an infected person.

  A firm, nontender, raised, red lesion *(chancre)* forms on the penis, cervix, vaginal wall, or anus; this will heal even without therapy.

  Treponemes are present at the chancre surface and in the associated exudate (demonstrable by special techniques); there is an underlying infiltrate of plasma cells, macrophages, and lymphocytes, with a proliferative endarteritis.

- *Secondary syphilis* occurs 2 to 10 weeks later in 75% of untreated patients, with cutaneous spread of spirochetes (causing maculopapular, scaly, or pustular lesions and superficial erosions in mucocutaneous tissues).

  Superficial lesions are painless and contain infectious spirochetes.

  Lymphadenopathy, mild fever, malaise, and weight loss are common.

  Mucocutaneous lesions show plasma cell infiltrates and obliterative endarteritis.

- *Tertiary syphilis* occurs in one third of untreated patients, after a long latent period (>5 years).

  Cardiovascular syphilis (>80% of tertiary syphilis) involves aortitis (due to endarteritis of the aortic vasa vasorum) and causes aortic root and arch dilation, with resulting aneurysms and aortic valve insufficiency.

  Neurosyphilis can be symptomatic (meningovascular disease, *tabes dorsalis,* and a generalized brain parenchymal disease) or asymptomatic (CSF abnormalities only, with pleocytosis, increased protein, decreased glucose).

"Benign" tertiary syphilis is associated with necrotic, rubbery masses *(gummas)*, which form in various sites (bone, skin, oral mucosa).

- *Congenital syphilis* usually occurs with maternal primary or secondary syphilis.

  Intrauterine and perinatal death each occur in 25% of untreated cases.

  Early congenital syphilis includes nasal discharge, skin sloughing, hepatomegaly, and skeletal abnormalities.

  Late manifestations include notched central incisors, deafness, and interstitial keratitis with blindness *(Hutchinson triad)*.

- Serologic tests for syphilis:

  Treponemal antibody tests measure antibodies reactive with *T. pallidum.*

  Nontreponemal tests (VDRL, RPR) measure antibody to cardiolipin phospholipid.

  Both tests become positive about 6 weeks after infection and are positive during secondary syphilis; nontreponemal test may become negative with time or treatment, but treponemal antibody tests remain positive.

Relapsing Fever (p. 391)

Relapsing fever is caused by *Borrelia* species, and is characterized by chills, fever, headache, and fatigue, followed by disseminated intravascular coagulation and multiorgan failure.

- Epidemic relapsing fever is caused by body louse-transmitted *Borrelia recurrentis*, often in conditions of poverty or overcrowding.
- Endemic relapsing fever is caused by several different *Borrelia* species, transmitted from small animals to humans by *Ornithodorus* (soft-bodied) ticks.
- Spirochetes are found in blood smears obtained during febrile periods; relapses are due to ongoing variation of the major surface protein, allowing the organism to repeatedly escape host antibody responses.

Lyme Disease (p. 392)

Lyme disease is caused by *B. burgdorferi* transmitted to people from rodents by *Ixodes* ticks.

- In the United States, Lyme disease incidence doubled from 1991 to 2000; most cases occur in the Northeast and Midwest.
- Lyme disease is divided into three stages.

  Stage 1: Spirochetes multiply at the site of the tick bite, causing an expanding area of redness, often with a pale center *(erythema chronicum migrans)*, fever, and lymphadenopathy.

  Stage 2: Spirochetes spread hematogenously, causing secondary skin lesions, lymphadenopathy, migratory joint and muscle pain, cardiac arrhythmias, and meningitis.

  Stage 3: A few years later, borreliae can cause encephalitis and a chronic, occasionally destructive, arthritis.

- *B. burgdorferi* evades antibody-mediated immunity through antigenic variation.
- A distinctive feature of Lyme arthritis is an arteritis resembling that seen in lupus erythematosus.

Anaerobic Bacteria (p. 393)

Existing within sites of the body normally exhibiting relatively low oxygen tension (intestine, vagina, oral recesses), these organisms cause disease when introduced into sterile sites, or when they overgrow and exceed the natural balance of microbial flora (e.g., *C. difficile* colitis following antibiotic treatment). Environmental anaerobes also cause disease.

Abscesses (p. 393)

Abscesses are caused by mixed bacteria flora, averaging 2.5 species of bacteria, 1.6 of which are anaerobic and 0.9 of which are aerobic or facultative. Commensal bacteria from adjacent sites are the usual cause of abscesses, so the species in the abscess are typically those found in the normal flora.

- Head and neck abscesses derive from oral flora *(Prevotella* and *Porphyromonas*, mixed with *S. aureus* and *S. pyogenes).*
- Abdominal abscesses derive from gastrointestinal tract species *(Bacteroides fragilis, Peptostreptococcus* and *Clostridium* species, and facultative *E. coli).*
- Genital tract abscesses in women (e.g., Bartholin's cyst abscesses and tubo-ovarian abscesses) are caused by anaerobic gram-negative bacilli, including *Prevotella* species, often mixed with *E. coli* or *S. agalactiae.*
- *Fusobacterium necrophorum*, an oral commensal, causes *Lemierre syndrome,* an infection of the lateral pharyngeal space with septic jugular vein thrombosis.

Clostridial Infections (p. 393)

Clostridium species are gram-positive bacillary anaerobes that produce spores in the soil.

- *C. perfringens* and *Clostridium septicum* cause cellulitis and muscle necrosis in wounds *(gas gangrene),* food poisoning, and small bowel infection in ischemic or neutropenic patients.

  C. perfringens α-toxin has multiple activities (phospholipase C, sphingomyelinase, and release of phospholipid derivatives such as inositol triphosphate, prostaglandins, and thromboxanes).

  Histologically, gangrene exhibits gas bubbles, myonecrosis, hemolysis, and thrombosis; it resembles an infarct but lacks inflammatory cells.

- *Clostridium tetani* in wounds (or the umbilical stump of newborns) releases a neurotoxin (tetanospasmin) that causes tetanus (convulsive contractions of skeletal muscles).

  Tetanus toxoid (formalin-fixed tetanospasmin) is part of DPT (diphtheria, pertussis, and tetanus) immunization.

  Tetanus toxin causes spastic paralysis because it blocks release of the γ-aminobutyric acid neurotransmitter that is responsible for inhibiting motor neuron activity.

- *Clostridium botulinum* grows in canned foods and releases a neurotoxin that causes flaccid paralysis of respiratory and skeletal muscles *(botulism).*

  Botulism toxin binds to motor neuron gangliosides; after entering cells, an A fragment cleaves synaptobrevin, promoting fusion of neurotransmitter vesicles with the neuron membrane and blocking acetylcholine release.

- *C. difficile* overgrows other intestinal flora in antibiotic-treated patients and releases toxins, causing *pseudomembranous colitis*.

  C. difficile produces two glucosyl transferase toxins; toxin A stimulates chemokine production, and toxin B (used in the diagnosis of *C. difficile* infections) causes cytopathic effects in cultured cells.

Obligate Intracellular Bacteria (p. 394)

These bacteria are adapted to the intracellular environment with membrane transporters to capture amino acids and ATP; they only proliferate within host cells.

Chlamydial Infections (p. 394)

Specific *Chlamydia trachomatis* diseases are attributable to particular serotypes: urogenital infections and conjunctivitis (serotypes D through K), *lymphogranuloma venereum* (serotypes L1, L2, and L3), and *trachoma,* an ocular infection of children (serotypes A, B, and C).

- *C. trachomatis* exists in two forms:

  The infectious *elementary body* (EB) is an inactive, spore-like structure.

  Inside host cell endosomes, the EB differentiates into the metabolically active *reticulate body* (RB), that replicates to form new EBs for release.

- Chlamydial infection is the most common bacterial sexually transmitted infection in the world; there are 780,000 cases annually in the United States.

  Although frequently asymptomatic, infections may cause epididymitis, prostatitis, pelvic inflammatory disease, pharyngitis, conjunctivitis, perihepatic inflammation, and proctitis.

  Infections exhibit a mucopurulent discharge containing neutrophils, but no visible organisms by Gram stain.

  CDC recommendations call for treatment of both *C. trachomatis* and *N. gonorrhoeae* when either is diagnosed, due to frequent coinfections.

- Lymphogranuloma venereum is a sporadic genital infection in the United States and western Europe, but is endemic in parts of Asia, Africa, the Caribbean, and South America.

  Lesions contain a mixed granulomatous and neutrophilic response; chlamydial inclusions can be seen in epithelial or inflammatory cells.

Rickettsial Infections (p. 395)

Rickettsiae are insect-transmitted obligate intracellular bacteria causing typhus, spotted fevers, and ehrlichiosis (see Table 8–10 in *Robbins and Cotran Pathologic Basis of Disease,* 7th ed., p. 396).

- *Epidemic typhus (Rickettsia prowazekii)* lesions range from a rash with small hemorrhages, to skin necrosis and gangrene with internal organ hemorrhages.
- CNS typhus nodules show microglial proliferations with T-cell and macrophage infiltration.

- *Rocky Mountain spotted fever (Rickettsia rickettsii)* occurs in the southeastern and south-central United States. A hemorrhagic rash extends over the entire body, including the palms of the hands and soles of the feet.
- Typhus and spotted fever organisms proliferate in endothelial cells, causing endothelial swelling, thrombosis, and vessel wall necrosis, with a perivascular cuff of mononuclear inflammatory cells.
- *Ehrlichiosis* results from infection of neutrophils *(Anaplasma phagocytophila* and *Ehrlichia ewingii)* or macrophages *(Ehrlichia chaffeensis);* it is characterized by fever, headache, and malaise, progressing to respiratory insufficiency, renal failure, and shock.

MYCOLOGIC INFECTIONS (p. 397)

Fungi are eukaryotes that grow mainly by budding (yeasts) or by filamentous extensions called *hyphae* (molds). Some fungi, such as *Candida albicans,* grow mainly as yeast, but also form hyphae. Dimorphic fungi have both a yeast form (at human body temperature) and mold form (at room temperature).

Yeasts (p. 397)

Candidiasis (p. 397)

Candida species, including *C. albicans* and *Candida tropicalis,* are part of the normal flora of the skin, mouth, and gastrointestinal tract; they can cause superficial infections in healthy individuals and disseminated visceral infections in neutropenic patients.

- *Candida* virulence factors include adhesins that mediate binding to host cells, enzymes that contribute to invasiveness, and catalases that aid intracellular survival by resisting phagocyte oxidative killing.
- *Candida* grows best on warm, moist surfaces; it frequently causes vaginitis (particularly during pregnancy), diaper rash, and oral thrush.
- *Candida* infections of the mouth and vagina produce superficial curdy white patches; these are easily detached to reveal a reddened, irritated mucosa.
- Microscopically, lesions contain yeast, hyphae, and pseudohyphae with acute and chronic inflammation, and (sometimes) granulomas.
- Chronic mucocutaneous candidiasis occurs in persons with AIDS, with defective T-cell immunity, or with polyendocrine deficiencies (hypoparathyroidism, hypoadrenalism, and hypothyroidism).
- Severe, invasive candidiasis occurs via blood-borne dissemination in neutropenic persons; typically, microabscesses (with fungi in the center) are surrounded by areas of tissue necrosis.

Cryptococcosis (p. 399)

Cryptococcus neoformans causes meningoencephalitis in patients with AIDS, leukemia or lymphoid malignancies, lupus, sarcoidosis, or organ transplants, or those receiving high-dose corticosteroids.

- Virulence is associated with the capsular polysaccharide; in tissues, the capsule stains bright red with mucicarmine, and in cerebrospinal fluid, it is negatively stained with India ink.
- In healthy individuals, *C. neoformans* can form a solitary pulmonary granuloma; in immunosuppressed patients, it produces small cysts within the gray matter of the brain ("soap bubble lesions"), occasionally with no inflammatory response.

Molds (p. 399)

Aspergillosis (p. 399)

Aspergillus fumigatus is a ubiquitous mold causing allergies and colonization in otherwise healthy persons; in neutropenic persons, it can cause severe sinusitis, pneumonia, and disseminated disease.

- *Aspergillus* species growing on peanuts can secrete the carcinogen *aflatoxin,* a major cause of liver cancer in Africa.
- Allergic bronchopulmonary aspergillosis is a hypersensitivity reaction, associated with asthma.
- Preexisting pulmonary lesions caused by tuberculosis, bronchiectasis, old infarcts, or abscesses may develop local *Aspergillus* colonies *(aspergillomas)* without tissue invasion.
- Invasive aspergillosis is an opportunistic infection of immunosuppressed hosts; primary lesions manifest as necrotizing pneumonia with sharply delineated, rounded gray foci within hemorrhagic borders (target lesions).
- Invasive aspergilli exhibit septated hyphae branching at acute angles; occasionally, lung cavity lesions will exhibit spore-producing fruiting bodies.
- Aspergilli invade blood vessels with resulting thrombosis; consequently, areas of hemorrhage and infarction are superimposed on necrotizing inflammation.

Zygomycosis (Mucormycosis) (p. 400)

An opportunistic infection in neutropenic patients and ketoacidotic diabetics, zygomycosis is caused by *Zygomycetes* molds *(Mucor, Absidia, Rhizopus,* and *Cunninghamella).*

- The primary site (nasal sinuses, lungs, or gastrointestinal tract) depends on whether the spores (widespread in dust and air) are inhaled or ingested.
- In diabetics, fungus may spread from nasal sinuses to the orbit or brain.
- Zygomycetes are nonseptate with right-angle branching, invade arterial walls, and cause necrosis.

PARASITIC INFECTIONS (p. 401)

Protozoa (p. 401)

Unicellular, eukaryotic organisms, parasitic protozoa are transmitted by insects or by the fecal-oral route. In humans, they mainly occupy the intestine or blood (extracellular or intracellular).

Malaria (p. 401)

Malaria affects 300 million people worldwide, killing 1 million annually. *Plasmodium falciparum* causes severe malaria; three other *Plasmodium* species *(vivax, ovale,* and *malariae)* cause less severe malaria. All species are transmitted by *Anopheles* mosquitoes.

The *Plasmodium* life cycle is schematized in Figure 8–1:

- *Sporozoites* injected by female mosquitoes invade hepatocytes by binding to thrombospondin and properdin receptors.
- Parasites multiply, causing hepatocyte rupture and release of up to 30,000 *merozoites*. *P. vivax* and *P. ovale* also form latent liver *hypnozoites* that can cause late relapses.
- Merozoites bind by a lectin-like molecule to erythrocyte surface glycophorin molecules.
- In erythrocytes, parasites grow as *trophozoites* hydrolyzing red blood cell hemoglobin to generate characteristic *hemozoin* pigment; trophozoites divide to form *schizonts* that form new merozoites that lyse host erythrocytes and release parasites for another round of red blood cell infection.
- A small fraction of the parasites develop into sexual forms *(gametocytes)* that infect mosquitoes when they feed.

P. falciparum has unique virulence factors:

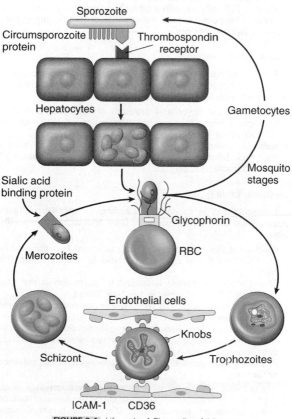

FIGURE 8–1 Life cycle of *Plasmodium falciparum.*

- Infects erythrocytes of any age, leading to high parasitemia; other species infect only new or old red blood cells.
- Causes ischemia by making infected erythrocytes adhere to small vessel endothelium leading to vascular occlusion (*P. falciparum* erythrocyte membrane protein 1 [PfEMP1] binds to CD36, thrombospondin, VCAM-1, ICAM-1, and E-selectin on endothelial cells).
- Endothelial adhesion causes splenic congestion and enlargement, progressing to fibrosis. The liver also becomes enlarged and pigmented with Kupffer cells laden with hemozoin pigment, parasites, and cellular debris.
- Significantly, endothelial adhesion leads to cerebral malaria (main cause of malarial death in children) in which vessels are plugged with parasitized red blood cells with surrounding hemorrhage and ischemia.

Resistance to *Plasmodium* is facilitated by heritable erythrocyte traits:

- Sickle cell trait (HbS) and hemoglobin C (HbC) lessen malaria severity by reducing parasite proliferation.
- Many Africans are not susceptible to *P. vivax* infection because they lack the erythrocyte Duffy blood group antigen that permits parasite binding.
- *P. falciparum* evades the immune response by antigenic variation of PfEMP1; repeated infections frequently produce an immune response repertoire capable of minimizing subsequent disease severity.

Babesiosis (p. 403)

Babesia microti is a malaria-like protozoan transmitted from white-footed mice to humans by *Ixodes* ticks, or rarely contracted through blood transfusion.

- *Babesiae* cause fever and, through erythrocyte parasitization, cause hemolytic anemia that is particularly severe in debilitated or splenectomized individuals.
- *Babesiae* resemble *P. falciparum* schizont stages, although they lack hemozoin pigment, are more pleomorphic, and form characteristic tetrads.

Leishmaniasis (p. 403)

Leishmaniasis is caused by *Leishmania* species, obligate intracellular parasites transmitted from host to host by sandfly bites.

- *Cutaneous disease* is caused by *L. major* and *L. aethiopica* in the Old World and *L. mexicana* and *L. braziliensis* in the New World.
- *Mucocutaneous disease* is caused by *L. major* in the Old World and *L. braziliensis* in the New World.
- *Visceral disease* is caused by *L. donovani* in the Old World and *L. chagasi* in the New World.
- After transmission, *Leishmania promastigotes* are phagocytosed by macrophages; the acidic phagolysosome stimulates development into *amastigotes*.
- Promastigotes produce two glycoconjugates that enhance virulence:

    Lipophosphoglycan forms a glycocalyx that activates complement (leading to C3b deposition on the parasite surface and increasing phagocytosis) but also inhibits complement action (by preventing membrane attack complex assembly).

gp63 cleaves complement and lysosomal antimicrobial enzymes, and also binds fibronectin to promote promastigote adhesion to macrophages.

- Activation of macrophages by IFN-γ is probably necessary for adequate host defense; activated macrophages kill parasites through toxic metabolites of oxygen and nitric oxide.

African Trypanosomiasis (p. 405)

African trypanosomes are extracellular parasites transmitted by tsetse flies.

- *Trypanosoma brucei rhodesiense* (East Africa) is acute and virulent, and *Trypanosoma brucei gambiense* (West Africa) is chronic.
- African trypanosomes have a variant surface glycoprotein (VSG) that undergoes antigenic variation to evade the host response.
- A chancre forms at the insect bite site; large numbers of parasites are surrounded by a dense, largely mononuclear, inflammatory infiltrate.
- Trypanosomes proliferate in the blood, causing intermittent fevers, lymphadenopathy, splenomegaly, brain dysfunction *(sleeping sickness)*, cachexia, and death.
- Lymph nodes and spleen enlarge as a result of hyperplasia and infiltration by lymphocytes, plasma cells, and parasite-laden macrophages.

Chagas Disease (p. 405)

Chagas disease occurs in South America and is caused by *Trypanosoma cruzi,* an intracellular protozoan.

- *T. cruzi* is transmitted between animals (cats, dogs, rodents) and humans by "kissing bugs" (triatomids) that pass parasites in their feces as they bite.
- *T. cruzi* requires exposure to acidic phagolysosome to stimulate *amastigote* development; the organism therefore elicits increased cytosolic calcium in infected cells to promote phagosome-lysosome fusion.
- Acute Chagas disease may be mild or severe (high parasitemia, fever, or progressive cardiac dilation and failure).
- In 20% of patients, chronic Chagas disease occurs years later; manifestations include:

  Myocardial inflammation causing cardiomyopathy and arrhythmias.

  Damage to the myenteric plexus causing colon and esophageal dilation.

Metazoa (p. 406)

Metazoa are multicellular, eukaryotic organisms, typically contracted by eating undercooked meat, through insect bites, or by direct invasion of the host through the skin. Depending on the organism, they may ultimately dwell in the host intestine, skin, lung, liver, muscle, blood vessels, or lymphatics.

Strongyloidiasis (p. 406)

Strongyloides stercoralis larvae live in the soil, penetrate the skin of humans, and travel in the circulation to the lungs, then up the trachea to be swallowed; finally adult female worms produce eggs in the mucosa of the small intestine.

- In mild strongyloidiasis, larvae are present in the duodenal crypts with an underlying eosinophil-rich infiltrate.
- In immunocompromised hosts, larvae hatched in the gut can invade colonic mucosa and reinitiate infection; such hyperinfection results in larval invasion of the colonic submucosa, lymphatics, blood vessels, and other organs.

Tapeworms (Cestodes): Cysticercosis and Hydatid Disease (p. 406)

The tapeworms *Taenia solium* (cysticercosis) and *Echinococcus granulosus* (hydatid disease) have life cycles requiring two hosts: a definitive host in which the worm reaches sexual maturity and an intermediate host.

- *T. solium* can be transmitted to humans in two ways with distinct outcomes:

  Larval cysts (cysticerci) ingested in pork attach to the intestinal wall where they mature and produce egg-laden proglottids (segments) that are passed in stool.

  Intermediate hosts (pigs or humans) can ingest eggs in feces-contaminated food or water; when larvae hatch, they penetrate the gut wall, and disseminate to encyst in many organs, including the brain (causing severe neurologic manifestations).

- *T. saginata* (beef) and *Diphyllobothrium latum* (fish) are acquired by eating undercooked meat; in humans, these parasites live only in the gut.
- Humans are accidental hosts for *E. granulosus* and *E. multilocularis;* these are normally passed only between the definitive (dog or fox) and intermediate (sheep and rodents) hosts.
- Hydatid disease is caused by ingestion of echinoccal eggs in food contaminated with dog or fox feces; the eggs hatch in the duodenum and invade the liver, lungs, or bones, where they form cysts.

Trichinosis (p. 407)

Trichinella spiralis is acquired by ingestion of larvae in undercooked meat from pigs that have themselves been infected by eating infected rats or pork.

- In the gut, larvae develop into adults that release new larvae, that disseminate hematogenously and penetrate muscle cells causing fever, myalgias, eosinophilia, and periorbital edema.
- *T. spiralis* stimulates T-helper type 2 cells, which activate eosinophils and mast cells (typical inflammatory response to nematodes, see Chapter 6) and increase gut contractility to expel worms.
- Cysts form in striated skeletal muscle characterized by coiled larvae surrounded by membrane-bound vacuoles in myocytes, which are in turn surrounded by an eosinophil-rich infiltrate.

Schistosomiasis (p. 408)

Schistosomiasis is caused by *Schistosoma mansoni* (Latin America, Africa, and the Middle East), *S. haematobium*

(Africa), and *S. japonicum* or *S. mekongi* (East Asia); it is transmitted from freshwater snails.

- Larvae penetrate human skin, migrate through the vasculature and settle in the pelvic *(S. haematobium)* or portal (all others) venous systems, where females produce eggs that are released in urine or stool.
- The immune response to *S. mansoni* and *S. japonicum* eggs in the liver causes eosinophil-rich granulomas and fibrosis.
- The early immune response involves T-helper type 1 cells; in chronic infections, T-helper type 2 responses predominate.

Lymphatic Filariasis (p. 409)

Lymphatic filariasis is caused by two nematodes, *Wuchereria bancrofti* (90% of cases) and *Brugia malayi*.

- Larvae are contracted from mosquitoes and develop into adults in lymphatic channels, where they mate and release microfilariae that enter the bloodstream.
- Filariasis can manifest as asymptomatic microfilaremia, chronic lymphadenitis with swelling of the dependent limb or scrotum *(elephantiasis),* or tropical pulmonary eosinophilia.
- Endosymbiotic rickettsia-like *Wolbachia* bacteria infect filaria and are needed for nematode development and reproduction.
- *Brugia malayi* produces numerous molecules to evade or inhibit immune defenses:

  Antioxidant glycoproteins protect from oxygen radical injury.

  Homologues of cystatins, cysteine protease inhibitors, impair antigen presentation.

  Serpins (serine protease inhibitors) inhibit neutrophil proteases.

  Homologues of TGF-β bind to host TGF-β receptors, and down-regulate inflammatory responses.

Onchocerciasis (p. 410)

Onchocerca volvulus is a filarial nematode transmitted by black flies; it affects more than 17 million people in Africa, South America, and Yemen.

- Nematodes mate in the host dermis, surrounded by host inflammatory cells that produce a subcutaneous nodule *(onchocercoma).*
- Female worms release large numbers of microfilariae that accumulate in the skin and eye chambers, causing pruritic dermatitis and blindness.
- Treatment includes doxycycline to kill the symbiotic *Wolbachia* bacteria that live inside *O. volvulus* and are required for worm fertility.

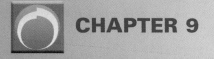

CHAPTER 9

Environmental and Nutritional Pathology

ENVIRONMENT AND DISEASE (p. 415)

Environmental and occupational health encompasses the diagnosis, treatment, and prevention of injuries and illnesses resulting from exposure to exogenous chemical or physical agents. Such exposure may occur in the workplace, as a result of personal habits (e.g., drug or alcohol abuse, or cigarette smoking), or involuntarily (e.g., fetuses exposed *in utero* or children exposed to second-hand smoke). Chronic exposures to low-level contaminants in air, water, and food are also important.

Recognition of Occupational and Environmental Diseases (p. 416)

The magnitude of adverse health effects (accidents, illness, and premature deaths) attributable to occupational and environmental exposures is enormous, affecting 130 million workers in the United States, and tallying an annual workplace fatality rate of 4.8 deaths per 100,000 people. In addition to injuries, occupational exposures contribute to a wide range of illnesses that may lead to premature death (Table 9–1).

Environmental exposure to chemicals is also substantial; more than 80,000 chemicals are currently used in the United States, including some 1500 pesticides and 5500 food additives that can affect water and food supplies. Industrial chemicals and metals are common at hazardous waste sites, and there are 11,300 Superfund-designated waste sites in the United States. To date, only 600 or so chemicals have been formally tested, with 10% shown to cause cancer in rodents.

TABLE 9–1 **Reported Occupational Diseases in the United States in 1997**

Disease	Number of Workers	Percentage
Repeated trauma	276,600	64
Skin disorders	57,900	13
Lung conditions due to toxic exposures	20,300	5
Physical injury	16,600	4
Poisoning	5100	1
Lung disease due to dusts	2900	1
All other illnesses	50,600	12
Total	430,000	100

Data from Levy BS, Wegman DH: Occupational health—An overview. In Levy BS, et al. (eds): Occupational Health. Recognizing and Preventing Work-Related Disease and Injury, 4th ed. Philadelphia, Lippincott Williams & Wilkins, 2000, p 3; Bureau of Labor Statistics, U.S. Department of Labor, *www.hls.gov*

Mechanisms of Toxicity (p. 417)

Toxicology studies the detection, effects, and mechanisms of action of poisons and toxic chemicals. The toxicity of a given compound depends on its structural properties as well as the administered dose. Dose-response curves are produced by exposing laboratory animals to various amounts of a test substance and assaying outcomes. From this information, it is possible to establish the *daily (or annual) threshold limit* or the *permissible exposure level* for occupational exposures:

- *No observed effect level* is a dose that produces no measurable response.
- *Threshold dose* is the amount of chemical producing a measurable response.
- *Ceiling effect* is a plateau at which the response is no longer increased.

Several important toxicologic principles apply (Fig. 9–1):

- Exogenous chemicals are absorbed after ingestion, inhalation, or skin contact, then distributed to various organs.
- Chemicals are metabolized to products that may be more or less toxic than the parent compound. These products then interact with a target molecule, resulting in a toxic effect.
- The site of toxicity is usually where metabolism or excretion of toxic metabolites occurs.
- The dose administered (external dose) may not be the same as the biologic effective dose delivered to the target organ and target macromolecule.

There are several basic principles of *xenobiotic* (meaning chemicals foreign to the biologic system) metabolism (Fig. 9–2):

- Most xenobiotics are *lipophilic* (fat soluble), facilitating bloodstream transport and cell membrane penetration.
- Lipophilic xenobiotics are metabolized to hydrophilic metabolites by two steps:

  Phase I reactions: Polar functional groups are added to the parent compound.

  Phase II reactions: Endogenous substances are conjugated to the phase I metabolite to produce compounds that are more water soluble and therefore more readily excreted.

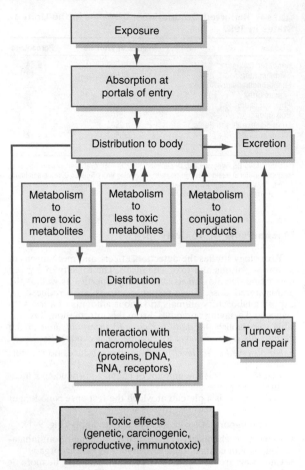

FIGURE 9–1 Absorption and distribution of toxicants. (From Hodgson E, Levi PE: Absorption and distribution of toxicants. In Hodgson E, Levi PE [eds]: A Textbook of Modern Toxicology. Stamford, CT, Appleton & Lange, 1997, p 52.)

- There are genetic variations in the level of activity of xenobiotic-metabolizing enzymes, such as the cytochrome P-450–dependent monooxygenase (P-450) system. People with alleles of the P-450 gene *CYP1A1* that confer higher activity and inducibility may be at increased risk for developing certain cancers.
- Metabolizing enzymes not only modify endogenous compounds, but can also activate xenobiotics to form reactive intermediates and carcinogens. Thus, benzo[a]pyrene, one of several chemical carcinogens present in cigarette smoke, is converted by cytochrome P-450 to a secondary metabolite that binds covalently to DNA and causes lung and skin tumors.
- Multiple pathways may be involved in metabolizing a xenobiotic, and dominance of one pathway over another

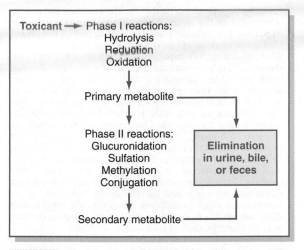

FIGURE 9–2 Biotransformation of lipophilic toxicants to hydrophilic metabolites. (Adapted from Hodgson E: Metabolism of toxicants. In Hodgson E, Levi PE [eds]: A Textbook of Modern Toxicology. Stamford, CT, Appleton & Lange, 1997, p 57.)

may account for individual differences in toxicity and carcinogenicity.

- Endogenous factors, such as nutritional and hormonal status, alter enzyme activities involved in xenobiotic metabolism.
- Exogenous factors, such as drugs or ethanol, can inhibit or induce activities of metabolizing enzymes.
- Repair pathways may modify interactions between active metabolites and target molecules.

Phase I reactions involve the following:

- The P-450 system is located in smooth endoplasmic reticulum, with greatest activity in hepatocytes; it is composed of a complex containing a heme protein (P-450), NADPH–P-450 reductase, and phosphatidylcholine. Different P-450 isozymes have specific tissue distributions and show preferential activity toward different substrates.
- A flavin-containing monooxygenase system is located in liver smooth endoplasmic reticulum. It oxidizes nicotine in cigarette smoke, as well as other amines.
- Peroxidase-dependent co-oxidation, catalyzed by prostaglandin H synthase, occurs in the smooth endoplasmic reticulum of seminal vesicles, kidneys, and urinary bladder. This pathway is involved in the metabolism of 2-naphthylamine, a chemical found in dyes and associated with bladder cancer.

All the oxidative reactions generate oxygen-derived free radicals as byproducts. Reduced glutathione and the mammalian thioredoxin system are the major defense mechanisms against oxygen free radicals and toxic metabolites of xenobiotics. Oxidant stress and tissue injury can occur when these defense mechanisms are overwhelmed.

Phase II reactions involve the following:

- *Glucuronidation:* An alternate pathway for naphthylamine metabolism involves oxidation by cytochrome P-450 followed by hepatic glucuronidation. The resulting glucuronide is excreted in the urine, where it can form a carcinogen, explaining the increased incidence of cancer of the urinary bladder in workers exposed to synthetic dyes.

- *Biomethylation:* Occupational exposure to inorganic mercury ($HgCl_2$) occurs during the manufacture of germicides, fungicides, electronics, and plastics, and can cause necrosis of the renal proximal convoluted tubule. Mercury can also be methylated by aquatic microorganisms; these organisms are subsequently ingested by herbivorous fish, which, in turn, are consumed by carnivorous fish, which may be eaten by humans. This is an example of *bioaccumulation* of a toxic chemical in the environment. Industrial discharge of mercury into a bay in Minamato, Japan, resulted in a *million-fold* bioaccumulation of the toxicant in fish. Methyl mercury is readily absorbed from the gastrointestinal tract; individuals who ingested the fish developed paralysis and subsequently died. In addition, the developing fetus is especially susceptible to even low-level mercury injury, resulting in brain damage, mental retardation, or death.

- *Glutathione conjugation:* A common pathway for xenobiotic metabolism involves conjugation to reduced glutathione. These resulting water-soluble metabolites are readily excreted in bile and urine.

COMMON ENVIRONMENTAL AND OCCUPATIONAL EXPOSURES (p. 419)

Personal Exposures

Tobacco Use (p. 419)

Use of cigarettes, cigars, pipes, and snuff is associated with more deaths and diseases than any other personal, environmental, or occupational exposure.

- Tobacco use is estimated to contribute to 440,000 deaths per year in the United States and is associated with 10 million cases of chronic diseases.
- Smoking is a major risk factor for lung cancer; it is also interacts synergistically with other environmental and occupational exposures.
- Cigarette smoke consists of a particulate phase and a gas phase. The smoke has more than 4000 constituents:
  Chemical carcinogens (at least 43 known) and *carcinogenic metals* (e.g., arsenic, nickel, cadmium, chromium)
  Tumor promoters (e.g., acetaldehyde)
  Irritants (e.g., nitrogen dioxide)
  Cilia toxins (e.g., hydrogen cyanide)
  Carbon monoxide (binds to hemoglobin with high affinity and decreases oxygen delivery to peripheral tissues)
- Cigarette smoke contains nicotine, an alkaloid that readily crosses the blood-brain barrier and stimulates neuronal nicotine receptors. Nicotine is responsible for tobacco addiction.
- Inhaled compounds in cigarette smoke can act directly on the mucous membranes, can be swallowed in saliva, or be absorbed from alveolar capillaries into the bloodstream. They can therefore act locally or on distant target organs, causing diseases ranging from lung cancer and chronic

obstructive pulmonary disease to coronary atherosclerosis and cardiac ischemia. Smoking cessation reduces but does not eliminate the risks of lung cancer and coronary artery disease.

- The fetus is especially vulnerable to the consequences of maternal smoking: As few as 10 cigarettes per day can cause fetal hypoxia, resulting in low birth weight, prematurity, increased incidence of spontaneous abortion, and complications at delivery.
- Cigarette smoking can facilitate transport of other hazardous agents, and exacerbate particulate-associated bronchitis, asthma, and pneumoconiosis (e.g., due to silica or coal dust).
- Tobacco use also increases the prevalence of peptic ulcers, impairs their healing, and increases the likelihood of recurrences.
- *Second-hand* smoke *(passive smoking* or *environmental tobacco smoke)* also increases the risk of lung cancer, ischemic heart disease, and acute myocardial infarction. Maternal smoking increases the risk of sudden infant death syndrome, and children in homes with smokers have increased rates of respiratory and ear infections and asthma exacerbations.

Alcohol Abuse (p. 421)

Ethanol is the most widely used and abused agent throughout the world.

- There are 15 million to 20 million alcoholics in the United States, and approximately 100,000 deaths attributed to alcohol abuse each year.
- The effects of drinking depend on the amount of ethanol consumed per unit of body weight and the time period over which it is ingested. Approximately 12 oz (340 mL) of beer, 4 oz (115 mL) of nonfortified wine, or 1.5 oz (43 mL) of an 86 proof beverage each contain approximately 10 gm of ethanol. A blood alcohol concentration of 80 mg/dL is the legal definition for drunk driving in many states.
- Chronic alcohol use results in psychological and physical dependence, although the biologic basis for this is unknown; there may be a genetic component.
- Ethanol is metabolized by alcohol dehydrogenase in the gastric mucosa and liver, and by cytochrome P-450 and catalase in the liver to produce acetaldehyde. Acetaldehyde is converted to acetic acid by aldehyde dehydrogenase. Genetic polymorphisms in aldehyde dehydrogenase—resulting in delayed ethanol metabolism—are encountered in about 50% of certain Asian populations.

The metabolism of ethanol is directly responsible for most of its toxic and chronic effects (Table 9–2):

- *Liver:* Ethanol can cause *fatty change, acute alcoholic hepatitis,* or *cirrhosis* (Chapter 18). Fatty change is an acute but reversible accumulation of lipid in hepatocytes. Alcoholic hepatitis can produce fever, liver tenderness, and jaundice due to direct ethanol toxicity. Cirrhosis (irreversible damage) occurs in 10% to 15% of alcoholics; it is characterized by a hard, shrunken liver with nodules of regenerating hepatocytes surrounded by dense bands of collagen.

TABLE 9–2 **Mechanisms of Disease Caused by Ethanol Abuse**

Organ System	Lesion	Mechanism
Liver	Fatty change	Toxicity
	Acute hepatitis	
	Alcoholic cirrhosis	
Nervous system	Wernicke syndrome	Thiamine deficiency
	Korsakoff syndrome	Toxicity and thiamine deficiency
	Cerebellar degeneration	Nutritional deficiency
	Peripheral neuropathy	Thiamine deficiency
Cardiovascular system	Cardiomyopathy	Toxicity
	Hypertension	Vasopressor
Gastrointestinal tract	Gastritis	Toxicity
	Pancreatitis	Toxicity
Skeletal muscle	Rhabdomyolysis	Toxicity
Reproductive system	Testicular atrophy	?
	Spontaneous abortion	?
Fetal alcohol syndrome	Growth retardation	Toxicity
	Mental retardation	
	Birth defects	

Data from Rubin E: Alcohol abuse. In Craighead JE (ed): Pathology of Environmental and Occupational Disease. St. Louis, Mosby–Year Book, 1996, p 249; Lewis DD, Woods SE: Fetal alcohol syndrome. Am Fam Physician 50:1025, 1994.

- *Nervous system:* The acute depressive effects and addiction produced by ethanol are attributed to altered membrane fluidity and signal transduction. Thiamine deficiency, common in chronic alcoholics, contributes to neuronal degeneration, reactive gliosis, and cerebellar and peripheral nerve atrophy. The outcome is the ataxia, disturbed cognition, ophthalmoplegia, and nystagmus characteristic of *Wernicke syndrome.* Some alcoholics with poor nutrition develop severe memory loss characteristic of *Korsakoff syndrome.*
- *Cardiovascular system:* Chronic ethanol abuse can cause a dilated cardiomyopathy.
- *Gastrointestinal tract:* Acute gastritis is a direct toxic effect of ethanol.
- *Skeletal muscle:* Direct ethanol toxicity can injure skeletal myocytes, leading to weakness, pain, and myoglobin catabolism.
- *Reproductive system:* Ethanol abuse leads to testicular atrophy in men and decreased fertility in both sexes.
- *Fetal alcohol syndrome:* As little as one maternal drink per day can result in fetal alcohol syndrome. First recognized in 1968, it is characterized by growth and developmental defects, including microcephaly, facial dysmorphology, and malformations of the brain, cardiovascular system, and genitourinary system. Fetal alcohol syndrome is the most common type of preventable mental retardation in the United States, affecting 1200 children per year.
- *Ethanol and cancer:* Alcohol use is associated with increased cancer rates in the oral cavity, pharynx, esophagus, liver, and possibly breast. Although ethanol is not a direct-acting carcinogen, its acetaldehyde metabolite may act as a tumor promoter. Ethanol also induces the P-450 complex enhancing metabolic activation of other carcinogens.
- *Methanol and ethylene glycol* may be ingested accidentally or as inexpensive substitutes for ethanol. Both cause initial

intoxication. However, methanol is metabolized by alcohol dehydrogenase to formaldehyde or formic acid and can cause blindness; ethylene glycol is metabolized to aldehydes and glycolic and oxalic acids and results in renal failure from calcium oxalate obstruction of renal tubules.

Drug Abuse (p. 424)

Drug abuse, addiction, and overdose are serious public health problems. Commonly abused drugs can be classified as sedative hypnotics, psychomotor stimulants, narcotics, or hallucinogens.

- *Sedative hypnotics:* Barbiturates *(downers)* and ethanol both induce sedation and decrease anxiety. Tolerance develops rapidly, causing drug users to increase the dose.
- *Psychomotor stimulants:* Cocaine produces a rapid, short-duration effect characterized by euphoria and increased energy; it inhibits neurotransmitter (dopamine and norepinephrine) reuptake in the central nervous system (and peripheral nervous system), resulting in excess catecholamine stimulation. Acute cocaine overdose produces seizures, cardiac arrhythmias, and respiratory arrest. Chronic abuse causes insomnia, increased anxiety, paranoia, and hallucinations, and is associated with hypertension, strokes, and sudden death. Amphetamines are also potent central nervous system stimulants. Overdose causes sweating, tremors, restlessness, and confusion that may progress to delirium, convulsions, coma, and death.
- *Narcotics:* These drugs relieve pain, but also cause sedation and altered mood. Heroin suppresses anxiety, and induces sedation, mood changes, nausea, and respiratory depression. Chronic abuse leads to tolerance, as well as psychological dependence. Overdose can cause convulsions, cardiorespiratory arrest, and death. Intravenous drug users are susceptible to infections of the skin and subcutaneous tissue, heart valves (particularly tricuspid), liver, and lungs; most infections are caused by staphylococci. Viral hepatitis and AIDS (acquired immunodeficiency syndrome) are common among drug addicts and are acquired by using contaminated needles.
- *Hallucinogens:* Both natural and chemical substances have hallucinogenic properties. Natural hallucinogens include the alkaloid mescaline (isolated from the peyote cactus), and marijuana (isolated from the hemp plant *Cannabis sativa*). The active ingredient in marijuana is tetrahydrocannabinol, which produces a state of relaxation and heightened sensation. Synthetic hallucinogens include phencyclidine (PCP), which causes inebriation, disorientation, and numbness, and lysergic acid diethylamide (LSD), which is absorbed rapidly and causes psychic effects and visual illusions.

Therapeutic Drugs (p. 426)

Adverse reactions refer to untoward effects of drugs given in conventional therapeutic settings (Table 9–3). Some commonly used herbal medicines can also produce adverse effects and potentially serious interactions with prescription drugs (see Table 9–8, in *Robbins and Cotran Pathologic Basis of Disease,* 7th ed., p. 427).

TABLE 9–3　**Mechanisms of Adverse Drug Reactions**

Mechanism	Example	Adverse Effect
Toxicity due to overdose	Acetaminophen	Liver necrosis and failure
Predictable reaction based on pharmacologic mechanism	Nonselective, nonsteroidal anti-inflammatory drugs	Peptic ulcer
Altered drug metabolism related to:		
Thiopurine S-methyltransferase deficiency	Azathioprine	Bone marrow failure
Cytochrome P-450 CYP2C9 variants	Oral anticoagulants	Bleeding
Cytochrome P-450 CYP2D6 variants	Some antipsychotic drugs	Excessive sedation; parkinsonism
N-acetyltransferase, slow acetylator phenotype	Hydralazine	Lupus
Idiopathic	Chloramphenicol	Aplastic anemia

Oral Contraceptives and Hormone Replacement Therapy (p. 427)

Estrogens and oral contraceptives are discussed separately because (i) estrogens for postmenopausal syndrome may be given alone and are usually natural estrogens; and (ii) oral contraceptives contain synthetic estrogens, which are almost always given with progesterone.

- *Oral contraceptives:* Oral contraceptives usually contain a synthetic estradiol and variable amounts of a progestin (combined oral contraceptives). Currently prescribed oral contraceptives contain smaller amounts of estrogens and are associated with fewer side effects. The various pros and cons of oral contraceptives must be balanced against the risk of an unwanted pregnancy.

  Breast carcinoma: Two recent epidemiologic studies showed that past or current use of oral contraceptives was not associated with an increased risk of breast cancer.

  Endometrial cancer: There is no increased risk of endometrial cancer, and these drugs may exert a protective effect.

  Cervical cancer: Although the risk of cervical cancer may be somewhat increased, it could be correlated with increased sexual activity rather than the contraceptives.

  Ovarian cancer: Oral contraceptives protect against ovarian cancer.

  Thromboembolism: Oral contraceptives increase the risk of thrombosis and embolism, especially in carriers of mutations in factor V or prothrombin.

  Hypertension: Newer formulations cause only a slight increase in blood pressure.

  Cardiovascular disease: Nonsmoking, healthy women younger than 45 years of age who use the newer low-estrogen formulations do not incur an increased risk of ischemic heart disease; risk *is* increased in women over age 35 who smoke.

  Hepatic adenoma: There is a well-defined association between oral contraceptives and this benign tumor.

- *Hormone replacement therapy (HRT):* HRT has been used to reduce perimenopausal or postmenopausal hot flashes, vaginal dryness, and sleep disturbances. Long-term therapy may slow the onset of osteoporosis. Recent epidemiologic studies revealed the following risks of HRT:

  Endometrial carcinoma: Unopposed estrogen therapy increases the risk of endometrial cancer three-fold to six-fold after 5 years and more than 10-fold after 10 years, compared with the risk of untreated women. This risk is substantially reduced when progestins are added to the therapeutic regimen.

  Breast carcinoma: There is an increased risk of breast cancer with HRT combined therapy administered for 5 or more years.

  Thromboembolism: The risk of a thromboembolic event is increased two-fold in HRT users, especially within the first year.

  Cholecystitis: The risk of gallbladder disease increases over time.

Acetaminophen (p. 428)

Acetaminophen is a commonly used nonprescription analgesic and antipyretic. When taken in large doses, it causes hepatic necrosis and liver failure.

Aspirin (Acetylsalicylic Acid) (p. 428)

Aspirin overdoses occur from accidental ingestion by young children and in suicide attempts by adults. Initial consequences of an overdose are respiratory alkalosis, followed by metabolic acidosis that can prove fatal. *Chronic aspirin toxicity (salicylism)* may develop in persons who take 3 gm or more daily for chronic inflammatory conditions. Aspirin toxicity is manifested by headache, dizziness, ringing in the ears (tinnitus), difficulty in hearing, mental confusion, drowsiness, nausea, vomiting, and diarrhea. More serious is the development of acute erosive gastritis. Proprietary analgesic mixtures containing aspirin and phenacetin when taken for years have been associated with potentially fatal renal papillary necrosis *(analgesic nephropathy)*.

Outdoor Air Pollution (p. 428)

Epidemiologic research, as well as clinical and toxicologic studies provide evidence for the adverse health effects of air pollutants in the United States and most other industrial countries. Major sources of air pollution are:

- Combustion of fossil fuels in motor vehicles and power plants
- Photochemical reactions producing ozone as a secondary pollutant
- Factories, waste incinerators, smelters

The lung is the major organ affected by outdoor air pollution. Decreased pulmonary function, lung inflammation, increased airway reactivity, diminished mucociliary clearance, and increased infections are all common effects. Especially vulnerable are children and individuals with chronic lung or heart disease. The following major outdoor air pollutants can cause problems:

- *Ozone:* Ozone is a major component of smog. Exposure to as little as 0.08 ppm produces cough, chest discomfort, and inflammation in the lungs. Ozone is highly reactive and oxidizes polyunsaturated lipids to hydrogen peroxide and lipid aldehydes, which act as irritants and induce the release of inflammatory mediators.
- *Nitrogen dioxide:* Nitrogen dioxide is less reactive than ozone. It dissolves in water in the airways to form acids that damage the airway lining.
- *Sulfur dioxide:* Sulfur dioxide is absorbed in the airways where it releases products that cause local irritation.
- *Acid aerosols:* Combustion products of fossil fuels are released into the atmosphere, where the sulfur and nitrogen dioxide are oxidized to sulfuric acid and nitric acid. These products are dissolved in water droplets or absorbed onto particulates and become irritants to the airway epithelium.
- *Particulates:* The deposition and clearance of inhaled particulates depend on their size and shape (Chapter 15). Although it is unclear exactly how these cause injury, it is suspected that the effects are related to free radical generation at the surface of ultrafine particles.

Intense industrial activity and economic growth in Western and developing countries have resulted in serious air pollution. A layer of ozone normally present in the upper atmosphere is important because it prevents solar ultraviolet (UV) light from penetrating the environment where it causes injury by generating free radicals or damaging DNA. Unfortunately, many chemicals destroy ozone; the major offenders are chlorofluorocarbons (CFCs) used as aerosols and refrigerants, and nitrogen dioxide, produced by internal combustion engines. The consequences of the ozone depletion include an increased incidence of skin cancers in humans and injury to other life forms. A closely related problem is global warming. The accumulation of carbon dioxide and other gases in the atmosphere traps the earth's infrared radiation while permitting entrance of visible light and warming solar radiation. The result is accumulation of heat at the earth's surface, the so-called *greenhouse effect.*

Indoor Air Pollution (p. 430)

Levels of indoor air pollutants have increased during the last 30 years owing to improved insulation and fewer air leaks in homes, coupled with increasing reliance on air conditioning rather than open window ventilation. Effects range from increased skin, eye, and airway irritation to respiratory infections to the cancers associated with radon or asbestos exposures. The following are some of the major indoor air pollutants:

- *Carbon monoxide* is an odorless, colorless gas byproduct of combustion of gasoline, oil, coal, wood, or natural gas. Carbon monoxide levels in ambient air should not exceed 9 ppm. Poisoning (displacing oxygen from hemoglobin and thereby causing asphyxia) manifests as headaches, dizziness, loss of motor control, and coma.
- *Nitrogen dioxide* is produced by gas stoves and kerosene heaters; it impairs lung defenses.

- *Wood smoke* is a complex mixture of particulates and other toxic components that can increase the incidence of respiratory infections, especially in children.
- *Formaldehyde* is a soluble, volatile chemical used in the manufacture of many consumer products; it can cause acute irritation of the eyes and upper respiratory tract.
- *Radon* is a radioactive gas formed as a decay product of uranium found naturally in the soil. Radon gas emanating from the earth is prevalent in some mines and homes and may cause lung cancer.
- *Asbestos* was used in homes and public buildings before the 1970s; low levels of fibers have been found in indoor air. Workers who repair or remove asbestos-containing materials are at risk for lung cancer and mesothelioma if respirators are not used.
- *Manufactured mineral fibers,* such as fiberglass, are used for home insulation and can cause skin and lung irritation.
- *Bioaerosols*, such as the bacterial aerosols responsible for *Legionella* pneumonia, are associated with contaminated heating and cooling systems (Chapter 8).

Industrial Exposures (p. 430)

Occupational exposures contribute to diseases that can affect almost all organ systems and result in acute toxicity, hypersensitivity reactions, chronic toxicity, and cancer (Table 9–4).

Volatile Organic Compounds (p. 431)

These compounds typically are used in homes and in industry. High levels of exposure cause headaches, dizziness, and liver or kidney toxicity.

- *Aliphatic hydrocarbons,* such as chloroform and carbon tetrachloride, are widely used as industrial solvents and cleaning agents. These compounds are readily absorbed through the lungs, skin, and gastrointestinal tract. In addition to acute central nervous system depression, they can cause liver and kidney toxicity.
- *Petroleum products,* such as gasoline and kerosene, are quite volatile and are a common cause of poisoning in children. Inhalation of these products causes dizziness, incoordination, and central nervous system depression.
- *Aromatic hydrocarbons,* such as benzene and toluene, are widely used solvents that are hazardous when inhaled. Benzene causes bone marrow toxicity, aplastic anemia, and acute leukemia.

Polycyclic Aromatic Hydrocarbons (p. 431)

Polycyclic aromatic hydrocarbons (three or more fused benzene rings) are produced during fossil fuel combustion and by iron and steel foundries. Benzo[a]pyrene is the prototype of this class of compounds; it is metabolized to reactive intermediates capable of binding DNA. Occupational exposure is associated with an increased risk of lung and bladder cancers. Cigarette smoking is another important source of benzo[a]pyrene.

TABLE 9–4 **Human Diseases Associated with Occupational Exposures**

Organ	Effect	Toxicant
Cardiovascular system	Heart disease	Carbon monoxide, lead, solvents, cobalt, cadmium
Respiratory system	Nasal cancer	Isopropyl alcohol, wood dust
	Lung cancer	Radon, asbestos, silica, bis(chloromethyl)ether, nickel, arsenic, chromium, mustard gas
	Chronic obstructive lung disease	Grain dust, coal dust, cadmium
	Hypersensitivity	Beryllium, isocyanates
	Irritation	Ammonia, sulfur oxides, formaldehyde
	Fibrosis	Silica, asbestos, cobalt
Nervous system	Peripheral neuropathies	Solvents, acrylamide, methyl chloride, mercury, lead, arsenic, DDT
	Ataxic gait	Chlordane, toluene, acrylamide, mercury
	Central nervous system depression	Alcohols, ketones, aldehydes, solvents
	Cataracts	Ultraviolet radiation
Urinary system	Toxicity	Mercury, lead, glycol ethers, solvents
	Bladder cancer	Naphthylamines, 4-aminobiphenyl, benzidine, rubber products
Reproductive system	Male infertility	Lead, phthalate plasticizers
	Female infertility	Cadmium, lead
	Teratogenesis	Mercury, polychlorinated biphenyls
Hematopoietic system	Leukemia	Benzene, radon, uranium
Skin	Folliculitis and acneiform dermatosis	Polychlorinated biphenyls, dioxins, herbicides
	Cancer	Ultraviolet radiation
Gastrointestinal tract	Liver angiosarcoma	Vinyl chloride

Data from Leigh JP, et al: Occupational injury and illness in the United States. Estimates of costs, morbidity, and mortality. Arch Intern Med 157:1557, 1997; Mitchell FL: Hazardous waste. In Rom WN (ed): Environmental and Occupational Medicine, 2nd ed. Boston, Little, Brown, 1992, p 1275; Levi PE: Classes of toxic chemicals. In Hodgson E, Levi PE (eds): A Textbook of Modern Toxicology, Stamford, CT, Appleton & Lange, 1997, p 229.

Plastics, Rubber, and Polymers (p. 432)

Occupational exposure to vinyl chloride monomers used to produce polyvinyl chloride resins is associated with angiosarcoma of the liver. Rubber workers exposed to 1,3-butadiene have an increased risk of leukemia.

Metals (p. 432)

Occupational exposure to metals in mining and manufacturing is associated with acute and chronic toxicity, as well as carcinogenicity (Table 9–5). Although exposure to cobalt, cadmium, chromium, and nickel may present significant occu-

TABLE 9–5　Toxic and Carcinogenic Metals

Metal	Disease	Occupation
Lead	Renal toxicity Anemia, colic Peripheral neuropathy Insomnia, fatigue Cognitive deficits	Battery and ammunition workers, foundry workers, spray painting, radiator repair
Mercury	Renal toxicity Muscle tremors, dementia Cerebral palsy Mental retardation	Chlorine-alkali industry
Arsenic	Cancer of skin, lung, liver	Miners, smelters, oil refinery workers, farm workers
Beryllium	Acute lung irritant Chronic lung hypersensitivity ? Lung cancer	Beryllium refining, aerospace manufacturing, ceramics
Cobalt and tungsten carbide	Lung fibrosis Asthma	Toolmakers, grinders, diamond polishers
Cadmium	Renal toxicity ? Prostate cancer	Battery workers, smelters, welders, soldering
Chromium	Cancer of lung and nasal cavity	Pigment workers, smelters, steel workers
Nickel	Cancer of lung and nasal sinuses	Smelters, steel workers, electroplating

Data from Levi PE: Classes of toxic chemicals. In Hodgson E, Levi PE (eds): A Textbook of Modern Toxicology. Stamford, CT, Appleton & Lange, 1997, p 229; Sprince NL: Hard metal disease. In Rom WN (eds): Environmental and Occupational Medicine, 2nd ed. Boston, Little, Brown, 1992, p 791.

pational hazards, exposure to lead continues to be the most serious public health problem.

Lead is used in the production of batteries, alloys, and ammunition. In some parts of the world, tetraethyl lead is used as a gasoline additive. Environmental sources of lead are urban air from leaded gasoline, soil and house dusts contaminated with leaded paint, and water supplies when there is lead plumbing. Although inhalation is the most important route of occupational exposure, ingested lead from contaminated food and beverages can be absorbed in the gastrointestinal tract. Absorbed lead accumulates in bones and teeth, particularly in children. Lead toxicity is due to the following:

- High affinity for sulfhydryl groups, inhibiting enzyme functions such as those involved in the incorporation of iron into the heme molecule (patients develop hypochromic anemia)
- Competition with calcium ions for storage in bone
- Inhibition of membrane-associated enzymes leading to impaired red blood cell survival (hemolysis), renal damage, and hypertension
- Impaired metabolism of 1,25-dihydroxyvitamin D

Lead contributes to multiple chronic health effects:

- Injury to the central and peripheral nervous systems causes headache, dizziness, and memory deficits in the adult; encephalopathy with acute cerebral edema and mental deterioration occurs in children.

- Changes include a characteristic punctate basophilic stippling of erythrocytes, microcytic hypochromic anemia, and hemolysis.
- Gastrointestinal changes include abdominal pain and anorexia.
- Infants and children are particularly vulnerable to lead toxicity. Up to 10% of preschool children in urban areas have significant blood lead levels (>10 µg/dL). Even at low levels, intellectual impairment, behavioral abnormalities, and learning deficits have been described.

Agricultural Hazards (p. 434)

Agricultural productivity has increased through the use of fertilizers and pesticides; agricultural pesticides are divided into categories depending on the target pest (e.g., insecticides, herbicides, fungicides, rodenticides). All pesticides are toxic to some plant or rodent species and, at higher doses, can also be toxic to farm animals, pets, and humans (Table 9–6). The acute toxicity of pesticides has been established, but the chronic toxicity of these chemicals is less certain; of note, pesticide residues frequently persist in soil and water supplies, and can be routinely found on foods.

- *Organochlorine* insecticides such as *DDT* (dichlorodiphenyltrichloroethane) and *dioxins*, such as TCDD (2,3,7,8-tetrachlorodibenzo-p-dioxin), have low acute toxicity for humans; however, they bioaccumulate and persist in the environment and in adipose tissue. DDT may cause reproductive dysfunction and cancer in humans, although this is controversial. In animals, TCDD is highly toxic, immunosuppressive, teratogenic, and carcinogenic; the defoliant agent orange used in the Vietnam War was contaminated with TCDD.
- *Organophosphate* insecticides, such as malathion, are irreversible inhibitors of cholinesterases and cause abnormal neural synaptic transmission. These chemicals are absorbed through the skin, gastrointestinal tract, and lungs and can cause neurotoxicity and delayed neuropathy.

Natural Toxins (p. 435)

Potent toxins and carcinogens are present in the natural environment, including mycotoxins (e.g., ergot alkaloids) and phytotoxins (e.g., cycasin) that can contaminate foods. Aflatoxin B_1 produced by fungi that contaminate stored peanuts, corn, and other grains is a potent carcinogen, and contributes to the high incidence of hepatocellular carcinoma in Africa and the Far East. *Amanita phalloides* mushrooms may cause hepatic necrosis or even death. Animal toxins include venoms produced by snakes and bees. Dinoflagellate toxins (e.g., ciguatoxin or saxitoxin) may be ingested by consuming fish, snails, or mollusks that have eaten the dinoflagellates.

Radiation Injury (p. 436)

Radiation is energy distributed across the electromagnetic spectrum as waves (long wavelengths, low frequency) or particles (short wavelengths, high frequency). Approximately 80%

TABLE 9–6 **Health Effects of Agricultural Pesticides**

Category	Example	Effects and Disease Associations
Insecticides	Organochlorines DDT Chlordane Lindane Methoxychlor	Neurotoxicity; hepatotoxicity
	Organophosphates Parathion Diazinon Malathion	Neurotoxicity; delayed neuropathy
	Carbamates Aldicarb Carbaryl	Neurotoxicity (reversible)
	Botanical agents Nicotine Pyrethrins Rotenone	Paresthesia; lung irritant; allergic dermatitis
Herbicides	Arsenic compounds	Hyperpigmentation; gangrene; anemia; sensory neuropathy; cancer
	Dinitrophenols	Hyperthermia; sweating
	Chlorophenoxy herbicides 2,4-D and 2,4,5-T TCDD	? Lymphoma; sarcoma Fetotoxicity; immunotoxicity; cancer
	Paraquat	Acute lung injury
	Atrazine	? Cancer
	Alachlor	? Cancer
Fungicides	Captan Maneb Benomyl	? Reproductive toxicity
Rodenticides	Fluoroacetate	Cardiac and respiratory failure
	Warfarin	Hemorrhage
	Strychnine	Respiratory failure
Fumigants	Carbon disulfide	Cardiac toxicity
	Ethylene dibromide	Neurotoxicity
	Phosphine	Lung edema; brain damage
	Chloropicrin	Eye irritation; lung edema; arrhythmias

Data from Hodgson E: Introduction to toxicology. In Hodgson E, Levi PE (eds): A Textbook of Modern Toxicology. Stamford, CT, Appleton & Lange, 1997, p 1; Levi PE: Classes of toxic chemicals. In Hodgson E, Levi PE (eds): A Textbook of Modern Toxicology. Stamford, CT, Appleton & Lange, 1997, p 229.

of radiation is derived from natural sources, including cosmic radiation, UV light, and natural radioisotopes, especially radon gas. The remaining 20% is derived from manmade sources, such as medical and dental diagnostic and therapeutic procedures, consumer products, and occupational exposures.

Electromagnetic radiation characterized by long wavelengths and low frequencies (e.g., radio waves and microwaves) produces vibration and rotation of atoms in biologic molecules and is described as *nonionizing radiation.* Radiation energy of short wavelengths and high frequency can ionize biologic target molecules and eject electrons; x-rays, gamma rays, and cosmic rays are forms of such *ionizing radiation. Particulate radiation* is classified by the type of particles emitted (e.g., alpha or beta particles). The energy of these particles is typically measured in million electron volts (MeV). The decay of radioisotopes is expressed by the *curie*—3.7 × 10^{10} disintegrations per second (Ci)—or the *becquerel*—1 disintegration per second (Bq). The rate of decay of radioisotopes is usually expressed as the *half-life* and ranges from a few seconds to centuries.

Ionizing Radiation (p. 436)

The dose of ionizing radiation is measured in several units:

- *Roentgen:* Unit of charge produced by x-rays or gamma rays that ionize a specific volume of air.
- *Rad:* The dose of radiation that produces absorption of 100 ergs of energy per gram of tissue.
- *Gray* (Gy): The dose of radiation that produces absorption of 1 joule of energy per kilogram of tissue. 1 Gy corresponds to 100 rad.
- *Rem:* The dose of radiation that causes a biologic effect equivalent to 1 rad of x-rays or gamma rays.

These measurements do not directly quantify energy absorbed per unit of tissue and therefore do not predict the biologic effects of radiation. These effects depend on several factors, in addition to the physical properties of the radioactive material and the dose:

- Dose rate is important; a single dose can cause greater injury than divided or fractionated doses that allow time for cellular repair.
- A single dose of external radiation administered to the whole body is potentially more lethal than regional doses with shielding.
- Different cell types differ in the extent of their adaptive and reparative responses to radiation.
- Ionizing radiation can penetrate tissue and ionize atoms or molecules within cells with secondary generation of ions and free radicals, such as reactive oxygen species derived from water (Chapter 1). Free radical scavengers and antioxidants protect against radiation injury.
- Because DNA is the most important subcellular target of ionizing radiation, rapidly dividing cells (e.g., hematopoietic cells, gastrointestinal epithelium) are more radiosensitive than quiescent cells (e.g., bone, muscle).
- Cells in the G_2 and mitotic phases of the cell cycle are most sensitive to ionizing radiation.

Cellular Mechanisms of Radiation Injury (p. 437)

The acute effects of ionizing radiation range from overt necrosis at high doses (>10 Gy), killing of proliferating cells at intermediate doses (1 to 2 Gy), and no histopathologic effect at doses less than 0.5 Gy. If cells undergo extensive DNA damage or if they are unable to repair this damage, they may undergo apoptosis. Surviving cells may show delayed effects of radiation injury: mutations, chromosomal aberrations, and genetic instability. These genetically damaged cells may become malignant and cause cancers.

- *Acute effects:* Ionizing radiation produces a variety of lesions in cellular DNA, including DNA-protein cross-links and

DNA strand breaks. DNA damage stimulates expression of several genes involved in DNA repair. The tumor-suppressor gene *p53* is activated after DNA damage and increases expression of several downstream effector genes. These, in turn, induce cell cycle arrest and DNA repair, or in some cases, apoptosis.

- *Chronic effects:* Chronic effects are caused by a combination of atrophy of parenchymal cells, ischemia as a result of vascular damage, and fibrosis resulting in scarring.
- *Carcinogenesis:* Exposure to ionizing radiation produces an increased incidence of skin, thyroid, and lung cancers as well as leukemia and osteogenic sarcomas. Notable examples are the increased rates of thyroid cancer in children exposed to radiation from atomic bombs or from the Chernobyl nuclear accident. The delayed carcinogenic effect of ionizing radiation may be due to *induced genetic instability,* in which mutations persist and accumulate.
- *Heritable mutations* may also follow exposure to ionizing radiation.

Clinical Manifestations of Exposure to Ionizing Radiation (p. 439)

Acute, whole-body exposure can be described as the *acute radiation syndrome* or *radiation sickness*. Depending on the dose, four syndromes are produced: subclinical, hematopoietic, gastrointestinal, and central nervous system. These syndromes are summarized in Table 9–7.

Effects of Radiation Therapy (p. 439)

External radiation is delivered to malignant neoplasms at fractionated doses, with shielding of normal tissues. Patients may experience transient fatigue, vomiting, and anorexia.

Effects on Growth and Developmental Stages (p. 439)

Developing fetuses and young children are highly sensitive to growth and developmental abnormalities induced by ionizing radiation. Four susceptible phases can be defined:

- *Preimplantation embryo:* Irradiation of the mother before implantation can be lethal to the embryo.
- *Organogenesis:* Critical stages of organogenesis are from implantation to 9 weeks of gestation.
- *Fetal period:* From 6 weeks of gestation until birth, functional abnormalities of the central nervous system and reproductive systems may be produced by maternal irradiation.
- *Postnatal period:* Infants and young children exposed to radiation may cease bone growth and maturation. Development of the central nervous system, eyes, and teeth may also be perturbed.

Delayed Radiation Injury (p. 439)

Months to years after irradiation, delayed complications may occur; the following sites are the most vulnerable:

- *Blood vessels:* Blood vessels in the radiation field show subintimal and medial fibrosis, degeneration of the internal elastic lamina, and severe lumenal narrowing.

TABLE 9–7 **Clinical Features of the Acute Radiation Syndrome**

Category	Whole-Body Dose (rem)	Symptoms	Prognosis
Subclinical	<200	Mild nausea and vomiting Lymphocytes <1500/μL	100% survival
Hematopoietic	200–600	Intermittent nausea and vomiting Petechiae, hemorrhage Maximum neutrophil and platelet depression in 2 wk Lymphocytes <1000/μL	Infections May require bone marrow transplant
Gastrointestinal	600–1000	Nausea, vomiting, diarrhea Hemorrhage and infection in 1–3 wk Severe neutrophil and platelet depression Lymphocytes <500/μL	Shock and death in 10–14 days even with replacement therapy
Central nervous system	>1000	Intractable nausea and vomiting Confusion, somnolence, convulsions Coma in 15 min–3 hr Lymphocytes absent	Death in 14–36 hr

- *Skin:* Atrophy of the epidermis, dermal fibrosis, and dilation and weakening of the subcutaneous vessels are changes collectively called *radiation dermatitis.*
- *Heart:* Chest radiotherapy (e.g., for malignancy) may damage myo- and pericardium.
- *Lungs:* Radiation causes acute injury as well as delayed radiation pneumonitis with intra-alveolar and interstitial fibrosis.
- *Kidneys and urinary bladder:* Renal peritubular fibrosis, vascular damage, and hyalinization of glomeruli develop gradually, leading to hypertension and atrophy. The bladder is sensitive to radiation injury, with acute necrosis of the epithelium followed by submucosal fibrosis, contracture, bleeding, and ulceration.
- *Gastrointestinal tract:* Esophagitis, gastritis, enteritis, colitis, and proctitis can result from local irradiation.
- *Eyes and central nervous system:* Radiation gives rise to cataracts. The brain may show focal necrosis and demyelination of white matter. Irradiation of the spinal cord can damage small blood vessels, leading to necrosis, demyelination, and paraplegia, called *transverse myelitis.*

Ultraviolet Radiation (p. 441)

UV radiation is divided into UVA, UVB, and UVC; 3% to 5% of the total solar radiation that penetrates to the earth's surface is UV. Ozone in the atmosphere is an important protection against UV radiation: it completely absorbs all UVC and partially absorbs UVB. By increasing UV radiation at the earth's surface, ozone depletion by atmospheric pollutants is predicted to contribute to a 2% to 4% increase in skin cancer incidence.

- The acute effects of UVA and UVB are short-lived and reversible; they include erythema, pigmentation, and injury to epidermal Langerhans cells and keratinocytes. Erythema, edema, and acute inflammation are mediated by release of histamine from dermal mast cells.
- Tanning induced by UVA and UVB is due to increased melanin synthesis by melanocytes, elongation and extension of dendritic processes, and transfer of melanin to keratinocytes. To a lesser extent, UVA and UVB also increase melanocyte number.
- Repeated exposures to UV radiation produce changes in the skin characteristic of premature aging such as wrinkling, solar elastosis, and irregularities in pigmentation.
- Skin damage induced by UVB may be mediated by reactive oxygen species. UV radiation also directly damages DNA and generates pyrimidine dimers. A series of molecular changes (collectively referred to as the *UV response pathway*) leads to a protective cellular response consisting of DNA repair, cell cycle arrest, or apoptosis. The importance of DNA repair as a defense mechanism against skin cancer is illustrated by the increased incidence of UV-induced cutaneous malignancies in patients with defective DNA repair mechanisms (e.g., *xeroderma pigmentosum*).

Electromagnetic Fields (p. 442)

Nonionizing electromagnetic fields range between less than 1 cycle/sec (Hertz, or Hz) for DC power lines up to 100 GHz for long-distance microwaves and radar. Epidemiologic studies showed that residential exposure to ambient 50- to 60-Hz magnetic fields is not a health threat and does not cause any increased incidence of childhood leukemia.

Physical Environment (p. 442)

Human injury, death, and disability are major public health problems in modern industrialized societies. Injuries potentially result from human activities as well as external forces.

Mechanical Force (p. 443)

Mechanical force may injure soft tissues, bones, or head. Soft tissue injuries can be superficial, involving mainly the skin, or deep, associated with visceral damage:

- *Abrasion:* Typically a scrape, in which the superficial epidermis is avulsed by friction or force. Regeneration without scarring usually occurs unless infection complicates the process.
- *Laceration and incision:* A laceration is an irregular tear in the skin produced by overstretching. It may be linear or

stellate, depending on the tearing force, and typically heals with some scarring. In contrast, an incision is made by a sharp cutting object, such as a knife (scalpel) or a piece of glass, and can usually be neatly approximated by sutures, leaving little or no scar. Deep tissues and organs may sustain lacerations from an external blow even without apparent superficial injury.

- *Contusion:* A contusion is caused by blunt force trauma that injures small blood vessels and causes interstitial bleeding, usually without disruption of the continuity of the tissue.
- *Gunshot wounds* (p. 444) are part of forensic pathology, a subspecialty dealing with trauma and associated medicolegal issues. The character of a gunshot wound at entry and exit and the extent of injury depend on the type of gun used (handgun or rifle) and on a large number of variables, including the caliber of the bullet, the type of ammunition, the distance of the firearm from the body, the locus of the injury, the trajectory of the missile (at right angles to the skin or oblique), and the gyroscopic stability of the bullet (the presence or absence of wobbling or tumbling). Guns fired at close range (within a foot of the skin surface) leave a gray-black discoloration about the wound of entrance (fouling) produced by the heat, smoke, and burned powder deposits exiting with the bullet from the muzzle. When firearms are held more than a foot away but within 3 feet, there may be only stippling without fouling. At greater distances, neither is present. Cutaneous exit wounds are generally larger and more irregular than entrance wounds because in passing through the tissues bullets almost inevitably develop wobbling trajectories.

Thermal Injuries (p. 444)

Cutaneous burns are responsible for about 4500 deaths annually in the United States, a large proportion involving children and the elderly. The clinical significance of a burn depends on:

- Depth of the burn
- Percentage of body surface involved
- Possible internal injuries from inhalation of hot gases and fumes
- Promptness and efficacy of the postburn therapy, in particular, fluid and electrolyte management, prevention of shock, and prevention or control of wound infection

Any burn exceeding 50% of the total body surface, whether superficial or deep, is potentially fatal. In *partial-thickness burns*, characterized by blistering, the dermis and its skin appendages are spared, and complete regeneration is possible. By contrast, a *full-thickness burn* results in total destruction of the entire epidermis, extending into the dermis and sometimes even more deeply; regeneration of the epidermis is possible only from the margins or spared deeper appendages.

Burn patients present a set of complex clinical problems that require specialized care; the *systemic consequences* of a burn are far more important than the local injury. In large burns, neurogenic shock may appear almost immediately, followed by hypovolemic shock, owing to copious exudative losses from the burn surface. Secondary *infection* is an important complication in all burn patients. Following burn injury, a *hypermetabolic state* also develops; together with plasma protein loss, this may induce serious fluid, electrolyte, and nutritional imbalances.

Hyperthermia

Prolonged exposure to elevated ambient temperatures can result in the following conditions:

- *Heat cramps* occur from loss of electrolytes through sweating.
- *Heat exhaustion* is the most common heat syndrome. It results from a failure of the cardiovascular system to compensate for hypovolemia, secondary to water depletion. Its onset is sudden with prostration and collapse.
- *Heat stroke* is associated with high ambient temperatures and high humidity. Thermoregulatory mechanisms fail, sweating ceases, and core body temperature rises to high (e.g., 106°F) levels. This situation results in a marked generalized peripheral vasodilation with peripheral pooling of blood and a decreased effective circulating blood volume. Necrosis of muscles and myocardium may occur associated with systemic effects, such as arrhythmias and disseminated intravascular coagulation. Heat stroke typically occurs in individuals undergoing intense physical training and in people with cardiovascular disease.

Hypothermia

Prolonged exposure to low ambient temperature leads to hypothermia. At a core temperature of 90°F, loss of consciousness occurs; at lower temperatures, bradycardia and atrial fibrillation occur. Freezing of cells and tissues causes direct injury through the crystallization of intracellular and extracellular water, and indirect effects secondary to circulatory changes. Slowly falling temperatures may induce vasoconstriction and increased vascular permeability, leading to edematous changes (e.g., *trench foot*). Persistent low temperatures may cause ischemic injury.

Electrical Injuries (p. 446)

The passage of an electric current through the body may be without effect; may cause sudden death by disruption of neural regulatory impulses, producing cardiac arrest; or may cause thermal injury to organs interposed in the pathway of the current. Several variables are involved in electrical injuries:

- *Resistance of the tissues* to the conductance of the electric current affects the outcome. Tissue resistance to the flow of electricity varies inversely with water content. Dry skin is particularly resistant, but when skin is wet or immersed in water, its resistance is greatly decreased. The greater the resistance of tissues, the greater the heat generated. Thus, an electric current may cause a surface burn of dry skin but may cause death by disruption of nerve pathways when it is transmitted through wet skin.
- *Intensity of the current* also affects the thermal effects of the passage of electricity. High-intensity current, such as lightning, may course along the skin producing linear arborizing burns known as *lightning marks*, or be conducted around the victim (*flashover*).

Injuries Related to Changes in Atmospheric Pressure (p. 446)

Depending on the direction of change (increase or decrease), as well as the rate and magnitude of change, four syndromes occur:

- *High-altitude illness* is encountered in mountain climbers in the rarefied atmosphere encountered at altitudes above 4000 m. The lowered oxygen tension produces progressive mental obtundation and may be accompanied by increased capillary permeability with cerebral and pulmonary edema.
- *Blast injury* implies a violent increase in pressure either in the atmosphere (air blast) or in water (immersion blast).
- *Air or gas embolism* may occur as a complication of scuba diving, mechanical positive-pressure ventilatory support, or hyperbaric oxygen therapy. Abnormal increases in intra-alveolar air pressure cause entrance of air into the interstitium and small blood vessels. Pulmonary, mediastinal, and subcutaneous emphysema may result. In some instances, the coalescence of numerous small air emboli in the arterial circulation may lead acutely to strokelike syndromes or myocardial ischemia.
- *Decompression disease* is classically encountered in deep-sea divers who spend long periods of time at depth under increased atmospheric pressure; injury occurs after too-rapid decompression. As the underwater depth and consequent atmospheric pressure increase, progressively larger amounts of oxygen and accompanying gases (mostly nitrogen) dissolve in the blood and tissue fluids. With too-rapid ascent, the dissolved gases come out of solution and form minute bubbles in the bloodstream and tissues. Coalescence of these bubbles produces even larger masses capable of becoming significant emboli in the bloodstream. Periarticular bubbles produce painful *bends;* bubbles within the lung vasculature cause severe substernal pain and impair respiration, referred to as the *chokes.* Days after decompression *caisson disease of bone* may appear, attributed to embolic occlusion of the vascular supply of femoral and humeral heads and forming foci of aseptic necrosis.

NUTRITION AND DISEASE (p. 446)

Food Safety: Additives and Contaminants (p. 446)

Food contains numerous natural constituents as well as additives that can threaten human health. A wide range of compounds are natural constituents of foods, including carcinogens and natural pesticides. Food may also be contaminated by natural toxicants or microorganisms, such as hepatitis A, *Salmonella enteritidis, Escherichia coli,* or *Cryptosporidium.*

Additional chemicals are added to foods either directly (chemical sweeteners, preservatives, food colors) or indirectly (agricultural pesticides, residues of drugs or hormones given to animals, industrial contaminants). Low levels of metals, chlorinated hydrocarbons, and polychlorinated biphenyls are also present in the food supply.

Nutritional Deficiencies (p. 447)

In developing countries, undernutrition or protein-energy malnutrition (PEM) is common; it also occurs even in affluent societies in low socioeconomic communities. In industrialized societies, the most common diseases (atherosclerosis, cancer, diabetes, and hypertension) have all been linked to some form of dietary indiscretion.

Adequate diets should provide:

* Energy, in the form of carbohydrates, fats, and proteins
* Essential (and nonessential) amino acids and fatty acids
* Vitamins and minerals

In *primary malnutrition,* one or all of these components are missing from the diet. By contrast, in *secondary* or *conditional malnutrition,* the supply of nutrients is adequate, but malnutrition results from nutrient malabsorption, impaired nutrient use or storage, excess nutrient losses, or increased need for nutrients. Undernutrition in affluent societies is associated with the following:

* *Ignorance and poverty:* The homeless, elderly, and children of the poor demonstrate the effects of undernutrition.
* *Chronic alcoholism:* Alcoholics can have vitamin deficiencies as well as PEM.
* *Acute and chronic illnesses:* In some illnesses, the basal metabolic rate becomes elevated (e.g., burns).
* *Self-imposed dietary restriction:* Eating disorders such as anorexia nervosa and bulimia nervosa affect a population concerned about body image.

Protein-Energy Malnutrition (p. 447)

PEM refers to a range of clinical syndromes characterized by a dietary intake of protein and calories inadequate to meet the body's needs. The diagnosis of PEM is usually made by comparing the body weight for a given height with a standard table, although evaluation of fat stores, muscle mass, and serum proteins can also be helpful. The most common victims of PEM worldwide are children. Severe PEM is common in developing countries, where up to 25% of children may be affected. A child whose weight falls to less than 80% of normal is considered to be malnourished.

The major features of PEM include:

* Growth failure
* Peripheral edema
* Loss of body fat and atrophy of muscle
* Enlarged and fatty liver in kwashiorkor but not in marasmus
* Hypoplastic bone marrow in both kwashiorkor and marasmus because of decreased numbers of red blood cell precursors

When the level falls to 60% of normal weight for sex and age, the child is considered to have *marasmus:*

* Growth retardation and loss of muscle mass occur.
* Subcutaneous fat is mobilized.
* Extremities are emaciated, and the head appears too large for the body.
* Serum albumin levels are near normal.
* Immune deficiency results in concurrent infections.

The other form of severe malnutrition is *kwashiorkor*, which occurs when protein deprivation is relatively greater than the reduction in total calories. *Kwashiorkor is a more severe form of malnutrition than marasmus:*

- There are two protein compartments in the body: the *visceral protein compartment*, consisting of protein stores in visceral organs (e.g., liver), and the *somatic protein compartment*, represented by skeletal muscles. These two compartments are regulated differently. The visceral compartment is depleted more severely in kwashiorkor, whereas the somatic compartment is affected more severely in marasmus. The marked loss of the visceral protein compartment in kwashiorkor results in hypoalbuminemia, giving rise to a generalized or dependent edema.
- Skin lesions give a *flaky paint* appearance.
- Hair changes include loss of normal color and texture.
- Fatty liver results from decreased synthesis of carrier proteins.
- Immune defects and secondary infections occur.
- Kwashiorkor is most commonly seen in impoverished African and Southeast Asian children.

Secondary PEM occurs in chronically ill or hospitalized patients. Both marasmus-like and kwashiorkor-like syndromes (with intermediate forms) may develop. Secondary PEM is common in advanced cancer and AIDS patients. The malnutrition in these settings is sometimes called *cachexia.*

Anorexia Nervosa and Bulimia (p. 449)

Anorexia nervosa is self-induced starvation, resulting in marked loss of weight; bulimia is a condition in which the patient binges on food and then induces vomiting. These eating disorders occur primarily in previously healthy young women who obsess over their body image. The clinical findings are similar to those in severe PEM.

Vitamin Deficiencies (p. 450)

Thirteen vitamins are necessary for health; four—vitamins A, D, E, and K—are fat soluble, and the remainder are water soluble. A summary of all the essential vitamins along with their functions and deficiency syndromes is shown in Table 9–8.

Vitamin A (p. 450)

Vitamin A includes a group of related chemicals with hormone-like function. *Retinol* is the transport and also the storage form of vitamin A. Carotenoids, found in yellow and leafy green vegetables, are metabolized to active vitamin A. About 90% of the body's vitamin A reserve is found in the perisinusoidal stellate (Ito) cells in the liver. Functions include:

- Maintaining normal vision in reduced light
- Potentiating the differentiation of mucus-secreting epithelial cells
- Enhancing immunity to infections, particularly in children
- Acting as photoprotective and antioxidant agents

Vitamin A deficiency results in the following:

- Impaired vision occurs, particularly night blindness.
- *Xerophthalmia* (dry eye) refers to a collection of ocular changes, including dryness of the conjunctivae (xerosis),

TABLE 9–8 Vitamins: Major Functions and Deficiency Syndromes

Vitamin	Functions	Deficiency Syndromes
Fat-Soluble		
Vitamin A	A component of visual pigment	Night blindness, xerophthalmia, blindness
	Maintenance of specialized epithelia	Squamous metaplasia
	Maintenance of resistance to infection	Vulnerability to infection, particularly measles
Vitamin D	Facilitates intestinal absorption of calcium and phosphorus and mineralization of bone	Rickets in children
		Osteomalacia in adults
Vitamin E	Major antioxidant; scavenges free radicals	Spinocerebellar degeneration
Vitamin K	Cofactor in hepatic carboxylation of procoagulants—factors II (prothrombin), VII, IX, and X; and protein C and protein S	Bleeding diathesis
Water-Soluble		
Vitamin B₁ (thiamine)	As pyrophosphate, is coenzyme in decarboxylation reactions	Dry and wet beriberi, Wernicke syndrome, ? Korsakoff syndrome
Vitamin B₂ (riboflavin)	Converted to coenzymes flavin mononucleotide and flavin adenine dinucleotide, cofactors for many enzymes in intermediary metabolism	Ariboflavinosis, cheilosis, stomatitis, glossitis, dermatitis, corneal vascularization
Niacin	Incorporated into nicotinamide adenine dinucleotide (NAD) and NAD phosphate, involved in a variety of redox reactions	Pellagra—three "D's": dementia, dermatitis, diarrhea
Vitamin B₆ (pyridoxine)	Derivatives serve as coenzymes in many intermediary reactions	Cheilosis, glossitis, dermatitis, peripheral neuropathy
Vitamin B₁₂	Required for normal folate metabolism and DNA synthesis	Combined system disease (megaloblastic pernicious anemia and degeneration of posterolateral spinal cord tracts)
	Maintenance of myelinization of spinal cord tracts	
Vitamin C	Serves in many oxidation-reduction (redox) reactions and hydroxylation of collagen	Scurvy
Folate	Essential for transfer and use of 1-carbon units in DNA synthesis	Megaloblastic anemia, neural tube defects
Pantothenic acid	Incorporated in coenzyme A	No nonexperimental syndrome recognized
Biotin	Cofactor in carboxylation reactions	No clearly defined clinical syndrome

formation of small opaque spots (Bitot spots) or ulcers on the corneal surface, and eventual destruction of the cornea (keratomalacia).

- Keratinizing metaplasia of epithelial surfaces results in respiratory tract infections due to airway squamous metaplasia and in renal and urinary bladder calculi due to desquamation of keratinized epithelium.
- Immune deficiency leading to increased risk of death from measles, pneumonia, and infectious diarrhea.

Vitamin A toxicity can cause several symptoms—both short- and long-term excesses produce clinical consequences (an issue resulting from the availability of large doses at health food stores):

- Acute toxic manifestations include headache, vomiting, stupor, and papilledema.
- Chronic toxicity is associated with weight loss, nausea and vomiting, lip dryness, and bone and joint pain.

Vitamin D (p. 452)

Vitamin D is critical for maintenance of normal plasma levels of calcium and phosphorus. Besides maintaining normal bone formation, vitamin D regulation of calcium levels prevents hypocalcemic tetany. Activities include the following:

- Stimulates intestinal absorption of calcium and phosphorus
- Collaborates with parathyroid hormone (PTH) in the mobilization of calcium from bone
- Stimulates PTH-dependent reabsorption of calcium in the distal renal tubules

Vitamin D metabolism is outlined in Figure 9–3*A*:

- Vitamin D is absorbed in the gut or synthesized from precursors in the skin.
- Vitamin D binds to a plasma α_1-globulin and is transported to liver.
- In the liver, it is converted to 25-hydroxyvitamin D (25(OH)D) by 25-hydroxylase.
- In the kidney 25(OH)D is converted to $1,25(OH)_2D$ by α_1-hydroxylase.
- Biologically, $1,25(OH)_2D$ is the most active form. It can be thought of as a steroid hormone that binds to a widely expressed receptor.
- The production of $1,25(OH)_2D$ by the kidney is regulated by three mechanisms:

  In a feedback loop, increased levels of $1,25(OH)_2D$ down-regulate synthesis of this metabolite by inhibiting the action of α_1-hydroxylase.

  Hypocalcemia stimulates secretion of PTH, which, in turn, augments the conversion of 25(OH)D to $1,25(OH)_2D$ by activating α_1-hydroxylase.

  Hypophosphatemia directly activates α_1-hydroxylase and thus increases formation of $1,25(OH)_2D$.

The effects of vitamin D deficiency are schematized in Figure 9–3*B*:

- Vitamin D deficiency causes *rickets* in growing children and *osteomalacia* in adults. Both forms of skeletal disease result from altered vitamin D absorption or metabolism or, less commonly, from disorders that affect the function of vitamin D or disturb calcium or phosphorus homeostasis.

NORMAL VITAMIN D METABOLISM

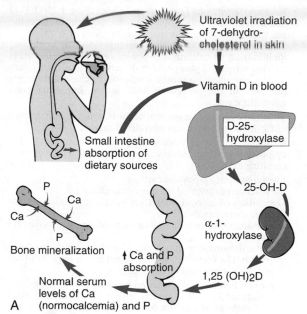

VITAMIN D DEFICIENCY

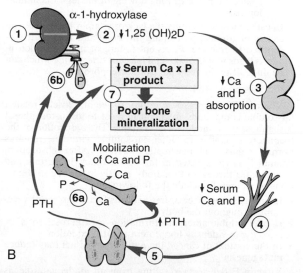

FIGURE 9–3 *A,* Schema of normal vitamin D metabolism. *B,* Vitamin D deficiency. There is inadequate substrate for the renal hydroxylase (1), yielding a deficiency of 1,25(OH)₂D (2), and deficient absorption of calcium and phosphorus from the gut (3), with consequent depressed serum levels of both (4). The hypocalcemia activates the parathyroid glands (5), causing mobilization of calcium and phosphorus from bone (6a). Simultaneously, the parathyroid hormone (PTH) induces wasting of phosphate in the urine (6b) and calcium retention. Consequently, the serum levels of calcium are normal or nearly normal, but the phosphate is low; hence mineralization is impaired (7).

- Inadequate vitamin D causes a deficiency of $1,25(OH)_2D$ and deficient absorption of calcium and phosphorus from the gut with consequent depressed serum levels of both.
- Hypocalcemia activates the parathyroid glands, causing mobilization of calcium and phosphorus from bone. PTH induces wasting of phosphate in the urine and calcium retention. Consequently, serum levels of calcium are nearly normal, but the phosphate level is low, impairing bone mineralization.

The morphologic changes that occur in vitamin D deficiency result from an excess of unmineralized matrix:

- In rickets in children, inadequate provisional calcification of epiphyseal cartilage deranges endochondral bone growth, resulting in:

    Overgrowth of epiphyseal cartilage
    Persistence of distorted masses of cartilage
    Deposition of osteoid matrix on poorly mineralized cartilaginous remnants
    Disruption of the orderly replacement of cartilage by osteoid matrix
    Skeletal deformation due to disordered endochondral bone growth. The skeletal changes depend on the severity of the rachitic process and its duration:

    Frontal bossing and a squared head occurs in infants.
    Deformation of the chest resulting from cartilage overgrowth at the costochondral junction produces the *rachitic rosary;* the sternum protrudes anteriorly causing a *pigeon breast* deformity.
    In ambulating children, deformities affect the long bones, spine, and pelvis causing bowing of the legs and lumbar lordosis.

- In osteomalacia in adults, the lack of vitamin D produces an excess of osteoid, weakening the bone and making it susceptible to fracture. Persistent failure of mineralization in adults leads to loss of skeletal mass, or *osteopenia,* which can be difficult to differentiate from osteoporosis.

Vitamin E (p. 455)

Vitamin E comprises a group of eight closely related fat-soluble compounds abundant in most foods; α-tocopherol is the most active and widely available. The absorption of the tocopherols, similar to other fat-soluble vitamins, requires normal biliary and pancreatic function. After absorption, vitamin E is transported in the blood by chylomicrons, and accumulates throughout the body, mostly in fat depots. Functions of vitamin E include the following:

- It acts as a scavenger of free radicals formed in redox reactions throughout the body.
- It may inhibit atheroma formation in atherosclerosis by reducing low-density lipoprotein (LDL) oxidation.
- In the context of cancer, the antioxidant effect may reduce mutagenesis.

Vitamin E deficiency resulting from an inadequate diet is uncommon and occurs in association with malabsorption syndromes, infants of low birth weight, developmental defects in the gastrointestinal tract, or lipoprotein disorders.

- The central nervous system is particularly vulnerable to vitamin E deficiency with degeneration of axons in the posterior columns of the spinal cord, loss of nerve cells in the dorsal root ganglia, and degenerative changes in the spinocerebellar tracts.

- Neurologic manifestations are absent tendon reflexes, ataxia, dysarthria, and loss of position sense and pain sensation.

Vitamin K (p. 456)

Vitamin K is a required cofactor for a liver enzyme that carboxylates specific glutamate residues found in a variety of proteins, including:

- Clotting factors VII, IX, and X and prothrombin, in which carboxylation facilitates calcium binding and interactions involved in the generation of thrombin (Chapter 4)
- Anticoagulant proteins C and S
- Osteocalcin, a protein made by osteoblasts, in which vitamin K appears to favor calcification

Vitamin K is converted from its reduced form to an oxidized state during interactions with its substrate proteins but then is rapidly recycled by the healthy liver to its original form. Additionally the endogenous intestinal bacterial flora synthesizes the vitamin. Despite both of these sources of the vitamin, there is a definite need for a small amount of the exogenous vitamin.

Vitamin K deficiency occurs in several situations:

- Fat malabsorption syndromes
- After destruction of the vitamin K–synthesizing flora by antibiotics
- In the neonatal period, because liver reserves are small, the bacterial flora has not developed, and the level of vitamin K in breast milk is small
- In diffuse liver disease

Vitamin K deficiency in adults causes development of a *bleeding diathesis,* characterized by hematomas, hematuria, melena, ecchymoses, and bleeding from the gums.

Thiamine (p. 456)

Thiamine is widely available in the diet, although refined foods, such as polished rice and white flour, contain little. Thiamine is absorbed from the gut and phosphorylated to produce the functionally active form of the vitamin, which is then used as an enzyme cofactor or for maintenance of neural membranes and nerve conductance.

- In underdeveloped countries, where a large part of the scant diet consists of polished rice (e.g., Southeast Asia), thiamine deficiency sometimes develops. In developed countries, *thiamine deficiency affects one fourth of chronic alcoholics admitted to general hospitals.* Because a subclinical deficiency state may be converted to an overt deficiency when refeeding chronically malnourished persons, such as alcoholics, adequate amounts of thiamine must be administered concurrently.
- The three major targets of thiamine deficiency are the peripheral nerves, the heart, and the brain, so persistent thiamine deficiency gives rise to three distinctive syndromes, which typically appear in sequence:

  A *polyneuropathy (dry beriberi)* is symmetric and takes the form of a nonspecific peripheral neuropathy with myelin degeneration of axons involving motor, sensory, and reflex arcs, leading to footdrop, wristdrop, and sensory changes.

A *cardiovascular syndrome (wet beriberi)* is associated with peripheral vasodilation, high-output cardiac failure, and a flabby four-chambered dilated heart.

Wernicke-Korsakoff syndrome (Chapter 28) is seen in protracted severe deficiency states, typically in chronic alcoholics. Wernicke encephalopathy is marked by ophthalmoplegia, nystagmus, ataxia of gait and stance, and derangement of mental function, typically confusion. Korsakoff psychosis consists of impairment of remote recall, confabulation, and inability to acquire new information. Lesions in the central nervous system take the form of hemorrhages into the mammillary bodies.

Riboflavin (p. 457)

Riboflavin is a critical component of the flavin-containing nucleotides, which participate in a range of oxidation-reduction reactions. Riboflavin is found in many meat and dairy products and in vegetables.

Riboflavin deficiency (ariboflavinosis) still occurs as a primary deficiency state among persons in economically deprived and developing countries. In developed nations, it is found in alcoholics and in individuals with debilitating diseases, such as cancer. It is associated with:

- Cheilosis, or fissures at the angles of the mouth, which tend to become infected
- Glossitis, in which the tongue becomes atrophic and magenta in color
- Ocular changes, in which an inflammatory reaction in the cornea can cause opacities and sometimes ulcerations
- Dermatitis, greasy and scaling skin involving the nasolabial folds, which may extend into a butterfly distribution to involve the cheeks

Niacin (p. 458)

Niacin is the generic designation for nicotinic acid, an essential component of nicotinamide adenine dinucleotide (NAD) and nicotinamide adenine dinucleotide phosphate (NADP). NAD is a coenzyme for multiple dehydrogenases involved in the metabolism of fat, carbohydrates, and amino acids; NADP participates in similar reactions, notably in the hexose-monophosphate shunt of glucose metabolism.

Niacin can be derived from the dietary grains or may be synthesized endogenously from tryptophan. Thus, *pellagra* may result from either a niacin or a tryptophan deficiency. Pellagra is identified by the *three Ds:* dermatitis, diarrhea, and dementia.

- *Dermatitis* is bilaterally symmetric and is found on exposed areas of the body and consists of sharply demarcated scaling and desquamation.
- *Diarrhea* is caused by atrophy of the gastrointestinal epithelium.
- *Dementia* results from neuronal degeneration in the brain, accompanied by similar changes in the spinal cord.

Pyridoxine (Vitamin B_6) (p. 458)

Pyridoxine comprises a group of naturally occurring substances that participate as cofactors for enzymes involved in the metabolism of lipids and amino acids. Vitamin B_6 is present in most foods; however, food processing may destroy pyridoxine and in the past was responsible for severe deficiency in infants fed dried milk preparations. Secondary hypovitaminosis B_6 is produced by a variety of drugs that act as pyridoxine antagonists, including isoniazid (used to treat tuberculosis).

Clinical findings in vitamin B_6–deficient patients may be related to those of concomitant riboflavin and niacin deficiency, including cheilosis, glossitis, dermatitis, and peripheral neuropathy.

Vitamin C (Ascorbic Acid) (p. 458)

Vitamin C is present in many foods and is abundant in fruits and vegetables, so that all but the most restricted diets provide adequate amounts. Functions include:

- Activating prolyl and lysyl hydroxylases, providing for hydroxylation of procollagen.
- Scavenging free radicals and acting indirectly by regenerating the antioxidant form of vitamin E. The synergistic antioxidant properties of both of these vitamins may retard atherosclerosis by reducing the oxidation of LDL.

Deficiency of vitamin C leads to the development of *scurvy*, characterized by bone disease in children and hemorrhages and healing defects in both children and adults. Scurvy in a growing child is more dramatic than in an adult.

Inadequately hydroxylated precursors cannot be appropriately cross-linked, and so collagen lacks tensile strength. Additionally, lack of vitamin C leads to suppression of the rate of synthesis of collagen peptides. The defects in collagen synthesis affect the integrity of blood vessels and account for the predisposition to hemorrhages in scurvy.

- *Hemorrhages* often appear in the skin and in the gingival mucosa and cause subperiosteal hematomas and bleeding into joint spaces after minimal trauma.
- *Skeletal changes* occur because of inadequate formation of osteoid matrix. There is no defect in mineralization.
- *Gingival* swelling and secondary bacterial periodontal infections occur.
- *Skin lesions* include a perifollicular, hyperkeratotic, papular rash.
- *Wound healing* is impaired.

Folates (p.459)

Folates are essential cofactors in the transfer and use of single-carbon units in DNA synthesis. They are found in whole wheat flour, beans, nuts, and leafy green vegetables. Folate is heat labile and depleted in cooked and processed foods.

In the United States, 15% to 20% of adults have low serum folate. In developing countries with diets based on corn, folate deficiency is even more common. Some drugs (e.g., anticonvulsants), personal habits (e.g., ethanol use), and chronic diseases (malabsorption syndromes) interfere with folate absorption and metabolism and are associated with folate deficiency.

- Folate deficiency is associated with megaloblastic anemia and neural tube defects in the developing fetus.
- Combined folate and vitamin B_{12} deficiency has been postulated to contribute to the development of colon cancer.

Mineral Deficiencies (p. 459)

A number of minerals are essential for health. Of the trace elements found in the body, *only five—iron, zinc, copper, selenium, and iodine—have been associated with well-characterized deficiency states* (Table 9–9). Three influences are particularly relevant to mineral deficiencies:

- Inadequate supplementation in preparations used for total parenteral nutrition
- Interference with absorption by dietary constituents
- Inborn errors of metabolism leading to abnormalities of absorption

Zinc deficiency is characterized by:

- A distinctive rash most often around the eyes, nose, mouth, and distal extremities called *acrodermatitis enteropathica*
- Growth retardation in children
- Diminished reproductive capacity

Selenium, similar to vitamin E, protects against oxidative damage of membrane lipids. Deficiency of this element is known in China as *Keshan disease,* presenting as a congestive cardiomyopathy in children and young women.

Obesity (p. 461)

Obesity is a massive problem in the United States, where 27% of the adult population is clinically obese. Fat accumulation is measured in several ways:

- Some expression of weight in relation to height (e.g., body mass index; the body mass index is closely correlated with body fat)
- Skinfold measurements
- Various body circumferences, particularly the ratio of the waist-hip circumferences

TABLE 9–9 **Functions of Trace Metals and Deficiency Syndromes**

Nutrient	Functions	Deficiency Syndromes
Iron	Essential component of hemoglobin as well as a number of iron-containing metalloenzymes	Hypochromic microcytic anemia
Zinc	Component of enzymes, principally oxidases	Acrodermatitis enteropathica, growth retardation, infertility
Iodine	Component of thyroid hormone	Goiter and hypothyroidism
Selenium	Component of glutathione peroxidase	Myopathy, rarely cardiomyopathy
Copper	Component of cytochrome *c* oxidase, dopamine β-hydroxylase, tyrosinase, lysyl oxidase, and unknown enzyme involved in cross-linking keratin	Muscle weakness, neurologic defects, hypopigmentation, abnormal collagen cross-linking
Manganese	Component of metalloenzymes, including oxidoreductases, hydrolases, and lipases	No well-defined deficiency syndrome
Fluoride	Mechanism unknown	Dental caries

A 20% excess in body weight imparts a health risk. The adverse health effects of obesity are related not only to the total body weight, but also to the distribution of stored fat. Central or visceral fat is associated with a much greater health risk than is excess accumulation of fat in subcutaneous tissue.

Obesity is a disorder of *energy balance*. When food-derived energy chronically exceeds energy expenditure, the excess calories are stored as triglycerides in adipose tissue. The balance between intake and expenditure is controlled by neural and hormonal mechanisms (Fig. 9–4). Adipocytes com-

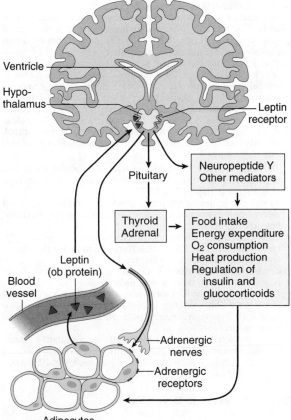

FIGURE 9–4 The hormonal and neural circuits that regulate body weight. Adipocytes secrete a hormone called *leptin* in response to increased fat stores and hormones such as insulin and glucocorticoids. Leptin is transported to the hypothalamus through the circulation, where it binds to the leptin receptor. This interaction regulates energy balance by affecting food intake and energy expenditure. Leptin decreases secretion of neuropeptide Y. In addition, through neuronal pathways, the activation of leptin receptor in the hypothalamus increases the release of norepinephrine from sympathetic nerve terminals that innervate adipose tissue leading to increased metabolism of fatty acids and dissipation of the energy as heat. (Modified from Scott J: New chapter for the fat controller. Nature 379:113, 1996. Reprinted with permission from Nature. Copyright ©1996 Macmillan Magazines Limited.)

municate with the hypothalamic centers that control appetite and energy expenditure by secreting a polypeptide hormone called *leptin*. Leptin acts as an antiobesity factor by binding to and activating leptin receptors in the hypothalamus. These receptors suppress appetite and increase energy expenditure, physical activity, and production of heat. Leptin decreases secretion of the appetite stimulant neurotransmitter neuropeptide Y. In addition, through neuronal pathways, hypothalamic leptin receptor activation increases norepinephrine release from sympathetic nerve terminals that innervate adipose tissue. Norepinephrine binds to the β_3-adrenergic receptors on fat cells and leads to increased metabolism of fatty acids with dissipation of the energy as heat.

Dysfunction of the leptin system likely plays a role in human obesity. The majority of obese patients have a high level of plasma leptin, indicating that there is some form of leptin resistance. Such resistance is most likely at the level of transport of leptin into the central nervous system or in abnormalities in hypothalamic pathways normally regulated by leptin. It is unlikely that mutational inactivation of the leptin gene or its downstream targets accounts for most instances of human obesity, although it is possible that polymorphisms in these genes cause subtle alterations resulting in obesity. It is clear that genetic influences play an important role in weight control.

Obesity increases the risk for a number of conditions, including the following:

- *Diabetes:* Obesity is associated with insulin resistance and hyperinsulinemia found in non–insulin-dependent, or type II, diabetes (Chapter 24).
- *Nonalcoholic steatohepatitis:* Fatty change and focal liver cell injury occur in obese adolescents and adults with type II diabetes (Chapter 18).
- *Cardiovascular disorders:* Hypertension, hypertriglyceridemia, and low HDL cholesterol all increase the risk of coronary artery disease (Chapter 12).
- *Cholelithiasis* (gallstones): Gallstones are six times more common in obese than in lean individuals.
- *Hypoventilation or Pickwickian syndrome:* This is a group of respiratory abnormalities in obese individuals. It is associated with hypersomnolence, polycythemia, and right-sided heart failure.
- *Osteoarthritis:* Osteoarthritis is due to the cumulative effects of added wear and tear on the joints.
- The relationships between *obesity and stroke* and between *obesity and cancer* are controversial.

Diet and Systemic Diseases (p. 465)

The composition of the diet can make a substantial contribution to the initiation and progression of disease:

- *Atherogenesis:* Reduction in the consumption of cholesterol and saturated animal fats (e.g., eggs, butter, beef) may reduce serum cholesterol levels and delay the development of atherosclerosis and coronary artery disease. Lowering the level of saturated fatty acids in the diet by substituting vegetable or fish oils for animal fat decreases serum cholesterol. People who consume diets that contain fresh fruits and vegetables, with a limited intake of meats and processed foods, have a lower risk of myocardial infarction.

- *Hypertension:* Hypertension is beneficially affected by restricting sodium intake.
- *Diverticulosis:* Dietary fiber increases fecal bulk and may have a preventive effect against diverticulosis.
- *Colon cancer:* High animal fat combined with low fiber intake has been implicated in the development of colon cancer.
- Calorie restriction has been demonstrated to increase life span in experimental animals (Chapter 2).

Chemoprevention of Cancer (p. 466)

Populations that consume large quantities of fruits and vegetables in their diets have a lower risk of some types of cancer. Although the mechanism for this effect is uncertain, it has been suggested that carotenoids, which are converted to vitamin A in the liver and intestine, may be important in the primary chemoprevention of cancer. The anticarcinogenic effect of the fruits and vegetables may be the result of the ability of retinoic acids to promote differentiation of some mucus-secreting epithelial tissue, scavenge free radicals and oxidants (thereby preventing DNA damage), and enhance immune responses. Despite the many trends and proclamations, to date there is no definite proof that diet can cause or protect against cancer.

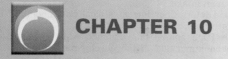

CHAPTER 10

Diseases of Infancy and Childhood

Conditions that afflict infants and children fall into one of four main categories (p. 469):

1. Consequences of organ or system immaturity (e.g., hyaline membrane disease)
2. Unique susceptibility of the fetus or infant to external or environmental factors
3. Genetic or inherited defects
4. Tumors and tumor-like conditions

The major causes of death in infancy and childhood are listed in Table 10–1.

CONGENITAL ANOMALIES (p. 470)

Congenital anomalies are morphologic defects present at birth; occasionally, these become apparent only later in life. About 3% of newborns have a major anomaly. Malformations represent a major cause of infant mortality and a significant cause of illness, disability, and death.

Definitions

Organ-Specific Terms
Agenesis Complete absence of an organ and its associated primordium.
Aplasia Absence of an organ due to failure of the developmental anlage.
Atresia Absence of an opening, usually of a hollow visceral organ (e.g., trachea or intestine).
Dysplasia In the context of malformations, refers to abnormal organization of individual cells.

Hyperplasia Overdevelopment of an organ associated with increased numbers of cells.

Hypoplasia Incomplete development or underdevelopment of an organ, with decreased numbers of cells (less severe form of aplasia).

Hypertrophy Increase in organ size or function related to an increase in cell size.

Hypotrophy Decrease in organ size or function related to a decrease in cell size.

Systemic Terms

Deformations Arise relatively late in fetal life and result from mechanical factors. Usually manifest as abnormalities in shape, form, or position (e.g., clubfeet). Most have a low risk of recurrence in subsequent siblings. Most common underlying factor is uterine constraint. Predisposing factors are both maternal (e.g., first pregnancy, uterine leiomyomas) and fetal/placental (e.g., oligohydramnios, multiple fetuses, abnormal fetal presentation).

Disruptions Secondary destruction or interference with a previously developmentally normal organ or body region. May be due to either external or internal interferences (e.g., amniotic bands). They are not heritable.

Malformations Intrinsic abnormalities occurring relatively early during development. May involve single or multiple organ systems. Risk of recurrence varies.

Sequence A series of multiple congenital anomalies resulting from a single localized aberration in organogenesis with secondary effects on other organs. The primary abnormality may be a malformation, deformation, or disruption. A good example is the *oligohydramnios* or *Potter sequence:* diverse factors, such as renal agenesis or an amniotic leak, result in decreased amniotic fluid (oligohydramnios), compression of the fetus, and a classic phenotype in the newborn infant (p. 472, Figs. 10–3 and 10–4 in *Robbins and Cotran Pathologic Basis of Disease,* 7th ed.).

Syndrome Several defects that cannot be readily explained on the basis of a single, localized initiating anomaly. Nevertheless, most often attributed to a specific etiologic agent (e.g., viral infection or chromosomal abnormality) that simultaneously affects several tissues.

Causes of Congenital Anomalies (p. 472)

The exact cause of a congenital anomaly is known in approximately half of cases; common causes are grouped into three major categories: genetic, environmental, and multifactorial (Table 10–2).

Genetic Causes

- *Karyotypic abnormalities* are present in approximately 10% to 15% of live-born infants with congenital anomalies. Most common abnormalities, listed in order of frequency, are trisomy 21, Klinefelter syndrome (47,XXY), Turner syndrome (45,XO), and trisomy 13. Most cytogenetic aberrations arise as defects in gametogenesis and are therefore not familial.
- *Single-gene mutations* are relatively uncommon but follow mendelian patterns of inheritance.

TABLE 10–1 Cause of Death Related with Age

Causes*	Rate[†]
Under 1 Year: All Causes	727.4
Congenital malformations, deformations, and chromosomal anomalies	
Disorders related to short gestation and low birth weight	
Sudden infant death syndrome (SIDS)	
Newborn affected by maternal complications of pregnancy	
Newborn affected by complications of placenta, cord, and membranes	
Respiratory distress of newborn	
Accidents (unintentional injuries)	
Bacterial sepsis of newborn	
Intrauterine hypoxia and birth asphyxia	
Diseases of the circulatory system	
1–4 Years: All Causes	32.6
Accidents and adverse effects	
Congenital malformations, deformations, and chromosomal abnormalities	
Malignant neoplasms	
Homicide and legal intervention	
Diseases of the heart[‡]	
Influenza and pneumonia	
5–14 Years: All Causes	18.5
Accidents and adverse effects	
Malignant neoplasms	
Homicide and legal intervention	
Congenital malformations, deformations, and chromosomal abnormalities	
Suicide	
Diseases of the heart	
15–24 Years: All Causes	80.7
Accidents and adverse effects	
Homicide	
Suicide	
Malignant neoplasms	
Diseases of the heart	

*Causes are listed in decreasing order of frequency. All causes and rates are preliminary 2000 statistics. (Minino AM, Smith BL: Deaths: Preliminary data for 2000. National Vital Statistics Report. 49:12, 2001).
[†]Rates are expressed per 100,000 population.
[‡]Excludes congenital heart disease.

Environmental Causes

The presence and nature of congenital anomalies due to environmental factors relates to the timing of the intrauterine exposure and the differential susceptibility of individual systems (p. 473, Fig. 10–5 in *Robbins and Cotran Pathologic Basis of Disease*, 7th ed.).

- Viruses

    Cytomegalovirus (most common fetal viral infection): Highest risk for malformations occurs with infection in second trimester when organogenesis is largely complete; commonly the virus affects the central nervous system resulting in mental retardation, microcephaly, and deafness.

    Rubella: Infection before 16 weeks' gestation can result in cataracts, heart defects, and deafness.

    Herpes simplex

TABLE 10–2 **Causes of Congenital Anomalies in Humans**

Cause	Frequency (%)
Genetic	
Chromosomal aberrations	10–15
Mendelian inheritance	2–10
Environmental	
Maternal/placental infections	2–3
Rubella	
Toxoplasmosis	
Syphilis	
Cytomegalovirus	
Human immunodeficiency virus (HIV)	
Maternal disease states	6–8
Diabetes	
Phenylketonuria	
Endocrinopathies	
Drugs and chemicals	1
Alcohol	
Folic acid antagonists	
Androgens	
Phenytoin	
Thalidomide	
Warfarin	
13-*cis*-retinoic acid	
Others	
Irradiations	1
Multifactorial (Multiple Genes? Environment)	20–25
Unknown	40–60

Adapted from Stevenson RE, et al (eds): Human Malformations and Related Anomalies. New York, Oxford University Press, 1993, p 115.

- *Drugs and chemicals:* Probably less than 1% of congenital anomalies are due to these substances. Agents suspected to be teratogenic include thalidomide, folate antagonists, androgenic hormones, alcohol, anticonvulsants, and 13-cis-retinoic acid.
- *Radiation:* Exposure to heavy doses during organogenesis can result in such defects as microcephaly, blindness, skull defects, and spina bifida.
- *Maternal diabetes:* Maternal hyperglycemia-induced fetal hyperinsulinemia causes increased body fat, muscle mass and organomegaly, cardiac anomalies, neural tube defects, and other central nervous system (CNS) malformations.

Multifactorial Causes

Anomalies may be due to the interaction of environmental factors with two or more genes (usually with minimal effect individually). Examples are cleft lip and palate, neural tube defects, and congenital hip dislocation.

Pathogenesis of Congenital Anomalies
(p. 474)

Although complex and frequently poorly understood, the following principles are important:

- Timing of the prenatal teratogenic insult will affect the occurrence and type of anomaly produced—a given agent

may produce distinct anomalies if exposure occurs at different times.
- Teratogens and genetic defects may act at several levels, including cellular proliferation, migration, or differentiation, or may damage already differentiated organs.
- Genetic defects may cause anomalies either directly or by influencing other genes. For example, morphogenesis genes (e.g., *HOX* and *PAX* genes) have proximal regulatory influences and distal target genes.

BIRTH WEIGHT AND GESTATIONAL AGE (p. 476)

Based on birth weight, infants are
- Appropriate for gestational age (10th to 90th percentiles)
- Small for gestational age (below 10th percentile)
- Large for gestational age (above 90th percentile)

Prematurity (p. 476)

Prematurity is defined as gestational age less than 37 weeks; major risk factors for prematurity are
- Preterm premature rupture of placental membranes: most common cause of prematurity (30%–40%).
- Intrauterine infection (25% of preterm births), with placental membrane inflammation (chorioamnionitis), and umbilical cord inflammation (funisitis). Most common microorganisms are *Ureaplasma urealyticum, Mycoplasma hominis, Gardnerella vaginalis, Trichomonas, gonorrhea,* and *Chlamydia.*
- Uterine, cervical, and placental structural abnormalities.
- Multiple gestation (twin pregnancy).

Fetal Growth Restriction (p. 477)

Infants with fetal growth restriction (FGR) are small for gestational age. Three main factors contribute:
- *Fetal:* chromosomal disorders (commonly trisomy 13, 18, and 21; live-born monosomy X; and triploidy); congenital anomalies; congenital infections, most commonly the TORCH group (*t*oxoplasmosis, *r*ubella, *c*ytomegalovirus, *h*erpesvirus, and *o*ther viruses and bacteria, such as syphilis).
- *Placental* (Chapter 22): abruptio placentae, placenta previa (low-lying placenta), placental thrombosis and infarctions, placental infections, umbilical-placental vascular anomalies, and multiple gestations. *Confined placental mosaicism* is another cause of FGR. Two genetic populations of cells (usually one normal and one abnormal—i.e., trisomic) are present in the placenta or fetus.
- *Maternal* (most common): underlying mechanism is decreased blood flow to the placenta. Causative factors are toxemia of pregnancy (Chapter 22), hypertension, nutritional status, narcotic or alcohol intake, heavy cigarette smoking, and certain drugs (may also be teratogens).

IMMATURITY OF ORGAN SYSTEMS (p. 478)

Structural and functional organ system immaturity is a major cause of morbidity and death in preterm infants, particularly those small for gestational age. Morphologic findings include the following:

- *Lungs:* The lungs may have thick-walled alveolar septa with increased connective tissue, physically separating vasculature from alveoli and hindering oxygenation. Alveolar spaces frequently contain eosinophilic proteinaceous precipitate and occasional squamous epithelial cells. Development of alveoli normally continues after birth, reaching the full complement of alveoli by age 8.

- *Kidneys:* Primitive glomeruli and tubules are present in the subcapsular zone (nephrogenic zone). However, deeper glomeruli and tubules are well formed and function is usually adequate.

- *Brain:* Grossly, the external surface is relatively smooth, with markedly simplified to absent convolutions (sulci and gyri). Both cell migration and myelination are incomplete; the brain is soft and gelatinous, and there is poor demarcation of white and gray matter. Vital brain centers are sufficiently developed to sustain normal function even in severe prematurity, although homeostasis of some systems (e.g., temperature, respiration) is imperfect.

- *Liver:* The liver is relatively large, partially as a result of extramedullary hematopoiesis. Many liver enzymes are poorly synthesized, including those responsible for biliary excretion; when coupled with fetal erythrocyte breakdown, this causes *physiologic jaundice* in prematurity.

APGAR SCORE (p. 479, Table 10–4 in *Robbins and Cotran Pathologic Basis of Disease*, 7th ed.)

The Apgar score is a measure of the physiologic condition and responsiveness of the newborn infant; it correlates with survival. It is calculated at 1 and 5 minutes of life using heart rate, respiratory effort, muscle tone, response to noxious stimulus, and skin color, each scored 0, 1, or 2. The higher the score, the better the outlook.

BIRTH INJURIES (p. 479)

The risk and nature of birth injuries vary with gestational age and size; injuries commonly involve the head, skeleton, liver, adrenals, and peripheral nerves.

- Intracranial hemorrhage is the most common important birth injury. Predisposing factors include prolonged labor, hypoxia, hemorrhagic disorders, and intracranial vascular anomalies. Consequences of intracranial hemorrhage include increased intracranial pressure, damage to brain substance, and herniation into the foramen magnum, with depression of vital medullary center function.

- *Caput succedaneum* is an accumulation of interstitial fluid in the scalp soft tissue; it causes circular areas of edema, congestion, and swelling where the head enters the lower uterine canal. If hemorrhage occurs, it is called *cephalohematoma*. Both caput succedaneum and cephalohematoma are of little clinical significance unless accompanied by skull fracture.

PERINATAL INFECTIONS (p. 480)

Specific infections are discussed in Chapter 8.

Transcervical (Ascending) Infections

Most bacterial and a few viral infections occur via the cervicovaginal route. Infection may be acquired *in utero* by inhaling infected amniotic fluid into the lungs, or at parturition by passing through an infected birth canal. Chorioamnionitis and funisitis are usually present. Pneumonia, sepsis, and meningitis are the most common sequelae.

Transplacental (Hematologic) Infections

Most parasites and viral infections (fewer bacterial infections) enter the fetal bloodstream via chorionic villi. Infection may occur at any time during gestation or, occasionally, at parturition. Sequela are highly variable, depending on the gestational timing and microorganism.

NEONATAL RESPIRATORY DISTRESS SYNDROME (p. 481)

There are many causes of respiratory distress in the newborn, including aspiration of blood or amniotic fluid during birth, brain injury affecting respiratory centers, an umbilical cord around the infant's neck, or excessive maternal sedation. The most common cause, however, is respiratory distress syndrome (RDS), also known as *hyaline membrane disease*.

Etiology and Pathogenesis (Fig. 10–1).

RDS occurs primarily in the immature lung. It is caused by a deficiency of the pulmonary surfactant synthesized by type II pneumocytes (Chapter 15). Type II pneumocytes are most abundant after 35 weeks' gestation; consequently, the incidence of RDS is 60% in infants born before 28 weeks' gestation and less than 5% in infants born after 37 weeks' gestation. Decreased surfactant results in increased alveolar surface tension, progressive alveolar atelectasis, and increasing inspiratory pressures required to expand alveoli. Hypoxemia results in acidosis, pulmonary vasoconstriction, pulmonary hypoperfusion, capillary endothelial and alveolar epithelial damage, and plasma leakage into alveoli; plasma proteins combine with fibrin and necrotic alveolar pneumocytes to form hyaline membranes. *Corticosteroids* help prevent RDS by inducing formation of surfactant lipids and apoprotein in fetal lung.

Morphology

Grossly, lungs are solid, airless, and reddish purple. Microscopically, alveoli are poorly developed and frequently collapsed; proteinaceous "membranes" line respiratory bronchioles, alveolar ducts, and random alveoli.

Clinical Presentation

The typical infant with RDS is preterm but appropriate for gestational age. RDS is associated with maternal diabetes

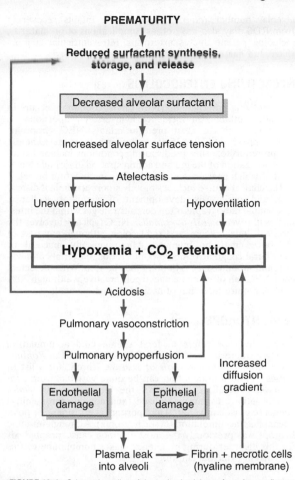

PREMATURITY

↓

Reduced surfactant synthesis, storage, and release

↓

Decreased alveolar surfactant

↓

Increased alveolar surface tension

↓

Atelectasis

Uneven perfusion | Hypoventilation

↓

Hypoxemia + CO₂ retention

↓

Acidosis

↓

Pulmonary vasoconstriction

↓

Pulmonary hypoperfusion

Increased diffusion gradient

Endothelial damage | Epithelial damage

↓

Plasma leak into alveoli → Fibrin + necrotic cells (hyaline membrane)

FIGURE 10–1 Schematic outline of the pathophysiology of respiratory distress syndrome (see text).

(surfactant synthesis is suppressed by high insulin levels) and cesarean section delivery.

Before delivery, amniotic fluid phospholipids (lecithin/sphingomyelin ratio) may be measured to assess fetal surfactant synthesis. If delivery cannot be delayed until the fetus is capable of adequate surfactant synthesis, therapy involves surfactant replacement and oxygen therapy. Prophylactic administration of surfactant at birth to extremely premature neonates (26–28 weeks) and symptomatic administration to older premature newborns is highly beneficial; it is now uncommon for infants to die of acute RDS. In uncomplicated cases, recovery begins in 3 to 4 days, but infants are at risk for developing *retinopathy of prematurity* (Chapter 29) and *bronchopulmonary dysplasia* (BPD), both due to high-concentration oxygen therapy. The major histopathologic abnormality in BPD is decreased alveolar number *(alveolar hypoplasia)*. Infants recovering from RDS may also have other complications of prematurity, including patent ductus arteriosus, intraventricular hemorrhage, and necrotizing enterocolitis.

NECROTIZING ENTEROCOLITIS (p. 483)

Necrotizing enterocolitis (NEC) most commonly occurs in premature infants; the incidence is inversely proportional to gestational age. In most preterm infants, NEC symptoms do not appear until 10 to 15 days after birth. Intestinal ischemia is a prerequisite; other predisposing conditions include bacterial colonization of the gut and administration of formula feeds, both of which aggravate mucosal injury in immature bowel.

The clinical course includes bloody stools, abdominal distention, and, ominously, development of circulatory collapse. Abdominal radiographs often demonstrate gas within the intestinal wall *(pneumatosis intestinalis)*. NEC typically involves the terminal ileum, cecum, and right colon, although any part of the bowel may be involved. Microscopically, mucosal or transmural coagulative necrosis, ulceration, bacterial colonization, and submucosal gas bubbles may be seen. When detected, early NEC can often be managed conservatively, although 20% to 60% require resection of necrotic bowel segments.

FETAL HYDROPS (p. 484)

Fetal hydrops refers to fetal edema fluid accumulation during intrauterine growth (see Table 10–5, p. 484 in *Robbins and Cotran Pathologic Basis of Disease*, 7th ed., for a list of causes). Fluid accumulation can be quite variable, from progressive, generalized edema of the fetus *(hydrops fetalis,* usually lethal), to more localized (and non–life-threatening) edema (e.g., isolated pleural and peritoneal effusions), or post-nuchal fluid accumulation (cystic hygroma). Although immune hydrops was previously the most common cause, prophylaxis for this disorder during pregnancy makes nonimmune causes the current principal culprits.

Immune Hydrops (Hemolytic Disease of the Newborn) (p. 485)

Immune hydrops occurs as a consequence of blood group incompatibility between mother and fetus.

Etiology and Pathogenesis

Immune hydrops occurs when the fetus inherits erythrocyte antigens from the father (e.g., Rh group D antigen) that the mother lacks. A small transplacental bleed (i.e., at the time of delivery) allows fetal erythrocytes to enter the maternal circulation where they induce antibody production. The first exposure to the specific antigenic stimulus elicits immunoglobulin M (IgM) antibodies that do not cross the placenta; however, subsequent exposure to the same antigen (usually small transplacental bleeds during subsequent pregnancies) elicit maternal IgG antibodies that do cross the placenta and bind to fetal red blood cells, resulting in erythrocyte lysis (p. 485, Fig. 10–14 in *Robbins and Cotran Pathologic Basis of Disease*, 7th ed.).

Only a minority of foreign blood group antigens are immunogenic; D antigen is the major cause of Rh incompatibility (the presence of D antigen is denoted Rh-positive; absence of D antigen is Rh-negative). In Rh-negative mothers, prophylaxis with anti-D immunoglobulin at the time of the initial delivery usually prevents sensitization and subsequent hemolytic disease of the newborn. Although ABO incompatibility is more common than Rh incompatibility, hemolytic disease severe enough to require treatment is rare in such mismatches because:

- Most anti-A and anti-B antibodies are IgM and do not cross the placenta.
- Neonatal red blood cells poorly express A and B blood group antigens.
- Many cells in addition to red blood cells express A and B antigens and therefore adsorb antibody that enters the fetal bloodstream.

Nonimmune Hydrops: Etiology and Pathogenesis (p. 486)

The three major causes of nonimmune hydrops are cardiovascular defects, chromosomal anomalies (Turner syndrome, trisomies 21 and 18), and fetal anemia unrelated to immune hemolysis (e.g., homozygous α-thalassemia). Transplacental infection by parvovirus B19 is also rapidly emerging as an important cause of hydrops; the virus enters and replicates within erythroid precursors (normoblasts), leading to erythrocyte maturation arrest and aplastic anemia. Approximately 10% of cases of nonimmune hydrops are related to monozygous twin pregnancies and twin-twin transfusions via anastomoses between the two circulations.

The anatomic findings in fetuses with intrauterine fluid accumulation vary with both the severity of the disease and the underlying cause. In hydrops associated with fetal anemia, both fetus and placenta are characteristically pale; the liver and spleen are enlarged from cardiac failure and congestion. Bone marrow demonstrates compensatory hyperplasia of erythroid precursors (except in parvovirus-associated aplastic anemia), and extramedullary hematopoiesis occurs in liver, spleen, and occasionally other tissues (kidneys, lungs, and heart). The increased hematopoiesis results in large numbers of immature red blood cells in the peripheral blood, including reticulocytes, normoblasts, and erythroblasts (hence the name *erythroblastosis fetalis*). The basis for hydrops in fetal anemia of both immune and nonimmune causes is tissue ischemia, with secondary myocardial dysfunction and circulatory failure. Liver failure may ensue, with loss of synthetic function contributing to hypoalbuminemia, reduced oncotic pressure, and exacerbating the edema. In severely jaundiced infants, elevated levels of unconjugated bilirubin cross the blood-brain barrier; these bind to lipids and are toxic to the brain, causing central nervous system damage *(kernicterus)*.

INBORN ERRORS OF METABOLISM AND OTHER GENETIC DISORDERS (p. 487)

Phenylketonuria (p. 487)

Approximately 50% of dietary phenylalanine is required for protein synthesis; the remainder is converted into tyrosine by the *phenylalanine hydroxylase* system. Homozygotes for one of several different mutations in the *phenylalanine hydroxylase* gene have variable enzymatic deficiencies and consequently variably elevated phenylalanine. The most frequent mutation, classic phenylketonuria (PKU), is relatively common in people of Scandinavian descent and uncommon in blacks and Jews.

Although normal at birth, affected infants exhibit rising plasma phenylalanine within the first few weeks of life, followed by impaired brain development and mental retardation. Fortunately, screening at birth for abnormally elevated urinary levels of various phenylalanine metabolites allows early diagnosis; subsequent phenylalanine dietary restriction prevents most clinical sequelae. Phenylalanine and its metabolites are teratogenic—most heterozygous infants born to PKU mothers with high phenylalanine levels are microcephalic and mentally retarded.

Some mutations in the *phenylalanine hydroxylase* gene result in a partial enzyme deficiency and therefore only moderately elevated phenylalanine levels. Such patients suffer no neurologic sequelae and the condition is called *benign hyperphenylalaninemia.* Other PKU variants result from deficiencies in other enzymes of the phenylalanine hydroxylase system; these patients have problems metabolizing other amino acids in addition to phenylalanine (such as tyrosine and tryptophan) and require specific recognition because phenylalanine restriction alone is not sufficient treatment.

Galactosemia (p. 488)

Dietary lactose, present in milk, is split into glucose and galactose in the intestinal mucosa by lactase; galactose is then converted to glucose by three additional enzymes. The most common and clinically significant form of galactosemia is autosomal recessive, resulting from mutation in *galactose-1-phosphate uridyl transferase (GALT);* affected patients accumulate galactose-1-phosphate.

The clinical picture of galactosemia is variable, corresponding to distinct mutations in *GALT.* Overall, infants fail to thrive and present with vomiting and diarrhea after milk ingestion. Liver, eyes, and brain are most severely affected; changes include hepatomegaly due to hepatic fat accumulation, followed by cirrhosis, cataracts, and nonspecific alterations in the central nervous system (including mental retardation).

Urinary screening at birth reveals the presence of an abnormal reducing sugar. Removal of dietary galactose for at least the first 2 years of life prevents most of the clinical and morphologic sequelae. Nevertheless, older patients may exhibit speech disorders and gonadal failure, possibly related to elevated levels of galactitol and other metabolites that accrue despite dietary compliance.

Cystic Fibrosis (p. 489)

With an incidence of 1 in 3200 live births in the United States, cystic fibrosis (CF) is the most common lethal genetic disease affecting whites. It affects epithelial ion transport resulting in abnormal fluid secretion in exocrine glands and in respiratory, gastrointestinal, and reproductive mucosa.

Etiology and Pathogenesis

The gene responsible for CF encodes the CFTR *(cystic fibrosis transmembrane conductance regulator)* protein. CFTR regulates the movement of multiple ions, as well as affecting other cellular processes; however, CFTR is primarily a chloride channel, and mutations in the *CFTR* gene disrupt epithelial chloride transport. Thus, normal sweat duct epithelia require CFTR for *resorption* of chloride; inability to resorb chloride causes increased sweat chloride concentration (hence the sweat chloride test used for clinical diagnosis). Conversely, normal airway and gastrointestinal epithelia require CFTR for *secretion* of chloride. The inability to secrete chloride into the lumen—combined with increased sodium absorption—causes osmotic resorption of water from the lumen and dehydration of the mucus layer coating the mucosal cells. Defective mucociliary action and the accumulation of hyperconcentrated, viscous secretions ultimately obstruct ductal outflow from the organs (the disease is also called *mucoviscidosis*). In addition, changes in secretion composition prevents activation of antibacterial "defensins" produced by epithelium, and predisposes patients to recurrent infections.

CFTR has two transmembrane domains, two nucleotide-binding domains, and a regulatory domain that contains protein kinase phosphorylation sites (p. 490, Fig. 10–20 in *Robbins and Cotran Pathologic Basis of Disease,* 7th ed.). Various mutations in the *CF* gene affect different regions of CFTR, resulting in distinct functional consequences and differing severity of clinical sequelae. At least 800 disease-causing mutations of *CFTR* have been identified; the most common is a three-nucleotide deletion normally coding for phenylalanine at position 508 (delta F508); this results in defective intracellular CFTR processing with degradation before it reaches the cell surface. Patients homozygous for the delta F508 mutation (or a combination of any two "severe" mutations) have virtual absence of CFTR function; they present with severe clinical disease (*classic* CF), including early pancreatic insufficiency and various degrees of pulmonary damage. Other combinations may present with features of *atypical* or *variant CF,* including isolated chronic pancreatitis, late-onset chronic pulmonary disease, or with infertility only (caused by bilateral absence of the vas deferens). Both environmental and genetic modifiers in addition to *CFTR* mutations modulate the frequency and severity of disease.

Morphology

Morphologic features are variable depending on the affected epithelium and the severity of involvement. Numerous areas may be involved:

- *Pancreas:* Abnormalities occur in 85% to 90% of patients; they range from mucus accumulation in small ducts with mild dilation to total atrophy of the exocrine pancreas, leaving only islets within fibrofatty stroma. Absence of pancreatic exocrine secretions impairs fat absorption; resulting avitaminosis A partly explains the squamous metaplasia frequently observed in ductal structures.
- *Intestine:* Thick viscous plugs of mucus (*meconium ileus*) may cause small intestinal obstruction (5%–10% of affected infants).
- *Liver:* Plugging of bile canaliculi by mucinous material (5% of patients) results in diffuse hepatic cirrhosis.
- *Salivary glands:* These glands are commonly involved with progressive duct dilation, ductal squamous metaplasia, and glandular atrophy.

- *Lungs:* The lungs are involved in most cases and such changes are the most serious complication of CF. Mucus-secreting cells hyperplasia and viscous secretions block and dilate bronchioles. Superimposed infections and pulmonary abscesses are common. *Staphylococcus aureus, Haemophilus influenzae,* and *Pseudomonas aeruginosa* are the three most common organisms; *Burkholderia cepacia* is associated with fulminant illness.
- *Male genital tract:* Azoospermia and infertility occur in 95% of males surviving to adulthood, frequently with congenital bilateral absence of the vas deferens.

Clinical Course (p. 494, Table 10–7 in *Robbins and Cotran Pathologic Basis of Disease,* 7th ed.)

The different molecular variants as well as the presence of secondary modifiers result in highly variable clinical manifestations. In classic CF, pancreatic exocrine insufficiency is universal, associated with malabsorption that presents as large, foul-smelling stools, abdominal distention, and poor weight gain. Poor fat absorption results in fat-soluble vitamin deficiencies (A, D, and K). Cardiorespiratory complications, such as chronic cough, persistent lung infections, obstructive pulmonary disease, and *cor pulmonale*, are the most common causes of death (~80%). Median life expectancy is 30 years, but may be modified by gene therapy in the future (transfer of the *CFTR* gene to correct the chloride defect). CF is the most common diagnosis in children receiving bilateral lung transplants.

SUDDEN INFANT DEATH SYNDROME (p. 495)

Sudden infant death syndrome (SIDS) is officially defined by the National Institute of Clinical Health and Human Development as the "sudden death of an infant less than 1 year of age, that remains unexplained after a thorough case investigation, including performance of a complete autopsy, examination of the death scene, and review of the clinical history." Most SIDS deaths occur between 2 and 4 months of life; the infant usually dies while asleep, without evidence of distress or struggle. SIDS is the leading cause of death in children between 1 month and 1 year of age in the United States, and the third leading cause of infant death overall.

Pathogenesis is poorly understood; SIDS is most likely a heterogeneous, multifactorial disorder. Potential risk factors include infant sleeping prone, prematurity and low birth weight, SIDS in a prior sibling, young maternal age, short intergestational interval, inadequate prenatal care, low socioeconomic status, and maternal smoking or drug abuse. Most SIDS babies have an immediate prior history of a mild respiratory tract infection, but no single causative organism has been isolated. Developmental immaturity of critical brain stem regions (e.g., arcuate nucleus) involved in arousal and cardiorespiratory control may play a role.

Autopsy findings are usually subtle and of uncertain significance. Multiple petechiae (thymus, visceral and parietal pleura, epicardium) and histologic evidence of recent infection in the upper respiratory tract are common. The central nervous system demonstrates astrogliosis of the brain stem and cerebellum; hypoplasia of the arcuate nucleus is reported. SIDS is a diagnosis of exclusion, and a thorough autopsy must be performed to exclude other causes of sudden death (infections, metabolic disorders, and trauma).

TUMORS AND TUMOR-LIKE LESIONS OF INFANCY AND CHILDHOOD (p. 498)

Benign tumors are much more common than malignant tumors; however, cancer is the leading cause of death from disease in U.S. children ages 4 to 14 years.

Benign Tumors and Tumor-Like Lesions (p. 498)

Distinguishing between true tumors and tumor-like lesions in the infant and child is difficult because displaced cells and masses of tissue may be present from birth; these are frequently histologically normal and grow at approximately the same rate as the infant.

- *Heterotopia* represents microscopically normal cells or tissues present in abnormal locations; these cells are usually of little significance but may be clinically confused with true neoplasms.
- *Hamartomas* are excessive (but focal) overgrowth of cells and tissues native to the organ or site in which they occur; they may be considered a link between malformations and neoplasms.

Hemangiomas

Hemangiomas are the most common tumors of infancy; most are cutaneous, particularly on the face and scalp. They may enlarge along with the growth of the child, but commonly spontaneously regress (p. 498, Fig. 10–25 in *Robbins and Cotran Pathologic Basis of Disease,* 7th ed.); they rarely become malignant. Hemangiomas may represent one facet of hereditary disorders such as *von Hippel–Lindau disease* (Chapter 28).

Lymphangiomas

Lymphangiomas may occur on the skin but also within deeper regions of the neck, axilla, mediastinum, and retroperitoneal tissue. They tend to increase in size and, depending on location, become clinically significant if they encroach on vital structures. Histologically, lymphangiomas are composed of cystic and cavernous lymphatic spaces, with variable numbers of associated lymphocytes.

Fibrous Tumors

Histologically, fibrous tumors range from sparsely cellular proliferations (fibromatosis) to richly cellular lesions indistinguishable from adult fibrosarcomas. In contrast to fibrous tumors occurring in adults, the histologic picture does not predict the biology of an individual tumor (e.g., congenital-infantile fibrosarcomas may spontaneously regress). A characteristic chromosomal translocation t(12;15)(p13;q25), producing an *ETV6-NTRK3* fusion gene, has been described in congenital-infantile fibrosarcomas.

Teratomas

Teratoma incidence has two peaks: at age 2, and again in late adolescence. Those occurring in infancy and childhood tend to arise in the sacrococcygeal region.

- Approximately 10% of sacrococcygeal teratomas are associated with congenital anomalies, primarily defects of the hindgut and cloacal region and other midline defects.
- Sacrococcygeal teratomas are histologically similar to other teratomas; mesodermal, endodermal, and ectodermal elements are present (Chapter 22). Approximately 75% contain mature tissues only and are benign; approximately half of the remainder are mixed with other germ cell malignancies (e.g., endodermal sinus tumor) and are malignant. The rest, designated immature teratomas, contain mature and immature tissue, with malignant potential correlating with the extent of immature tissues.

Malignant Tumors (p. 499)

Malignant tumors not discussed here are covered in the appropriate organ system chapter. Childhood malignancies differ biologically and histologically from their adult counterparts by:

- A close relationship between abnormal development (teratogenesis) and tumor induction (oncogenesis)
- A greater prevalence of underlying familial or genetic germline aberrations
- A tendency for some malignancies in the fetal or neonatal period to regress spontaneously or cytodifferentiate

The most frequent childhood cancers arise in the hematopoietic system (leukemia, some lymphomas), central nervous system (astrocytoma, medulloblastoma, ependymoma), adrenal medulla (neuroblastoma), retina (retinoblastoma), soft tissue (rhabdomyosarcoma), bone (Ewing sarcoma, osteogenic sarcoma), and kidney (Wilms tumor). Leukemia accounts for more deaths in children younger than 15 years of age than all other tumors combined (Table 10–3).

Histologically, many pediatric cancers tend to have a more primitive (embryonal) rather than anaplastic/pleomorphic appearance, frequently exhibiting features of organogenesis specific to the site of origin. Some pediatric tumors with a primitive appearance are collectively referred to as "small, round blue cell tumors" (e.g., neuroblastoma, lymphoma, rhab-

TABLE 10–3 **Common Malignant Neoplasms of Infancy and Childhood**

0 to 4 Years	5 to 9 Years	10 to 14 Years
Leukemia	Leukemia	
Retinoblastoma	Retinoblastoma	
Neuroblastoma	Neuroblastoma	
Wilms tumor		
Hepatoblastoma	Hepatocarcinoma	Hepatocarcinoma
Soft tissue sarcoma (especially rhabdomyosarcoma)	Soft tissue sarcoma	Soft tissue sarcoma
Teratomas		
Central nervous system tumors	Central nervous system tumors	
	Ewing sarcoma	
	Lymphoma	
		Osteogenic sarcoma
		Thyroid carcinoma
		Hodgkin disease

domyosarcoma, Ewing sarcoma/peripheral neuroectodermal tumor [PNET]).

Neuroblastic Tumors (p. 500)

Most neuroblastic tumors occur in children younger than 5 years of age, and arise in the adrenal medulla or various sympathetic ganglia. Neuroblastoma is the most common histologic subtype, characterized by sheets of small, round blue neuroblasts within a neurofibrillary background (neuropil) and characteristic *Homer-Wright pseudorosettes* (p. 501, Fig. 10–28 in *Robbins and Cotran Pathologic Basis of Disease,* 7th ed.). Some tumors display variable differentiation toward ganglion cells, accompanied by the appearance of a so-called *"schwannian stroma"* (organized fascicles of neuritic processes, Schwann cells, and fibroblasts). Depending on the degree of differentiation, these latter tumors are called *ganglioneuroblastomas* or *ganglioneuromas*.

In addition to local infiltration and lymph node spread, there is a pronounced tendency for hematogenous spread involving the liver, lungs, bones, and marrow. Depending on the pattern of metastases, tumors are stage I (confined to the organ of origin) through IV (disseminated metastases). Stage IV/S tumors are unique, usually occurring in infants or neonates; there is a primary adrenal tumor, a markedly enlarged liver from extensive liver metastases, and tumor nodules within the skin and bone marrow (without bony destruction). Infants with these disseminated tumors have a greater than 80% 5-year survival rate with minimal to no therapy.

About 90% of neuroblastomas produce catecholamines; elevated blood or urine catecholamine metabolites are important diagnostic features. Stage and age are the most important determinants of outcome. Infants (<12 months) have an excellent prognosis regardless of stage, but children older than 5 years usually have extremely poor outcomes. Additional prognostic indicators include histologic features (schwannian stroma is favorable), tumor ploidy (diploidy, near-diploidy, or near-tetraploidy are unfavorable), *N-myc* amplification (unfavorable), 17q gain and 1p loss (unfavorable), telomerase overexpression (unfavorable), and *TrkA* expression (favorable).

Wilms Tumor (p. 504)

Wilms tumor of the kidney is usually diagnosed between ages 2 and 5 years. Although malignant, the overall survival rate is greater than 90%. Although 90% are sporadic, there are associations with three groups of malformation syndromes, all involving chromosome 11p:

- *WAGR* (Wilms tumor, aniridia, genital anomalies, mental retardation): Patients have a 33% chance of developing Wilms tumor; WAGR involves deletion on chromosome 11p band 13 of the Wilms tumor 1 *(WT1)* gene and also the aniridia gene *PAX6* just distal to this locus. The *WT1* gene is critical to normal renal and gonadal development, and transgenic mice lacking functional *WT1* have agenesis of both organs.

- *Denys-Drash syndrome:* Patients have gonadal dysgenesis and nephropathy leading to renal failure; most develop Wilms tumors. The genetic abnormality is a dominant negative mutation in the *WT1* gene that affects DNA binding.

- *Beckwith-Wiedemann syndrome:* Patients have enlarged body organs, hemihypertrophy, renal medullary cysts, adrenal cytomegaly, and a predisposition to developing Wilms and other primitive tumors; the genetic abnormality is localized to chromosome 11 band p15.5 (the Wilms tumor 2 *[WT2]* locus). Several candidate genes map to this locus, including insulin-like growth factor 2 *(IGF2); IGF2* is normally imprinted (transcribed from only one parental allele) but demonstrates loss of imprinting (biallelic expression) in tumors.

Morphology. Wilms tumors are soft, large, well-circumscribed renal masses characterized by triphasic histologic features: (1) blastema, (2) immature stroma, and (3) tubules—an attempt to recapitulate nephrogenesis (p. 506, Fig. 10–32 in *Robbins and Cotran Pathologic Basis of Disease,* 7th ed.). Histologic anaplasia (cells with large, hyperchromatic, pleomorphic nuclei and abnormal mitoses) is associated with a worse prognosis (approximately 5% of tumors). *Nephrogenic rests* are putative precursor lesions of Wilms tumors, and are seen in renal parenchyma adjacent to approximately 40% of unilateral tumors; with bilateral Wilms tumors, this frequency rises to nearly 100%. With appropriate chemotherapy, prognosis is now excellent.

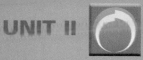

DISEASES OF
ORGAN SYSTEMS

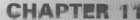

CHAPTER 11

Blood Vessels

Pathologic changes in blood vessels have the following general consequences (p. 516):

- Narrowing and obstructing the vessel lumen—either slowly (e.g., by atherosclerosis) or precipitously (e.g., by thrombosis)—thereby restricting blood flow to the downstream tissues. Restricted flow can cause tissue atrophy or infarction, depending on the severity of the narrowing and the rate at which it develops.
- Weakening the vessel walls, leading to dilation, dissection, or rupture.
- Causing thrombotic deposits that can embolize and obstruct downstream vessels.

CONGENITAL ANOMALIES (p. 515)

- Anomalous (e.g., aberrant, reduplicated) vessels, principally of interest to surgeons.
- *Berry aneurysms* are vascular outpouchings resulting from areas of congenital wall weakness. Occurring in cerebral vessels, they occasionally rupture catastrophically (Chapter 28).
- *Arteriovenous fistulas* are abnormal communications between arteries and veins. They may be congenital or secondary to trauma, inflammation, or a healed ruptured aneurysm. Fistulas can cause left-to-right vascular shunts, increasing venous return and predisposing to high-output heart failure.

ARTERIOSCLEROSIS (p. 515)

Arteriosclerosis denotes arterial wall thickening and loss of elasticity. Three patterns are recognized:

- Atherosclerosis (most important).
- *Arteriolosclerosis* (primarily associated with hypertension).

267

- *Mönckeberg medial calcific sclerosis*: Characterized by medial calcification in small to medium-sized muscular arteries (commonly femoral, tibial, radial, ulnar, and genital arteries), typically occurring after age 50. The pathogenesis is unknown, but is not related to atherosclerosis. The calcific deposits are nonobstructive and not usually clinically significant.

ATHEROSCLEROSIS (p. 515)

Atherosclerosis is a slowly progressive disease of large to medium-sized muscular and large elastic arteries; principal sites include the abdominal aorta, coronary arteries, popliteal arteries, descending thoracic aorta, internal carotid arteries, and circle of Willis (in descending frequency). Atherosclerosis is characterized by elevated intimal-based *fibrofatty plaques* composed of lipids, proliferating smooth muscle cells (SMCs), and increased extracellular matrix (ECM). Lesions are initially focal, with patchy vessel involvement both circumferentially and longitudinally.

Morphology (p. 517)

The characteristic atheromatous plaque *(atheroma or fibrofatty plaque)* is a raised white-yellow intimal-based lesion, protruding into the vessel lumen. *Histologically,* plaques are composed of superficial *fibrous caps* containing SMCs, leukocytes, and dense connective tissue ECM overlying *necrotic cores,* containing dead cells, lipid, cholesterol clefts, lipid-laden foam cells (macrophages and SMCs), and plasma proteins; small blood vessels proliferate at the intimal-medial interface. Two common variants are recognized:

- *Fatty streaks:* Early lesions composed of intimal collections of lipid-laden macrophages and SMCs in patients as young as 1 year old. A causal relationship between fatty streaks and atheromatous plaques is suspected but remains unproved.
- *Complicated plaques:* Calcified, hemorrhagic, fissured, or ulcerated atheromas, predisposing to local thrombosis, medial thinning, cholesterol microemboli, and aneurysmal dilation.

Epidemiology and Risk Factors (p. 520)

Risk of developing atherosclerosis increases with age, family history, hypertension, cigarette smoking, hypercholesterolemia, and diabetes—the last five designated *major risk factors.* Lesser influences on atherosclerosis risk include obesity, sedentary or high-stress life style, type A personality, and other factors listed in Table 11–1.

Risk correlates with levels of serum low-density lipoprotein (LDL); because LDL carries 70% of the total serum cholesterol, increased level implies increased circulating cholesterol that can deposit in vessel walls. Risk is *inversely* related to high-density lipoprotein (HDL) levels, in part because HDL helps clear cholesterol from vessel wall lesions. Hereditary defects involving the LDL receptor (e.g., *familial hypercholesterolemia*) or LDL apoproteins cause elevated LDL, hypercholesterolemia, and accelerated atherosclerosis.

TABLE 11-1   **Risk Factors for Atherosclerosis**

Major	Lesser, Uncertain, or Nonquantitated
Nonmodifiable	
Increasing age	Obesity
Male gender	Physical inactivity
Family history	Stress ("type A" personality)
Genetic abnormalities	Postmenopausal estrogen deficiency
	High carbohydrate intake
Potentially Controllable	
Hyperlipidemia	Lipoprotein Lp(a)
Hypertension	Hardened (trans)unsaturated fat intake
Cigarette smoking	*Chlamydia pneumoniae*
Diabetes	

Several markers of hemostatic/thrombotic function and inflammation are also predictive; for example, C-reactive protein (CRP), an indicator of systemic inflammation levels, correlates with atherosclerosis risk.

Pathogenesis (p. 521)

Most models of atherosclerosis invoke endothelial (or medial) damage as an initiator. Causes of endothelial cell (EC) injury include hyperlipidemia, hemodynamic disturbances (e.g., disturbed flow), smoking, hypertension, toxins, and infectious agents. In turn, EC injury causes increased endothelial permeability, white blood cell and platelet adhesion, and coagulation activation. These events induce chemical mediator (e.g., growth factors and inflammatory mediators) release and activation, followed by recruitment and subsequent proliferation of SMC in the intima to produce the atheroma. This contemporary view of pathogenesis is called the *response to injury hypothesis: atherosclerosis is considered to be a chronic inflammatory response of the arterial wall to some form of EC injury* (Fig. 11-1):

- Focal EC injury, usually subtle, causes endothelial dysfunction, increasing endothelial permeability and expression of leukocyte adhesion molecules.
- Blood monocytes and other leukocytes adhere to the altered ECs.
- Monocytes migrate into the intima and transform into macrophages; these can accumulate lipid to become *foam cells*.
- Lipoproteins (mainly LDL with its high cholesterol content and very low density lipoproteins [VLDL]) insudate into vessel walls at foci of EC injury.
- Macrophages oxidize the lipoproteins.
- Platelets adhere to areas of EC injury (or loss), or to leukocytes.
- Activated platelets, macrophages, or vascular wall cells release factors (e.g., platelet-derived growth factor [PDGF]) that cause medial SMCs to migrate into the intima.
- SMCs proliferate in the intima and elaboration of ECM lead to collagen and proteoglycan accumulation.
- Lipids accumulate both within cells (macrophages and SMC) and extracellularly.
- Ongoing inflammation mediates lesion progression and *subsequent complications* (see also Chapter 12). Although

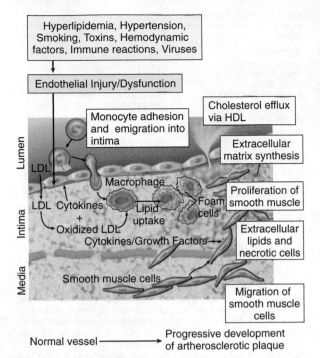

FIGURE 11–1 Schematic diagram of hypothetical sequence of cell-level events and cellular interactions in atherosclerosis. Hyperlipidemia and other risk factors are thought to cause endothelial injury, resulting in adhesion of platelets and monocytes and release of growth factors, including platelet-derived growth factor (PDGF), which lead to smooth muscle cell migration and proliferation. Foam cells of atheromatous plaques are derived from both macrophages and smooth muscle cells—from macrophages via the very low density lipoprotein (VLDL) receptor and low-density lipoprotein (LDL) modifications recognized by scavenger receptors (e.g., oxidized LDL), and from smooth muscle cells by less certain mechanisms. Extracellular lipid is derived from insudation from the vessel lumen, particularly in the presence of hypercholesterolemia, and also from degenerating foam cells. Cholesterol accumulation in the plaque reflects an imbalance between influx and efflux, and high-density lipoprotein (HDL) likely helps clear cholesterol from these accumulations. Smooth muscle cells migrate to the intima, proliferate, and produce extracellular matrix, including collagen and proteoglycans.

monocyte recruitment and foam cell formation is initially protective (by removing potentially harmful lipid metabolites), activated macrophages produce cytokines that recruit more monocytes and T cells to the intima, induce growth factor production (contributing to SMC proliferation), and induce synthesis of reactive oxygen species (that can oxidize LDL). Macrophage and T-cell cross-talk also causes cellular immune activation characteristic of a chronic inflammatory state.

Clinical Features (p. 516)

Atherosclerosis can begin in childhood but is typically asymptomatic for decades until it finally manifests itself via one of the following mechanisms (Fig. 11–2):

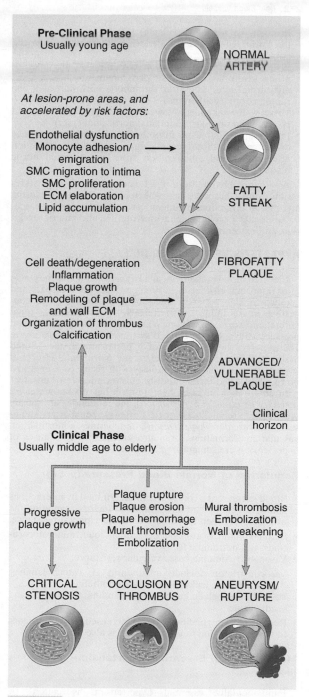

Pre-Clinical Phase
Usually young age

NORMAL ARTERY

At lesion-prone areas, and accelerated by risk factors:

Endothelial dysfunction
Monocyte adhesion/ emigration
SMC migration to intima
SMC proliferation
ECM elaboration
Lipid accumulation

FATTY STREAK

Cell death/degeneration
Inflammation
Plaque growth
Remodeling of plaque and wall ECM
Organization of thrombus
Calcification

FIBROFATTY PLAQUE

ADVANCED/ VULNERABLE PLAQUE

Clinical horizon

Clinical Phase
Usually middle age to elderly

Progressive plaque growth

Plaque rupture
Plaque erosion
Plaque hemorrhage
Mural thrombosis
Embolization

Mural thrombosis
Embolization
Wall weakening

CRITICAL STENOSIS

OCCLUSION BY THROMBUS

ANEURYSM/ RUPTURE

FIGURE 11–2 Schematic summary of the morphologic features, pathogenetic events, and clinical complications and natural history of atherosclerosis in the coronary arteries. ECM, extracellular matrix; SMC, smooth muscle cells.

- Insidious narrowing of vascular lumens (e.g., gangrene of the lower leg because of stenosing atherosclerosis in the popliteal artery)
- Plaque rupture or superficial erosion followed by superimposed thrombus causing sudden luminal occlusion (e.g., myocardial infarction after thrombotic occlusion of a disrupted coronary atheroma)
- Vessel wall weakening followed by aneurysm formation and possible rupture (e.g., abdominal aortic aneurysm)
- Providing a source of thromboemboli or atheroembolic debris causing distal organ damage (e.g., renal infarction after cholesterol embolization from an ulcerated aortic plaque)

Approximately one third of all deaths in the United States result from atherosclerosis, which is significant in causing myocardial infarction or sudden cardiac death, cerebrovascular accidents (strokes), aneurysm rupture, mesenteric occlusion, and extremity gangrene.

HYPERTENSIVE VASCULAR DISEASE (p. 525)

Elevated blood pressure is called *hypertension;* it is the single most important risk factor in both coronary heart disease and cerebrovascular accidents and can also directly cause congestive heart failure (hypertensive heart disease), renal failure, and aortic dissection. When defined as diastolic blood pressure above 90 mm Hg and systolic blood pressure above 140 mm Hg, the prevalence of hypertension in the United States is about 25%. Nevertheless, the detrimental effects of hypertension increase continuously with rising pressures and no rigidly defined threshold distinguishes safe versus unsafe.

In about 90% of cases hypertension has no known cause *(primary* or *essential hypertension);* the remainder are mostly secondary to renal disease or (less often) to renal artery stenosis *(renovascular hypertension),* endocrine abnormalities, vascular malformations, or neurogenic disorders. Causes of hypertension are summarized in Table 11–2.

Regulation of Normal Blood Pressure (p. 526)

Blood pressure is a complex trait determined by interactions of multiple genetic and environmental factors regulating the relationship between blood volume and peripheral resistance.

- Blood volume is affected by sodium load, mineralocorticoids, and natriuretic factors
- Vasoconstriction increases vascular resistance:

   Vasoconstrictors include angiotensin II, catecholamines, thromboxane, leukotrienes, and endothelin.
   Vasodilators include kinins, prostaglandins, nitric oxide, and adenosine.

- Regional autoregulation, wherein increased blood flow leads to vasoconstriction (and vice versa), is also important.

Mechanisms of Essential Hypertension (p. 527)

Fundamentally, essential hypertension is caused by increased blood volume (e.g., due to reduced renal sodium

TABLE 11–2   **Types and Causes of Hypertension**

Essential Hypertension

Secondary Hypertension

Renal
  Acute glomerulonephritis
  Chronic renal disease
  Polycystic disease
  Renal artery stenosis
  Renal artery fibromuscular dysplasia
  Renal vasculitis
  Renin-producing tumors
Endocrine
  Adrenocortical hyperfunction (Cushing syndrome, primary
    aldosteronism, congenital adrenal hyperplasia, licorice ingestion)
  Exogenous hormones (glucocorticoids, estrogen [including pregnancy-
    induced and oral contraceptives], sympathomimetics and tyramine-
    containing foods, monoamine oxidase inhibitors)
  Pheochromocytoma
  Acromegaly
  Hypothyroidism (myxedema)
  Hyperthyroidism (thyrotoxicosis)
  Pregnancy-induced
Cardiovascular
  Coarctation of aorta
  Polyarteritis nodosa (or other vasculitis)
  Increased intravascular volume
  Increased cardiac output
  Rigidity of the aorta
Neurologic
  Psychogenic
  Increased intracranial pressure
  Sleep apnea
  Acute stress, including surgery

excretion) or increased peripheral resistance (e.g., due to increased release of vasoconstrictor agents, increased sensitivity of vascular smooth muscle cells, or neurogenic factors), or both. Abnormalities in renal blood pressure regulation can also contribute to essential hypertension by affecting either of two systems:

- The renin-angiotensin system (e.g., hypertension in individuals with specific genetic variants of *angiotensinogen,* the physiologic substrate for renin)
- Sodium homeostasis

Although single gene disorders can *rarely* cause severe hypertension, it is unlikely that mutations in a single gene locus are major sources of essential hypertension in the larger population. It is much more likely that essential hypertension is a heterogeneous and multifactorial disorder in which the combined effect of mutations or polymorphisms at several gene loci influence blood pressure in concert with multiple nongenetic variables. Thus, environmental factors (e.g., stress, salt intake) can also contribute, but usually only in genetically predisposed individuals.

Vascular Pathology in Hypertension (p. 529)

Hypertension accelerates atherogenesis and causes structural changes that potentiate both aortic dissection and cerebrovascular hemorrhage. In addition, hypertension is associated with *arteriolosclerosis,* primarily affecting arterioles and small arteries, particularly in the kidney. The two basic types of arteriolosclerosis, *hyaline* and *hyperplastic,* are characterized by diffuse arteriolar wall thickening, luminal narrowing, and resultant distal tissue ischemia.

Morphology (p. 529)

- *Hyaline arteriolosclerosis* typically occurs in elderly patients, particularly those with mild hypertension and mild diabetes, and is the major microscopic feature of benign nephrosclerosis (see Chapter 20). The lesion probably reflects EC injury, with subsequent plasma leakage into arteriolar walls and ECM synthesis by SMCs. Microscopically, there is diffuse, pink, hyaline arteriolar thickening.

- *Hyperplastic arteriolosclerosis* is characteristic of malignant hypertension (acute, severe elevations in blood pressure; see Chapter 20). There is concentric laminated *(onionskin)* arteriolar thickening with reduplicated basement membrane and SMC proliferation, frequently associated with fibrin deposition and wall necrosis, so-called *necrotizing arteriolitis.*

ANEURYSMS AND DISSECTIONS (p. 530)

Aneurysms are focal abnormal vascular dilations. A *true aneurysm* is bounded by all three vessel wall layers (intima, media, and adventitia), although they may be attenuated. In contrast, a *false aneurysm* (also called *pseudoaneurysm* or *pulsating hematoma*) is an extravascular hematoma that communicates with the intravascular space; part of the vessel wall is missing. Morbidity and death due to aneurysms are secondary to:

- Rupture
- Impingement on adjacent structures
- Occlusion of proximal vessels by extrinsic pressure or superimposed thrombosis
- Embolism from a mural thrombus

Causes of aneurysms include atherosclerosis and *cystic medial degeneration* (the two most common causes), syphilis, trauma, polyarteritis nodosa, congenital defects, and infections (called *mycotic aneurysms*). Atherosclerosis causes arterial wall thinning through medial destruction secondary to expansion of the intimal plaque. *Atherosclerotic aneurysms usually (but not exclusively) occur in the abdominal aorta, most frequently between the renal arteries and the iliac bifurcation or in the common iliac arteries.*

Abdominal Aortic Aneurysms (p. 531)

Abdominal aortic aneurysms (AAAs) are true aneurysms typically found in men over age 50. Risk of rupture increases with the maximal diameter of the AAA: minimal risk if smaller than 5 cm but a risk of 5% to 10% annually when greater than 5 cm. Operative mortality rate is 5% for unruptured aneurysm but more than 50% after rupture. Because aortic atherosclerosis is usually accompanied by severe coronary atherosclerosis, patients with AAA have a high incidence of ischemic heart disease.

Syphilitic (Luetic) Aneurysms (p. 532)

Arising in the tertiary stage of syphilis, these aneurysms are typically confined to the ascending aorta and arch. They may extend retrograde to the aortic valve ring with dilation leading to valvular insufficiency. With time, chronic left ventricular volume overload produces massive cardiac hypertrophy (often to 1000 gm), called *cor bovinum*.

Syphilitic aortitis begins as adventitial inflammation involving the vasa vasorum, with resultant *obliterative endarteritis;* affected vasa vasora have a perivascular infiltrate of lymphocytes and plasma cells, with hyperplastic thickening of the walls that severely restricts blood supply to the outer two thirds of the medial wall. The result is aortic medial ischemia and patchy elastic fiber and SMC loss, with wall weakening and scarring.

Symptoms occur as a consequence of the valvular insufficiency, impingement of the aneurysm on surrounding thoracic organs, or—rarely—rupture.

Aortic Dissection (Dissecting Hematoma) (p. 532)

Dissection of blood along the laminar planes of the aortic media, forming an intramural blood-filled channel, is an ominous event, as it often ruptures, causing massive hemorrhage that may produce sudden death. Aortic dissection is not usually associated with marked preexisting aortic dilation. Although it can be a complication of therapeutic or diagnostic arterial cannulation or other trauma, aortic dissection occurs principally in two groups:

- Men 40 to 60 years old, in whom hypertension is almost invariably an antecedent (>90% of dissections). Hypertensive patients have nonspecific degenerative histologic changes, including mild-moderate elastic fragmentation and excess amorphous ECM.
- Younger individuals with connective tissue defects that affect the aorta (e.g., *Marfan syndrome*). In Marfan syndrome, there is marked elastic tissue fragmentation and disruption with focal cleftlike or "cystic" spaces filled with amorphous ECM, so-called *cystic medial degeneration.* The defect in Marfan syndrome is a genetic deficiency of an elastic tissue microfibrillary protein called *fibrillin* (see Chapter 5).

The risk of serious complications following dissection depend strongly on the portion of the aorta affected. Complications include rupture of the dissection into a body cavity, extension into the great arteries of the neck or other major branches of the aorta, and retrograde dissection that disrupts the aortic valve or coronary arteries. Aortic dissections are classified into two types:

- The more common (and dangerous) *proximal* lesions, involving the ascending aorta (called *type A*)
- *Distal lesions not involving the ascending part* and usually beginning distal to the subclavian artery *(type B)*

The classic clinical presentation of aortic dissection is the sudden onset of excruciating pain, usually beginning in the anterior chest, radiating to the back, and moving downward as the dissection progresses. In type A dissections, there is typically an intimal tear (a portal of entry of blood) in the ascending aorta within 10 cm of the aortic valve. When an intimal tear is not present, rupture of an intramural portion of the vasa vasorum is the likely source of hemorrhage.

INFLAMMATORY DISEASE: THE VASCULITIDES
(p. 534)

Vasculitis (i.e., vascular inflammatory injury, often with necrosis) may be localized, due to direct injury (e.g., infection, trauma, toxins), or systemic, characterized by multifocal necrosis *(necrotizing vasculitis)* and thrombosis. Most systemic vasculitides probably have an immune etiology, resulting from:

- Deposition of circulating antigen-antibody complexes (e.g., acute arteritis in systemic lupus erythematosus, see Chapter 6)
- Antibody to fixed tissue antigens (e.g., Goodpasture syndrome, see Chapters 15 and 20)
- Delayed-type hypersensitivity reactions, especially in lesions with granulomas (e.g., temporal arteritis, see below)

In many patients with small vessel vasculitis, there are circulating antibodies reactive with neutrophil cytoplasmic antigens (demonstrable by immunofluorescence assays), so-called *antineutrophilic cytoplasmic autoantibodies (ANCA).* The pattern of immunofluorescent staining is either perinuclear (*P-ANCA*), in which the major antigen is *myeloperoxidase,* or cytoplasmic (*C-ANCA*), in which the antigen is *proteinase 3.* Either specificity can occur in patients with ANCA-associated vasculitis, but C-ANCA is characteristically associated with *Wegener granulomatosis,* and P-ANCA is found in most cases of *microscopic polyangiitis* or *Churg-Strauss syndrome.* It is worth emphasizing that the assay is neither 100% sensitive nor specific for these entities; 10% of cases of otherwise characteristic small vessel vasculitis do not have demonstrable ANCA, and P- and C-ANCA are found in other entities. A close association between ANCA titers and disease activity (particularly C-ANCA in Wegener granulomatosis) suggests they are important in pathogenesis, although the mechanisms by which ANCA induces injury are unknown.

Vasculitides are classified according to vessel size and site, lesion histology, clinical manifestations, and pathogenesis (Table 11–3).

Giant Cell (Temporal) Arteritis (p. 536)

The most common form of vasculitis, this is characterized by focal granulomatous inflammation of medium-sized and small arteries, chiefly cranial vessels and most commonly the temporal arteries in elderly people. It may rarely involve the aortic arch *(giant cell aortitis).* The cause is unknown.

Morphology

There are three general histologic types, likely reflecting stages in a continuum; there often is associated thrombosis. Biopsy may be negative in one-third of patients, presumably owing to lesion focality.

- Granulomatous vasculitis with fragmented internal elastic lamina and a giant cell reaction (two-thirds of cases)

TABLE 11–3 **Classification and Characteristics of Selected Types of Vasculitis**

Large Vessel Vasculitis*†	
Giant cell (temporal) arteritis	Granulomatous arteritis of the aorta and its major branches, with a predilection for the extracranial branches of the carotid artery. Often involves the temporal artery. Usually occurs in patients older than age 50 and often is associated with polymyalgia rheumatica.
Takayasu arteritis	Granulomatous inflammation of the aorta and its major branches. Usually occurs in patients younger than age 50.
Medium-Sized Vessel Vasculitis‡	
Polyarteritis nodosa (classic polyarteritis nodosa)	Necrotizing inflammation of medium-sized or small arteries without glomerulonephritis or vasculitis in arterioles, capillaries, or venules
Kawasaki disease	Arteritis involving large, medium-sized, or small arteries and associated with mucocutaneous lymph node syndrome. Coronary arteries are often involved. Aorta and veins may be involved. Usually occurs in children.
Small Vessel Vasculitis§	
Wegener granulomatosis″	Granulomatous inflammation involving the respiratory tract and necrotizing vasculitis affecting small to medium-sized vessels (e.g., capillaries, venules, arterioles, and arteries). Necrotizing glomerulonephritis is common.
Churg-Strauss syndrome″	Eosinophil-rich and granulomatous inflammation involving the respiratory tract and necrotizing vasculitis affecting small to medium-sized vessels associated with asthma and blood eosinophilia.
Microscopic polyangiitis (microscopic polyarteritis)″	Necrotizing vasculitis with few or no immune deposits affecting small vessels (i.e., capillaries, venules, or arterioles). Necrotizing arteritis involving small and medium-sized arteries may be present. Necrotizing glomerulonephritis is common. Pulmonary capillaritis often occurs.

*Note that some small and large vessel vasculitides may involve medium-sized arteries, but large and medium-sized vessel vasculitides do not involve vessels smaller than arteries.
†Aorta and its largest branches to extremities and head and neck.
‡Main visceral arteries and their branches.
§Arterioles, venules, capillaries (occasionally small arteries).
″Strongly associated with antineutrophil cytoplasmic autoantibodies (ANCA), predominantly cytoplasmic (antiproteinase 3) C-ANCA in Wegener granulomatosis, and perinuclear (antimyeloperoxidase) P-ANCA in microscopic polyangiitis and Churg-Strauss syndrome.
Modified from Jennette JC, et al: Nomenclature of systemic vasculitides: The proposal of an international consensus conference. Arthritis Rheum 37:187, 1994.

- Nonspecific leukocytic infiltration of vessel walls
- Intimal fibrosis with wall thickening and luminal narrowing

Clinical Features

Temporal arteritis typically presents with headache and facial pain; 50% of patients have systemic symptoms, including a flu-like syndrome with myalgias, arthralgias, and fever, called *polymyalgia rheumatica*. It may cause visual disturbances and even blindness (an acute emergency). The disease responds well to steroids.

Takayasu Arteritis (p. 538)

This form of granulomatous vasculitis of medium-sized to large arteries is characterized by fibrous thickening of the aortic arch and virtual obliteration of the great vessel branches. The cause and pathogenesis are unknown.

Morphology

Grossly, there is irregular aortic thickening with intimal wrinkling. *Microscopically*, early stages show adventitial perivascular (vasa vasorum) mononuclear cell infiltrates, followed in later stages by medial fibrosis, occasionally with granulomas and acellular intimal thickening; the changes may be indistinguishable from those of giant cell arteritis.

Clinical Features

This disease causes ocular disturbances, neurologic deficits, and markedly attenuated upper extremity pulses (hence the alternate name *pulseless disease*). In a third of cases, the disease affects the remainder of the aorta and its branches; hypertension occurs secondary to renal artery involvement. Another variant causes proximal aortic dilation and valvular insufficiency. The condition is most common in Asian women less than 45 years old.

Polyarteritis Nodosa (p. 539)

Polyarteritis nodosa (PAN) is a systemic disease characterized by necrotizing vasculitis involving small to medium-sized arteries. The diagnosis is made by biopsy of affected arterial segments.

Morphology

PAN lesions are sharply demarcated and often induce thrombosis, causing distal ischemic injury. Lesions at different histologic stages may be present concurrently.

- *Acute* lesions are characterized by sharply circumscribed arterial fibrinoid necrosis, with associated neutrophilic infiltrates that may extend into the adventitia.
- *Healing* lesions show fibroblast proliferation superimposed on ongoing fibrinoid necrosis.
- *Healed* lesions show only marked fibrotic thickening of the artery, with associated elastic lamina fragmentation and occasionally aneurysmal dilation.

Clinical Features

PAN is largely a disease of young adults, with protean and nonspecific clinical presentation related to whatever tissue is involved (e.g., hematuria, albuminuria, and hypertension [kidneys]; abdominal pain and melena [gastrointestinal tract]; diffuse myalgias; and peripheral neuritis). The most common systemic manifestations include fever, malaise, and weight loss. PAN may be associated with *hepatitis B antigenemia,* and deposited immune complexes may play a role in pathogenesis. Untreated, the disease is generally fatal, but a 90% remission rate is achieved with immunosuppressive therapy.

Kawasaki Disease (Mucocutaneous Lymph Node Syndrome) (p. 539)

An acute illness of infants and children, patients have numerous immunoregulatory disturbances, including T-cell activation, autoantibodies to EC, and circulating immune complexes; the pathogenesis is unknown. It is endemic in Japan but considerably less common in the United States.

Morphology

Lesions resemble those of PAN.

Clinical Features

The disease is characterized by fever, lymphadenopathy, skin rash, oral or conjunctival erythema, and (in 20% of cases) coronary arteritis, often leading to aneurysm formation. The disease is usually self-limited but rarely is fatal owing to the coronary arteritis and aneurysm formation, with subsequent thrombosis, or rupture leading to myocardial infarction. Aspirin and intravenous gamma globulin reduce the long-term sequelae.

Microscopic Polyangiitis (Microscopic Polyarteritis or Leukocytoclastic Vasculitis) (p. 539)

This entity can be distinguished from PAN by involvement of smaller vessels (arterioles, capillaries, and venules), with lesions typically all at the same histologic stage. This synchronization suggests an acute inciting agent (e.g., drugs, microorganisms, heterologous protein) forming immune complexes in a previously sensitized host. In general, the disease responds to removal of the offending agent.

Morphology

Lesions may be confined to skin (cutaneous vasculitis) or may involve other sites, including lung, brain, heart, and kidneys. Fibrinoid necrosis often occurs, but affected vessels may show only fragmented neutrophilic nuclei within and around vessel walls *(leukocytoclastic angiitis).*

Clinical Features

A variant is *allergic granulomatosis and angiitis (Churg-Strauss syndrome),* characterized by eosinophilia and bronchial asthma, with pulmonary and splenic vessel involvement and intravascular and extravascular granulomas. Specific syndromes with systemic hypersensitivity angiitis include *Henoch-Schönlein purpura, essential mixed cryoglobulinemia,* and *vasculitis of malignancy* (typically lymphoproliferative disorders). There is a strong association of disease activity with ANCA, particularly P-ANCA.

Wegener Granulomatosis (p. 541)

Classically, this form consists of the following triad:
- Focal necrotizing vasculitis of the lung and upper airway
- Necrotizing granulomas of the upper and lower respiratory tract
- Necrotizing glomerulitis

Although immune complexes are occasionally seen in lesional tissue, no causative agent has been identified.

Morphology

Vascular lesions resemble those of acute PAN but are frequently accompanied by granuloma formation.

Clinical Features

Peak incidence is from ages 40–50 years. Without treatment, 80% of patients die within 1 year; in contrast, 90% respond to immunosuppression, particularly with cyclophosphamide. C-ANCA is present in more than 90% of patients with active disease, and is a good marker of disease activity.

Thromboangiitis Obliterans (Buerger Disease) (p. 542)

Typically encountered in heavy smokers less than 35 years old, thromboangiitis obliterans is marked by segmental, thrombosing, acute, and chronic inflammation of intermediate and small *arteries and veins* in the extremities. The cause is unknown.

Morphology

Acute lesions consist of arterial neutrophilic infiltrates with mural thrombi containing microabscesses, often with giant cell formation and secondary involvement of the adjacent vein and nerve. Late lesions show organization and recanalization.

Clinical Features

It begins with nodular phlebitis, followed by Raynaud-like cold sensitivity and leg claudication. The vascular insufficiency can lead to excruciating pain and ultimately gangrene of the extremities.

RAYNAUD PHENOMENON (p. 542)

Raynaud disease and Raynaud phenomenon are distinguished as follows:
- *Raynaud disease* is paroxysmal pallor or cyanosis of hand or foot digits (and infrequently nose or ear tips), caused by

intense vasospasm of local small arteries or arterioles. It occurs principally in young, otherwise healthy women. Of uncertain etiology, Raynaud disease reflects exaggerated vasomotor responses to cold or emotion.

- *Raynaud phenomenon* is extremity arterial insufficiency *secondary to arterial narrowing induced by other conditions* (e.g., atherosclerosis, systemic lupus erythematosus, systemic sclerosis [scleroderma], or Buerger disease).

VEINS AND LYMPHATICS (p. 543)

Vein disorders are common clinical problems; 90% involve *varicose veins* or *thrombophlebitis/phlebothrombosis*.

Varicose Veins (p. 543)

These abnormally dilated, tortuous veins (typically, lower extremity *superficial* veins) result from chronically elevated intraluminal pressure. Vessel walls are markedly thinned at points of maximal dilation. Although luminal thrombosis is common, superficial vein varicosities are rarely sources of clinically significant emboli.

Varicose veins occur in 10% to 20% of the general population; they occur in women more often than men, presumably due to venous stasis occurring in pregnancy. Other pathogenetic influences include hereditary defects in the vein wall, obesity, prolonged dependent leg position, proximal thrombosis, and compressive tumor masses.

Vein dilation or deformation renders the valves incompetent, with consequent stasis, persistent edema, and trophic skin changes, ultimately resulting in stasis dermatitis and ulceration *(varicose ulcers)*. Affected tissues may have impaired circulation and poor healing.

Thrombophlebitis and Phlebothrombosis (p. 544)

The terms *thrombophlebitis* and *phlebothrombosis* are largely interchangeable; vein thrombosis *(phlebothrombosis)* incites venous inflammation *(thrombophlebitis)*. Predisposing factors for *deep vein thrombosis* include congestive heart failure, neoplasia, pregnancy, postoperative state, prolonged immobilization, or local infection. Although 90% occur in deep leg veins, periprostatic plexus in men and ovarian and pelvic veins in women are other important sites. *In contrast to superficial vein thromboses, deep vein thromboses are common sources of pulmonary emboli.*

Migratory thrombophlebitis (Trousseau syndrome) is an entity consisting of multiple evanescent venous thrombi cropping up sporadically in multiple sites. It is attributed to malignancy-associated hypercoagulability (particularly adenocarcinomas, see Chapter 4), and may be associated with nonbacterial thrombotic endocarditis.

Superior and Inferior Vena Caval Syndromes (p. 544)

The superior vena cava (SVC) syndrome is usually caused by neoplasms compressing or invading the SVC (e.g., primary bronchogenic carcinoma or mediastinal lymphoma). The resulting obstruction produces a distinctive complex manifested by dusky cyanosis and marked dilation of head, neck, and arm veins.

The inferior vena cava (IVC) syndrome is caused by similar processes. Moreover, certain neoplasms, particularly hepatocellular carcinoma and renal cell carcinoma, show a striking tendency to grow within veins, extending into the IVC and occasionally up to the heart. IVC obstruction induces marked leg edema, distention of the lower abdominal superficial collateral veins, and—when renal veins are involved—massive proteinuria.

Lymphangitis and Lymphedema (p. 544)

Lymphangitis denotes infection of the lymphatics draining a locus of inflammation, frequently (but not exclusively) resulting from β-hemolytic streptococci. Lymphangitis presents as painful subcutaneous red streaks along involved lymphatics, with regional lymphadenopathy.

Dilated lymphatics are filled with neutrophils and histiocytes. Inflammation frequently extends into perilymphatic tissue and can develop into cellulitis or frank abscess. Lymph node involvement *(acute lymphadenitis)* may lead to septicemia.

Lymphedema is due to lymphatic obstruction and dilation, with interstitial fluid accumulation in the affected drainage site.

- The most common causes of obstruction are:

  Malignancy
  Surgical resection of regional lymph nodes
  Post-radiation fibrosis
  Filariasis
  Postinflammatory thrombosis with lymphatic scarring

- When prolonged, lymphedema causes interstitial fibrosis.
- When cutaneous tissues are involved, lymphedema gives a *peau d'orange* (orange peel) appearance to the skin, with associated ulcers and brawny induration.
- Chylous accumulations in any body cavity may occur secondary to rupture of obstructed, dilated lymphatics.

TUMORS (p. 545)

Primary tumors of blood vessels and lymphatics run the spectrum from benign *hemangiomas* (some regarded as hamartomas), to intermediate, locally aggressive (but infrequently) metastasizing lesions, to relatively rare, highly malignant *angiosarcomas*. Congenital or developmental malformations (e.g., *Sturge-Weber syndrome*) and non-neoplastic reactive vascular proliferations (e.g., *bacillary angiomatosis*) may also present as tumor-like lesions.

Classically, benign vascular neoplasms are composed of *well-formed vascular channels lined by ECs;* frankly malignant tumors show few or poorly developed vascular channels with solid, cellular, anaplastic endothelial proliferation. A few entities fall into an intermediate group.

Benign Tumors and Tumor-like Conditions
(p. 545)

Hemangioma (p. 545)

These are common lesions, especially in childhood, accounting for 7% of all benign tumors. They encompass several histologic and clinical variants:

- *Capillary hemangiomas* are the most common type of vascular tumor; they occur primarily in skin or mucous membranes, but also in viscera. Tumors range from 1 to 2 mm to several centimeters in diameter. All are well defined, unencapsulated lesions composed of closely packed aggregates of capillary-sized, thin-walled vessels. They may be partially or completely thrombosed.

- *Juvenile capillary (strawberry) hemangiomas* are a specific variant that are present at birth, grow rapidly for a few months, and begin regressing at age 1 to 3 years. Almost all disappear by age 7.

- *Cavernous hemangiomas* are characterized by *large, cavernous* vascular channels, forming unencapsulated but discrete lesions, usually 1 to 2 cm in diameter (with rare giant forms). They have the same distribution as capillary hemangiomas but are also common in liver, where imaging modalities may detect them as small tumors; they may also involve the central nervous system and other viscera. They can be locally destructive and generally do not regress. Cavernous hemangiomas in the cerebellum, brain stem, or eye grounds are associated with angiomatous or cystic neoplasms in pancreas and liver in *von Hippel–Lindau disease*.

- *Pyogenic granulomas (lobular capillary hemangiomas)* are an ulcerated polypoid variant of capillary hemangiomas on skin or oral mucosa, often following trauma. Composed of proliferating capillaries with interspersed edema and inflammatory infiltrates, they resemble exuberant granulation tissue. Pregnancy tumor *(granuloma gravidarum)* is essentially the same lesion, occurring in gingiva of 1% to 5% of pregnant women and regressing postpartum.

Lymphangioma (p. 547)

Lymphangiomas are the benign lymphatic analog of hemangiomas.

- *Capillary lymphangiomas* are composed of small lymphatic channels; they are typically 1 to 2 cm in diameter, exudate-filled blister-like blebs, with a predilection for head, neck, and axillary subcutaneous tissue. Grossly, these are cutaneous nodules or pedunculated lesions, or well-demarcated, compressible gray-pink visceral masses. *Microscopically*, they are networks of EC-lined spaces, identifiable as lymphatics only by the absence of erythrocytes. Variants include lymphangiomyomas containing SMC in the vessel walls.

- Analogous to the cavernous hemangioma, *cavernous lymphangioma* (or *cystic hygroma*) occurs in children in the neck or axilla (and rarely retroperitoneally). They occasionally achieve considerable size, up to 15 cm in diameter, and may fill the axilla or produce gross deformities in the neck area. These lesions are not well encapsulated, and complete surgical resection can be difficult. *Microscopically*, they are composed of hugely dilated cystic spaces lined by endothelium with scant stroma.

Glomus Tumor (Glomangioma) (p. 547)

A benign, albeit extremely painful tumor of modified smooth muscle cells arising from the glomus body, a temperature-sensitive neuromyoarterial receptor regulating arteriolar flow. Receptors (and thus their tumors) are most commonly found in the distal phalanges, especially beneath nail beds. Excision is curative.

Grossly the tumors are less than 1 cm in diameter and may be pinpoint. *Histologically,* they consist of branching vascular channels separated by stroma dominated by aggregates, nests, and masses of specialized glomus cells resembling SMC on electron microscopy.

Vascular Ectasias (p. 547)

Aggregates of abnormally prominent capillaries, venules, and arterioles in skin or mucous membranes; these are acquired dilations of existing vessels.

- *Nevus flammeus* is the term used for classic birthmarks. It is a macular cutaneous lesion that histologically shows only dermal vessel dilation. A special variety is the *port-wine stain,* which persists and grows along with the child, thickening the involved skin. Most eventually regress. Facial port-wine nevi with associated leptomeningeal angiomatous masses, mental retardation, seizures, hemiplegia, and skull radiopacities comprise the *Sturge-Weber syndrome.*
- *Spider telangiectasias* are minute subcutaneous arterioles, often pulsatile, arranged in radial fashion around a central core. They typically occur above the waist and are associated with hyperestrogenic states, such as pregnancy and cirrhosis.
- *Hereditary hemorrhagic telangiectasia (Osler-Weber-Rendu disease)* is a rare, mendelian dominant disorder characterized by multiple small (<5 mm) aneurysmal telangiectasias on skin and mucous membranes. The syndrome typically presents with epistaxis, hemoptysis, or gastrointestinal or genitourinary bleeding, worsening with advancing age.

Bacillary Angiomatosis (p. 548)

A potentially fatal infectious disease caused by a rickettsia-like bacillus *(Bartonella* species*),* bacillary angiomatosis induces a distinctive non-neoplastic small blood vessel proliferation in skin, lymph nodes, and visceral organs of immunocompromised patients, especially those with acquired immunodeficiency syndrome (AIDS). In immunocompetent individuals, *Bartonella henselae* causes cat-scratch disease, and *B. quintana* causes *trench fever.* Grossly, skin lesions have one or more red papules or nodular subcutaneous masses; *microscopically,* these are tumor-like capillary proliferations composed of atypical ECs. In contrast to pyogenic granuloma, Kaposi sarcoma, or angiosarcoma, there are also numerous neutrophils, nuclear dust, and purplish granular material (bacteria). Treatment with erythromycin is curative.

Intermediate-Grade (Borderline, Low-Grade Malignant) Tumors (p. 548)

Kaposi Sarcoma (p. 548)

Four forms of Kaposi sarcoma (KS) are recognized, based largely on epidemiology:

- *Chronic/classic/European KS* occurs typically in elderly men of Eastern European (especially Ashkenazi Jew) or Mediterranean descent. Lesions consist of multiple red-purple cutaneous plaques and nodules on the lower extremities, rarely with visceral involvement. Infrequently this form causes death but more often is marked by relapses and remissions.
- *Lymphadenopathic/African KS* is clinically similar to the classic form but occurs in younger men in equatorial Africa, composing 10% of all tumors. This disease is largely restricted to the lymph node, but is aggressive.
- *Transplant-associated KS* occurs in patients undergoing immunosuppressive therapy. There is both cutaneous and visceral systemic involvement; lesions may regress when immunosuppression is discontinued.
- *Acquired immunodeficiency syndrome (AIDS)-associated (epidemic) KS* occurs more commonly in homosexuals than in other AIDS risk groups. Lesions may occur anywhere in the skin and mucous membranes, lymph nodes, gastrointestinal tract, or viscera. Wide visceral dissemination occurs early and frequently, but lesions respond to cytotoxic chemotherapy or α-interferon.

Microscopically, the characteristic lesions consist of sheets of plump, spindle-shaped cells creating slit-like vascular spaces filled with red blood cells, intermingled with vascular channels lined by recognizable ECs. Three stages of KS are recognized grossly: patch, plaque, and nodule:

- *Patches* comprise pink-red to purple macules usually confined (in classic disease) to the distal lower extremities. Microscopic examination discloses only dilated, irregular and angulated blood vessels lined by ECs, with interspersed infiltrates of lymphocytes, plasma cells, and macrophages (sometimes containing hemosiderin)—lesions are difficult to distinguish from granulation tissue.
- *Raised plaques* have dilated, jagged vascular channels lined by somewhat plump spindle cells accompanied by perivascular aggregates of similar spindled cells.
- *Nodular lesions* are more distinctly neoplastic. This stage is often accompanied by lymph node and visceral involvement, particularly in the African and AIDS-associated diseases.

Nearly all KS lesions are infected with human herpesvirus 8 (HHV-8), also known as KS-associated herpesvirus (KSHV); this agent is both necessary and sufficient for KS development, although immunosupression is an important cofactor in disease pathogenesis and clinical expression.

Hemangioendothelioma (p. 550)

These neoplasms lie at the interface between benign and malignant and must be distinguished from the much more aggressive angiosarcomas. Most lesions are cured by excision, although up to 40% may recur, and 20% eventually metastasize. *Microscopically,* vascular channels may be evident or inconspicuous, with dominant masses and sheets of somewhat pleomorphic, spindle-shaped to large, plump cells (especially in the *epithelioid* variant) of endothelial origin.

Malignant Tumors (p. 550)

Angiosarcoma (p. 550)

Among vascular tumors, angiosarcomas are the most malignant. Spontaneous angiosarcomas tend to arise in skin, soft tissue, breast, liver, and spleen. They begin as small, well-demarcated red nodules evolving into large, fleshy, gray-white, soft tissue masses. *Microscopically,* all degrees of differentiation are found, from plump, anaplastic ECs in a highly vascularized variety, to quite undifferentiated lesions with marked cellular atypia (including giant cells) without vascular lumens. Angiosarcomas metastasize widely and are frequently fatal.

Hepatic angiosarcomas are associated with exposure to arsenicals (in some pesticides), polyvinylchloride (used in plastic manufacture), and Thorotrast (radiocontrast material used from 1928 to 1950); in the setting of such exposures, the angiosarcomas are frequently multicentric, and arise concomitantly in the spleen.

Angiosarcomas may also develop in the setting of chronic lymphedema—classically up to a decade after radical mastectomy for breast cancer. In such cases, the tumor presumably arises from dilated lymphatic vessels *(lymphangiosarcomas).* Angiosarcomas may also be induced by radiation in the absence of lymphedema and are associated with chronically indwelling foreign materials.

Hemangiopericytoma (p. 551)

Hemangiopericytoma is a tumor of pericytes, most commonly arising on the lower extremities or in the retroperitoneum; 50% metastasize. Most are small, but can grow to 8 cm. *Microscopically* they are composed of numerous capillary channels encased by nests and masses of spindle-shaped to round cells extrinsic to the EC basement membrane (resembling pericytes).

PATHOLOGY OF VASCULAR INTERVENTIONS
(p. 551)

Balloon Angioplasty and Related Techniques
(p. 551)

Angioplasty involves dilating arterial atheromatous stenoses (most commonly in coronary arteries) using a balloon catheter. Balloon dilation of an atherosclerotic vessel characteristically causes plaque fracture, medial dissection, and stretching of the media of the dissected segment. Complications of balloon angioplasty and related techniques include abrupt reclosure (small percentage of patients) and proliferative restenosis in one third of patients within the first 4 to 6 months.

Coronary stents are expandable tubes of metallic mesh inserted percutaneously to preserve luminal patency at sites of balloon angioplasty. They are currently used in >70% of angioplasty procedures. Stents may ameliorate the untoward effects of angioplasty by providing a larger and more regular lumen, acting as a scaffold to support the intimal flaps and dissections that occur during angioplasty, limiting elastic recoil, mechanically preventing vascular spasm, and increasing blood flow. Nevertheless, both early thrombosis and late intimal thickening may occur and lead to in-stent restenosis, the major limitation of coronary stenting. Approaches to inhibiting in-stent restenosis include local irradiation at the time of angioplasty or incorporation of antiproliferative drugs in the stents (*drug elating stents*).

Vascular Replacement (p. 551)

Large-diameter (>10 cm) Dacron grafts in the aorta perform well. In contrast, small-diameter vascular conduits (<6 to 8 mm)—whether using autologous saphenous vein or fabricated from expanded polytetrafluoroethylene—perform less well. Graft failure is related to thrombotic occlusion or intimal fibrous hyperplasia, either generalized (vein grafts) or anastomoses only (synthetic graft).

The patency of saphenous veins used as coronary artery bypass grafts is 60% or less at 10 years, owing to thrombosis (usually early), intimal thickening (several months to years), and atherosclerosis (>2 or 3 years postoperatively). In comparison, internal mammary arteries used as coronary bypass grafts have over 90% patency at 10 years. Late symptom (e.g., angina) recurrence results most frequently from either graft occlusion or progression of atherosclerosis in the native vessels distal to the grafts.

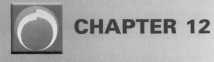

CHAPTER 12

The Heart

Heart disease is the leading cause of morbidity and death in industrialized nations, accounting for approximately 30% of deaths in the United States.

- About 80% of cardiac deaths are attributable to *ischemic heart disease*.
- From 5% to 10% of cardiac deaths are also individually attributable to:

  Hypertensive heart disease (including *cor pulmonale*)
  Congenital heart disease
  Valvular diseases

  Cardiac disease occurs as a consequence of one (or more) of the following general mechanisms:

- *Disruption of the continuity of circulation* (e.g., rupture of a major vessel) with hemorrhage
- *Abnormal cardiac conduction* (e.g., complete heart block) or other arrhythmia (e.g., ventricular fibrillation) leading to uncoordinated myocardial contractions
- *Blood flow obstruction* (e.g., coronary atherosclerosis, thrombosis, or aortic valvular stenosis)
- *Regurgitant flow* (e.g., mitral or aortic regurgitation) causing output from each contraction to be directed backward (thus causing volume overload and diminishing forward flow)
- *Shunts* that allow abnormal blood flow either right-to-left (bypassing the lungs) or left-to-right (causing volume overload)
- Failure of the myocardium itself (*congestive heart failure*)

HEART FAILURE (p. 560)

Congestive heart failure (CHF) is the common end point of many forms of heart disease; it is a pathologic state in which impaired cardiac function renders the heart unable to maintain output sufficient for the metabolic requirements of the body. CHF is characterized by diminished cardiac output (forward failure), accumulation of blood in the venous system (backward failure), or both.

- With the exception of frank myocyte death, the *mechanisms* of myocardial decompensation in CHF are not well understood.
- Most instances of heart failure are the consequence of progressive deterioration of myocardial contractile function *(systolic dysfunction),* frequently due to ischemic injury, pressure or volume overload, or dilated cardiomyopathy. The damaged muscle contracts weakly or inadequately, and the chambers cannot empty properly.
- Because adult myocytes cannot proliferate, the heart characteristically responds to pressure or volume overload by increasing myocyte size *(myocyte hypertrophy);* the mechanism(s) that translate physical stress into cellular changes is uncertain. The ultimate result is increased heart size. However, although hypertrophy is initially adaptive, it can make myocytes vulnerable to injury.
- Occasionally, failure results from inability of the heart chambers to relax sufficiently during diastole so that the ventricles can properly fill *(diastolic dysfunction)*. This can occur with massive left ventricular hypertrophy, myocardial fibrosis, deposition of amyloid, or constrictive pericarditis.

Regardless of the causes of heart failure, the cardiovascular system attempts to compensate for inadequate cardiac output in CHF by:

- Ventricular dilation (improves contraction by myofiber stretching, according to the Frank-Starling law)
- Blood volume expansion by salt and water retention
- Tachycardia

Unfortunately, these compensatory changes ultimately impose further burdens on cardiac function. They combine with both the original cardiac disease and the secondary hypertrophy to induce dilation in excess of the optimal tension-generating point; the outcome is progressive CHF.

Left-Sided Heart Failure (p. 562)

The major causes of left-sided heart failure are ischemic heart disease, hypertension, aortic and mitral valve disease, and myocardial disease. Left-sided failure is manifested by:

- Classically, *pulmonary congestion and edema* due to impaired pulmonary outflow
- Reduced renal perfusion (due to diminished cardiac output) causing:

  Salt (and attendant water) retention to expand blood volume

  Ischemic acute tubular necrosis (ATN)

  Impaired waste excretion, causing prerenal azotemia

- Reduced central nervous system perfusion, often causing *hypoxic encephalopathy,* with symptoms ranging from irritability to coma

Right-Sided Heart Failure (p. 563)

Right-sided heart failure is most commonly caused by left-sided failure. Pure right-sided heart failure can be caused by tricuspid or pulmonary valvular disease, or by intrinsic pulmonary or pulmonary vasculature disease causing functional right ventricular outflow obstruction *(cor pulmonale)*. Right-sided failure is manifested by:

- Portal, systemic, and dependent peripheral (e.g., feet, ankles, sacrum) congestion and edema, with effusions
- Hepatomegaly with centrilobular congestion and atrophy of central hepatocytes, producing a *nutmeg* appearance *(chronic passive congestion)*

  With severe hypoxia, *centrilobular necrosis* can occur; with high right-sided pressure, sinusoidal rupture causes *central hemorrhagic necrosis*.
  Subsequent central fibrosis creates *cardiac sclerosis*.

- Congestive splenomegaly with sinusoidal dilation, focal hemorrhages, hemosiderin deposits, and fibrosis
- Renal congestion, hypoxic injury, and ATN (more marked in right- *versus* left-sided CHF)

CONGENITAL HEART DISEASE (p. 564)

Congenital heart disease refers to cardiac or great vessel abnormalities that are present at birth; most are attributable to faulty embryogenesis during gestational weeks 3 through 8, when major cardiovascular structures develop. The most severe anomalies may be incompatible with intrauterine survival; defects that permit embryologic maturation and birth generally involve only specific chambers or regions of the heart, while the remainder of the heart develops normally. Congenital disorders constitute the most common cardiac disease among children, with an incidence of 1% of live births. The most frequent disorders are listed in Table 12–1.

Etiology

Congenital heart disease likely has a strong developmental basis; multifactorial genetic, environmental, and maternal factors probably account for the majority of cases. Well-defined

TABLE 12–1 **Frequencies of Congenital Cardiac Malformations***

Malformation	Incidence per Million Live Births	%
Ventricular septal defect	4482	42
Atrial septal defect	1043	10
Pulmonary stenosis	836	8
Patent ductus arteriosus	781	7
Tetralogy of Fallot	577	5
Coarctation of aorta	492	5
Atrioventricular septal defect	396	4
Aortic stenosis	388	4
Transposition of great arteries	388	4
Truncus arteriosus	136	1
Total anomalous pulmonary venous connection	120	1
Tricuspid atresia	118	1
Total	9757	

*Presented as upper quartile of 44 published studies. Percentages do not add to 100% owing to rounding.
Source: Hoffman JIE, Kaplan S: The incidence of congenital heart disease. J Am Coll Cardiol 39:1890, 2002.

genetic or environmental influences are thus far identifiable in 10% of cases; trisomy 21 (i.e., *Down syndrome*) is the most common known genetic cause, and congenital rubella infection or teratogens are common environmental factors.

Clinical Features

Children with congenital anomalies not only have direct hemodynamic sequelae, but also have cyanosis, retarded development, and failure to thrive. They are at increased risk of chronic or recurrent illness and of infective endocarditis (due to abnormal valves or endocardial injury from jet lesions). The various congenital anomalies are of two types: *shunts* or *obstructions*.

Shunt Congenital Anomalies (p. 566)

Shunts denote abnormal communications between heart chambers, between vessels, or between chambers and vessels. Depending on pressure relationships, blood is shunted either from left to right (more common) or from right to left. Left-to-right shunts cause chronic volume overload; right-to-left shunts bypass the lungs, leading to hypoxia and tissue *cyanosis*. Right-to-left shunts also allow venous emboli to enter the systemic circulation *(paradoxical emboli)*.

Left-to-Right Shunts (p. 566)

Left-to-right shunts induce chronic right-sided volume overload with secondary pulmonary hypertension and right ventricle hypertrophy; eventually, right-sided pressures exceed left-sided pressures, and the shunt becomes right to left. *Hence, cyanosis appears late.* Once significant pulmonary hypertension develops, the underlying structural defects are no longer candidates for surgical correction.

The major congenital left-to-right shunts are:

- Atrial septal defect (ASD)
- Ventricular septal defect (VSD)
- Patent ductus arteriosus (PDA)

Atrial Septal Defect (p. 567). Abnormal openings in the atrial septum allowing shunting of blood, ASDs are the most common congenital cardiac anomaly *seen in adults:*

- *Primum type:* Only 5% of ASDs, but common in Down syndrome, this type occurs low in the atrial septum, and occasionally is associated with mitral valve deformities.
- *Secundum type:* ninety percent of ASDs; this type occurs at the foramen ovale, may be any size (generating a single atrial chamber if large), and may be single, multiple, or fenestrated. Secundum type usually is not associated with other anomalies.
- *Sinus venosus type:* five percent of ASDs; this type occurs high in the septum near the superior vena cava (SVC) entrance. It can be associated with anomalous right pulmonary vein drainage into the SVC or right atrium.

Even large ASDs are usually asymptomatic until adulthood, when either right-sided heart failure occurs or gradually increasing right-sided hypertrophy and pulmonary hypertension finally induce right-to-left shunting with cyanosis. Early surgical correction is advocated to prevent pulmonary vascular changes.

Ventricular Septal Defect (p. 568). Abnormal openings in the ventricular septum allowing shunting of blood, VSDs are the most common congenital cardiac anomaly overall.

- VSDs are frequently associated with other anomalies, particularly *tetralogy of Fallot* (see later discussion), but 30% are isolated; 90% involve the membranous septum *(membranous VSD)* near the aortic valve, while the remainder are muscular.
- With small to moderate-sized VSDs, patients are at increased risk of infective endocarditis.

Depending on VSD size, the clinical picture ranges from fulminant CHF to late cyanosis, to asymptomatic holosystolic murmurs, to spontaneous closure (50% of those <0.5 cm diameter). Surgical correction is desirable before right-sided heart overload and pulmonary hypertension develop.

Patent Ductus Arteriosus (p. 568). In the fetus, the ductus arteriosus (located distal to the left subclavian artery) permits blood flow between the aorta and pulmonary artery. At birth, under the influence of higher oxygen tensions and reduced local prostaglandin E synthesis, muscular contraction normally closes the ductus within 1 or 2 days of life. Persistent patency beyond that point is generally permanent.

- About 85% to 90% of PDAs occur as isolated defects; length and diameter (up to 1 cm) are variable. Left ventricular hypertrophy and pulmonary artery dilation occur secondary to ductus patency.
- Although initially asymptomatic (but notable for a prominent *machinery-like* heart murmur), long-standing PDA causes pulmonary hypertension followed by right ventricle hypertrophy and eventually right-to-left shunting with late cyanosis.
- Early PDA closure (either surgically or with prostaglandin synthesis inhibitors) is advocated.

Right-to-Left Shunts (p. 568)

Right-to-left shunts *(cyanotic congenital heart disease)* cause *cyanosis from the outset* by allowing poorly oxygenated blood to flow directly into the systemic circulation (they also permit *paradoxical embolism*). Secondary findings in long-standing cyanotic heart disease include:

- Fingers and toe *clubbing*
- Hypertrophic osteoarthropathy
- Polycythemia

The major congenital right-to-left shunts are:

- Tetralogy of Fallot
- Transposition of the great arteries (TGA)
- Truncus arteriosus

Tetralogy of Fallot (p. 568). Owing to anterosuperior displacement of the infundibular septum, the cardinal findings (other anomalies may also be present) of tetralogy are:

- VSD
- Dextroposed aorta overriding the VSD
- Pulmonary stenosis with right ventricle outflow obstruction
- Right ventricular hypertrophy

Symptom severity is directly related to the extent of right ventricle outflow obstruction. With a large VSD and mild pulmonary stenosis, there is minimal left-to-right shunt without cyanosis. More severe pulmonary stenosis produces a cyanotic right-to-left shunt.

With complete pulmonary obstruction, survival can occur only by flow through a PDA or dilated bronchial arteries. Surgical correction can be delayed provided that the child can tolerate the level of oxygenation; when present, pulmonary valvular stenosis protects the lung from volume and pressure overload, and right ventricular failure is rare because it can pump excess volume into the left ventricle and aorta.

Transposition of the Great Arteries (p. 569). Systemic and pulmonary venous return—to the right and left atria, respectively—are normal; however, the aorta arises from the right ventricle and the pulmonary artery from the left, so that the pulmonary and systemic circulations are functionally separated. TGA is particularly common in children of diabetic mothers.

- Normal fetal development occurs because venous and systemic blood mixes through the ductus arteriosus and a patent foramen ovale.
- Postnatal life critically depends on some mechanism of blood mixing (e.g., a PDA, VSD, ASD, or patent foramen ovale).
- Prognosis depends on the severity of tissue hypoxia and the ability of the right ventricle to maintain systemic aortic pressures. Untreated, most infants die within months.

Truncus Arteriosus (p. 569). Associated with numerous concomitant cardiac defects, truncus arteriosus is basically a failure of the aorta and pulmonary artery to separate. It results in an infundibular VSD with a single vessel receiving blood from both right and left ventricles.

- Right-to-left shunting causes early cyanosis.
- Eventually the flow reverses, and patients develop right ventricle hypertrophy and pulmonary hypertension. The anomaly carries a poor prognosis.

Obstructive Congenital Anomalies (p. 570)

Obstructions include aortic coarctation, and valvular stenoses and atresias; none of these cause cyanosis.

Aortic Coarctation (p. 570)

Aortic coarctation is a constriction of the aorta; 50% occur as isolated defects, the remainder with other anomalies.

- In most cases, cardiac hypertrophy occurs due to chronic pressure overload.
- Clinical manifestations depend on the location and severity of the constriction; most coarcts occur just distal to the ductus or ligamentum arteriosus (*postductal*).

   Preductal coarctation manifests early in life and may be rapidly fatal. Survival depends on the ability of the ductus arteriosus to provide adequate systemic blood flow; there is frequently lower body cyanosis. Preductal coarctation usually involves a 1- to 5-cm segment of the aortic root and is associated with fetal right ventricle hypertrophy and right-sided heart failure.

   Postductal coarctation is generally asymptomatic unless severe. It leads to upper extremity hypertension but lower extremity hypotension with arterial insufficiency (claudication, cold sensitivity). Collateral flow around the coarctation generally develops via internal mammary and axillary artery dilation, with intercostal rib notching notable on x-rays.

- Untreated, mean life span is 40 years; death is secondary to CHF, aortic dissection proximal to the coarctation, intracranial hemorrhage, or infection of the coarctation.

Pulmonary Stenosis and Atresia (p. 571)

Pulmonary stenosis and atresia, usually with an intact interventricular septum, occurs in isolation or associated with other anomalies (e.g., transposition or tetralogy).

- Pulmonary outflow obstructions may involve the valve, or be subvalvar, supravalvar, or even multiple.
- *Pulmonary stenosis,* generally due to cuspal fusion, varies from mild to severe.
- Mild stenosis is generally asymptomatic. Progressively more severe stenoses cause increasing cyanosis with earlier onset.
- In *complete pulmonary atresia* surviving to birth, the right ventricle is hypoplastic and there is an ASD with blood entering the lungs via a PDA.

Aortic Stenosis and Atresia (p. 571)

- Survival with congenital *aortic valvular stenosis* (three types—subvalvar, valvar, and supravalvuar) depends on the severity of the lesion.
- Consequences include infective endocarditis, left ventricle hypertrophy (pressure overload), post-stenotic dilation of the aortic root, and (rarely) sudden death.
- *Congenital complete aortic atresia* is rare and incompatible with neonatal survival.
- Infants with severe stenosis or atresia can survive, but only if a PDA permits flow to the aorta and coronary arteries; fetal under development of the left ventricle in this setting causes the *hypoplastic left heart syndrome.*
- *Congenital bicuspid aortic valve* is a common anomaly but is generally functionally unimportant throughout early life. It is prone to calcific degeneration in middle age and has increased risk of infective endocarditis.
- Rare, single-cusp aortic valves are also seen, and are commonly associated with early sudden death.

ISCHEMIC HEART DISEASE (p. 571)

Ischemic heart disease (IHD) comprises a group of closely related syndromes resulting from *ischemia*—essentially a mismatch between cardiac demand and vascular supply of oxygenated blood. In most cases, ischemia not only causes oxygen insufficiency *(hypoxia, anoxia)*, but also reduces nutrient availability and metabolite removal.

Ischemia can be caused by:

- *Reduced coronary blood flow* (the cause in >90%) due to some combination of coronary atherosclerosis, vasospasm, and thrombosis. Uncommon causes of reduced coronary flow include arteritis, emboli, cocaine-induced vasospasm, and shock (causing systemic hypotension).
- *Increased myocardial demand* (e.g., tachycardia, hypertrophy).
- *Hypoxia due to diminished oxygen transport* (overall a less serious cause of ischemia than reduced flow because nutri-

ent supply and metabolite removal are not affected). Nevertheless, hypoxia can exacerbate ischemia due to other causes. Hypoxia occurs secondary to severe anemia, advanced lung disease, cyanotic congenital heart disease, carbon monoxide poisoning, or cigarette smoking.

There are four overlapping ischemic syndromes, differing in severity and rate of onset (and described in greater detail later):

1. *Myocardial infarction (MI)* is the most important form of IHD; MI occurs when duration and severity of ischemia is sufficient to cause death of heart muscle.

2. *Angina pectoris* is characterized by paroxysmal substernal pain; the duration and severity of ischemia are not sufficient to cause infarction. Three patterns of angina are recognized based on the nature of the provocation and severity of the pain:

   Stable angina: Anginal symptoms reliably occur with the same level of exertion and go away with rest; typically seen when there is 75% or greater chronic stable stenosis in a coronary artery.

   Prinzmetal angina: Due to vasospasm, angina typically occurs without fixed atherosclerotic disease.

   Unstable angina: Due to atherosclerotic plaque disruption with variable, usually incomplete, mural thromboses; the angina is therefore not clearly related to exertion. Since the mechanism is similar to that of MI, unstable angina is frequently a harbinger of myocardial infarction.

3. *Chronic ischemic heart disease* is seen typically in elderly patients with moderate to severe multivessel coronary atherosclerosis who insidiously develop CHF; it may result from postinfarction cardiac decompensation or slow ischemic myocyte degeneration.

   Microscopically, the myocardium has variable myocyte atrophy with perinuclear deposition of lipofuscin, myocytolysis of single cells or clusters, diffuse perivascular and interstitial fibrosis, and patchy to confluent replacement fibrosis (scarring).

   Diagnosis depends on excluding other CHF causes. Death can result from slowly progressive CHF, a superimposed acute MI, or an arrhythmic event.

4. *Sudden cardiac death is defined as unexpected cardiac death within 1 hour of symptom onset.* Greater than 300,000 cases of sudden cardiac death occur annually in the United States. It is predominantly caused by ischemic heart disease, and 75% to 95% of victims have significant atherosclerotic stenoses, often with acute plaque disruption. Sudden cardiac death is infrequently a consequence of aortic valvular stenosis, hereditary or acquired conduction system abnormalities, electrolyte derangements, mitral valve prolapse, dilated or hypertrophic cardiomyopathy, myocardial deposition, myocarditis, or intrinsic electrical instability. In patients who survive sudden death (by cardiac resuscitation), only 25% to 50% actually develop an MI, indicating that a fatal arrhythmia (e.g., asystole or ventricular fibrillation) is the most common etiology. Arrhythmias are presumably triggered by conduction system scarring, acute ischemic injury, or electrical instability resulting from an ischemic focus or electrolytic imbalance.

Myocardial Infarction (p. 575)

There are two interrelated types of MI, with different morphology, pathogenesis, and clinical significance:

- *Transmural infarct* is an MI involving the full thickness of the ventricular wall; it is usually caused by severe coronary atherosclerosis, with acute plaque rupture and superimposed occlusive thrombosis.
- *Subendocardial infarct* is typically limited to the inner one third of the ventricular wall; it is caused by increased cardiac demand in the setting of limiting supply due to fixed atherosclerotic disease; alternatively, subendothelial infarction can occur in an evolving transmural infarct when the coronary obstruction is relieved in sufficient time to prevent transmural necrosis.

Pathogenesis (p. 576)

The pathogenesis of irreversible ischemic myocardial injury is summarized in Figure 12–1.

Transmural Infarcts

Transmural infarcts are largely a consequence of coronary atherosclerosis and one (or more) disrupted plaques. Signifi-

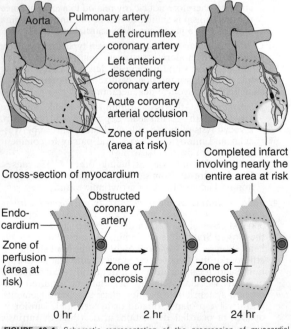

FIGURE 12–1 Schematic representation of the progression of myocardial necrosis after coronary artery occlusion. Necrosis begins in a small zone of the myocardium beneath the endocardial surface in the center of the ischemic zone. This entire region of myocardium *(shaded)* depends on the occluded vessel for perfusion and is the area at risk. Note that a very narrow zone of myocardium immediately beneath the endocardium is spared from necrosis because it can be oxygenated by diffusion from the ventricle. The end result of the obstruction to blood flow is necrosis of the muscle that was dependent on perfusion from the obstructed coronary artery. Nearly the entire area at risk loses viability. The process is called *myocardial infarction*, and the region of necrotic muscle is a *myocardial infarct.*

cant plaques typically occur in the proximal 2 cm of the left anterior descending and left circumflex coronary arteries and in the proximal and distal thirds of the right coronary artery. In a few cases, vasospasm and platelet aggregation cause MIs without atherosclerotic stenoses. With sufficient collateral blood flow, even complete vessel occlusion will not necessarily result in an MI.

- The initial event in most transmural MIs is erosion, ulceration, fissuring, rupture, or hemorrhagic expansion (collectively called *acute plaque change* or *disruption*) of an atherosclerotic plaque.
- Plaques involved in coronary events typically have a large lipid pool, a thin fibrous cap, and macrophage-rich inflammation; plaques with such features are considered susceptible to rupture, and are termed *vulnerable*. Patients at risk of cardiovascular events may have multiple vulnerable plaques.
- Transient changes in blood pressure and platelet reactivity (both occur upon morning awakening), affected by exercise and smoking (both are associated with catecholamine release), and may increase the risk of plaque rupture and thrombosis.
- High levels of serum markers of inflammation (e.g., C-reactive protein [CRP]) and hypercoagulability (e.g., protein C or S deficiency, factor V Leiden) also affect a patient's risk of acute cardiovascular events.
- Thrombosis follows the acute plaque change and occludes flow to distal tissues.
- The time interval between onset of complete myocardial ischemia and the initiation of irreversible injury is 20 to 40 minutes.
- If the patient survives, thrombi may either lyse spontaneously or after fibrinolysis; alternatively, vasospasm may relax. In both cases, flow is reestablished and some myocardium is spared from necrosis.
- Reflow to (*reperfusion* of) precariously injured cells may restore viability but leave the cells poorly contractile (*stunned*) for 1 to 2 days.
- Nearly all transmural MIs affect the left ventricle; 15% simultaneously involve the right ventricle, particularly in posterior-inferior left ventricle infarcts. Isolated right ventricle infarction occurs in 1% to 3% of cases.

Subendocardial Infarcts

Subendocardial infarcts are usually caused by:

- Diffuse coronary atherosclerosis and global borderline perfusion made transiently critical by increased demand, vasospasm, or hypotension but without superimposed thrombosis.
- Plaque disruption with overlying thrombus that spontaneously lyses (or is removed by therapeutic intervention), thereby limiting the extent of myocardial injury. Myocardial injury is usually less than in a transmural infarct and often multifocal.

Morphology (p. 577)

MIs undergo a characteristic sequence of gross and microscopic changes (Fig. 12–2).

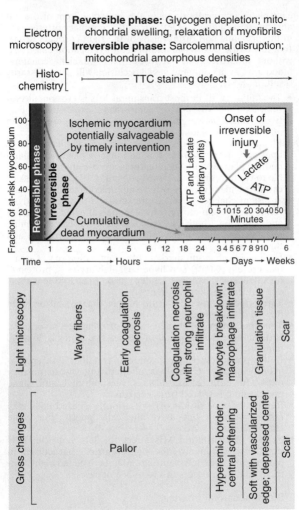

Electron microscopy
- **Reversible phase:** Glycogen depletion; mitochondrial swelling, relaxation of myofibrils
- **Irreversible phase:** Sarcolemmal disruption; mitochondrial amorphous densities

Histochemistry ⟶ TTC staining defect ⟶

FIGURE 12–2 Temporal sequence of biochemical, ultrastructural, histochemical, and histologic findings after onset of severe myocardial ischemia. For approximately $1/2$ hour following the onset of even the most severe ischemia, myocardial injury is potentially reversible. Thereafter, progressive loss of viability occurs and is complete by 6 to 12 hours. The benefits of reperfusion are greatest when it is achieved early, with progressively smaller benefit occurring as reperfusion is delayed. TTC, triphenyl tetrazolium chloride. (From Schoen FJ: Pathologic Considerations of the Surgery of Adult Heart Disease. In Edmunds LH (ed): Cardiac Surgery in the Adult. New York: McGraw-Hill, 1997, p. 85.)

Gross Changes

- Before 6 to 12 hours, MIs are usually inapparent; however, changes occurring as early as 3 to 6 hours after injury can be highlighted by histochemical techniques (e.g., triphenyl tetrazolium chloride is a substrate for lactate dehydrogenase; it colors viable myocardium red-brown but leaves non-viable areas pale).

- By 18 to 24 hours, infarcted tissue is generally readily apparent as discrete pale to cyanotic areas.
- In the first week, lesions become progressively more defined, yellow, and softened.
- Hyperemic granulation tissue appears by 7 to 10 days at the edges of the infarct; with time, granulation tissue progressively fills in the area of the MI.
- White fibrous scar is usually well established by 6 weeks.

Microscopic Changes

- Within 1 hour of an MI, there is intercellular edema, and myocytes at the edge of the infarct become wavy and buckled (attributable to stretching of noncontractile dead fibers by adjacent viable contracting myocytes). Coagulative necrosis is not yet evident.
- From 12 to 72 hours after MI, dead myocytes become hypereosinophilic with loss of nuclei *(coagulative necrosis);* neutrophils also progressively infiltrate the necrotic tissue.
- From 3 to 7 days after injury, dead myocytes are digested by invading macrophages.
- After 7 to 10 days, granulation tissue progressively replaces necrotic tissue, ultimately generating a dense fibrous scar.

Clinical Features (p. 583)

Diagnosis of an MI is based mainly on symptoms (chest pain, nausea, diaphoresis, dyspnea), electrocardiographic changes, and elevation in the serum of cardiomyocyte-specific proteins released from dead cells (e.g., creatine kinase MB isoform or various troponins). Angiography, echocardiography, and perfusion scintigraphy are diagnostic adjuncts.

- About 25% of patients experience sudden death after infarction (presumably secondary to a fatal arrhythmia), most before reaching a hospital.
- Of those surviving, the risk of death within 1 month after MI is 7% to 10%, and 80% to 90% will develop complications (cited in next section).
- Early restoration of flow (thrombolysis or balloon angioplasty) through occluded vessels responsible for the infarction yields a better prognosis.

Complications

Complications of an MI depend on the size and location of injury, as well as functional myocardial reserves. Overall mortality rate in the first year after MI is 30% and thereafter 5% to 10% per year. Typical complications include:

- Arrhythmias.
- CHF.
- Cardiogenic shock (usually seen when ≥40% of the left ventricle is infarcted).
- Ventricular rupture (1%–2% of transmural MIs), which typically occurs within the first 10 days (median, 4–5 days). Rupture of the free wall causes pericardial tamponade and rupture of the septum causes a left-to-right shunt with right-sided volume overload.
- Rarely, papillary muscle infarction with or without rupture can cause severe mitral regurgitation.

- Fibrinous pericarditis is common 2 to 3 days after MI (but is not usually clinically significant).
- Mural thrombosis adjacent to a noncontractile area, with risk of peripheral embolization.
- Stretching of a large area of transmural infarction (*expansion*) that may heal into a *ventricular aneurysm*; both are prone to mural thrombosis.
- Repetitive infarction (*extension*).

HYPERTENSIVE HEART DISEASE (p. 587)

Systemic (Left-Sided) Hypertensive Heart Disease (p. 587)

Diagnosis

Diagnostic criteria:

- A history or extracardiac anatomic evidence of hypertension
- Left ventricular hypertrophy, typically concentric
- Absence of other lesions that induce cardiac hypertrophy (e.g., aortic valve stenosis, aortic coarctation)

Pathogenesis

Myocyte hypertrophic enlargement occurs in response to increased work; because myocytes cannot divide, this is the only way that these cells can augment contractile proteins. Thickened myocardium reduces left ventricle compliance, impairing diastolic filling while increasing oxygen demand; individual myocyte hypertrophy increases the distance for oxygen and nutrient diffusion from adjacent capillaries. Coronary atherosclerosis accompanying hypertension can add an element of ischemia.

Morphology

The left ventricular wall is thickened (>2 cm) and heart weight is increased (>500 gm). Myocytes and nuclei are enlarged. Long-term, diffuse interstitial fibrosis and focal myocyte atrophy and degeneration may develop, with resulting left ventricle chamber dilation and wall thinning.

Clinical Features

CHF is the cause of death in one third of hypertensive patients; hypertensive hypertrophy also increases the risk of sudden cardiac death. The remainder die of renal disease, stroke, or unrelated causes. Therapeutic control of blood pressure may, in time, lead to regression of the myocyte hypertrophy and to restoration of heart size.

Pulmonary (Right-Sided) Heart Disease (Cor Pulmonale) (p. 588)

Cor pulmonale is the right-sided counterpart to systemic hypertensive heart disease; basically, pulmonary hypertension (caused by disorders affecting lung structure or function) causes right ventricular hypertrophy or dilation. Right ventricular enlargement due to congenital heart disease or left ventricular pathology is excluded.

- *Acute cor pulmonale* refers to right ventricular dilation after massive pulmonary embolization.
- *Chronic cor pulmonale* results from chronic right ventricular pressure overload.
- Hypoxemia and acidosis (e.g., in the setting of pneumonia or pulmonary emboli) cause vasoconstriction in the pulmonary vasculature that exacerbates any baseline pulmonary hypertension.

Morphology

Right ventricular hypertrophy (often ≥1 cm), dilation, or both are present; right ventricular dilation can cause tricuspid regurgitation. The left side of the heart is essentially normal. Pulmonary arteriolar wall thickening and atherosclerosis occur, secondary to the increased right-sided pressures.

Clinical Features

Chronic cor pulmonale is fairly common because chronic obstructive pulmonary disease is widespread. It can precipitate cardiac decompensation, with the cardiac symptoms being masked by those of the underlying lung disease.

VALVULAR HEART DISEASE (p. 588)

Valvular heart disease in adults is typically caused by degeneration (e.g., calcific aortic stenosis, mitral annular calcification, mitral valve prolapse), immunologic inflammatory processes (e.g., rheumatic heart disease), or infection (e.g., infective endocarditis).

Degenerative Calcific Aortic Valve Stenosis (p. 590)

Degenerative calcific aortic valve stenosis is a common age-related lesion that typically becomes clinically important over the age of 70. Earlier onset (patients aged 50–60 years) of degenerative calcific stenosis occurs most commonly in congenitally bicuspid valves (occurring in 1%–2% of the population).

Morphology

Nodular, rigid calcific subendothelial masses on the outflow surface of the valve cause cuspal thickening and immobility, thus impeding aortic outflow. In contrast to rheumatic stenosis, there is no commissural fusion and the thickening spares the cuspal free edges. Concentric left ventricular hypertrophy commonly occurs as a result of the chronic pressure overload.

Clinical Features

The failure of compensatory hypertrophy mechanisms is heralded by angina (reduced perfusion in hypertrophied myocardium), syncope (and increased risk of sudden death), or CHF. With onset of such symptoms, and if left untreated, there is a 50% risk of death within 2 to 5 years; urgent surgical valve replacement is clearly indicated.

Mitral Annular Calcification (p. 591)

These degenerative, noninflammatory calcific deposits are found within the mitral annulus, usually in the elderly.

- Regurgitation can occur from inadequate systolic contraction of the mitral valve ring.
- Stenosis can occur because leaflets are unable to open over bulky deposits.
- Nodular calcific deposits can impinge on conduction pathways, causing arrhythmias.
- Rarely, these deposits become a focus for infective endocarditis.

Mitral Valve Myxomatous Degeneration (Mitral Valve Prolapse) (p. 591)

One or both mitral valve leaflets are enlarged, myxomatous, and floppy; they balloon back (prolapse) into the left atrium during systole, causing midsystolic clicks and regurgitation. The disease occurs in 5% to 10% of the U.S. population, typically between ages 20 and 40, in a female-male ratio of 7:1. The etiology is uncertain; a high frequency in Marfan syndrome suggests a developmental anomaly or abnormal extracellular matrix synthesis.

Morphology

Grossly, redundancy and ballooning of the mitral valve leaflets is seen with elongated, attenuated, or occasionally ruptured chordae tendineae. *Microscopically,* the *fibrosa* layer (on which the strength of the leaflet depends) shows thinning and degeneration with myxomatous expansion of the *spongiosa.* Similar changes occur in the chordae.

Secondary changes include:

- Fibrous thickening of valve leaflets, especially at points of contact
- Thickened ventricular endocardium at sites of contact with prolapsing leaflets or chordae
- Atrial thrombosis behind the ballooning cusps, a potential source of emboli
- Mitral annular calcification

Clinical Features

Some patients also have aortic, tricuspid, or pulmonary valve myxomatous degeneration. *Mitral valve prolapse is generally asymptomatic* and discovered only as a midsystolic click on auscultation. It can be associated with atypical chest pain, dyspnea, fatigue, or psychiatric manifestations (e.g., depression, anxiety). Importantly, there is a somewhat increased risk of:

- Infective endocarditis
- Gradual mitral valvular insufficiency to produce CHF
- Arrhythmias
- Sudden death

Rheumatic Fever and Rheumatic Heart Disease (p. 592)

Rheumatic fever is an acute inflammatory disease classically occurring in children (5–15 years old) within 5 weeks following group A streptococcal infection (usually pharyngitis). It is attributed to host antistreptococcal antibodies that cross-react with cardiac antigens. Diagnosis is based on clinical history, and two of five major (Jones) criteria (minor criteria include fever, arthralgia, and leukocytosis):

- *Erythema marginatum:* Macular skin lesions with erythematous rims and central clearing, typically in a *bathing suit* distribution
- *Sydenham chorea:* A neurologic disorder with rapid, involuntary, purposeless movements
- *Carditis:* 50% to 75% of children and 35% of adults; can involve myocardium, endocardium, or pericardium
- *Subcutaneous nodules*
- *Migratory large joint polyarthritis:* 90% of adults; less common in children

Death (most frequently secondary to *myocarditis*) occurs rarely in acute rheumatic fever. Typically, myocarditis and arthritis are transient and resolve without complications; however, valvular involvement can deform and scar the valve causing permanent dysfunction *(chronic rheumatic heart disease)* and subsequent CHF. Chronic rheumatic heart disease is most likely when the first attack is in early childhood or is particularly severe, or with recurrent attacks.

Morphology

Characteristic features in the acute phase:

- *Aschoff bodies* are pathognomonic; these are foci of fibrinoid necrosis typically found in the myocardium. Initially surrounded by lymphocytes, macrophages, and plasma cells, they are slowly replaced by scar.
- Transient fibrinous pericarditis may contain Aschoff bodies.
- Inflammatory valvulitis is characterized by beady fibrinous vegetations *(verrucae)* that can contain Aschoff bodies.

Characteristic features of the chronic (or healed) valve:

- Fibrous thickening of leaflets
- Bridging fibrosis across valve commissures *(commissural fusion),* generating *fishmouth* or *buttonhole* stenoses
- Thickened, fused, and shortened chordae
- Calcification occurring deep in the fibrous leaflets
- Subendocardial collections of Aschoff nodules, usually in the left atrium, forming thickened *MacCallum plaques*

Solitary mitral involvement occurs in 65% to 70% of cases, with combined aortic and mitral involvement in 20% to 25%; tricuspid and pulmonary valves are less frequently affected.

Clinical Features

Changes secondary to mitral stenosis (the most frequent chronic result):

- Left atrial hypertrophy and enlargement, occasionally with mural thrombi
- Atrial fibrillation secondary to atrial dilation
- CHF with chronic pulmonary congestive changes
- Right ventricular hypertrophy
- Increased risk of infective endocarditis

ENDOCARDITIS (p. 595)

A few cardiac disorders are marked mainly by valve vegetations; major examples are:

- Infective endocarditis
- Nonbacterial thrombotic endocarditis
- Endocarditis associated with systemic lupus erythematosus (*Libman-Sacks endocarditis*)

Infective Endocarditis (p. 595)

Microbial colonization of heart valves results in friable, infected vegetations, frequently causing valve damage. Traditionally, *acute* and *subacute* forms of infective endocarditis are described:

- *Acute infective endocarditis* is caused by highly virulent organisms (e.g., *Staphylococcus aureus*), often seeding a previously normal valve to produce necrotizing, ulcerative, and invasive infections. Clinically, there is a rapidly developing fever with rigors, malaise, and weakness. Larger vegetations can cause embolic complications; splenomegaly is common. Even with treatment, death occurs in days to weeks in 50% to 60% of patients.
- *Subacute infective endocarditis* is typically caused by moderate to low virulence organisms (frequently *Streptococcus viridans*) seeding an abnormal or previously injured valve; there is less valvular destruction than acute infective endocarditis. This pattern occurs insidiously with nonspecific malaise, low-grade fever, weight loss, and a flulike syndrome. Vegetations tend to be small so that embolic complications occur less frequently. The disease tends to have a protracted course even without treatment and has a lower mortality rate than acute infective endocarditis.

Pathogenesis

Blood-borne organisms, usually bacteria *(bacteremia),* are prerequisites for infective endocarditis. They can come from infections elsewhere in the body, intravenous drug abuse, dental or surgical procedures, or otherwise trivial injury to gut, urinary tract, oropharynx, or skin. Contributory conditions include neutropenia and immunosuppression.

Although endocarditis can occur on normal valves, certain valvular and other cardiovascular conditions provide more favorable conditions for infection:

- Cardiac congenital anomalies, particularly tight shunts (e.g., VSD) or stenoses with jet streams
- Chronic rheumatic heart disease
- Mitral valve prolapse
- Degenerative calcific stenosis
- Bicuspid aortic valve
- Prosthetic valves
- Indwelling catheters

Morphology

- Friable, 0.5- to 2.0-cm, microbe-laden vegetations on one or more valves.
- Acute infective endocarditis is commonly associated with bulky (1–2 cm) vegetations causing erosions or leaflet perforations, with invasion into adjacent myocardium or aorta to produce abscesses.
- Subacute infective endocarditis has smaller vegetations that rarely erode or penetrate the leaflets.

- In nonvalvular endocarditis, vegetations are typically on the downstream margin of a jet lesion.
- In prosthetic valves, ring abscess is typically present.
- With intravenous drug abuse, the organism is most often *S. aureus;* vegetations are typically on right-sided valves, although left-sided valves can be involved.

Clinical Features

- Direct injury to valves (causing insufficiency with CHF) or myocardium and aorta (causing ring abscess or perforation).
- Emboli from vegetations to spleen, kidneys, heart, and brain with infarction or metastatic infection
- Renal injury, including embolic infarction or infection and antigen-antibody complex–mediated glomerulonephritis (with nephrotic syndrome, renal failure, or both).

Diagnosis is confirmed by the Duke criteria, summarized in Table 12–2; blood cultures are critically important for directing therapy (positive in 80%–95% of cases).

TABLE 12–2 **Diagnostic Criteria for Infective Endocarditis***

Pathologic Criteria

Microorganisms, demonstrated by culture or histologic examination, in a vegetation, embolus from a vegetation, or intracardiac abscess

Histologic confirmation of active endocarditis in vegetation or intracardiac abscess

Clinical Criteria

Major

Positive blood culture(s) indicating characteristic organism or persistence of unusual organism

Echocardiographic findings, including valve-related or implant-related mass or abscess, or partial separation of artificial valve

New valvular regurgitation

Minor

Predisposing heart lesion or intravenous drug use

Fever

Vascular lesions, including arterial petechiae, subungual/splinter hemorrhages, emboli, septic infarcts, mycotic aneurysm, intracranial hemorrhage, Janeway lesions[†]

Immunologic phenomena, including glomerulonephritis, Osler nodes,[‡] Roth spots,[§] rheumatoid factor

Microbiologic evidence, including single blood culture showing uncharacteristic organism

Echocardiographic findings consistent with but not diagnostic of endocarditis, including new valvular regurgitation, pericarditis

*Diagnosis by these guidelines, often called the Duke Criteria, requires either pathologic or clinical criteria; if clinical criteria are used, 2 major, 1 major + 3 minor, or 5 minor criteria are required for diagnosis.

[†]Janeway lesions are small erythematous or hemorrhagic, macular, nontender lesions on the palms and soles and are the consequence of septic embolic events.

[‡]Osler nodes are small, tender subcutaneous nodules that develop in the pulp of the digits or occasionally more proximally in the fingers and persist for hours to several days.

[§]Roth spots are oval retinal hemorrhages with pale centers.

Modified from Durack DT, et al: Am J Med 96:200, 1994 and Karchmer AW, In Braunwald E, et al. (eds): Heart Disease. A Textbook of Cardiovascular Medicine, 6th ed. Philadelphia, WB Saunders, 2001, p 1723.

Nonbacterial Thrombotic Endocarditis
(p. 598)

Nonbacterial thrombotic endocarditis, also called *marantic endocarditis*, characteristically occurs in settings of cancer (particularly adenocarcinomas) or prolonged debilitating illness (e.g., renal failure, chronic sepsis), and is attributed to disseminated intravascular coagulation or other hypercoagulable states.

• Small (1–5 mm) sterile, bland fibrin and platelet thrombi are loosely adherent to valve leaflets (typically mitral) along closure lines, without significant inflammation or valve damage.
• Vegetations can embolize systemically.

Endocarditis Associated with Systemic Lupus Erythematosus (Libman-Sacks Endocarditis) (p. 598)

This type of endocarditis can occur in systemic lupus erythematosus and in antiphospholipid syndrome; the pathogenesis is uncertain. Mitral and tricuspid valves are most often affected; findings include fibrinoid necrosis, mucoid degeneration, and small, fibrinous, sterile vegetations on *either* side of valve leaflets. Valve deformations can result from vegetation healing.

Carcinoid Heart Disease (p. 599)

Carcinoid tumors (Chapter 17) can elaborate bioactive products (e.g., serotonin, kallikrein, bradykinins, histamine, prostaglandins, and tachykinins P and K) that can cause cardiac lesions. The precise agent responsible is uncertain, although it is presumably rapidly metabolized in the lung, because right-sided heart lesions predominate.

Morphology

Plaque-like intimal thickening of the tricuspid and pulmonary valves, and right ventricular outflow tract, is superimposed on otherwise unaltered endocardium. The left side of the heart is usually unaffected except in primary pulmonary carcinoid tumors. Similar valve lesions are reported in the setting of fenfluramine and phentermine (fen-phen) use; these are appetite suppressants (for treating obesity) that may affect systemic serotonin metabolism.

Complications of Artificial Valves (p. 600)

Prosthetic valves are of two basic types: mechanical (rigid, synthetic) and bioprosthetic (glutaraldehyde-treated animal valves). Various complications can ensue:

• *Paravalvular leak:* Sewing ring may separate from the valve annulus.
• *Thrombosis, thromboembolism,* or both: These events can hinder valve function or embolize and can cause morbidity and death. Such complications are more common with mechanical valves.
• *Hemorrhage* can occur from the anticoagulation used to prevent thrombosis in mechanical valves.

- *Infective endocarditis* occurs in 5% of patients within 5 years of valve replacement; the infection is difficult to treat without removing the valve.
- *Structural deterioration:* Uncommon with most mechanical valves, but 20% to 30% of bioprosthetic valves require replacement for degeneration within 10 years.
- *Occlusion* may be due to tissue overgrowth.
- *Hemolysis* can occur from mechanical trauma to erythrocytes.

CARDIOMYOPATHIES (p. 601)

Although myocardial dysfunction can occur secondary to ischemic, valvular, hypertensive, or other heart diseases, the term *myocardial disease* implies *principal* cardiac dysfunction. Causes of myocardial disease include:

- Inflammatory disorders *(myocarditis)*
- Immunologic and systemic metabolic disorders
- Genetic abnormalities in cardiomyocytes

When the abnormality is primary in and localized to the myocardium, the condition is called *cardiomyopathy*. Cardiomyopathy is not synonymous with CHF; the latter represents a consequence of many forms of cardiac disease. Cardiomyopathy is divided into three main categories: *dilated, hypertrophic,* and *restrictive* (Table 12–3).

Dilated Cardiomyopathy (p. 601).

Characterized by gradual four-chamber hypertrophy and dilation, dilated cardiomyopathy (DCM) can occur at any age as slow, progressive CHF. Only 25% of patients survive more than 5 years. Although the cause is frequently unknown *(idiopathic DCM),* certain pathologic mechanisms may contribute (see also Fig. 12–3):

- *Genetic defect:* DCM has a familial occurrence in 25% to 35% of cases; autosomal dominant inheritance is most common; X-linked, autosomal recessive, and mitochondrial inheritance are less frequent. The known genetic abnormalities largely involve cytoskeletal proteins, such as dystrophin in X-linked cardiomyopathy (Duchenne and Becker muscular dystrophies). Others involve mutations of enzymes involved in fatty acid β-oxidation, or mitochondrial gene deletions causing abnormal oxidative phosphorylation. These defects typically cause childhood-onset DCM.
- *Alcohol toxicity:* DCM is attributed to direct toxicity of alcohol or a metabolite (especially acetaldehyde) on the myocardium. No morphologic features distinguish alcohol-induced cardiac damage from associated idiopathic DCM or chronic thiamine deficiency.
- *Peripartum cardiomyopathy:* DCM discovered within several months before or after delivery. Although the mechanism is uncertain, the association with pregnancy suggests possible etiologies of chronic hypertension, volume overload, nutritional deficiency, metabolic derangement, or immunologic response.
- *Postviral myocarditis* (see later discussion): Myocarditis (even after resolution of the infection) can progress to DCM.

TABLE 12–3 **Cardiomyopathy and Indirect Myocardial Dysfunction: Functional Patterns and Causes**

Functional Pattern	Left Ventricular Ejection Fraction*	Mechanisms of Heart Failure	Causes	Indirect Myocardial Dysfunction (Not Cardiomyopathy)
Dilated	<40%	Impairment of contractility (systolic dysfunction)	Idiopathic; alcohol; peripartum; genetic; myocarditis; hemochromatosis; chronic anemia; doxorubicin (Adriamycin); sarcoidosis	Ischemic heart disease; valvular heart disease; hypertensive heart disease; congenital heart disease
Hypertrophic	50–80%	Impairment of compliance (diastolic dysfunction)	Genetic; Friedreich ataxia; storage diseases; infants of diabetic mothers	Hypertensive heart disease; aortic stenosis
Restrictive	45–90%	Impairment of compliance (diastolic dysfunction)	Idiopathic; amyloidosis; radiation-induced fibrosis	Pericardial constriction

*Normal, approximately 50–65%.

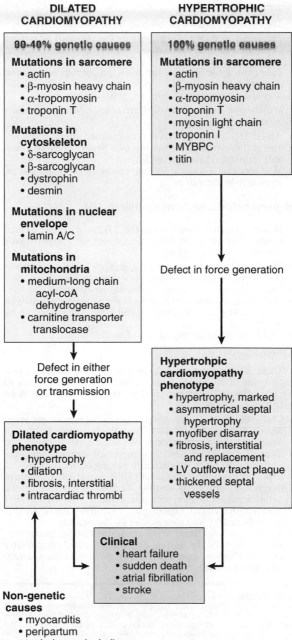

DILATED CARDIOMYOPATHY

30-40% genetic causes

Mutations in sarcomere
- actin
- β-myosin heavy chain
- α-tropomyosin
- troponin T

Mutations in cytoskeleton
- δ-sarcoglycan
- β-sarcoglycan
- dystrophin
- desmin

Mutations in nuclear envelope
- lamin A/C

Mutations in mitochondria
- medium-long chain acyl-coA dehydrogenase
- carnitine transporter translocase

Defect in either force generation or transmission

Dilated cardiomyopathy phenotype
- hypertrophy
- dilation
- fibrosis, interstitial
- intracardiac thrombi

Non-genetic causes
- myocarditis
- peripartum
- toxic (e.g., alcohol)
- idiopathic

HYPERTROPHIC CARDIOMYOPATHY

100% genetic causes

Mutations in sarcomere
- actin
- β-myosin heavy chain
- α-tropomyosin
- troponin T
- myosin light chain
- troponin I
- MYBPC
- titin

Defect in force generation

Hypertrohpic cardiomyopathy phenotype
- hypertrophy, marked
- asymmetrical septal hypertrophy
- myofiber disarray
- fibrosis, interstitial and replacement
- LV outflow tract plaque
- thickened septal vessels

Clinical
- heart failure
- sudden death
- atrial fibrillation
- stroke

For legend see following page.

Morphology

The following *gross changes* may be observed:

- The heart is flabby. Cardiomegaly (to 900 gm) is typical, although wall thickness may not reflect the degree of hypertrophy due to dilation.
- Poor contractile function and stasis can predispose to mural thrombi.
- Valves and coronary arteries are generally normal.

Microscopic changes in DCM are often subtle and entirely nonspecific:

- About 25% of patients have no significant alterations.
- The remainder have diffuse myocyte hypertrophy and variable interstitial myocardial fibrosis.
- Mild-moderate endocardial thickening is sometimes seen, especially in the ventricles.

Hypertrophic Cardiomyopathy (p. 604).

Hypertrophic cardiomyopathy (HCM) has also been termed *idiopathic hypertrophic subaortic stenosis* and *hypertrophic obstructive cardiomyopathy.*

- HCM is characterized by heavy, muscular, *hypercontractile,* poorly compliant hearts with poor diastolic relaxation.
- Over 50% have autosomal dominant inheritance.
- Symptomatic disease presents usually in young adults with dyspnea, angina, near-syncope, and CHF, but HCM can be asymptomatic.
- HCM carries an increased risk of sudden death.

Morphology

There is no discernible difference between familial and sporadic cases of HCM; all show marked cardiomegaly owing to hypertrophy, left ventricle greater than right ventricle, often with atrial dilation.

- Classically, there is disproportionate thickening of the interventricular septum (asymmetric septal hypertrophy), although many cases have concentric or symmetric hypertrophy.
- The left ventricular cavity is compressed into a *banana-like configuration* by the asymmetric bulging of the septum.
- Septal thickening at the level of the mitral valve compromises left ventricular systolic outflow by contact of the anterior mitral leaflet with the septum *(systolic anterior motion);* this causes *hypertrophic obstructive cardiomyopathy,* reflected by a fibrous plaque on the septum.
- *Microscopically,* there is marked myofiber hypertrophy; 25% to 50% of the septum classically shows helter-skelter *myocyte disarray,* accompanied by myofilament disorganization within muscle cells.

FIGURE 12–3 Pathways of dilated and hypertrophic cardiomyopathy, emphasizing several important concepts. Some forms of dilated cardiomyopathy (others are caused by myocarditis, alcohol and other toxic injury, or the peripartum state) and virtually all forms of hypertrophic cardiomyopathy are genetic in origin. The genetic causes of dilated cardiomyopathy involve a wide variety of proteins predominantly of the cytoskeleton, but also the sarcomere, mitochondria, and the nuclear envelope. In contrast, the several mutated genes that cause hypertrophic cardiomyopathy encode proteins of the sarcomere. Although these two phenotypes of cardiomyopathy differ greatly in subcellular basis and morphologic phenotypes, they share a common pathway of clinical complications. A and C are components of the nuclear membrane; LV, left ventricle.

- There are abnormal thick-walled intramyocardial arterioles, as well as patchy replacement fibrosis, the latter presumably due to focal ischemic injury.

Pathogenesis

HCM is caused by mutations in any of several genes that encode sarcomeric proteins, the contractile components of striated muscle. Thus, HCM is a disease of force generation within the cardiac myocyte. Familial cases are typically autosomal dominant with variable expression; remaining cases appear to be sporadic. Mutated proteins include β-myosin heavy chain (most frequently), cardiac troponin T, α-tropomyosin, and myosin binding protein-C. Although these genetic defects are critical to the etiology, the sequence of events leading from mutations to HCM remain ill defined (see also Fig. 12–3).

Clinical Features

The course of HCM is highly variable, but certain mutations have characteristic prognoses. Most patients remain unchanged for years, but some progressively worsen. Major complications include:

- Atrial fibrillation with mural thrombus and embolization
- Infective endocarditis
- Left ventricular outflow tract obstruction
- CHF
- Sudden death

Restrictive Cardiomyopathy (p. 606)

Relatively rare and with multiple etiologies, this entity is marked by a restriction of ventricular filling leading to reduced cardiac output. Interstitial myocardial fibrosis is usually present. Specific entities include:

- *Endomyocardial fibrosis* is typically seen in African children and young adults; the basic cause is unknown. It is characterized by ventricular subendocardial fibrosis extending from the apex to the ventricular inflow tracts, often with superimposed mural thrombus; the atrioventricular valves may be involved. Restrictive physiology results with reduced ventricular chamber volume.
- *Loeffler endocarditis* is morphologically similar to endomyocardial fibrosis but occurs in temperate zones. Loeffler endocarditis is classically associated with peripheral eosinophilia, eosinophilic infiltration of multiple organs (especially the heart), and a rapidly fatal course. The cardiac changes are probably due to toxic products of eosinophils.
- *Endocardial fibroelastosis* is an uncommon disorder of obscure etiology (and possibly the end point of different causes of injury), characterized by focal to diffuse, *fibroelastic* thickening of the endocardium, left ventricle more than right ventricle. It occurs at all ages but is most common in patients younger than 2 years old. Congenital cardiac anomalies are present in a third of cases.

Arrhythmogenic Right Ventricular Cardiomyopathy (Arrhythmogenic Right Ventricular Dysplasia) (p. 604)

Arrhythmogenic right ventricular cardiomyopathy is a recently recognized cardiomyopathy with distinct presentation and morphology. It is typically a familial disorder characterized by predominantly right-sided failure (occasionally left-sided) and various rhythm disturbances, particularly ventricular tachycardia and sudden death. Morphologically, the right ventricular wall is severely thinned with myocyte loss, and profound fatty infiltration. Death occurs secondary to progressive CHF, embolism of mural thrombi, or fatal arrhythmias.

Myocarditis (p. 607)

Myocarditis is characterized by myocardial inflammation as the principal feature.

* The clinical spectrum is broad, from entirely asymptomatic to abrupt onset of arrhythmia, CHF, or even sudden death; most patients recover quickly and without sequelae, although postviral DCM can occur (see earlier discussion).
* Most cases are thought to be of viral origin (e.g., coxsackievirus A and B, echovirus). Cardiac involvement occurs days to weeks after a primary viral infection, which can be in the heart or solely at another site.
* The cardiac involvement can be a direct infection or an immunological reaction to a myocardial antigen triggered by the infectious agent.
* Rare cases are secondary to bacteremia (e.g., staphylococcal, tuberculous).
* Myocarditis occurs in approximately two-thirds of patients with Lyme disease *(Borrelia burgdorferi)*. Lyme myocarditis is usually mild and reversible, but occasionally requires a temporary pacemaker for atrioventricular block.
* *Trypanosoma cruzi* (causal organism in Chagas disease) causes myocarditis in up to 50% of the population in endemic areas of South America.
* Noninfectious myocarditis may be immune mediated (e.g., associated with rheumatic fever, systemic lupus erythematosus, or drug allergies).
* In some cases, the cause is unknown (e.g., sarcoidosis, giant cell myocarditis) or the microbe is unidentifiable.

Morphology

Gross manifestations include a flabby heart often with four-chamber dilation and patchy hemorrhagic mottling.

* Mural thrombi can form in dilated chambers.
* Endocardium and valves are unaffected.
* After the acute stage, there may be residual dilation or hypertrophy.

Microscopically, there is a myocardial inflammatory infiltrate with associated myocyte necrosis or degeneration. Lesions are typically focal (and may be missed by routine *endomyocardial biopsy*).

* In *viral infections,* isolated myofiber necrosis is seen with interstitial edema and a mononuclear cell infiltrate. After the acute stage, inflammatory lesions may resolve, leaving either no residua or variable interstitial and replacement fibrosis.
* *Bacteria and other larger parasites* produce reactions characteristic of the lesions they cause in other tissues (e.g., neutrophilic infiltrate, abscesses, granulomas).
* In *Lyme myocarditis,* spirochetes can be occasionally demonstrated.

- In *Chagas disease,* trypanosomes parasitize myocytes and produce acute and chronic inflammation, including eosinophils.
- In *hypersensitivity reactions,* there are predominantly perivascular mononuclear and eosinophilic infiltrates, occasionally with acute vasculitis and spotty myofiber necrosis. This variant is often induced by therapeutic drugs.
- In *giant cell myocarditis,* there is focal myocyte necrosis associated with granulomatous inflammation, including multinucleated giant cells. This variant of myocarditis has a poor prognosis.

Other Specific Causes of Myocardial Disease (p. 609)

Cardiotoxic agents commonly cause myofiber swelling, fatty change, and individual cell lysis. Electron microscopy shows mitochondrial abnormalities, smooth endoplasmic reticulum swelling and fragmentation, and myofibril lysis. With time, delicate interstitial fibrosis and focal replacement scarring occur.

- Anthracycline chemotherapeutic agents doxorubicin (Adriamycin) and daunorubicin induce dose-dependent cardiotoxicity, attributed primarily to lipid peroxidation of myofiber membranes. Both the physiologic and the morphologic patterns may be indistinguishable from those of idiopathic DCM.
- *Iron overload* with myocyte hemosiderin deposits occurs in hereditary hemochromatosis and hemosiderosis from multiple blood transfusions. Patients with iron storage disease present most commonly with DCM.
- *Amyloidosis* occurs as patchy and perivascular hyaline deposits; it can be part of systemic amyloidosis (Chapter 6) or may be isolated (e.g., senile cardiac amyloidosis, occurring in some individuals more than 70 years old). Often, cardiac involvement is incidental, but can induce arrhythmias or restrictive physiology.
- *Catecholamines,* either administered exogenously (e.g., epinephrine) or produced endogenously (e.g., by pheochromocytomas), induce tachycardia and vasomotor constriction (with superimposed platelet aggregation); this can result in diffuse but patchy ischemic necrosis. *Cocaine* can have a similar effect by blocking catecholamine reuptake at adrenergic nerve terminals.

PERICARDIAL DISEASE (p. 610)

Pericardial disease is typically secondary to diseases of adjacent structures or part of a systemic disorder; it is rarely primary.

Pericardial Effusion and Hemopericardium (p. 611)

The normal pericardial sac contains 30 to 50 mL of serous, *noninflammatory* fluid. Slow fluid accumulation can be well tolerated, resulting in collections greater than 500 mL; rapid accumulating fluids can cause fatal tamponade with as little as 200 mL.

- *Serous* effusions are the most common form; the serosa is smooth and glistening. Fluid accumulates slowly and is therefore well tolerated until large volumes compromise diastolic filling. The most common causes are CHF and hypoproteinemia.

- *Serosanguineous* effusions usually result from blunt chest trauma (e.g., cardiopulmonary resuscitation), and are rarely clinically significant.
- *Chylous* accumulations are due to lymphatic obstruction (benign or malignant), and are rarely clinically significant.
- *Hemopericardium* refers to accumulation of pure, often clotted blood in the pericardium without an inflammatory component. It is usually due to traumatic perforation, myocardial rupture after a transmural MI, rupture of the intrapericardial aorta, or hemorrhage from an abscess or tumor metastasis. Escaping blood rapidly fills the sac under high pressure, and as little as 200 to 300 mL can cause tamponade.

Pericarditis (p. 611)

Pericarditis is usually secondary to disorders involving the heart or adjacent mediastinal structures (e.g., MI, surgery, trauma, radiation, tumors, infections) or, less frequently, systemic abnormalities (e.g., uremia, autoimmune diseases). Acute pericarditis is most often viral in origin. Chronic reactions also occur (e.g., with tuberculosis and fungi), and healing can lead to damaging adhesions.

Acute Pericarditis (p. 611)

- *Serous pericarditis:* From 50 to 200 mL of exudate slowly accumulates; although the etiology is frequently unknown, it is characteristically induced by nonbacterial causes (e.g., rheumatic fever, systemic lupus erythematosus, tumors, uremia, and primary viral infections). Microscopically, there is scant pericardial acute and chronic inflammatory infiltration (mostly lymphocytes). The fluid resorbs if the underlying disease remits, rarely leaving any residual change.
- *Fibrinous and serofibrinous pericarditis:* The most common clinical form, this is seen with MI, and is associated with a pericardial friction rub; it can also be caused by any of the etiologies for serous pericarditis. Exudates can be completely resolved or can organize, leaving delicate, stringy adhesions *(adhesive pericarditis)* or plaquelike thickening, both usually inconsequential.
- *Purulent (suppurative) pericarditis:* This form usually signifies bacterial, fungal, or parasitic infection, reaching the pericardium by direct extension, by hematogenous or lymphatic spread, or during cardiotomy. Common organisms include staphylococci, streptococci, and pneumococci. Purulent pericarditis is typically composed of 400 to 500 mL of a thin-to-creamy pus with erythematous, granular serosal surfaces. It presents with high fevers, rigors, and a friction rub, and can organize to produce *mediastinopericarditis* or *constrictive pericarditis* (see following discussion).
- *Hemorrhagic pericarditis* denotes an exudate of blood admixed with fibrinous-to-suppurative effusion. Most commonly, it follows cardiac surgery or is associated with tuberculosis or malignancy. It usually organizes with or without calcification.
- *Caseous pericarditis* is due to tuberculosis (typically by direct extension from neighboring lymph nodes) or, less commonly, mycotic infection. This pattern is the most frequent antecedent to fibrocalcific constrictive pericarditis.

Chronic or Healed Pericarditis (p. 612)

Healing of acute lesions can lead to resolution or pericardial fibrosis ranging from a thick, pearly, nonadherent epicardial plaque (*soldier's plaque*), to thin, delicate adhesions, to massive adhesions.

- *Adhesive mediastinopericarditis* is clinically significant; the pericardial sac is obliterated, and the parietal layer is tethered to mediastinal tissue. The heart thus contracts against all the surrounding attached structures, with subsequent hypertrophy and dilation.
- *Constrictive pericarditis* is clinically significant; it is marked by thick (up to 1 cm), dense, fibrous obliteration, often with calcification of the pericardial sac encasing the heart, limiting diastolic expansion and restricting cardiac output.

Rheumatoid Heart Disease (p. 612)

Rheumatoid arthritis involves the heart in 20% to 40% of severe chronic cases. The typical finding is pericarditis, with a mixture of fibrin and necrotic debris derived from pericardial rheumatoid granulomas that can progress to form dense, fibrous, and potentially restrictive adhesions. Less frequently, granulomatous rheumatoid nodules occur in the myocardium, endocardium, aortic root, or valves, where they are particularly damaging. Rheumatoid valvulitis can produce changes similar to those seen in rheumatic heart disease but classically without commissural fusion.

TUMORS OF THE HEART (p. 613)

Cardiac metastases (usually hematogenous) occur much more frequently than primary heart tumors; metastases involve the pericardium or penetrate into the myocardium. The heart can also be *indirectly* affected by tumors at other sites; the spectrum of cardiac effects of noncardiac tumors is summarized in Table 12–4.

The following are primary cardiac tumors:

- *Myxomas: the most common primary cardiac tumor in adults.* Usually isolated, 90% arise in the left atria in the region of the fossa ovale (20% occur in the right atrium).

TABLE 12–4 **Cardiovascular Effects of Noncardiac Neoplasms**

Direct Consequences of Tumor
Pericardial and myocardial metastases
Large vessel obstruction
Pulmonary tumor emboli
Indirect Consequences of Tumor (Complications of Circulating Mediators)
Nonbacterial thrombotic endocarditis (NBTE)
Carcinoid heart disease
Pheochromocytoma-associated heart disease
Myeloma-associated amyloidosis
Effects of Tumor Therapy
Chemotherapy
Radiation therapy

Modified from Schoen FJ, et al: Cardiac effects of non-cardiac neoplasms. Cardiol Clin 2:657, 1984.

Grossly, they are 1- to 10-cm sessile-to-pedunculated masses varying from globular and hard to papillary and myxoid. They may cause symptoms by physical obstruction, by trauma to the atrioventricular valves, or by peripheral embolization.

Histologically, they are composed of stellate or globular multipotential mesenchymal myxoma cells, admixed with endothelial cells, smooth muscle cells, and inflammatory cells, all in an acid mucopolysaccharide matrix.

- *Lipomas:* Lipomas are circumscribed but poorly encapsulated, often subendocardial large polypoid accumulations of adipose tissue, more commonly in the left ventricle, right atrium, or septum. Symptoms depend on location and on encroachment on valve function or conduction pathways. These are probably hamartomas.

- *Papillary fibroelastomas:* Papillary fibroelastomas can cause emboli but are usually incidental findings at autopsy. They are characteristically found on right-sided valves in children and left-sided valves in adults. They are composed of clusters of 2- to 5-mm hairlike filaments. *Microscopically,* filaments have a core of myxoid connective tissue with smooth muscle cells and fibroblasts, covered by endothelium. Most probably derive from organized thrombi.

- *Rhabdomyomas:* Rhabdomyomas are much less common than myxomas but are the most common primary heart tumor in children. Rhabdomyomas may cause valvular or outflow tract obstruction; they are probably hamartomas and may be associated with tuberous sclerosis.

  Grossly, they are left- or right-sided gray-white ventricular wall masses up to several centimeters in diameter.

  Microscopically, they are composed of large, rounded, or polygonal cells rich in glycogen and containing myofibrils. Fixation and histologic processing leaves characteristic artifactual cytoplasmic stranding radiating from the central nucleus to plasma membrane, forming so-called *spider cells.*

- *Angiosarcomas and rhabdomyosarcomas:* These malignant neoplasms resemble their counterparts in other locations.

CARDIAC TRANSPLANTATION (p. 615)

Cardiac transplantation is performed most commonly for DCM and ischemic heart disease (approximately 3000 cases annually worldwide). The 1-year survival is 70% to 80%, with 5-year survival rates greater than 60%.

Acute allograft rejection is characterized by interstitial lymphocytic inflammation with associated myocyte damage; severe rejection is accompanied by extensive myocyte necrosis and frequently inflammatory vascular injury. Other issues in the immunosuppressed transplant recipients include opportunistic infections and malignancies, particularly lymphomas (commonly related to Epstein-Barr virus). The major current limitation to the long-term success of cardiac transplantation is progressive, diffuse intimal proliferation of the coronary arteries *(graft arteriosclerosis)* causing downstream myocardial ischemia.

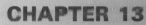

CHAPTER 13

Red Blood Cell and Bleeding Disorders

ANEMIAS (p. 622)

Anemia is a reduction in blood oxygen transport capacity, usually due to reduced circulating red blood cell mass; it is reflected by low hematocrit and hemoglobin concentrations. In most anemias, increased erythropoietin production induces erythroid marrow hyperplasia. Classification of anemias in Table 13–1 is based on the mechanisms of production. Anemias can also be classified on the basis of red blood cell indices, such as mean cell volume, mean cell hemoglobin concentration, etc. (Table 13–2).

Anemias of Blood Loss (p. 623)

Clinical and morphologic reactions depend on the rate of hemorrhage:
- *Acute blood loss:* Alterations principally reflect loss of blood volume (may lead to shock and death). After 4 to 5 days, if the patient survives, increased erythropoietin leads to compensatory increases in marrow production (reticulocytosis).
- *Chronic blood loss:* Anemia results when iron reserves are depleted—iron deficiency anemia. With iron replenishment, increased marrow production (reticulocytosis) appears in several days.

Hemolytic Anemias (p. 624)

Hemolytic anemias are characterized by premature red blood cell destruction, accumulation of hemoglobin catabolites (e.g., bilirubin), and markedly increased erythropoiesis with associated reticulocytosis.

Hemolysis can occur intravascularly or extravascularly:

TABLE 13–1 **Classification of Anemia According to Underlying Mechanism**

Blood Loss
Acute: trauma
Chronic: lesions of gastrointestinal tract, gynecologic disturbances

Increased Rate of Destruction (Hemolytic Anemias)
Intrinsic (intracorpuscular) abnormalities of red blood cells
   Hereditary
   Red blood cell membrane disorders
      Disorders of membrane cytoskeleton: spherocytosis, elliptocytosis
      Disorders of lipid synthesis: selective increase in membrane lecithin
   Red blood cell enzyme deficiencies
      Glycolytic enzymes: pyruvate kinase deficiency, hexokinase deficiency
      Enzymes of hexose monophosphate shunt: G6PD, glutathione synthetase
   Disorders of hemoglobin synthesis
      Deficient globin synthesis: thalassemia syndromes
      Structurally abnormal globin synthesis (hemoglobinopathies): sickle cell anemia, unstable hemoglobins
   Acquired
   Membrane defect: paroxysmal nocturnal hemoglobinuria
Extrinsic (extracorpuscular) abnormalities
   Antibody mediated
      Isohemagglutinins: transfusion reactions, erythroblastosis fetalis
      Autoantibodies: idiopathic (primary), drug-associated, systemic lupus erythematosus, malignant neoplasms, mycoplasmal infection
   Mechanical trauma to red blood cells
      Microangiopathic hemolytic anemias: thrombotic thrombocytopenic purpura, disseminated intravascular coagulation
      Cardiac traumatic hemolytic anemia
   Infections: malaria, hookworm
   Chemical injury: lead poisoning
   Sequestration in mononuclear phagocyte system: hypersplenism

Impaired Red Blood Cell Production
Disturbance of proliferation and differentiation of stem cells: aplastic anemia, pure red blood cell aplasia, anemia of renal failure, anemia of endocrine disorders
Disturbance of proliferation and maturation of erythroblasts
   Defective DNA synthesis: deficiency or impaired use of vitamin B_{12} and folic acid (megaloblastic anemias)
   Defective hemoglobin synthesis
   Deficient heme synthesis: iron deficiency
   Deficient globin synthesis: thalassemias
Unknown or multiple mechanisms: sideroblastic anemia, anemia of chronic infections, myelophthisic anemias due to marrow infiltrations

TABLE 13–2 **Adult Reference Ranges for Red Blood Cells***

Measurement (units)	Men	Women
Hemoglobin (gm/dL)	13.6–17.2	12.0–15.0
Hematocrit (%)	39–49	33–43
RBC count ($10^6/\mu$L)	4.3–5.9	3.5–5.0
Reticulocyte count (%)	0.5–1.5	
Mean cell volume (fL)	82–96	
Mean corpuscular hemoglobin (pg)	27–33	
Mean corpuscular hemoglobin concentration (gm/dL)	33–37	
RBC distribution width	11.5–14.5	

*Reference ranges vary among laboratories. The reference ranges for the laboratory providing the result should always be used in interpreting the test result.
RBC, red blood cell.

- *Intravascular hemolysis:* Red blood cells are damaged by mechanical injury (e.g., microangiopathic hemolytic anemia) or complement (e.g., mismatched blood transfusion). Patients exhibit hemoglobinemia; hemoglobinuria; hemosiderinuria; jaundice (conjugated hyperbilirubinemia); reduced serum haptoglobin (a protein that binds hemoglobin).
- *Extravascular hemolysis* occurs in mononuclear phagocytes of spleen (and other organs). Predisposing factors include red blood cell membrane injury, reduced deformability, or opsonization. Manifestations are similar to intravascular hemolysis but without hemoglobinemia and hemoglobinuria.

Hereditary Spherocytosis (p. 625)

Hereditary spherocytosis (HS) is a predominantly autosomal dominant disorder (75%) in which red blood cell cytoskeletal membrane protein defects render erythrocytes spheroidal, less deformable, and vulnerable to splenic sequestration and destruction.

Pathophysiology

Defects in several different membrane skeletal proteins can cause HS; all lead primarily or secondarily to deficiencies in spectrin, a meshwork protein associated with the inner red blood cell membrane. Spectrin-deficient red blood cells have unstable membranes and spontaneously lose fragments. The resulting surface area reduction causes red blood cells to assume a spheroidal shape; such spherocytes have diminished membrane flexibility and are trapped and destroyed in the splenic cords.

Morphology

In the peripheral blood, spherocytic red blood cells appear small and lack central pallor. There is marked congestion and prominent erythrophagocytosis in the splenic cords of Billroth. Bone marrow exhibits normoblastic hyperplasia.

Clinical Features

Clinical features are variable, although anemia, moderate splenomegaly, and jaundice are characteristic. Infections can trigger *hemolytic crisis* (with massive hemolysis) or *aplastic crisis* (transient suppression of erythropoiesis by parvovirus infection). Half of adults develop gallstones from chronic hyperbilirubinemia. Diagnosis depends on family history, hematologic findings, and laboratory evidence of spherocytosis including increased red blood cell osmotic fragility. The mean cell hemoglobin concentration is increased as a result of cellular dehydration.

Glucose-6-Phosphate Dehydrogenase Deficiency (p. 627)

Glucose-6-phosphate dehydrogenase (G6PD) is an enzyme in the hexose monophosphate shunt that produces reduced glutathione, a molecule that protects red blood cells from oxidative injury. In G6PD-deficient cells oxidant stresses induce hemoglobin denaturation. The altered hemoglobin precipitates as Heinz bodies, which attach to the inner cell membrane, reduce deformability, and increase susceptibility to splenic macrophage destruction. Heinz bodies damage cell membranes sufficiently to cause both intravascular and extravascular hemolysis.

G6PD deficiency is an X-linked disorder; although there are several G6PD variants, only two, G6PD A⁻ and G6PD Mediterranean, lead to clinically significant hemolysis. A⁻ is present in about 10% of American blacks, and is associated with progressive loss of G6PD in older red blood cells. These older cells hemolyze after exposure to oxidant drugs (such as antimalarials) or to oxidant stress resulting from inflammatory responses. Because younger red blood cells are unaffected, hemolytic episodes are self-limited. In the Mediterranean form, G6PD levels are much lower and hemolytic episodes are more severe. Ingestion of fava beans can cause hemolysis in G6PD deficiency *(favism)* because these legumes generate oxidants.

Sickle Cell Disease (p. 628)

Sickle cell disease is a hereditary hemoglobinopathy resulting from substitution of valine for glutamic acid at the sixth position of the β-globin chain, transforming normal hemoglobin A ($\alpha_2\beta_2$) to the mutant hemoglobin S ($\alpha_2\beta^s_2$). Approximately 8% of American blacks are heterozygous for hemoglobin S (HbS).

Sickling Phenomenon

Deoxygenated HbS undergoes aggregation and polymerization into long, stiff chains that deform (sickle) red blood cells. In the homozygous state, irreversibly sickled cells can be readily identified in peripheral blood. Many factors influence sickling of the red blood cells:

- *The amount of HbS and its interaction with other hemoglobin chains in the cell (the most important factor).* In heterozygotes, approximately 40% of hemoglobin is HbS; the rest is HbA, which interacts weakly with HbS and thereby interferes with aggregation. Therefore, heterozygotes have little tendency to sickle *(sickle cell trait).* In contrast, *homozygotes have mostly HbS and will have full-blown sickle cell anemia.* β-Globin chains other than HbA also influence sickling. Because fetal hemoglobin (HbF, with γ-globin chains) also interacts weakly with HbS, newborns do not manifest disease complications until 5 to 6 months of age; at that time, red blood cell HbF content approaches adult levels. HbC, another mutant hemoglobin, has a greater tendency to aggregate with HbS than HbA; patients heterozygotic for both HbS and HbC have more severe disease (HbSC) than patients with sickle cell trait alone.
- *The mean corpuscular hemoglobin concentration (MCHC).* High HbS concentrations increase the rate of contact and interaction between individual HbS molecules. Dehydration is one factor that increases MCHC, thereby facilitating sickling and occlusion of small blood vessels. Conversely, concurrent diseases that reduce MCHC (e.g., α-thalassemia) lessen sickling severity.
- *Capillary bed transit times.* Normally, the capillary transit rate is so great that significant deoxygenation (and therefore sickling) cannot occur; consequently, sickling is usually confined to tissues with intrinsically sluggish blood flow (e.g.,

spleen, bone marrow) or those involved by inflammation, where blood flow is retarded and cell retention is enhanced.

Consequences of Sickling

- *Chronic hemolysis:* Repeated episodes of sickling damages red blood cell membranes so that cells become irreversible sickled. These rigid, nondeformable cells are prone to sequestration and destruction. Average red blood cell survival is shortened to 20 days; the severity of the anemia correlates with the percentage of circulating irreversibly sickled cells.
- *Microvascular occlusions:* Because of inelasticity and propensity to adhere to capillary endothelium, sickle cells occlude small blood vessels. The resultant hypoxia and infarction is the most clinically important and debilitating component of the disease.

Morphology

- The *spleen* is enlarged in early childhood due to sickled cell trapping in splenic cords. By adulthood, repeated episodes of vaso-occlusion have caused progressive scarring and shrinkage *(autosplenectomy)*.
- *Bone marrow* shows normoblastic hyperplasia. When hyperplasia is severe, expansion of the marrow can cause bone resorption.
- *Microvascular occlusions* produce tissue damage and infarction in several organs.

Clinical Features

- Chronic hemolytic anemia is seen with its associated features (e.g., chronic hyperbilirubinemia and propensity for gallstones).
- Vaso-occlusive crises present as painful episodes of ischemic necrosis, most commonly involving bones, lungs, liver, brain, penis, and spleen.
- Aplastic crisis due to transient suppression of erythropoiesis is triggered by parvovirus infections. Folate deficiency due to increased requirements can also impair erythropoiesis.
- Progressive splenic fibrosis and impairment of the alternate complement pathway predispose to infections, particularly *Salmonella* osteomyelitis, and others involving encapsulated organisms such as *Streptococcus pneumoniae* and *Haemophilus influenzae*.

Diagnosis

Diagnosis is based on clinical findings, sickle cells in the peripheral blood smear, and detection of HbS by hemoglobin electrophoresis. Prenatal detection of heterozygotes and homozygotes is possible through fetal DNA analysis.

Thalassemia Syndromes (p. 632)

Thalassemia syndromes are a heterogeneous group of mendelian disorders, characterized by defects that lead to reduced synthesis of α- or β-globin chains. β chains are encoded by a single gene on chromosome 11; α chains are encoded by two closely linked genes on chromosome 16.

Genetic Defects

- β-*Thalassemia syndromes* are characterized by deficient synthesis of β-globin:

In β°-thalassemia, there is total absence of β-globin chains in the homozygous state.

In β⁺-thalassemia, there is reduced (but detectable) β-globin synthesis in the homozygous state.

Several different point mutations affecting transcription, processing, or translation of β-globin mRNA can cause β°-thalassemia or β⁺-thalassemia; mutations causing aberrant mRNA splicing are most common.

- *α-Thalassemia* is characterized by reduced α-globin synthesis due to deletion of one or more α-globin genes.

Pathophysiology

The consequences of diminished synthesis of one globin chain derive from both low intracellular hemoglobin (hypochromia) and a relative excess of the other chain.

- *β-Thalassemia:* With decreased β-globin synthesis, excess unbound α chains form highly unstable aggregates that result in cell membrane damage; in turn, red blood cell precursors are destroyed in the marrow (ineffective erythropoiesis) and abnormal red blood cells are removed by phagocytes in the spleen (hemolysis). Severe anemia causes marked compensatory expansion of the erythropoietic marrow, ultimately encroaching on cortical bone and causing skeletal abnormalities in growing children. Ineffective erythropoiesis is also associated with excessive absorption of dietary iron; along with repeated blood transfusions this leads to severe iron overload.
- *α-Thalassemia* is due to imbalanced synthesis of α and non-α chains (γ chains in infancy, β chains after 6 months of age). Free β chains form unstable tetramers (HbH) that damage red blood cells and their precursors. Free γ chains form stable tetramers (HbBarts) that bind O_2 with excessive avidity, resulting in tissue hypoxia.

Clinical Classification

β-Thalassemia. Classification of β-thalassemia is based on the severity of anemia; severity is based on the genetic defect (β⁺ or β°), as well as gene dosage (homozygous or heterozygous).

- *Thalassemia major:* Homozygotes for β-thalassemia genes have severe, transfusion-dependent anemia; hemoglobin levels are 3 to 6 gm/dL. This form is most common in Mediterranean countries, parts of Africa, and Southeast Asia. Peripheral blood shows severe abnormalities, including marked anisocytosis (variability in cell size) with many microcytic, hypochromic red blood cells, target cells, and stippled or fragmented red blood cells. The clinical course of β-thalassemia major is generally brief; without transfusions, death occurs at an early age from profound anemia. Blood transfusions lessen the anemia and suppress secondary changes related to excessive erythropoiesis (bone deformities). In multiply transfused patients, morbidity and fatality are related to cardiac failure resulting from progressive iron overload and secondary hemochromatosis.
- *Thalassemia minor:* Heterozygotes are usually asymptomatic due to sufficient β-globin synthesis. This form is more common than thalassemia major and affects the same ethnic groups. Peripheral blood shows minor abnormalities, including hypochromia, microcytosis, basophilic stippling, and target cells. Hemoglobin electrophoresis shows increased

HbA$_2$ ($\alpha_2\delta_2$ hemoglobin), up to 4% to 8% of the total hemoglobin. Recognition of β-thalassemia trait is important for genetic counseling.

● *Thalassemia intermedia*: Clinical features and severity are intermediate between the major and minor forms. These patients are genetically heterogeneous.

α-Thalassemia. Classification—and the severity of the anemia—is related to the number of α-globin genes deleted. The clinical and genetic features of thalassemia are summarized in Table 13–3, on p. 634 of *Robbins and Cotran Pathologic Basis of Disease*, 7th ed.

- *Silent carrier state:* This type is completely asymptomatic, resulting from a single α-globin gene deletion; reduction in α-globin chain synthesis is barely detectable.
- *α-Thalassemia trait:* Either one chromosome has both α-globin genes or each chromosome has a deletion of one gene; the clinical picture is comparable to β-thalassemia minor. Although these two genotypes are clinically identical, they differ in whether offspring are at risk for severe α-thalassemia (≥ three α chains deleted).
- *Hemoglobin H (HbH) disease:* Deletion of three α-globin genes causes marked suppression of α chain synthesis, and formation of unstable tetramers of excess β-globin (HbH). Clinically, HbH disease resembles β-thalassemia intermedia.
- *Hydrops fetalis:* Deletion of all four α-globin genes. In the fetus, excess γ-globin chains form tetramers (HbBarts) with extremely high oxygen affinity and inability to release O$_2$ to tissues. This form is not compatible with life.

Paroxysmal Nocturnal Hemoglobinuria (p. 636)

Paroxysmal nocturnal hemoglobinuria (PNH) is a rare disorder, characterized by chronic intravascular hemolysis. It is the only hemolytic anemia resulting from an acquired (rather than inherited) membrane defect. Red blood cells have increased sensitivity to complement-mediated lysis due to deficient expression of a family of proteins normally anchored into the cell membrane via glycosylphosphatidylinositol (GPI). Mutations in the X-linked gene phosphatidylinositol glycan A (*PIGA*) prevents the synthesis of the GPI anchor. Among the GPI-linked proteins affected are several that regulate complement inactivation: decay-accelerating factor (CD55), membrane inhibitor of reactive lysis (CD59), and C8-binding protein. Their deficiency renders red blood cells hypersensitive to complement, which is activated spontaneously at low rates. Granulocyte and platelet GPI-proteins are also affected, resulting in a predisposition to thrombosis, particularly in portal, cerebral, and hepatic veins.

PNH may arise due to an autoimmune response to GPI-linked proteins on hematopoietic stem cells. In this scenario, rare clones harboring a mutated *PIGA* gene have a selective advantage and eventually "take over" the marrow. This pathogenic basis explains the association of PNH with aplastic anemia, which sometimes precedes the development of PNH. PNH also rarely transforms to acute leukemia.

Immunohemolytic Anemias (p. 636)

Hemolysis in immunohemolytic anemias is due to anti–red cell antibodies. The major diagnostic criterion is the direct

Coombs test, which detects antibodies and complement on red blood cells. Classification is based on the nature of the antibodies and the presence or absence of an underlying disorder (Table 13–3).

Warm Antibody Hemolytic Anemia

This anemia is idiopathic in 60% of cases. IgG anti–red blood cell antibodies coat the red blood cells; they do not fix complement, but do act as opsonins. Red blood cells are spherocytic due to membrane fragment loss through macrophage phagocytosis; they are eventually sequestered and destroyed in the spleen. Splenomegaly is characteristic. The mechanism of antibody formation is best understood in drug-induced hemolytic anemias:

- *Hapten model:* Drugs (e.g., penicillin, cephalosporins, quinidine) bind to the red blood cell surface; antibodies then interact with the drug or the red blood cell–drug complex.
- *Autoantibody model:* Drugs (e.g., α-methyldopa) initiate production of antibodies directed against intrinsic red blood cell antigens.

Cold Agglutinin Immune Hemolytic Anemia

Anemia is caused by IgM antibodies that agglutinate red blood cells at low temperatures.

- *Acute* hemolysis occurs during recovery from certain infections (e.g., *Mycoplasma* pneumonia and Epstein-Barr virus infection). It is usually self-limited and rarely induces significant hemolysis.
- *Chronic* hemolysis occurs with lymphoproliferative disorders or may be idiopathic. Clinical symptoms result from red blood cell agglutination and complement fixation in areas of the body that are 30°C or lower. The hemolytic anemia is of variable severity; vascular obstruction in areas exposed to cold temperatures results in pallor, cyanosis, and Raynaud phenomenon.

TABLE 13–3 **Classification of Immunohemolytic Anemias**

Warm Antibody Type
IgG antibodies that do not fix complement and are active at 37°C.
Primary (idiopathic)
Secondary
   Lymphomas and leukemias
   Other neoplastic diseases
   Autoimmune disorder (particularly systemic lupus erythematosus)
Drugs

Cold Agglutinin Type
IgM antibodies that dissociate from red blood cells at 30°C or above; agglutination of cells by IgM and complement fixation occurs only in peripheral cool parts of the body (e.g., fingers, ears, and toes).
Acute (mycoplasmal infection, infectious mononucleosis)
Chronic
   Idiopathic
   Associated with lymphoma

Cold Hemolysins (Paroxysmal Cold Hemoglobinuria)
IgG antibodies bind red blood cells at low temperature, fix complement, and cause hemolysis when the temperature is raised above 30°C.

Cold Hemolysin Hemolytic Anemia

This anemia occurs in *paroxysmal cold hemoglobinuria,* manifesting as acute intermittent massive intravascular hemolysis after exposure to cold. Autoantibodies are IgG (Donath-Landsteiner antibody) directed against the P blood group antigen. They attach to the red blood cells and fix complement at low temperatures; when the temperature is elevated, hemolysis occurs. Most cases follow infections (e.g., *Mycoplasma* pneumonia, measles, mumps, and influenza).

Hemolytic Anemias Resulting from Trauma to Red Blood Cells (p. 638)

Significant trauma to red blood cells results in fragmentation and intravascular hemolysis. The peripheral blood reveals fragmented red blood cells (schistocytes). Underlying conditions include:

- Prosthetic heart valves with turbulent flow and shear forces
- Diffuse narrowing of the microvasculature owing to fibrin deposition, for example, in disseminated intravascular coagulation (DIC)

Anemias of Diminished Erythropoiesis

Impaired red blood cell production may be due to various disorders, including deficiency of a vital nutrient (iron, vitamin B_{12}, folate) or stem cell failure.

Megaloblastic Anemias (p. 638)

Megaloblastic anemias are most commonly due to deficiency of vitamin B_{12} or folate.

Morphology

- Abnormally large erythroid precursors (megaloblasts) in which nuclear maturation lags behind cytoplasmic maturation
- Ineffective erythropoiesis (megaloblasts dying in the marrow) with compensatory megaloblastic hyperplasia
- Prominent anisocytosis, reflecting abnormal erythropoiesis, and abnormally large and oval red blood cells (macro-ovalocytes); the mean corpuscular volume is usually 110 fL or greater
- Abnormal granulopoiesis with giant metamyelocytes and hypersegmented neutrophils

Pathophysiology

Vitamin B_{12} and folate are essential for the production of thymidine, a building block of DNA. Deficiency results in deranged or inadequate DNA synthesis, but normal RNA and protein synthesis. Cytoplasmic enlargement and maturation are normal, but lag behind nuclear maturation. Anemia results from a combination of ineffective erythropoiesis, and abnormal red cells that are unusually susceptible to premature removal by phagocytes. Besides affecting red blood cell production, vitamin B_{12} and folate deficiencies also impact all rapidly dividing cells, including myeloid precursors and gastrointestinal epithelium. Ineffective granulopoiesis and thrombopoiesis often results in pancytopenia.

Anemias of Vitamin B$_{12}$ Deficiency: Pernicious Anemia (p. 639)

Vitamin B$_{12}$ deficiency can happen via several mechanisms. The ultimate source of vitamin B$_{12}$ is dietary animal products (see Fig. 13–20, p. 640 in *Robbins and Cotran Pathologic Basis of Disease,* 7th ed.):

- Peptic digestion releases dietary vitamin B$_{12}$; it is bound to salivary proteins called *R binders*.
- R-B$_{12}$ complexes are digested in the duodenum by pancreatic proteases; released vitamin B$_{12}$ binds to intrinsic factor (IF), a protein secreted by parietal cells of the gastric fundus.
- IF-B$_{12}$ complexes bind to IF receptors in the distal ileum epithelium; absorbed vitamin B$_{12}$ complexes with transcobalamin II and is transported to tissues.

Deficiencies in vitamin B$_{12}$ therefore result from impaired absorption, which has several causes:

- Achlorhydria (in elderly individuals), which impairs vitamin B$_{12}$ release from the R protein-bound form
- Gastrectomy, which leads to loss of IF
- Pernicious anemia (see following discussion)
- Resection of the distal ileum, which prevents absorption of IF-B$_{12}$ complex
- Malabsorption syndromes
- Increased requirements (e.g., pregnancy)
- Inadequate diet (very uncommon, since the body has large vitamin B$_{12}$ reserves)

Pernicious anemia is likely due to an autoimmune response to gastric parietal cells resulting in chronic atrophic gastritis and marked parietal cell loss, followed by deficient IF production. Gastric injury is probably initiated by autoreactive T cells; secondarily generated autoantibodies to various components of the vitamin B$_{12}$ uptake pathway are also present in the serum and gastric secretions of most patients and will exacerbate the disease process:

- Type I antibodies block the binding of vitamin B$_{12}$ to IF.
- Type II antibodies prevent IF or IF-B$_{12}$ complex from binding to the ileal receptor.
- Antibodies against the gastric proton pump bind to parietal cells and affect acid secretion.

There is a significant association of pernicious anemia with other autoimmune disorders of the adrenal and thyroid glands.

Morphology

- *Bone marrow:* Changes include megaloblastic erythroid hyperplasia; giant myelocytes and metamyelocytes; hypersegmented neutrophils; large multilobed nuclei in megakaryocytes.
- *Alimentary canal:* Changes include atrophic glossitis—the tongue is shiny, glazed, and red; gastric fundal atrophy with virtual absence of parietal cells; atrophic gastric mucosa replaced by mucus-secreting goblet cells ("intestinalization").
- *Central nervous system:* Lesions are found in 75% of cases; they are characterized by demyelination of dorsal and lateral spinal cord tracts, and, if advanced, result in spastic paresis and sensory ataxia. The basis of this effect is obscure, but is likely distinct from the hematologic sequelae (thus, folate deficiency produces megaloblastic anemia, but no neurologic effect).

Clinical Features. Onset is insidious; patients are usually aged 40 to 60 with symptoms due to anemia and posterolateral spinal tract involvement. There is an increased risk of gastric cancer. Diagnosis is based on serum vitamin B_{12} levels, the detection of anti-IF antibodies (pernicious anemia), and hematologic responses (reticulocytosis) after parenteral vitamin administration.

Anemia of Folate Deficiency (p. 642)

Folate deficiency induces a megaloblastic anemia clinically and hematologically indistinguishable from that seen with vitamin B_{12} deficiency, *except* that gastric atrophy and the neurologic changes of vitamin B_{12} deficiency do not occur. Diagnosis of folate deficiency requires demonstration of reduced serum or red blood cell folate levels. Deficiency may be due to:

- Inadequate intake, usually in those living on marginal diets (e.g., chronic alcoholics, elderly, and the indigent)
- Malabsorption syndromes (e.g., tropical and nontropical sprue)
- Increased demand, as in pregnancy, infancy, or disseminated cancer
- Administration of folate antagonists, such as methotrexate (used in cancer chemotherapy)

Iron Deficiency Anemia (p. 643)

Iron Metabolism (Fig. 13–24, p. 645)

Iron deficiency is an extremely common cause of anemia worldwide. The normal Western diet includes 10 to 20 mg of iron daily, mostly in the form of heme found in animal products; the remainder is inorganic iron found in vegetables. The duodenum is the primary site of absorption; about 20% of heme iron is absorbable, in contrast to only 1% to 2% of nonheme iron. Heme iron enters mucosal cells directly, whereas nonheme iron must first be reduced to ferrous iron by membrane-bound cytochrome B and then transported into the cell by the transport protein DMT1. Some of the absorbed iron is transported across the basolateral membrane, where it is bound to plasma transferrin for distribution throughout the body; this basolateral transport involves ferriportin, a membrane transporter, and hephaestin, an iron oxidase. The remaining intracellular iron is bound to ferritin and subsequently excreted in feces when the epithelium is sloughed during normal turnover. Iron homeostasis is regulated in part by hepcidin, a small liver-derived polypeptide that blocks duodenal iron uptake by inhibiting ferroportin activity.

Total body iron content is about 2 gm for women and 6 gm for men; it is found in all tissues but particularly in liver, spleen, bone marrow, and skeletal muscle. About 80% of body iron is found in hemoglobin, myoglobin, and iron-containing enzymes (e.g., catalase and cytochromes); the remainder is in a storage pool bound to hemosiderin and ferritin. Because serum ferritin is largely derived from the storage pool of iron, its level is a good indicator of the adequacy of body iron stores.

Etiology

Negative iron balance and consequent anemia can result from low dietary intake, malabsorption, excessive demand, and chronic blood loss.

- *Low dietary intake* alone is rarely the cause of iron deficiency in the United States because the average daily intake of 10 to 20 mg is more than enough for men and adequate for most women.
- *Malabsorption* can occur with sprue and celiac disease or after gastrectomy.
- *Increased demands* not met by normal dietary intake can occur in pregnancy and infancy.
- *Chronic blood loss* is the most important cause of iron deficiency anemia in the Western world; loss can occur from the gastrointestinal tract (e.g., peptic ulcers, colonic cancer, hemorrhoids, hookworm disease) or the female genital tract (e.g., menorrhagia, metrorrhagia, cancers).

Clinical Features

- *Peripheral blood:* Red blood cells are pale (hypochromic), small (microcytic), and variable in shape (poikilocytosis).
- *Marrow:* There is a mild hyperplasia of normoblasts, but loss sideroblasts and stainable iron in marrow macrophages are absent.
- *Other organs:* In severe iron deficiency, depletion of essential iron-containing enzymes can cause alopecia, koilonychia, and atrophy of the tongue and gastric mucosa. The *Plummer-Vinson triad* of hypochromic microcytic anemia, atrophic glossitis, and esophageal webs may occur.

Diagnosis

Diagnosis rests on clinical and hematologic features, low serum iron and ferritin, increased total plasma iron-binding capacity, and reduced plasma transferrin saturation.

Anemia of Chronic Disease (p. 646)

Anemia is common in the setting of diverse chronic inflammatory mediators (such as tumor necrosis factor-α and interleukin-1), which increase the release of hepcidin from the liver. Hepcidin blocks ferroportin activity on macrophages; as a result, iron is sequestered away from erythroid progenators. Serum iron is low, but ferritin levels are high. Inflammatory mediators also reduce erythropoietin production, exacerbating the anemia. The anemia is normocytic/normochromic or microcytic/hypochromic. Treatment of the underlying condition corrects the anemia; erythropoietin therapy is partially effective.

Aplastic Anemia (p. 647)

Aplastic anemia is characterized by a failure or suppression of multipotent myeloid stem cells; neutropenia, anemia, and thrombocytopenia (pancytopenia) result.

Etiology

Aplastic anemia is idiopathic in 65% of cases; known causes are:

- Myelotoxic drugs or chemicals are the most common causes of secondary aplastic anemia. Marrow suppression may be dose related, predictable, and reversible (benzene, alkylating agents, and antimetabolites such as vincristine or busulfan)

or idiosyncratic, affecting only some exposed individuals in an unpredictable manner (chloramphenicol, chlorpromazine, and streptomycin).
● Total body irradiation.
● Infections (e.g., non-A, non-B, non-C, and non-G hepatitis).
● Inherited diseases (e.g., Fanconi anemia).

Pathogenesis

Stem cell alterations may be due to environmental insults, drug exposure, or infections. In idiopathic cases, stem cell failure may be due to:

● A primary defect in the number or function of stem cells, in some cases due to mutagen exposure. Occasionally, genetically damaged stem cells can transform to acute leukemias.
● Suppression of antigenically altered stem cells by T cell–mediated immune mechanisms.

Morphology

Hypocellular marrow (hematopoietic cells replaced by fat cells), with secondary effects due to granulocytopenia (infections) and thrombocytopenia (bleeding).

Clinical Features

Onset is insidious with symptoms related to loss of red blood cells, neutrophils, and platelets. Splenomegaly is absent. In cases of chemical exposure, withdrawal of the inciting agent can sometimes lead to recovery; more commonly, bone marrow transplantation or immunosuppression is required.

Pure Red Blood Cell Aplasia (p. 648)

A form of marrow failure due to absence of red blood cell precursors, this type of anemia may appear acutely and transiently in chronic hemolytic states due to parvovirus infection (*aplastic crisi*s). Rarely, anemia occurs in an immune-mediated chronic form that is either idiopathic or arises in association with neoplasms (e.g., large granular lymphocytic leukemia or thymoma). In the latter, the anemia may remit following tumor resection.

Other Forms of Marrow Failure (p. 648)

● *Myelophthisic anemia:* Space-occupying lesions that destroy or distort the marrow architecture depress productive capacity; associated with pancytopenia and frequently with the appearance of white and red blood cell precursors in peripheral blood. The most common cause is metastatic cancer.
● *Diffuse liver disease* (toxic, infectious, or cirrhotic): The anemia is primarily due to bone marrow failure, often exacerbated by variceal bleeding or folate deficiency.
● *Chronic renal failure:* Chronic renal failure is almost invariably associated with anemia. The basis is multifactorial, but inadequate erythropoietin production is most important. Treatment with recombinant erythropoietin usually yields significant improvement.

POLYCYTHEMIA (p. 649)

Polycythemia is a relative or absolute increase in the concentration of red blood cells in the peripheral blood. *Relative* increases may be due to decreased plasma volumes associated with dehydration (e.g., water deprivation, vomiting, or diarrhea) or due to *stress polycythemia,* an obscure condition of unknown cause also called *Gaisböck syndrome. Absolute* increases may be primary or secondary:

* *Primary:* Increased red blood cell mass is due to a myeloid neoplasm, *polycythemia vera,* in which red blood cell precursors proliferate in an erythropoietin-independent fashion.
* *Secondary:* Increased red blood cell mass is due to increased erythropoietin, which may be physiologic (lung disease, high-altitude living, cyanotic heart disease) or pathophysiologic (erythropoietin-secreting tumors, such as renal cell or hepatocellular carcinomas, cerebellar hemangioblastoma).

BLEEDING DISORDERS (p. 649)

Hemorrhagic diatheses may be caused by increased blood vessel fragility, platelet disorders, coagulation defects, or some combination. Evaluation requires laboratory testing:

* Bleeding time
* Platelet counts
* Prothrombin time
* Partial thromboplastin time
* Specialized tests (e.g., clotting factor levels)

Increased Vascular Fragility

Disorders of increased vascular fragility are relatively common but usually do not cause serious bleeding; they typically induce only petechial and purpuric hemorrhages. Platelet count and coagulation time are usually normal; bleeding time is variable. Several conditions cause increased vascula fragility:

* *Infections:* Especially meningococcus and rickettsia; underlying mechanisms are vasculitis or DIC (discussed later).
* *Drug reactions:* Often secondary to immune complex deposition in vessel walls with resulting hypersensitivity vasculitis.
* *Poor vascular support:* Abnormal collagen synthesis (e.g., scurvy or Ehlers-Danlos syndrome), loss of perivascular supporting tissue (e.g., Cushing syndrome), or vascular wall amyloid deposition.
* *Henoch-Schönlein purpura:* Systemic hypersensitivity reaction of unknown cause characterized by purpuric rash, abdominal pain, polyarthralgia, and acute glomerulonephritis; associated with vascular and glomerular mesangial deposition of immune complexes.

Thrombocytopenia

Decrease in platelet number is characterized principally by petechial bleeding, most often from small vessels of skin and mucous membranes. Thrombocytopenia must be severe

(10,000–20,000 platelets per mm^3; reference range, 150,000–300,000/mm^3) before bleeding becomes clinically evident. Causes of thrombocytopenia may be classified into five major categories:

- *Decreased production:* Thrombocytopenia is due to ineffective megakaryopoiesis (e.g., megaloblastic states) or to generalized marrow disease that also compromises megakaryocyte number (e.g., aplastic anemia, disseminated cancer).
- *Decreased survival:* Thrombocytopenia is due to immune-mediated platelet destruction, usually with a compensatory megakaryocytic marrow hyperplasia; it can follow drug exposure (e.g., quinine, quinidine, methyldopa, heparin) or infections (particularly human immunodeficiency virus infection [HIV]). Platelet deficiencies due to consumption often occur in systemic coagulopathies (DIC, hemolytic uremic syndrome, thrombotic thrombocytopenia purpura).
- *Sequestration:* Platelets are retained in the red pulp of enlarged spleens.
- *Dilution:* Massive whole blood transfusions can cause a relative reduction in the number of circulating platelets because storage for longer than 24 hours at 4°C results in rapid hepatic platelet sequestration upon infusion.
- *HIV:* Thrombocytopenia results from immune complex injury, antiplatelet antibodies, and HIV-induced suppression of megakaryocytes.

Immune Thrombocytopenia Purpura (p. 651)

Immune thrombocytopenia purpura (ITP) encompasses two forms of antibody-mediated platelet destruction:

- *Acute ITP:* This self-limited disorder is seen most often in children after a viral infection (e.g., rubella, cytomegalovirus infection, viral hepatitis, infectious mononucleosis). Platelet destruction is due to transient antiplatelet autoantibodies.
- *Chronic ITP:* Platelet autoantibodies (synthesized in the spleen) are usually directed toward one of two platelet antigens—the platelet membrane glycoprotein complexes IIb/IIIa or Ib/IX. Destruction of antibody-coated platelets occurs in the spleen. Splenectomy benefits 75% to 80% of patients.

Clinical Features

Chronic ITP typically occurs in adults, particularly women of childbearing age. There is usually a long history of easy bruising or nosebleeds, but sometimes the onset is sudden, with a shower of petechial hemorrhages or internal bleeding (melena, hematuria). Subarachnoid or intracerebral hemorrhage is rare but serious. The idiopathic form must be distinguished from that occurring in the context of systemic lupus erythematosus, AIDS, drug exposure, and lymphoid neoplasms.

Morphology

The spleen is normal in size but shows sinusoidal congestion and prominent germinal centers. Bone marrow megakaryocyte numbers are increased.

Diagnosis

Diagnosis is based largely on clinical features, such as petechiae and thrombocytopenia; bone marrow biopsy can be performed to confirm increased megakaryocyte numbers. The bleeding time is prolonged, while the prothrombin and partial thromboplastin times are normal. Tests for antiplatelet antibody are not reliable. Splenomegaly and lymphadenopathy are extremely uncommon; if present, a lymphoid neoplasm should be suspected.

DRUG-INDUCED THROMBOCYTOPENIA (p. 652)

A wide variety of drugs can cause immune-mediated platelet destruction by acting as haptens or participating in the formation of immune complexes that deposit on platelet membranes. In most instances, drug-induced antibodies cause rapid removal of platelets via the reticuloendothelial system and result in bleeding symptoms. An exception is thrombocytopenia caused by heparin, which sometimes stimulates the formation of antibodies directed against a complex of heparin and platelet factor 4. Antibody binding to this complex activates platelets, leading to thrombi in arteries and veins that can be limb- and life-threatening. In all forms of drug-induced thrombocytopenia, withdrawal of the offending drug leads to clinical improvement.

THROMBOTIC THROMBOCYTOPENIC PURPURA AND HEMOLYTIC UREMIC SYNDROME (p. 652)

Thrombotic thrombocytopenic purpura (TTP) and hemolytic uremic syndrome (HUS) are two related disorders within the spectrum of *thrombotic microangiopathies* characterized by thrombocytopenia, microangiopathic hemolytic anemia, fever, transient neurologic deficits (in TTP), or renal failure (in HUS). In some patients, there are overlapping symptoms. Most of the clinical manifestations are due to *widespread hyaline microthrombi* in arterioles and capillaries composed of dense aggregates of platelets and fibrin.

Pathophysiology

Although clinically similar to DIC, activation of the clotting system is not a prominent feature in the thrombotic angiopathies. TTP and HUS have similar clinical features and histologic findings but have different causes.

- TTP is associated with inherited or acquired deficiencies in ADAMTS13, a serum metalloprotease that limits the size of von Willebrand factor multimers in the plasma. In its absence, very high molecular weight von Willebrand factor multimers accumulate that are capable of promoting platelet aggregation throughout the microcirculation. In the case of acquired TTP, patients often have antibodies directed against ADAMTS13.
- HUS most commonly follows gastrointestinal infections with verotoxin-producing *Escherichia coli*. Verotoxin injures endothelial cells and thereby promotes dysregulated platelet activation and aggregation.

Clinical Features

Acquired TTP typically affects women; HUS often occurs in children and the elderly during outbreaks of food poisoning. Plasma exchange or plasmapheresis is effective in both, probably due to removal of antibodies (acquired TTP) or toxins (epidemic HUS). Endothelial injury mediated by other causes (e.g., toxic drugs, radiation) may cause chronic forms of HUS that are difficult to treat.

Hemorrhagic Disorders Related to Defective Platelet Functions (p. 653)

Hemorrhagic disorders related to defective platelet functions are characterized by prolonged bleeding time in association with normal platelet count. Disorders can be congenital or acquired.

Congenital Disorders

- *Defective platelet adhesion* is exemplified by the autosomal recessive Bernard-Soulier syndrome, caused by deficient platelet membrane glycoprotein complex GpIb/IX; this is the platelet receptor for von Willebrand factor (vWF) and is necessary for platelet-collagen adhesion.
- *Defective platelet aggregation* is exemplified by thrombasthenia, an autosomal recessive disorder caused by a deficiency of platelet membrane glycoprotein GpIIb/ GpIIIa, which is involved in binding fibrinogen.
- *Disorders of platelet secretion:* Initial platelet aggregation with collagen or adenosine diphosphate (ADP) is normal, but subsequent platelet responses are impaired (e.g., secretion of prostaglandins and granule-bound ADP).

Acquired Disorders

Two are clinically significant:

- *Aspirin ingestion:* Aspirin is a potent inhibitor of the enzyme cyclooxygenase and can suppress the synthesis of thromboxane A_2, necessary for platelet aggregation. The effect of aspirin on platelet aggregation forms the basis for its use in prevention of myocardial infarction.
- *Uremia:* The pathogenesis of bleeding in uremic patients is complex but includes defects in platelet function.

HEMORRHAGIC DIATHESES RELATED TO ABNORMALITIES IN CLOTTING FACTORS
(p. 653)

Bleeding in patients with clotting factor abnormalities differs from that encountered in patients with platelet deficiencies:

- The spontaneous appearance of petechiae or purpura is uncommon; more often, the bleeding manifests as large ecchymoses or hematomas after injury, or as prolonged bleeding after a laceration or surgical procedure.
- Bleeding into the gastrointestinal and urinary tracts, and particularly into weight-bearing joints, is common.

Clotting abnormalities can be acquired or hereditary in origin. *Acquired deficiencies* are usually associated with multiple clotting abnormalities. For example, vitamin K deficiency causes depressed synthesis of factors II, VII, IX, and X and protein C. Because the liver makes virtually all the clotting factors, severe parenchymal liver disease will also cause hemorrhagic diatheses. DIC also produces a deficiency of multiple coagulation factors.

Hereditary deficiencies typically affect a single clotting factor. The most common inherited disorders are hemophilia (A and B) and von Willebrand disease.

Plasma factor VIII-vWF is a complex made up of two separate proteins (factor VIII and vWF) distinguishable by functional, biochemical, and immunologic criteria (see Fig. 13–28, p. 654 in *Robbins and Cotran Pathologic Basis of Disease*, 7th ed.). One component required for factor X activation in the intrinsic coagulation pathway is *factor VIII procoagulant protein* (factor VIII). Factor VIII deficiency causes classic hemophilia (hemophilia A). Circulating factor VIII is carried in the plasma bound to vWF, which exist as a series of large multimers. vWF is necessary for platelet adhesion to subendothelial collagen, via interactions with platelet glycoprotein Ib. vWF may also promote platelet aggregation by binding to factor IIb/IIIa, particularly under conditions of high shear stress.

The two components of factor VIII-vWF complex are encoded by separate genes and synthesized by different cells. vWF is produced by endothelial cells and megakaryocytes. Liver endothelial cells and renal epithelial cells are the major sources of factor VIII.

von Willebrand Disease (p. 655)

von Willebrand disease is a relatively common disorder that is grouped into several categories:

- Type 1 and type 3 von Willebrand disease are associated with reduced levels of vWF. Type 1 is autosomal dominant and is the most common form; clinically, it is quite mild. Type 3 is a severe but uncommon autosomal recessive variant associated with more profound vWF deficiency.
- Type 2 is an autosomal dominant form caused by reduced amounts of the intermediate and large vWF multimers (the most active forms of vWF). In the most common form (2a disease), multimer assembly is defective; even though there is adequate vWF on an absolute basis, the failure to form the most active high-molecular-weight multimers leads to a functional deficit.

Levels of factor VIII are often reduced in von Willebrand disease because vWF stabilizes factor VIII in circulation. Therefore, patients have a compound defect involving platelet function and the coagulation pathway; this is reflected by a prolonged bleeding time (despite normal platelet counts) and a prolonged partial thromboplastin time.

Most commonly, von Willebrand disease presents with spontaneous bleeding from mucous membranes, excessive bleeding from wounds, and menorrhagia. Except in type 3 disease, factor VIII levels are only modestly depressed, and symptoms typical of hemophilia, such as bleeding into the joints, are uncommon.

Factor VIII Deficiency (Hemophilia A) (p. 655)

An X-linked recessive disorder primarily affecting males, hemophilia A is characterized by a reduced amount and activity of factor VIII. Clinical features develop only in the presence of severe deficiency (factor VIII levels <1% of normal). Mild or moderate degrees of deficiency (levels 1%–50% of normal) are asymptomatic, although post-traumatic bleeding may be excessive. The variable deficiency in factor VIII procoagulant protein results from different types of mutations in the factor VIII gene. Clinically, hemophilia is associated with the following:

- Massive hemorrhage after trauma or operative procedures
- *Spontaneous* hemorrhages in regions of the body normally subject to trauma, particularly the joints (hemarthroses); leads to progressive, crippling deformities
- Absence of petechiae
- Prolonged partial thromboplastin time and normal bleeding time

Diagnosis is possible by assay for factor VIII; the cloning of the factor VIII gene now allows antenatal diagnosis.

Treatment consists of replacement therapy with recombinant factor VIII or factor VIII concentrates. Before the routine screening of blood for HIV antibodies, transmission of HIV led to the development of AIDS in many hemophiliacs. With the current practice of using heat-treated factor VIII concentrates derived from the blood of HIV-seronegative donors (or recombinant factor VIII), the risk of HIV transmission has been eliminated.

Factor IX Deficiency (Hemophilia B) (p. 656)

Christmas disease, or hemophilia B, is an X-linked recessive disease caused by factor IX deficiency; it is clinically indistinguishable from hemophilia A. Identification of hemophilia B requires assay of factor IX levels.

Disseminated Intravascular Coagulation (p. 656)

DIC is an acute, subacute, or chronic thrombohemorrhagic disorder occurring as a *secondary complication in a variety of diseases* (Table 13–4). DIC is characterized by activation of the coagulation sequence, leading to the formation of microthrombi throughout the microcirculation. As a consequence of the thrombotic diathesis, there is consumption of platelets, fibrin, and coagulation factors and, secondarily, activation of fibrinolytic mechanisms. Thus, DIC may present with:

- Signs and symptoms relating to infarction caused by microthrombi
- A hemorrhagic diathesis resulting from activation of fibrinolytic mechanisms and depletion of the elements required for hemostasis

TABLE 13–4 **Major Disorders Associated with Disseminated Intravascular Coagulation**

Obstetric Complications
Abruptio placentae
Retained dead fetus
Septic abortion
Amniotic fluid embolism
Toxemia

Infections
Gram-negative sepsis
Meningococcemia
Rocky Mountain spotted fever
Histoplasmosis
Aspergillosis
Malaria

Neoplasms
Carcinomas of pancreas, prostate, lung, and stomach
Acute promyelocytic leukemia

Massive Tissue Injury
Traumatic
Burns
Extensive surgery

Miscellaneous
Acute intravascular hemolysis, snakebite, giant hemangioma, shock, heat stroke, vasculitis, aortic aneurysm, liver disease

Pathogenesis

DIC is triggered by two major mechanisms: release of tissue factor or thromboplastic substances into the circulation, and widespread endothelial cell injury (Fig. 13–1).

The *tissue factor or thromboplastic substances released into the circulation* can be derived from multiple sources (e.g., placenta in obstetric complications, granules of leukemic cells in acute promyelocytic leukemia); mucus released from certain adenocarcinomas can also be thromboplastic. In gram-negative sepsis, bacterial endotoxins activate monocytes to release interleukin-1 and tumor necrosis factor-α, both of which increase tissue factor expression on endothelial cell membranes while simultaneously decreasing thrombomodulin expression. This results in both activation of the clotting system and inhibition of coagulation control.

Endothelial injury initiates DIC by causing tissue factor release from endothelial cells, by promoting platelet aggregation, and by activating the intrinsic coagulation pathway by exposing subendothelial connective tissue. Widespread endothelial injury can occur through antigen-antibody complex deposition (e.g., systemic lupus erythematosus), temperature extremes (e.g., heatstroke, burns), or infections (e.g., meningococci, rickettsiae).

Morphology

Microthrombi, with infarctions and, in some cases, hemorrhages, are found in many organs and tissues. Clinically significant changes are encountered in several locations:

- *Kidneys:* Thrombi are found in renal glomeruli and may be associated with microinfarcts or renal cortical necrosis.

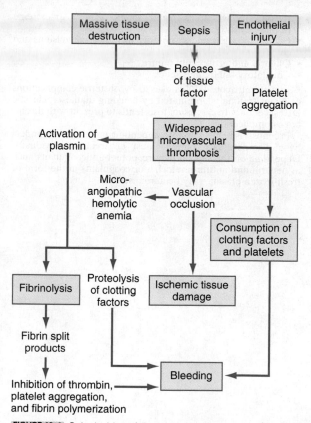

FIGURE 13–1 Pathophysiology of disseminated intravascular coagulation (DIC).

- *Lungs:* Microthrombi are found in alveolar capillaries and may be associated with histology resembling acute respiratory distress syndrome.
- *Brain:* Microinfarcts and fresh hemorrhages occur.
- *Adrenals:* Massive hemorrhages give rise to the Waterhouse-Friderichsen syndrome seen in meningococcemia.
- *Placenta:* Widespread thrombi occur, associated with cytotrophoblast and syncytiotrophoblast atrophy.

Clinical Features

About 50% of DIC occurs in obstetric patients with pregnancy complications; 33% of DIC occurs in the setting of carcinomatosis. Sepsis and major trauma are responsible for most of the remaining cases. Onset can be fulminant, as in endotoxic shock or amniotic fluid embolism, or insidious, as in cases of carcinomatosis or retention of a dead fetus. There are numerous clinical manifestations:

- Microangiopathic hemolytic anemia resulting from widespread microvascular occlusion

- Respiratory symptoms (e.g., dyspnea, cyanosis, or extreme respiratory difficulty)
- Neurologic signs and symptoms, including convulsions and coma
- Oliguria and acute renal failure
- Circulatory failure and shock

In general, acute DIC is caused by obstetric complications or major trauma is dominated by bleeding diatheses; chronic DIC secondary to carcinomatosis tends to present with thrombotic complications.

Prognosis is highly variable, depending largely on the underlying disorder; each patient must be treated individually. Depending on the clinical picture, potent anticoagulants, such as heparin and antithrombin III, or coagulants in the form of fresh-frozen plasma, may be administered.

CHAPTER 14

White Blood Cells, Lymph Nodes, Spleen, and Thymus

Disorders of white blood cells include deficiencies *(leukopenias)* or proliferations that can be reactive or neoplastic.

LEUKOPENIA (p. 662)

Leukopenia occurs because of decreased numbers of any of the specific leukocyte types; most often leukopenia involves neutrophils *(neutropenia,* granulocytopenia). *Lymphopenia* is less common; besides rare congenital immunodeficiency diseases, it occurs in specific settings (e.g., advanced human immunodeficiency virus [HIV] infection, after therapy with glucocorticoids or cytotoxic drugs, autoimmune disorders, malnutrition, certain acute viral infections).

Neutropenia (Agranulocytosis) (p. 662)

Clinically relevant neutropenia occurs with neutrophil counts at or below 1000 cells per mm³; counts at or below 500 cells per mm³ greatly increase the risk of severe bacterial and fungal infections. When counts are very low (<200–300 cells/mm³), the condition is called *agranulocytosis*.

Neutrophil half-life is 6 to 7 hours; consequently, insults that impair granulopoiesis quickly produce neutropenia. Mechanisms include the following:

- Inadequate or ineffective granulopoiesis

  Suppression of myeloid stem cells, as in aplastic anemia (Chapter 13) and various infiltrative marrow disorders (tumors, granulomatous disease)

Suppression of committed granulocytic precursors, such as after exposure to certain drugs

Disease states characterized by ineffective granulopoiesis (e.g., megaloblastic anemias [from vitamin B_{12} or folate deficiency] and myelodysplastic syndromes)

Rare inherited conditions (e.g., Kostmann syndrome)

- Accelerated removal or destruction of neutrophils

Injury to neutrophils by immunologic disorders (e.g., systemic lupus erythematosus) or drug exposures

Splenic sequestration

Increased peripheral utilization in overwhelming bacterial, fungal, or rickettsial infections

The most significant neutropenias are drug-induced:

- *Dose-related,* occurring in a predictable fashion (many chemotherapeutic cancer drugs, such as alkylating agents and antimetabolites, produce neutropenia)
- *Idiosyncratic and unpredictable* (implicated drugs include aminopyrine, chloramphenicol, sulfonamides, chlorpromazine, thiouracil, and phenylbutazone)

Morphology

Marrow anatomic alterations depend on the underlying basis of the neutropenia. In isolated neutropenia, only the granulocytic lineage is affected. If the insult also impairs erythroid and megakaryocytic progenitors, pancytopenia and aplastic anemia (empty marrow) may result.

- *Marrow hypercellularity* (due to increased numbers of granulocytic precursors) occurs with neutropenias caused by (1) increased destruction of mature neutrophils, or (2) ineffective granulopoiesis (e.g., megaloblastic anemias and myelodysplastic syndromes)
- *Marrow hypocellularity* occurs with neutropenias caused by agents (e.g., drugs) that suppress granulocyte progenitor cell growth and survival.

Clinical Course

Symptoms and signs relate to intercurrent bacterial or fungal infections and include malaise, chills, and fever, often with marked weakness and fatigability. Ulcerating necrotizing lesions of the gingiva, buccal mucosa, or pharynx are characteristic; these sites often show massive growth of microorganisms with relatively poor leukocytic response.

Prognosis

Infections in this setting are often fulminant; neutropenic patients are treated with broad-spectrum antibiotics at first sign of infection. Granulocyte-colony stimulating factor therapy decreases the duration and severity of the neutrophil nadir caused by chemotherapeutic drugs.

REACTIVE (INFLAMMATORY) PROLIFERATIONS OF WHITE BLOOD CELLS AND NODES (p. 663)

Leukocytosis (p. 663)

Leukocytosis occurs commonly in a variety of inflammatory states. The particular leukocyte series affected depends on the underlying cause:

- *Polymorphonuclear leukocytosis* (neutrophilic granulocytosis, neutrophilia) accompanies acute inflammation associated with infection or tissue necrosis. Sepsis or severe inflammatory disorders cause neutrophils to develop so-called "toxic changes":

  Abnormally coarse, dark neutrophilic granules (*toxic granulations*)

  Blue cytoplasmic patches of dilated endoplasmic reticulum (*Döhle bodies*)

  Cytoplasmic vacuoles

- *Eosinophilic leukocytosis* (eosinophilia) is seen in:

  Allergic disorders (e.g., asthma, hay fever, allergic skin diseases)

  Parasitic infestations

  Drug reactions

  Certain malignancies (e.g., Hodgkin lymphoma [HL] and some non-Hodgkin lymphomas [NHLs])

  Collagen vascular disorders and some vasculitides

  Atheroembolic disease (transiently)

- *Basophilic leukocytosis* is rare; it suggests an underlying myeloproliferative disease (e.g., chronic myelogenous leukemia).

- *Monocytosis* can be seen in:

  Chronic infections (e.g., tuberculosis, bacterial endocarditis, and malaria)

  Collagen vascular diseases (e.g., systemic lupus erythematosus)

  Inflammatory bowel diseases (e.g., ulcerative colitis)

- *Lymphocytosis* accompanies monocytosis in many disorders associated with chronic immunologic stimulation (e.g., tuberculosis, brucellosis), viral infections (e.g., hepatitis A, cytomegalovirus, Epstein-Barr virus), and *Bordetella pertussis* infections.

Pathogenesis

Elevation of circulating neutrophil counts (most common form of leukocytosis) occurs by various mechanisms:

- *Expansion of marrow neutrophilic progenitor cell and storage pools* occurs over hours to days secondary to elevated colony-stimulating factors released from marrow stromal elements. Stimulants of colony-stimulating factor production include sustained elevations of interleukin-1 (IL1) and tumor necrosis factor (TNF) (e.g., in infectious and inflammatory disorders).

- Increased release of mature neutrophils from bone marrow storage pool occurs rapidly following elevations in IL1 and TNF.

- Increased demargination of peripheral blood neutrophils is seen with acute stress or after glucocorticoids.

- Decreased extravasation of neutrophils into tissues is seen with glucocorticoid administration.

Other factors cause different forms of leukocytosis; IL5 causes eosinophilic leukocytosis, while c-kit ligand and IL7 induce lymphopoiesis.

Distinguishing reactive leukocytosis from neoplastic (leukemia) is problematic in two settings:

- Childhood acute viral infections, when atypical lymphocytes can appear in blood or bone marrow and simulate a lymphoid neoplasm
- Severe inflammatory states, when many immature granulocytes sometimes appear in the blood and simulate myelogenous leukemia (so-called *leukemoid reaction*)

Acute Nonspecific Lymphadenitis (p. 665)

Acute nonspecific lymphadenitis can be localized or systemic.

- The *localized* form is commonly caused by direct microbiologic drainage, most frequently in the cervical area associated with dental or tonsillar infections.
- The *systemic* form is associated with bacteremia and viral infections, particularly in children.

Morphology

Macroscopically the nodes are swollen, gray-red, and engorged. Histologically, there are large germinal centers with numerous mitotic figures. With pyogenic organisms, a neutrophilic infiltrate occurs and the follicular centers may undergo necrosis.

Clinical Features

Affected nodes are enlarged, tender, and (with extensive abscess formation) fluctuant. Overlying skin is frequently red; penetration of the infection to the skin surface produces draining sinuses. With control of the infection, lymph nodes can revert to their normal appearance, but scarring is common after suppurative reactions.

Chronic Nonspecific Lymphadenitis (p. 665)

Chronic nonspecific lymphadenitis occurs in the following patterns:

Follicular Hyperplasia

- Caused by inflammatory processes that activate B cells.
- Distinguished by prominent large, round or oblong germinal centers (secondary follicles) containing two distinct regions:
  A dark zone containing proliferating blastlike B cells (centroblasts)
  A light zone composed of B cells with irregular or cleaved nuclear contours (centrocytes)
- Can be confused morphologically with follicular lymphomas, although follicular hyperplasia typically shows:
  Preservation of the lymph node architecture
  Marked variation in the shape and size of lymphoid nodules
  Frequent mitotic figures, phagocytic macrophages, and recognizable light and dark zones
- Causes include rheumatoid arthritis, toxoplasmosis, and early stages of HIV infection; can be accompanied by *marginal zone B-cell hyperplasia,* especially in toxoplasmosis and early HIV infection.

Paracortical Lymphoid Hyperplasia

- Characterized by reactive changes within the T-cell regions of the lymph node.
- Activated parafollicular T cells (immunoblasts three to four times larger than resting lymphocytes) proliferate and partially efface B-cell follicles.
- Causes include immunologic reactions induced by drugs (especially phenytoin [Dilantin]) and acute viral infections (particularly infectious mononucleosis).

Sinus Histiocytosis (Reticular Hyperplasia)

- Characterized by distended, prominent lymphatic sinusoids due to marked hypertrophy of lining endothelial cells and infiltration with macrophages (histiocytes).
- Nonspecific, but often observed in lymph nodes draining tissues involved by epithelial cancers.

NEOPLASTIC PROLIFERATIONS OF WHITE BLOOD CELLS (p. 666)

White blood cell neoplasms are organized into three broad categories:

- *Lymphoid neoplasms*, encompassing tumors of B-cell, T-cell, or natural killer (NK) cell origin
- *Myeloid neoplasms*, originating from transformed hematopoietic stem cells that normally produce myeloid lineage cells (i.e., erythroid, granulocytic, or thrombocytic)
- *Histiocytoses*, representing proliferative lesions of histiocytes, including Langerhans cells

Etiologic and Pathogenetic Factors in White Blood Cell Neoplasia: Overview (p. 667)

Chromosomal Translocations and Oncogenes

Nonrandom karyotypic abnormalities, most commonly *translocations*, are present in most white blood cell neoplasms. They can cause inappropriate expression of normal proteins or synthesis of novel fusion oncoproteins.

- Translocations often involve antigen receptor genes and likely represent errors occurring during normal V(D)J recombination (early B and T cells) or immunoglobulin class switching (germinal center B cells). Germinal center B cells normally rely on genomic instability (class switching and somatic hypermutation) to generate antibody diversity; an increased risk of oncogenic events is a byproduct of this instability. Most human lymphoid neoplasms derive from B cells that have passed through germinal centers. The mechanisms that cause chromosome translocations in myeloid neoplasms are unknown.
- Some translocations are seen only in one type of tumor and are therefore diagnostic (e.g., t(15;17) is seen only in acute promyelocytic leukemia). In other cases, translocations occur in multiple neoplasms, perhaps due to more general effects on hematopoietic and lymphoid progenitors (e.g., t(9;22), the Ph[1] chromosome, occurs in acute lymphoblastic

leukemia, acute myelogenous leukemia, and chronic myelogenous leukemia).

- Expression of oncoproteins in mouse marrow cells often produces tumors resembling the human counterparts; such experiments demonstrate that the oncoproteins can be causal for development of the malignancies.

Inherited Genetic Factors

Genetic diseases that promote genomic instability (e.g., Bloom syndrome, Fanconi anemia, and ataxia telangiectasia) increase the risk of developing acute leukemia. Down syndrome (trisomy 21) and neurofibromatosis type I are also associated with an increased incidence of leukemia.

Viruses and Environmental Agents

- Three viruses, HTLV-1, Epstein-Barr virus (EBV), and HHV8, are implicated. Clonal episomal EBV genomes are found in tumor cells of some Burkitt lymphomas, Hodgkin lymphomas, diffuse large B-cell lymphomas occurring in the setting of T-cell immunodeficiency, and natural killer (NK) cell lymphomas. HTLV-1 is highly associated with adult T cell leukemia, and HHV8 is found in unusual large B-cell lymphomas presenting as lymphomatous effusions.
- Environmental agents that cause chronic immune stimulation can predispose to lymphoid neoplasia. The most clearcut associations are *H. pylori* infection with gastric marginal zone lymphoma, and gluten-sensitive enteropathy with intestinal T-cell lymphoma.

Iatrogenic Factors

Radiotherapy and certain forms of cancer chemotherapy increase the risk of white blood cell neoplasms (e.g., myelodysplastic syndrome, acute myelogenous leukemia, and lymphoma).

Lymphoid Neoplasms (p. 667)

Definitions (p. 667)

Leukemias   Usually exhibit widespread involvement of bone marrow, accompanied by large numbers of circulating tumor cells.

Lymphomas   Proliferations involving discrete tissue masses (e.g., within lymph nodes, the spleen, or extranodal tissues). Among the *lymphomas,* two broad categories are recognized:

  Hodgkin lymphoma (HL), with important clinical and histologic distinctions.

  Non-Hodgkin lymphoma (NHL), comprising all forms besides HL.

Plasma cell neoplasms   Tumors composed of terminally differentiated B cells.

Classification (p. 667)

Multiple classification schemes have been published, each with different merits. The *World Health Organization (WHO)*

Classification of Lymphoid Neoplasms defines entities based on clinical features, morphology, immunophenotype, and geno-type, and is currently favored. It includes lymphocytic leukemias, lymphomas, and plasma cell neoplasms sorted into four broad categories based on immunophenotype:

- Precursor B-cell neoplasms (immature B cells)
- Peripheral B-cell neoplasms (mature B cells)
- Precursor T-cell neoplasms (immature T cells)
- Peripheral T-cell and NK cell neoplasms (mature T cells and NK cells)

The salient features of the most common (or interesting) entities of the WHO classification are summarized in Table 14–1. The following general principles are relevant to lymphoid neoplasms:

TABLE 14–1 **Summary of the Lymphoid Neoplasms of the WHO Classification**

Types of Tumors	Salient Features
Tumors of Precursor B Lymphocytes	
Precursor B-cell acute lymphoblastic leukemia/lymphoma	Aggressive neoplasm of immature TdT+ B cells. Most common in childhood; usually presents with extensive marrow and blood involvement. Genetically heterogeneous.
Tumors of Precursor T Lymphocytes	
Precursor T-cell acute lymphoblastic leukemia/lymphoma	Aggressive neoplasm of immature TdT+ T cells. Most common in adolescent boys; often presents as a mediastinal mass. Genetically heterogeneous.
Tumors of Mature B Cells	
Small lymphocytic lymphoma/chronic lymphocytic leukemia	CD5+/CD23+ B-cell tumor of older adults; most commonly presents within marrow and blood; nodal and splenic enlargement also frequently observed. Indolent, but incurable.
Mantle cell lymphoma	Moderately aggressive tumor of CD5+/CD23– B cells. Presents in older adults within lymph nodes or at extranodal sites. Associated with cyclin D1 gene rearrangements.
Follicular lymphoma	CD10+ B-cell tumor of older adults associated with *BCL2* gene rearrangements; usually presents in lymph nodes. Typically indolent, but incurable.
Burkitt lymphoma	B-cell tumor of adolescents and young adults. Often appears at extranodal sites. Uniformly associated with rearrangements of the *cMYC* gene. Extremely aggressive, but curable.
Diffuse large B-cell lymphoma	Aggressive B-cell tumor; occurs at all ages but most common in adults. May appear at extranodal sites or within lymph nodes. Morphologically and genetically heterogeneous. Aggressive, but curable.
Marginal zone lymphoma	CD5–/CD10– B-cell tumor of adults; arises at extranodal sites of chronic inflammatory or autoimmune reactions. Often indolent, spreads late in its course.
Hairy cell leukemia	CD5–/CD10– B-cell tumor of older adults that presents in marrow and spleen; nodal disease almost never seen. Excellent prognosis.

Continued

TABLE 14–1 **Summary of the Lymphoid Neoplasms of the WHO Classification—cont'd**

Types of Tumors	Salient Features
Lymphoplasmacytic lymphoma	CD5–/CD10– tumor of mature B cells that show partial differentiation to IgM-producing plasma cells; presents in marrow, liver, and spleen.
	Seen in older patients; often associated with symptoms of serum hyperviscosity. Indolent, but incurable.
Multiple myeloma/ solitary plasmacytoma	Tumor of terminally differentiated B cells (plasma cells); presents in older adults as destructive bony lesions. Tumor cells usually secrete a complete or partial immunoglobulin.
	Poor prognosis.
Tumors of Mature T Cells and NK Cells	
Peripheral T-cell lymphoma, unspecified	Histologically and genetically heterogeneous tumors of mature T cells. Usually present in adults within lymph nodes. Aggressive, not usually curable.
Anaplastic large cell lymphoma	Aggressive tumor of mature T cells with characteristic morphologic features. Seen particularly in children and young adults, associated with rearrangements of the *ALK* gene. Good prognosis.
Adult T-cell leukemia/ lymphoma	Tumors of CD4+ mature T cells; presents in adults in marrow, skin, and lymph nodes. Associated with HTLV-1 infection. Very poor prognosis.
Mycosis fungoides/ Sezary syndrome	Tumor of CD4+ epidermotropic mature T cells. Occurs in adults; generally indolent course.
Large granular lymphocytic leukemia	Tumor of mature T cells or (less commonly) NK cells; presents in adults with marrow and blood involvement. Often complicated by anemia or neutropenia. Indolent.
Extranodal NK/T-cell lymphoma	Presents in adults as locally destructive masses, often in the sinonasal area. Tumor cells usually express NK cell markers and contain EBV genomes. Generally aggressive; poor prognosis.
Hodgkin lymphoma	
Classical subtypes (nodular sclerosis, mixed cellularity, lymphocyte-rich, and lymphocyte depletion subtypes)	Tumor cells express CD15 and CD30. Often associated with EBV. Subtypes defined by different patterns of cellular reaction. Good to excellent prognosis.
Lymphocyte predominance	Diagnostic RS cells rare; lymphocytic-histiocytic (L&H) variants present instead. Tumor cells express B-cell markers and are negative for CD15 and CD30. Not associated with EBV. Excellent prognosis.

EBV, Epstein-Barr virus; HTLV, human T-cell leukemia virus; NK, natural killer; TdT, terminal deoxytransferase; WHO, World Health Organization classification of lymphoid neoplasms.

- Diagnosis requires histologic examination of lymph nodes or other involved tissues.
- All lymphoid neoplasms are derived from a single transformed cell and are therefore monoclonal. In most lymphoid neoplasms, antigen receptor gene rearrangement precedes transformation; hence, daughter cells from a malignant progenitor share the same antigen receptor gene sequence and

synthesize identical antigen receptor proteins (either immunoglobulins or T-cell receptors).
- Most lymphoid neoplasms (80%–85%) are of B-cell origin, with most of the remainder being T-cell tumors; only rare tumors are of NK cell or histiocytic origin.
- Lymphoid neoplasms tend to disrupt normal immune regulatory mechanisms leading frequently to immunologic dysfunction.
- Neoplastic B and T cells circulate widely but tend to home to and grow in areas where their normal counterparts reside.

Precursor B-Cell and T-Cell Neoplasms (p. 670)

Acute Lymphoblastic Leukemia/Lymphoma (p. 670)

Acute lymphoblastic leukemias or lymphomas (ALLs) are neoplasms composed of immature, precursor B (pre-B), or precursor T (pre-T) lymphocytes *(lymphoblasts)*.

- Most (approximately 85%) are pre-B tumors manifesting as childhood acute leukemias with extensive marrow and peripheral blood involvement.
- The less common pre-T ALLs tend to present in adolescent boys as lymphomas involving the thymus (producing a mediastinal mass).

Morphology. Lymphoblasts in Wright-Giemsa stains have relatively condensed chromatin, lack conspicuous nucleoli, and have scant, agranular cytoplasm containing periodic acid–Schiff (PAS)-positive material. Pre-B and pre-T lymphoblasts are morphologically identical.

Immunophenotypic Subtypes. Leukemic blasts are analyzed for myeloid and lymphoid surface markers to distinguish ALL from acute myelogenous leukemia and to subclassify ALL. Terminal deoxytransferase (TdT), a specialized DNA polymerase expressed only by pre-B and pre-T lymphoblasts, is present in over 95% of cases. Subclassification is based on lymphoblast origin:

- Pre-B ALL cells are arrested at stages preceding surface immunoglobulin expression; the lymphoblasts express the pan B-cell antigen CD19.
- Pre-T ALL cells are arrested at early intrathymic stages of maturation; the lymphoblasts often express CD1a and variably express other T-cell markers.

Cytogenetics and Molecular Genetics. Approximately 90% of ALL have chromosomal changes. Pre-B and pre-T ALL are associated with distinctive recurrent chromosomal translocations, indicating that different molecular mechanisms underlie their pathogenesis. Important chromosomal or genetic aberrations include:

- *Hyperdiploidy (51 to 60 chromosomes):* Associated with pre-B cell phenotype and relatively good prognosis.
- *t(12;21):* Associated with early pre-B cell phenotype and good prognosis.
- *t(9;22), the Philadelphia chromosome:* Found in 5% of childhood pre-B ALL and up to 25% of adult cases; associated with poor prognosis.
- *Translocations involving chromosome 11 at band q23 (MLL gene):* Associated with early onset (<2 years of age), early pre-B phenotype, and poor prognosis.

Clinical Features. Approximately 2500 new cases of ALL are diagnosed each year in the United States; the age of peak incidence is approximately 4 years. ALL and acute myelogenous leukemia (AML) are immunophenotypically and genotypically distinct but have similar clinical features stemming from accumulation of neoplastic blast cells in the marrow. Major clinical features of both (and features that are more typical for ALL):

- *Abrupt stormy onset:* Patients present within days to weeks of symptom onset.
- *Symptoms related to depressed marrow function:* Fatigue due to anemia; fever, reflecting infections from the absence of mature leukocytes; and bleeding (petechiae, ecchymoses, epistaxis, gum bleeding) due to thrombocytopenia.
- *Bone pain and tenderness,* due to marrow expansion and infiltration of the subperiosteum by blasts.
- *Generalized lymphadenopathy, splenomegaly,* and *hepatomegaly* due to neoplastic infiltration; more common in ALL than in AML. In patients with pre-T cell ALL with thymic involvement, invasion of large vessels and airways can occur. Testicular involvement is also common in ALL.
- *Central nervous system manifestations* (e.g., headache, vomiting, and nerve palsies) due to meningeal spread; more common in ALL than AML.

Prognosis. With aggressive chemotherapy (including prophylactic treatment of the central nervous system), over 90% of children with ALL achieve complete remission; two thirds are cured. Features with worse prognosis:

- Age less than 2 (also associated with translocations involving the *MLL* gene).
- Age over 10.
- Presence of t(9;22) (Philadelphia chromosome). The high incidence of t(9;22) in adult cases may partially explain the poorer outcome in older patients; only a minority remain disease-free 5 years after diagnosis.

Peripheral B-Cell Neoplasms (p. 673)

Chronic Lymphocytic Leukemia/Small Lymphocytic Lymphoma (p. 673)

Chronic lymphocytic leukemia (CLL) and small lymphocytic lymphoma (SLL) are morphologically, phenotypically, and genotypically indistinguishable, differing only in the degree of peripheral blood lymphocytosis.

Morphology. Lymph node architecture is diffusely effaced by small lymphocytes containing round to slightly irregular nuclei mixed with variable numbers of larger cells actively dividing cells (prolymphocytes). These dividing cells often gather together in loose aggregates called *proliferation centers,* which are pathognomonic for CLL/SLL. In CLL, peripheral blood smears contain increased numbers of small lymphocytes that are disrupted, producing so-called *smudge cells.* Involvement of marrow, spleen, and liver is common.

Immunophenotype. CLL/SLL cells express pan-B cell markers (CD19 and CD20) and characteristically co-express CD5, a marker found on a small subset of normal B cells. Low-level surface expression of immunoglobulin (usually IgM) is typical.

Chromosomal Abnormalities and Molecular Genetics. Incidence varies from 25% to 67%. Most common are trisomy 12q, and deletions of 13q12-14, 11q, or 17p. Deletions of 13q and 17p correlate with higher-stage disease and portend a worse prognosis.

Clinical Features. CLL (defined as absolute lymphocyte count >4000 cells/mm³) is the most common adult leukemia in the Western world. A minority of cases do not have lymphocytosis and are classified as SLL (constitutes 4% of NHLs). Characteristic features:

- Onset after age 50 years (median, age 60)
- Male predominance (male-female ratio 2:1)
- Nonspecific symptoms (easy fatigability, weight loss, and anorexia)
- Generalized lymphadenopathy and hepatosplenomegaly (50%–60%)
- Lymphocytosis in CLL, up to 200,000 cells per mm³
- Immune abnormalities, including hypogammaglobulinemia (common) and autoantibodies against erythrocytes or platelets (10%–15%)

Prognosis. The prognosis is extremely variable, depending primarily on the clinical stage. Overall, the median survival is 4 to 6 years, but patients with minimal tumor burden often survive longer than 10 years. Hypogammaglobulinemia leads to increased susceptibility to bacterial infection. *Transformation* of CLL/SLL to a more aggressive histologic type is a common, ominous event; most patients survive less than 1 year. Two forms are seen:

- *Prolymphocytic transformation* (15%–30%) is heralded by worsening cytopenias, increasing splenomegaly, and large numbers of *prolymphocytes* in the circulation.
- *Transformation to diffuse large B-cell lymphoma,* so-called *Richter syndrome* (10% of patients), usually presents as a rapidly enlarging mass within a lymph node or spleen.

Follicular Lymphoma (p. 674)

Follicular lymphoma is the most common form of NHL in the United States (45% of adult lymphomas).

Morphology. In lymph nodes, follicular (nodular) and diffuse proliferations are composed of two principal cell types: *centrocytes,* which are small cells with irregular or cleaved nuclear contours and scant cytoplasm (small, cleaved cells); and *centroblasts,* which are larger cells with open nuclear chromatin, several nucleoli, and modest amounts of cytoplasm. Centrocytes predominate in most tumors. Involvement of spleen, liver, and marrow is common; peripheral blood involvement occurs in about 10%.

Immunophenotype. Neoplastic cells resemble normal follicular center B cells (CD19+, CD20+, CD10+, surface Ig+). Tumor cells also consistently express BCL2 protein (normal follicular center B cells are BCL2 negative).

Cytogenetics and Molecular Genetics. A characteristic (14;18) translocation juxtaposes the *IgH* locus on chromosome 14 and the *BCL2* locus on chromosome 18 leading to BCL2 protein overexpression; BCL2 prevents apoptosis and promotes tumor cell survival.

Clinical Features. Follicular lymphoma characteristically presents as painless, generalized lymphadenopathy in middle-aged adults, and follows an indolent waxing-waning course. While the overall median survival is 7 to 9 years, it is not curable with conventional chemotherapy. Histologic transformation to diffuse large B-cell lymphoma occurs in 30% to 50% of cases; after transformation, median survival is less than 1 year.

Diffuse Large B-Cell Lymphoma (p. 676)

Diffuse large B-cell lymphoma (DLBCL) is a heterogeneous group of tumors constituting 20% of NHLs and 60% to 70% of aggressive lymphoid neoplasms.

Morphology. All variants share a relatively large cell size (usually four to five times the diameter of a small lymphocyte) and a diffuse growth pattern obliterating the underlying architecture. The nuclear shape is variable and vesicular in appearance; it contains one to three prominent nucleoli. Cytoplasm is moderately abundant and can be pale or basophilic.

Immunophenotype. These mature B-cell tumors express the pan-B cell markers CD19 and CD20.

Cytogenetics and Molecular Genetics. Two chromosomal rearrangements are relatively common:

- *About 30% have translocations involving the BCL6 locus on chromosome 3. BLC6* encodes a zinc-finger transcription factor that regulates the development of germinal center B cells. Another group of tumors without translocations have somatic mutations in the *BCL6* promoter that leads to aberrant BCL6 expression.
- *From 10% to 20% have a (14;18) translocation* involving the *BCL2* gene. These tumors are sometimes associated with a typical follicular lymphoma at other sites (e.g., marrow); these likely represent *transformed* follicular lymphomas.

Special Subtypes. Several subtypes of DLBCL are described. Two—occurring in the setting of immunodeficiency states (e.g., AIDS)—merit a brief discussion.

- *Immunodeficiency-associated large B-cell lymphomas* occur in the setting of severe T-cell immunodeficiency. The neoplastic cells are often latently infected with EBV, which is thought to play a critical pathogenic role. In some settings, restoration of T-cell immunity leads to regression of the proliferations.
- *Body cavity–based large cell lymphomas* arise as malignant pleural or ascitic effusions; most occur in patients with advanced HIV infection, but some occur in elderly HIV-negative individuals. Tumor cells are infected with human herpesvirus 8 (HHV8), which plays a causal role.

Clinical Features. DLBCL can appear at any age but most frequently present in older adults (median age of 60) as a rapidly enlarging, symptomatic mass at a single nodal or extranodal site. Extranodal presentation (e.g., gastrointestinal tract, skin, bone, or brain) is relatively frequent. Involvement of liver, spleen, and marrow occurs but usually only late in the course.

Prognosis. DLBCL are aggressive, rapidly fatal tumors if left untreated. With intensive chemotherapy, complete remission is achieved in 60% to 80%, and 50% are cured. Patients with limited disease fare better than patients with widespread disease or a large bulky tumor mass.

Burkitt Lymphoma (p. 677)

Burkitt lymphomas (BLs) occur in three different settings; although they are histologically identical, they have distinct clinical, genotypic, and virologic features:

- African (endemic) BL
- Sporadic (nonendemic) BL
- A subset of aggressive lymphomas occurring in patients infected with HIV

Morphology. Involved tissues are diffusely effaced by intermediate-sized (10–25 μ diameter) tumor cells with round-oval nuclei, coarse chromatin, several nucleoli, and moderate amounts of faintly basophilic-amphophilic cytoplasm. A high mitotic index and apoptotic cell death is typical; apoptotic cells are devoured by scattered large, pale macrophages, producing a characteristic *starry sky* appearance. Occasionally, BL presents with a leukemic picture; marrow aspirates show tumor cells with slightly clumped nuclear chromatin, two to five distinct nucleoli, and royal blue cytoplasm containing multiple, clear cytoplasmic vacuoles.

Immunophenotype. Tumors comprise relatively mature B cells expressing surface IgM, monotypic κ or λ light chains, and CD19, CD20, and CD10.

Cytogenetic and Molecular Genetic Features. BLs are associated with c-*MYC* gene (chromosome 8) translocations; the partner is usually the IgH locus (t(8;14)) but can be the κ (t(2;8)) or λ (t(8;22)) light chain loci. African tumors are latently infected with EBV; it is also present in 25% of HIV-associated tumors and in a minority of sporadic cases. Molecular analysis shows that the viral DNA configuration is identical in all tumor cells within a given case, indicating that infection precedes cellular transformation.

Clinical Features. Both African and sporadic BLs occur largely in children or young adults; in the United States, BL accounts for 30% of childhood NHL. Most arise at extranodal sites as rapidly growing masses; African BL often presents in the mandible, whereas nonendemic BL most commonly occurs as an ileocecal or peritoneal mass.

Prognosis. BL is aggressive but responds well to short-term, high-dose chemotherapy, with many patients being cured.

Plasma Cell Neoplasms and Related Disorders (p. 678)

This is a group of neoplasms of terminally differentiated B cells. They have in common the expansion of a single clone of immunoglobulin-secreting plasma cells and a resultant increase in serum levels of a single homogeneous immunoglobulin or its fragments, hence the synonym *monoclonal gammopathies*. Monoclonal immunoglobulins identified in blood or urine are called *M components* in reference to *m*yeloma. The M component is usually a complete immunoglobulin; in some cases, it is secreted along with excess free light (L) or heavy (H) chains. Occasionally, only L or H chains are produced; because of their small size, free L chains are excreted in the urine *(Bence Jones protein)*.

A variety of clinicopathologic entities are associated with monoclonal gammopathies:

- Multiple myeloma (plasma cell myeloma)
- Solitary plasmacytoma

- Monoclonal gammopathy of undetermined significance
- Waldenström macroglobulinemia, commonly seen in patients with lymphoplasmacytic lymphoma
- Heavy-chain disease, a rare disorder characterized by the appearance of free heavy chains in the blood; commonly associated with unusual small bowel lymphomas in Middle Eastern populations
- Primary or lymphocyte-associated amyloidosis, commonly associated with multiple myeloma, and occasionally seen in patients without an overt plasma cell neoplasm

Multiple Myeloma (p. 679)

Multiple myeloma is the most common of the malignant gammopathies; it is a plasma cell neoplasm of older adults characterized by destructive bony lesions at multiple sites.

Etiology and Pathogenesis

- Tumors often secrete free light chains, which cause renal disease and sometimes lead to amyloidosis.
- Tumor cells produce various cytokines, particularly MIP1α and RANKL, that are osteoclast-activating factors and contribute to the characteristic bony destruction.
- Many cases involve translocations of the IgH gene and various partners, including the *FGFR3* receptor gene, and cell cycle regulatory genes cyclin D1 and cyclin D3.

Morphology

- Bony involvement is most common in the vertebral column, ribs, skull, pelvis, and femur. Skull lesions have a sharply defined, punched-out radiologic appearance; generalized osteoporosis can also be seen.
- Microscopic examination of marrow reveals increased numbers of plasma cells (>30% of total cells) often with abnormal features. The cells can diffusely infiltrate or occur as sheet-like masses that completely replace normal elements.
- Significant renal disease is seen in most patients, reflected by one (or more) of the following:

  Protein casts in the distal convoluted tubule and collecting ducts, consisting of immunoglobulin light chains, albumin, and Tamm-Horsfall protein; often surrounded by multinucleated giant cells (so-called *myeloma kidney*)

  Metastatic calcifications secondary to hypercalcemia

  Pyelonephritis, owing to predisposition to bacterial infections

  Amyloid deposition of the AL type (see Chapter 6), typically within glomeruli; most common with λ light-chain disease and usually associated with systemic amyloidosis, which appears in 10% of patients

  Nonamyloidotic light-chain deposition (glomerular and peritubular hyaline deposits that do not stain with Congo red); most common with κ light-chain disease

  Interstitial infiltrates of abnormal plasma cells or chronic inflammatory cells

- In advanced disease, plasma cell infiltrates in spleen, liver, lymph nodes, skin, and nerve roots can also occur.

Laboratory Findings

In 99% of patients electrophoresis reveals urine Bence Jones protein (immunoglobulin light chain) or high levels of a single immunoglobulin in the serum (M protein "spike"). IgG (55%) and IgA (25%) are the most common M proteins; IgM, IgD, and IgE are rare. Normal serum immunoglobulin levels are characteristically decreased. In 20% of patients, Bence Jones proteinuria is an isolated finding.

Clinical Features

Peak incidence is 50 to 60 years of age. Principal clinical features stem from organ infiltration (particularly bones) by neoplastic plasma cells, excess immunoglobulin production (often having abnormal physicochemical properties), and suppression of normal humoral immunity.

- *Bone infiltration, bone pain, and pathologic fractures due to bone resorption.* Secondary hypercalcemia contributes to renal disease and polyuria, and can cause neurologic manifestations, including confusion, weakness, lethargy, and constipation.
- *Recurrent bacterial infections* result from decreased production of normal immunoglobulins.
- *Hyperviscosity syndrome* (see following discussion) occurs occasionally as a result of excessive M protein production and aggregation.
- *Renal insufficiency* (up to 50% of patients) is multifactorial (see previous discussion). Bence Jones proteinuria is likely most important, as excreted light chains are toxic to tubular epithelial cells.
- *Extensive marrow involvement* causes normocytic, normochromic anemia, and occasionally moderate pancytopenia.

Prognosis

Prognosis depends on the stage at diagnosis. Patients with multiple bony lesions, increasing serum M protein, and high levels of urine Bence Jones protein have a grave prognosis. Chemotherapy induces remission in 50% to 70%, but median survival is still only 3 years. Infection and renal failure are the two most common causes of death.

Solitary Myeloma (Plasmacytoma) (p. 681)

From 3% to 5% of plasma cell neoplasms present as solitary lesions of either bone or soft tissue. Modest elevations of serum or urinary M proteins are found in a minority.

- Solitary bony lesions occur in similar locations as multiple myeloma; most progress to multiple myeloma in 5 to 10 years.
- Extraosseous lesions are often located in lungs, oronasopharynx, or nasal sinuses; they rarely disseminate and can be cured by local resection.

Monoclonal Gammopathy of Uncertain Significance (p. 681)

M proteins are detected in sera of 1% of asymptomatic healthy persons over 50 years old, and 3% of people over 70 years old.

- In general, such asymptomatic individuals have less than 3 gm/dL of monoclonal protein in the serum and no Bence Jones proteinuria. Nevertheless, other forms of monoclonal gammopathy, particularly indolent multiple myeloma, must be excluded.
- Most patients follow a completely benign clinical course; 1% of patients annually progress to a symptomatic monoclonal gammopathy, typically multiple myeloma.

Lymphoplasmacytic Lymphoma (p. 681)

Lymphoplasmacytic lymphoma is a B-cell neoplasm of older adults that usually secretes monoclonal IgM, often in amounts sufficient to cause a *hyperviscosity syndrome* known as *Waldenström macroglobulinemia.*

Morphology

Diffuse marrow infiltrates of neoplastic lymphocytes, plasma cells, and plasmacytoid lymphocytes, mixed with reactive mast cells, are seen. With disseminated disease, similar polymorphous infiltrates can occur in lymph nodes, spleen, or liver.

Clinical Features

These lymphomas tend to present after age 50 with nonspecific complaints, such as weakness, fatigue, and weight loss. Half of these patients have lymphadenopathy, hepatomegaly, and splenomegaly.

- Marrow infiltration causes anemias that are exacerbated by autoimmune hemolysis due to cold agglutinins of the IgM type (about 10% of patients).
- IgM-secreting tumors cause additional complications related to physicochemical properties of the protein (mostly, its large size), which results in increased blood viscosity. This leads to a *hyperviscosity syndrome* characterized by:

Visual impairment: there is a striking *tortuosity* and distention of retinal veins (assuming a *sausage-link* appearance at points of arteriovenous crossings) with retinal hemorrhages and exudates.

Neurologic problems: headaches, dizziness, deafness, and stupor are attributable to sluggish blood flow and sludging.

Bleeding: this is related to the formation of complexes containing macroglobulins and clotting factors, as well as interference with platelet function.

Cryoglobulinemia: precipitation of macroglobulins at low temperatures, produces symptoms such as Raynaud phenomenon and cold urticaria.

Prognosis

Lymphoplasmacytic lymphoma is an incurable progressive disease with a median survival time of 4 years. Symptoms related to IgM (such as hyperviscosity and hemolysis) can be treated with plasmapheresis.

Mantle Cell Lymphoma (p. 682)

Mantle cell lymphoma accounts for about 3% of NHLs in the United States and 7% to 9% of NHLs in Europe. Extranodal disease is relatively common; marrow and splenic involvement are not unusual, and there is frequently multifocal mucosal involvement of the small bowel and colon *(lymphomatoid polyposis)*. Peripheral blood lymphocytosis, usually less than 20,000 cells per mm^3, occurs in 20% to 40% of patients.

Morphology

In lymph nodes, tumor cells either accumulate about normal germinal centers or diffusely efface normal architecture; tumor infiltrates typically consist of homogeneous populations of small lymphocytes with irregular to deeply clefted nuclear contours, condensed nuclear chromatin, inconspicuous nucleoli, and scant cytoplasm.

Immunophenotype

This is a B-cell neoplasm expressing CD5 and *characteristically overexpressing cyclin D1*, which regulates G1-S phase progression during the cell cycle.

Cytogenetic Abnormalities and Molecular Genetics

A distinctive t(11;14), detected in more than 70% of cases, results in the juxtaposition of the cyclin D1 and IgH loci.

Clinical Features

Most patients are men over 50 presenting with generalized lymphadenopathy and marrow and liver involvement; splenomegaly is present in 50%. "B symptoms" (fever and weight loss) are observed in a minority of patients.

Prognosis

Generally poor response to therapy; the median survival is 3 to 4 years. Most patients succumb to complications of organ dysfunction due to tumor infiltration.

Marginal Zone Lymphomas (p. 683)

A heterogeneous group of B-cell tumors that can arise within lymph nodes, spleen, or extranodal tissues. Because mucosa is the usual extranodal site, these have been called *m*ucosa-*a*ssociated *l*ymphoid *t*umors (or MALToma). Notable clinicopathologic characteristics of the extranodal marginal zone lymphomas include the following:

- There is a strong tendency to occur at sites of *chronic immune or inflammatory reactions* (e.g., salivary glands in Sjögren disease, thyroid in Hashimoto thyroiditis, stomach in *H. pylori* infection).
- Once established, these lymphomas remain localized at sites of origin for long periods, spreading systemically only late in their course.
- Although composed of cells at various stages of B lymphoid differentiation, *the predominant population resembles a normal marginal zone B cell.*

Pathogenesis

Stepwise progression from a polyclonal immune response to a monoclonal neoplasm has been proposed as the pathogenetic mechanism.

- It begins as a reactive, polyclonal immune reaction, sometimes triggered by environmental agents (e.g., *Helicobacter* gastritis).

- Over time, a monoclonal B-cell neoplasm emerges, probably due to acquired genetic changes; cell growth is still dependent on local factors (e.g., factors produced by reactive T-helper cells) for growth and survival.
- With additional genetic aberrations (e.g., t(11;18) or t(1;14)), the neoplasm becomes factor-independent. Spread to distant sites and eventual transformation to DLBCL can occur.

Prognosis

Before dissemination, the prognosis is extremely good; patients may be cured with therapy targeted to tumor cells or inciting factors (e.g., *Helicobacter*).

Hairy Cell Leukemia (p. 683)

Hairy cell leukemia is a rare but distinctive B-cell neoplasm.

Morphology

The name derives from fine hairlike projections on the tumor cells (visible by phase-contrast microscopy). On routine blood smears, tumor cells have round, oblong, or reniform nuclei and modest amounts of pale blue cytoplasm, often with threadlike or bleblike extensions. Because tumor cells get trapped in extracellular matrix, they are frequently absent from marrow aspirate smears. Marrow biopsies show diffuse infiltrates of cells with oblong or reniform nuclei, condensed chromatin, and abundant pale cytoplasm. Splenic red pulp is preferentially infiltrated, leading to obliteration of white pulp and a beefy red gross appearance. Hepatic portal triads are frequently infiltrated.

Immunophenotype

Hairy cells express B-cell markers, surface immunoglobulin, CD11c (an adhesion molecule), CD25 (the IL2 receptor), and CD103. Most tumors have hypermutated Ig genes, suggesting origin from a postgerminal center memory B cell.

Clinical Features

Hairy cell leukemia constitutes about 2% of all leukemias; it is predominantly a disease of middle-aged white men (male-female ratio of 4:1). Clinical manifestations result from marrow, liver, or splenic infiltration. *Splenomegaly,* often massive, is the most common and sometimes only abnormal physical finding. *Hepatomegaly* is less common and not as marked; lymphadenopathy is distinctly rare. *Pancytopenia,* resulting from marrow infiltration and splenic sequestration, is seen in over 50%. *Infections* are the presenting feature in one third of cases. Monocytopenia may contribute to the high incidence of atypical mycobacterial infections.

Prognosis

This is an indolent disorder with good prognosis. It is exquisitely sensitive to certain chemotherapies, which produce long-lasting remission in most patients.

Peripheral T-Cell and Natural Killer (NK) Cell Neoplasms (p. 684)

Peripheral T-cell and NK cell neoplasms are a heterogeneous group united by phenotypes that resemble normal mature T or NK cells. Peripheral T-cell tumors account for 15% of NHLs in the United States and Europe, while NK cell tumors are rare. Both types of tumors are more common in Asia.

Peripheral T-Cell Lymphoma, Unspecified (p. 684)

Peripheral T-cell lymphomas are heterogeneous and not easily categorized; most fall into the "wastebasket" category *peripheral T-cell lymphoma, unspecified*.

Morphology. Certain findings are characteristic though not reliably diagnostic of T-cell phenotype. Tumor cells diffusely efface lymph nodes and are commonly composed of a mixture of small, intermediate-sized, and large malignant T cells. Infiltrates of reactive cells (e.g., eosinophils and macrophages) are recruited by T cell–derived cytokines; small-vessel proliferation is also often observed.

Immunophenotype. By definition, all peripheral T-cell lymphomas have a mature T-cell phenotype; they lack TdT and CD1a and express pan-T cell markers (e.g., CD2, CD3) and T-cell receptors.

Clinical Features and Prognosis. Most patients have generalized lymphadenopathy, sometimes with eosinophilia, pruritus, fever, and weight loss. Although cures are reported, the prognosis is worse than for aggressive mature B-cell neoplasms (e.g., DLBCL).

Anaplastic Large Cell Lymphoma (p. 684)

Morphology, Immunophenotype, and Cytogenetics. Tumor cells are large with characteristic reniform, embryoid, or horseshoe-shaped nuclei and voluminous cytoplasm. Most express several T-cell markers and have clonal T-cell receptor gene rearrangements. There is a strong association (particularly in children and young adults) with chromosomal rearrangements involving the *ALK* gene on chromosome 2p23. These rearrangements create several different *ALK* fusion genes, all of which encode constitutively active forms of ALK—a tyrosine kinase.

Clinical Features and Prognosis. Most patients present with disseminated disease. It is important to distinguish ALK-positive and -negative tumors; patients with *ALK* rearrangements have an excellent prognosis with aggressive chemotherapy. ALK-negative tumors usually arise in older adults and have a poor prognosis, similar to peripheral T-cell lymphoma, unspecified.

Adult T-Cell Leukemia/Lymphoma (p. 685)

This leukemia occurs in patients infected by *human T-cell leukemia virus type 1 (HTLV-1)*, and is thus most common where HTLV-1 is endemic (southern Japan and Caribbean basin). Tumor cells express CD4 and contain clonal HTLV-1 provirus, compatible with direct pathogenic involvement of the virus. Tumor cell appearance is highly variable although *cells with multilobular (cloverleaf) nuclei are most characteristic*. Clinical findings include skin involvement, generalized lymphadenopathy and hepatosplenomegaly, peripheral blood lymphocytosis, and hypercalcemia. This is an extremely aggressive disease that is refractory to treatment in most cases. The median survival is 8 months.

Mycosis Fungoides and Sezary Syndrome (p. 685)

These diseases are different manifestations of closely related tumors comprised of T cells that home to the skin (cutaneous T-cell lymphomas). In the vast majority of patients, the tumors are composed of CD4+ peripheral T cells. Median survival is 8 to 9 years.

- *Mycosis fungoides* presents with an inflammatory *premycotic phase* and progresses through a *plaque phase* to a *tumor phase.* Histologically, the epidermis and upper dermis are infiltrated by neoplastic T cells with *cerebriform* nuclei (marked infolding of the nuclear membrane). Circulating tumor cells are identified in 25% of cases of mycosis fungoides in the plaque or tumor phase. Disease progression involves extracutaneous spread, most commonly to lymph nodes and marrow.
- *Sezary syndrome* is a variant in which skin involvement is manifested as a generalized exfoliative erythroderma with an associated leukemia of *Sezary* cells (these also have cerebriform nuclei).

Large Granular Lymphocytic Leukemia (p. 685)

This rare neoplasm is known by a variety of names (e.g., Tγ lymphoproliferative disease, CD8 lymphocytosis, and CD8+ T-CLL).

- The cytologic hallmark is a population of lymphocytes in blood and marrow with abundant cytoplasm containing scattered coarse *azurophilic granules.* Marrow involvement is usually focal, without displacement of normal hematopoietic elements. The splenic red pulp and hepatic sinusoids are also usually infiltrated.
- Two variants are recognized: T-cell tumors (expressing surface CD3 and CD8) and NK cell tumors (expressing CD16 and CD56).
- Patients usually present with mild to moderate lymphocytosis and variable splenomegaly, neutropenia, and anemia.

    Neutropenia is more common; it is associated with arrested progenitor cell maturation in the marrow.
    Pure red blood cell aplasia occurs in a small minority of patients, stemming from a direct suppressive effect of tumor cells on erythroid progenitors.

- There is also an increased incidence of *rheumatologic disorders;* some patients present with Felty syndrome, characterized by the triad of rheumatoid arthritis, splenomegaly, and neutropenia.
- The course is variable, being largely dependent on the severity of the cytopenias.

Extranodal NK/T-Cell Lymphoma (p. 686)

This lymphoma (previously called *lethal midline granuloma* and *midline malignant reticulosis*) is rare in the United States and Europe but constitutes 3% of Asian NHLs.

- It presents as a destructive midline mass involving the nasopharynx or, less commonly, the skin or testis; tumor cell infiltrates surround and invade small vessels, leading to extensive ischemic necrosis.
- Histologic appearance is variable; tumor cells can contain large *azurophilic granules* resembling those in normal NK cells.

- Most tumors express NK cell markers and lack T-cell receptor rearrangements, supporting an NK cell origin. Tumor cells are latently infected with EBV in most cases.
- Although some cases follow an indolent course, most are aggressive and poorly responsive to therapy.

Hodgkin Lymphoma (p. 686)

A category of lymphoid neoplasia, HL is one of the most common malignancies in young adults; average age at diagnosis is 32 years.

Differences from NHL (Table 14–2):

- HL is characterized morphologically by the presence of scattered distinctive neoplastic giant cells called *Reed-Sternberg (RS) cells,* within a predominant background of reactive lymphocytes, macrophages, and granulocytes.
- It is associated with distinctive clinical features (see Table 14–2).
- The origin in almost all cases is from a germinal center or postgerminal center B cell, albeit one lacking expression of many B-cell antigens.
- As a result, the immunophenotype is unique among lymphoid neoplasms.

Morphology of Reed-Sternberg Cells and Variants. RS cells and their variants are the neoplastic element; their identification is essential for histologic diagnosis.

- *Classic, diagnostic RS cells* are quite large (15–45 µ diameter) and have either a single bilobed nucleus or multiple nuclei. Each nucleus or nuclear lobe has a large, inclusion-like nucleolus roughly the size of a small lymphocyte (5–7 µ diameter).
- *Mononuclear variants* contain only a single round or oblong nucleus with a large inclusion-like nucleolus.
- *Lacunar cells* have more delicate folded or multilobate nuclei surrounded by abundant pale cytoplasm that retracts during tissue processing, leaving the nucleus in an empty hole (the lacune).
- *Lymphocytic and histiocytic variants (L&H cells)* have polypoid nuclei resembling popcorn kernels, inconspicuous nucleoli, and moderately abundant cytoplasm.

Cells similar or identical in appearance to RS cells occur in other conditions (e.g., infectious mononucleosis, solid tissue cancers, and NHL). Thus, RS cells must be present in an appropriate background of reactive, non-neoplastic inflammation to make the diagnosis.

Immunophenotype of RS Cells and Variants. Classic RS cells, mononuclear variants, and lacunar variants have a similar

TABLE 14–2 **Clinical Differences Between Hodgkin and Non-Hodgkin Lymphomas**

Hodgkin Lymphoma	Non-Hodgkin Lymphoma
More often localized to a single axial group of nodes (cervical, mediastinal, para-aortic)	More frequent involvement of multiple peripheral nodes
Orderly spread by contiguity	Noncontiguous spread
Mesenteric nodes and Waldeyer ring rarely involved	Waldeyer ring and mesenteric nodes commonly involved
Extranodal involvement uncommon	Extranodal involvement common

phenotype, lacking B- and T-cell markers and expressing CD15 and CD30. L&H cells are usually positive for pan-B cell markers (e.g., CD20) and negative for CD15 and CD30. Immunophenotyping is helpful in subtyping HD, and in distinguishing HD from NHL and other conditions in which RS-like cells may be seen.

Classification. There are five subtypes of HL in the WHO classification. RS cells of the nodular sclerosis, mixed cellularity, lymphocyte-rich, and lymphocyte depletion subtypes share the same immunophenotype and are all associated with EBV infection. These subtypes are grouped together as *classical HL*, to distinguish them from the rare lymphocyte predominance subtype.

NODULAR SCLEROSIS TYPE. This most common form of HL, constituting 65% to 75% of cases is the only form of HL that is more common in women, typically affecting adolescents or young adults. It has a propensity to involve the lower cervical, supraclavicular, and mediastinal lymph nodes. The prognosis is excellent.

This type is characterized by the presence of:

- The *lacunar cell* RS cell variant (classic RS cells are uncommon but can be found).
- *Collagen bands* that divide the lymphoid tissue into circumscribed nodules.
- Neoplastic cells that occur in a polymorphous background of small T cells, eosinophils, plasma cells, and macrophages. EBV is found uncommonly in the RS cells.

MIXED CELLULARITY TYPE. This form constitutes about 25% of cases; it is more common in men, and is associated with EBV in 70% of cases. It is more likely to be associated with older age, so-called B symptoms (fever and weight loss), and advanced tumor stage. The overall prognosis is good.

This type is rendered distinctive by diffuse effacement of lymph nodes by a heterogeneous cellular infiltrate, including small lymphocytes, eosinophils, plasma cells, and benign macrophages admixed with the neoplastic cells. In addition, classic RS cells and mononuclear variants are usually plentiful.

LYMPHOCYTE-RICH TYPE. This uncommon variant is associated with EBV in about 40% of cases. Reactive lymphocytes make up the vast majority of the non-neoplastic portion of the infiltrate. It otherwise resembles the mixed cellularity type.

LYMPHOCYTE-DEPLETION TYPE. This rare variant is most common in immunosuppressed patients, is almost uniformly associated with EBV, and has a somewhat worse prognosis than other subtypes. RS cells and variants are frequent and reactive cells are relatively sparse.

LYMPHOCYTE PREDOMINANCE TYPE. This uncommon variant accounts for approximately 5% of all cases. A majority of patients are men, usually younger than 35 years old, with isolated cervical or axillary lymphadenopathy. The overall prognosis is excellent.

It is characterized by several features:

- Nodal effacement results from a nodular infiltrate of small lymphocytes admixed with variable numbers of benign macrophages and *L&H RS cell variants*. Unlike other RS cell variants, L&H variants always express B-cell markers such as CD20.
- Classic RS cells are extremely difficult to find.

- Other cells, such as eosinophils, neutrophils, and plasma cells, are scanty or absent, and there is little evidence of necrosis or fibrosis.

Etiology and Pathogenesis. The different kinds of tissue reaction observed around RS cells in various subtypes is partly due to cytokines secreted by the RS cells and reactive background cells. Cytokines released from RS cells likely induce the accumulation of reactive cells, which may, in turn, support the growth and survival of tumor cells:

- IL5 synthesized by RS cells correlates with eosinophil accumulation (a feature of mixed cellularity and nodular sclerosis subtypes).
- Transforming growth factor β, a fibrogenic cytokine, is produced almost exclusively in the nodular sclerosis variant (it is synthesized by infiltrating eosinophils).

ORIGIN OF RS CELLS. In lymphocyte predominance type HL the L&H variant RS cells definitively have a germinal center B-cell origin. In all other types, the RS cells lose the expression of many B-cell markers, a fascinating phenomenon without a known basis. Nevertheless, based on Ig gene analysis from single RS cells, it is now also accepted that RS cells in these types of HL are also neoplastic germinal center B cells. This wholesale change in gene expression pattern "camouflaged" the true identity of RS cells for many years and remains one of the central enigmas of HL.

ROLE OF EBV. Substantial evidence exists implicating EBV infection in the pathogenesis of classical forms of HL.

- Patients with a history of infectious mononucleosis or elevated antibody titers against EBV antigens have a slightly higher risk of HL.
- EBV is identified in RS cells in most cases of HL, as described previously in the various subtypes.
- The configuration of EBV DNA is the same in all tumor cells within a given case, indicating infection preceded cellular transformation.
- EBV-positive tumor cells express latent membrane protein-1 (LMP-1), encoded by the EBV genome and shown to have transforming activity.

ROLE OF NF-κB. Signals elicited by EBV LMP-1 activate NF-κB, a transcription factor that promotes B-cell survival and proliferation. Other surface membrane receptors expressed on RS cells (e.g., CD30) also activate NF-κB. Some tumors acquire inactivating mutations in IκB, an NF-κB inhibitor. Together, the findings suggest that NF-κB activation is a common, critical event in HL.

Clinical Features. HL typically presents with painless lymph node enlargement. Involvement of extranodal sites, Waldeyer ring lymphoid tissue, or mesenteric lymph nodes is unusual and suggests the diagnosis of NHL. Anatomic staging is clinically important (Table 14–3). Younger patients with more favorable histologic types tend to present in clinical stage I or II without systemic manifestations. Patients with disseminated disease (stages III and IV) and mixed cellularity or lymphocyte depletion types are more likely to present with B symptoms.

Staging. Because HL spreads predictably from its site of origin to contiguous lymphoid groups, patients with limited disease can be cured with local radiotherapy. For this reason,

TABLE 14–3 **Clinical Staging of Hodgkin and Non-Hodgkin Lymphomas (Ann Arbor Classification)**

Stage	Distribution of Disease
I	Involvement of a single lymph node region (I) or involvement of a single extralymphatic organ or site (IE).
II	Involvement of two or more lymph node regions on the same side of the diaphragm alone (II) or with involvement of limited contiguous extralymphatic organ or tissue (IIE).
III	Involvement of lymph node regions on both sides of the diaphragm (III), which may include the spleen (IIIS) and/or limited contiguous extralymphatic organ or site (IIIE, IIIES).
IV	Multiple or disseminated foci of involvement of one or more extralymphatic organs or tissues with or without lymphatic involvement.
All stages are further divided on the basis of the absence (A) or presence (B) of the following systemic symptoms: significant fever, night sweats, and/or unexplained weight loss of greater than 10% of normal body weight.	

Data from Carbone PT, et al: Symposium (Ann Arbor): Staging in Hodgkin's disease. Cancer Res 31:1707, 1971.

HL staging is not only prognostically important, but also guides therapy. It requires careful physical examination and several investigative procedures, including computed tomography of the abdomen and pelvis, chest radiography, and marrow biopsy.

Prognosis. Tumor burden (i.e., stage) rather than histologic type is the most important prognostic variable. The 5-year survival rate for stage I or IIA disease approaches 90%, and many are likely cured. Even with advanced disease (stage IVA or IVB), a 60% to 70% 5-year disease-free survival rate is typically achieved.

Complications of Therapy. Long-term HL survivors treated with chemotherapy and radiotherapy have an increased risk of developing second hematologic cancers (myelodysplastic syndromes, acute myelogenous leukemia, NHL) or solid cancers of the lung, breast, stomach, skin, or soft tissues. Non-neoplastic complications of radiotherapy include pulmonary fibrosis and accelerated atherosclerosis. New combinations of chemotherapeutic drugs and more judicious use of radiotherapy may alleviate these complications.

Myeloid Neoplasms (p. 690)

The feature uniting myeloid neoplasms is their common origin from progenitor cells that normally give rise to terminally differentiated cells of the myeloid series (erythrocytes, granulocytes, monocytes, and platelets). These neoplasms almost always primarily involve the marrow, and present with altered hematopoiesis; there is usually lesser involvement of the secondary hematopoietic organs (spleen, liver, and lymph nodes). There are three general forms:

- *Acute myelogenous leukemia,* characterized by marrow accumulation of immature myeloid cells
- The *myelodysplastic syndromes,* characterized by ineffective hematopoiesis and subsequent cytopenias
- The *chronic myeloproliferative disorders,* characterized by increased production of terminally differentiated myeloid cells

Acute Myelogenous Leukemia (p. 692)

In this heterogeneous group of disorders, relatively undifferentiated immature myeloid progenitor cells (blasts) accumulate in the marrow and displace normal elements, leading to hematopoietic failure.

Pathophysiology. AML is associated with acquired (or, rarely, inherited) genetic alterations that inhibit terminal differentiation (commitment). Most mutations interfere with transcription factor activities required for normal myeloid cell differentiation. Mutations in genes that promote proliferation and survival also likely synergize with transcription factor mutations to cause full-blown AML. For example, in acute promyelocytic leukemia (APML), translocations involving the retinoic acid receptor-α (a transcription factor gene) typically collaborate with activating point mutations in FLT3 (a tyrosine kinase) (see later discussion).

Classification. Histochemical stains (for peroxidase, specific esterase, and nonspecific esterase) and monoclonal antibodies against common and lineage-specific myeloid cell determinants distinguish AML from ALL and determine the myeloid lineage(s) of the leukemic cells. Despite the ability to reliably identify cells, AML classification is in flux. In the most widely used system (FAB), AML is divided into eight categories (M0 to M7), taking into account both the degree of maturation and the blast lineage:

- M0 to M3 subtypes denote increasing granulocytic differentiation
- M4 mixed myelomonocytic differentiation
- M5 monocytic differentiation
- M6 erythrocytic differentiation
- M7 megarkaryocytic differentiation.

A new WHO system takes into account the molecular lesions that cause AML and is gaining favor largely because it predicts clinical outcome more reliably. In this classification (Table 14–4), AML is divided into four categories based on the presence or absence of characteristic cytogenetic abnormalities, the presence of dysplasia, prior exposure to drugs known to induce AML, and the type and degree of differentiation.

TABLE 14–4 **Proposed WHO Classification of Acute Myelogenous Leukemias (AMLs)**

Class	Prognosis
I. AML with Recurrent Chromosomal Rearrangements	
AML with t(8;21)(q22;q22); *CBFα/ETO* fusion gene	Favorable
AML with inv(16)(p13;q22); *CBFβ/MYHII* fusion gene	Favorable
AML with t(15;17)(q22;11–12); *RARα/PML* fusion gene	Intermediate
AML with t(11q23;v); diverse *MML* fusion genes	Poor
II. AML with Multilineage Dysplasia	
With prior myelodysplastic syndrome	Very poor
Without prior myelodysplastic syndrome	Poor
III. AML, Therapy Related	
Alkylating agent related	Very poor
Epipodophyllotoxin related	Very poor
IV. AML, Not Otherwise Specified	
Subclasses defined by extent of differentiation and FAB classification (e.g., M0–M7)	Intermediate

Morphology. The number of leukemic cells in the circulation is highly variable, sometimes greater than 100,000 cells per µL, but less than 10,000 cells per µL in 50% of patients. Occasionally, the peripheral smear does not contain any blasts (aleukemic leukemia). AML diagnosis is based on finding greater than 20% myeloid blasts in the marrow (or >20% blasts and promyelocytes in APML). Immature myeloid cells have different morphologic features depending on the AML type.

- *Myeloblasts* have delicate nuclear chromatin, two to four nucleoli, and voluminous cytoplasm containing fine, azurophilic, peroxidase-positive granules or distinctive red-staining, peroxidase-positive, needle-like structures called *Auer rods.* When present, Auer rods are definitive evidence of myeloid differentiation.
- *Monoblasts* have folded or lobulated nuclei, lack Auer rods, and usually do not express peroxidase but can be identified by staining for nonspecific esterase.
- Neoplastic *progranulocytes*, which predominate in APML, have bilobed nuclei and contain abundant, abnormally coarse azurophilic granules that are intensely peroxidase positive. Auer rods are also often present.
- *Erythroblasts*, which rarely predominate in AML, have intensely basophilic cytoplasm and a round nucleus with a single bar-shaped nucleolus.
- *Megakaryoblasts* are often difficult to recognize morphologically, and staining for thrombocyte-specific markers is usually required.

Chromosomal Abnormalities. In 50% to 70% of AMLs, karyotypic changes can be detected by standard cytogenetic techniques; high-resolution banding techniques reveal chromosomal abnormalities in 90% of cases. Several associations have emerged:

- AML arising *de novo* in patients with no risk factors is often associated with balanced chromosomal translocations.
- AMLs that follow a myelodysplastic syndrome or occur after exposure to DNA-damaging agents (e.g., chemotherapy or radiation therapy) usually lack chromosomal translocations; instead they are commonly associated with deletions or monosomies involving chromosomes 5 and 7.
- AMLs occurring after treatment with drugs that inhibit the enzyme topoisomerase II are often associated with translocations involving the *MLL* gene on chromosome 11 at band q23.
- The t(15;17) translocation characteristic of APML is of particular pathogenetic and therapeutic interest:

    t(15;17) results in the fusion of the retinoic acid receptor-α gene on chromosome 17 to the *PML* (for *promyelocytic leukemia*) gene on chromosome 15.

    The fusion gene encodes an abnormal retinoic acid receptor that blocks myeloid cell differentiation, probably by interfering with the function of other retinoid receptors.

    The block in differentiation is overcome by pharmacologic doses of the vitamin A derivative *all-trans-retinoic acid*; this causes neoplastic promyelocytes to differentiate into neutrophils, which then rapidly die. *Death by differentiation* clears the marrow of neoplastic cells and allows for resumption of normal hematopoiesis.

Clinical Features. Although AML constitutes 20% of childhood leukemias, it primarily affects adults, with a peak incidence between ages 15 and 39. Clinical findings in AML are similar to ALL, although signs and symptoms related to tissue infiltration are generally less striking than in ALL.

- Most patients present within weeks to months of symptom onset with findings related to *anemia, neutropenia,* and *thrombocytopenia,* most notably fatigue, fever, and spontaneous mucosal and cutaneous bleeding.
- The *bleeding diathesis* caused by thrombocytopenia is often the most striking clinical feature; there are cutaneous petechiae and ecchymoses, as well as hemorrhages into serosal linings, gingiva, and the gastrointestinal and urinary tracts.
- *Procoagulants* released by leukemic cells, especially in APML, can produce *disseminated intravascular coagulation.*
- *Neutropenia leads to infections (frequently opportunistic, e.g., fungi),* particularly in the oral cavity, skin, lungs, kidneys, urinary bladder, and colon.
- Lymphadenopathy and organomegaly are generally mild.
- In AMLs with monocytic differentiation, infiltration of the skin *(leukemia cutis)* and the gingiva can be observed.
- Central nervous system spread is less common than in ALL but is still seen.
- Rarely, patients initially present with localized masses composed of myeloblasts (called *myeloblastomas, granulocytic sarcomas,* or *chloromas*). These inevitably progress to a typical AML picture, although it may take several years.

Prognosis. Prognosis is variable, depending on the underlying molecular pathogenesis. Overall, 60% achieve complete remission with chemotherapy, but only 15% to 30% remain disease-free for 5 years. The prognosis is especially dismal for patients with AML arising out of a myelodysplastic syndrome (see following section) or after previous chemotherapy, since *normal* hematopoietic stem cells in such patients have likely been damaged. Drugs directed at specific molecular targets (e.g., retinoic acid or FLT3 inhibitors in APML) represent exciting new rational therapeutic approaches.

Myelodysplastic Syndromes (p. 695)

Myelodysplastic syndromes (MDS) are a group of clonal stem cell disorders characterized by ineffective hematopoiesis and an increased risk of transformation to AML. The marrow is partly or wholly replaced by the clonal progeny of a mutant multipotent stem cell that retains the capacity to differentiate into red blood cells, granulocytes, and platelets but in a manner that is both ineffective and disordered. The marrow is usually hypercellular or normocellular, but the peripheral blood shows pancytopenia.

MDS arises in two distinct settings:

- *Idiopathic or primary MDS* occurs mainly in patients over age 50, often developing insidiously.
- *Therapy-related MDS* is a complication of previous myelosuppressive drug therapy or radiotherapy, usually appearing 2 to 8 years after treatment.

All forms of MDS can transform to AML; transformation occurs most rapidly and with highest frequency in patients with therapy-related MDS. Characteristic morphologic changes are seen in the marrow and peripheral blood (see later discussion); cytogenetic analysis can help confirm the diagnosis.

Pathogenesis

Although the pathogenesis is largely unknown, MDS typically arises in a background of stem cell damage. Both primary and therapy-related MDS are associated with similar clonal chromosomal abnormalities, including monosomy 5 and monosomy 7, deletions of 5q and 7q, trisomy 8, and deletions of 20q.

Morphology

The most characteristic finding is disordered (dysplastic) differentiation affecting all three lineages (erythroid, myeloid, and megakaryocytic).

* Erythroid lineage effects:

  Ringed sideroblasts, erythroblasts with iron-laden mitochondria visible as perinuclear granules on Prussian blue stain.

  Megaloblastoid maturation, resembling that seen in vitamin B_{12} or folate deficiency.

  Nuclear budding abnormalities, producing misshapen nuclei, often with polypoid outlines.

* Granulocytic lineage effects:

  Neutrophils with decreased numbers of secondary granules, toxic granulations, or Döhle bodies.

  Pseudo-Pelger-Huet cells (neutrophils with only two nuclear lobes).

  Myeloblasts may be increased, but by definition comprise less than 20% of overall marrow cellularity.

* *Megakaryocytic lineage effects:* Megakaryocytes with single nuclear lobes or multiple separate nuclei ("pawn ball" megakaryocytes).

* *Peripheral blood effects:* The peripheral blood often contains pseudo-Pelger-Huet cells, giant platelets, macrocytes, poikilocytes, and a relative or absolute monocytosis. Myeloblasts usually comprise less than 10% of peripheral leukocytes.

Clinical Course

Primary MDS typically affects individuals over 60 years of age. Half are asymptomatic at presentation, and the disease is discovered only incidentally by blood tests. The course is dominated by symptoms stemming from cytopenias, particularly thrombocytopenia. Progression to AML occurs in 10% to 40% of individuals, accompanied by the appearance of additional clonal cytogenetic changes.

Prognosis

The median survival varies from 9 to 29 months, but some individuals live 5 years or more. Factors portending a worse outcome include

* Development after cytotoxic therapy. Therapy-related MDS patients have more severe cytopenias, often progress rapidly to AML, and have an overall median survival of only 4 to 8 months.
* Increased numbers of blasts in the marrow or blood.

* Multiple clonal chromosomal abnormalities.
* Severe thrombocytopenia.

Chronic Myeloproliferative Disorders (p. 696)

Four chronic myeloproliferative disorders (MPDs) are recognized:

* Chronic myelogenous leukemia (CML)
* Polycythemia vera
* Essential thrombocytosis
* Myelofibrosis with myeloid metaplasia

In the latter three, the target of neoplastic transformation is a multipotent progenitor cell capable of giving rise to mature erythrocytes, platelets, granulocytes, and monocytes. In CML, the target is a pluripotent stem cell that can give rise to lymphoid and myeloid cells.

Chronic MPDs are similar to AML in that neoplastic cells flood the marrow and suppress residual normal progenitor cells. However, as opposed to AML, terminal differentiation is initially unaffected in MPDs. The combination of neoplastic cell proliferation and "normal" differentiation leads to marrow hypercellularity, increased hematopoiesis, and (often) elevated peripheral blood cell counts.

Certain features are common to all four chronic MPDs:

* Circulation and homing of neoplastic stem cells to secondary hematopoietic organs, particularly the spleen. Resultant *extramedullary hematopoiesis* leads to splenomegaly.
* A terminal spent phase characterized by *marrow fibrosis* and peripheral blood cytopenias.
* Progression over time to acute leukemia. This invariably occurs only with CML.

The pathologic findings in MPDs are not specific, with considerable overlaps between each other and with many reactive conditions. Diagnosis and classification require correlation of morphologic findings with other clinical and laboratory findings, particularly cytogenetics.

Chronic Myelogenous Leukemia (p. 697)

CML is a neoplasm of pluripotent hematopoietic stem cells leading to preferential proliferation of granulocytic progenitors.

Pathophysiology

CML is distinguished from other chronic MPDs by the presence of the t(9;22) Philadelphia chromosome (Ph[1]).

* The translocation leads to fusion of portions of the *BCR* gene from chromosome 22 and the *ABL* gene from chromosome 9.
* The resultant *BCR-ABL* fusion gene directs the synthesis of a 210-kD fusion protein with tyrosine kinase activity.
* Expression of the BCR-ABL fusion protein kinase in murine hematopoietic progenitor cells induces a syndrome resembling human CML, suggesting a critical role in stem cell transformation.
* In human CML and murine models, there is a marked increase in marrow neoplastic granulocytic precursors, coexisting with a smaller number of *BCR-ABL*-negative

(normal) progenitors. The basis for preferential proliferation of granulocytic precursors is not known.

Morphology

CML marrow specimens are usually 100% cellular, with most of the increased cellularity comprising maturing granulocytic precursors. Blood analyses reveal increased granulocytes, often more than 100,000 cells/mm³. A mixture of neutrophils, metamyelocytes, and myelocytes, with fewer than 10% myeloblasts, is typical. Peripheral blood eosinophilia, basophilia, and thrombocytosis are also common. Extramedullary hematopoiesis within the splenic red pulp produces marked splenomegaly, often complicated by focal infarction.

Laboratory Findings

CML is best differentiated from other chronic MPDs by detecting the *BCR-ABL* fusion gene, either by chromosomal analysis or polymerase chain reaction.

- In over 90% of cases, karyotyping reveals the Ph[1].
- In 5% to 10%, the rearrangement is complex or cytogenetically cryptic; in such cases, fluorescent in situ hybridization or reverse transcriptase polymerase chain reaction are required to detect the *BCR-ABL* fusion gene or transcript.
- The absence of leukocyte alkaline phosphatase in CML is also helpful because leukemoid reactions and other chronic MPDs are associated with an elevated leukocyte alkaline phosphatase.

Clinical Features

CML primarily occurs in adults between 25 and 60 years of age; peak incidence is between the ages of 30 and 50. Onset is insidious; initial symptoms (fatigability, weakness, weight loss, and anorexia) are due to mild to moderate anemia or hypermetabolism owing to increased cell turnover. Other presentations are related to splenomegaly or splenic infarction.

- After a variable *stable phase* period averaging 3 years, 50% of patients enter an *accelerated phase* marked by worsening anemia and thrombocytopenia, increased basophilia, and refractoriness to treatment. Additional clonal cytogenetic abnormalities (e.g., trisomy 8, isochromosome 17q, or duplication of the Ph[1]) may appear.
- Within 6 to 12 months, the accelerated phase terminates in acute leukemia *(blast crisis)*.
- In the remaining 50%, blast crises occur abruptly without an intermediate accelerated phase.
- In 70% of patients, blasts have the morphologic and cytochemical features of myeloblasts; in about 30%, blasts contain the enzyme TdT and express early B-lineage antigens, such as CD10 and CD19. Rarely, blasts resemble precursor T cells.
- Less commonly, patients may progress to a phase of diffuse marrow fibrosis.

Prognosis

CML is curable by allogeneic bone marrow transplantation during the stable phase. Patients who are ineligible for marrow transplantation can be treated effectively with Gleevec, a BCR-ABL kinase inhibitor. Once blast crisis appears, the disease is much more resistant to either therapy. It is not yet clear whether BCR-ABL inhibitors can prevent or delay the appearance of blast crisis.

Polycythemia Vera (p. 699)

Arises in a transformed multipotent myeloid stem cell and is characterized by increased proliferation and production of erythroid, granulocytic, and megakaryocytic elements. Increased marrow production is reflected in the circulation by erythrocytosis (polycythemia), granulocytosis, and thrombocytosis, but *the absolute increase in red blood cell mass is responsible for most of the clinical symptoms.*

Pathophysiology

Although the pathogenesis is largely unknown, polycythemia vera progenitor cells do have decreased requirements for erythropoietin and other growth factors. Since three lineages are affected, the growth factor independence is likely caused by mutations in a protein common to multiple hematopoietic growth factor signaling pathways.

Morphology

Early in disease, the following features are noted:

- *Bone marrow hypercellularity*, resulting from increased progenitors of all lineages (erythroid, granulocytic, and megakaryocytic).
- Peripheral blood basophilia and neutrophilia.
- Giant platelets and megakaryocyte fragments in peripheral smears.
- Mild organomegaly.

Late in disease, the following features appear:

- Marrow fibrosis *(spent phase)*, leading to displacement of hematopoietic cells (15%–20% of patients).
- Marrow fibrosis results in increased *extramedullary hematopoiesis* in the spleen and liver, producing more prominent organomegaly.
- Transformation to AML in 2% to 15% of patients.

Laboratory Findings

Polycythemia vera is associated with a constellation of findings that help establish the diagnosis:

- Hemoglobin concentrations range from 14 to 28 gm per dL; hematocrits are usually above 60%.
- White blood cell counts are typically elevated, ranging from 12,000 to 50,000 cells per mm^3, and platelet counts are often above 500,000 cells per mm^3.
- BCR-ABL fusion genes are absent.
- Platelets show defects in functional aggregation studies.

Clinical Course

Polycythemia vera appears insidiously, usually in late middle age (median onset at age 60). Symptoms are related to:

- *Erythrocytosis:* Increased red blood cell mass and the accompanying increase in total blood volume leads to abnormal blood flow, vascular distention, and vascular stasis. These cause a ruddy complexion (plethora), cyanosis, and hypertension (70% of patients).

- *Basophilia:* Histamine release may underlie gastrointestinal symptoms, increased tendency to peptic ulceration, and intense pruritus.
- *High cell turnover* causes hyperuricemia and symptomatic gout in 5% to 10% of cases.
- *Platelet dysfunction* coupled with abnormal blood flow leads to increased risk of both major bleeding and thrombotic events. About 25% of patients first come to clinical attention with thrombosis; life-threatening hemorrhages occur in 5% to 10% of cases.

Prognosis

With no treatment, death from bleeding or thrombosis occurs within months. With simple phlebotomy to maintain the hematocrit within normal range, median survival time is about 10 years.

Essential Thrombocytosis (p. 700)

Essential thrombocytosis is an MPD arising in multipotent stem cells, but the increased proliferation and production is confined to the megakaryocytic elements.

Pathogenesis

Pathogenesis is largely unknown, although essential thrombocytosis resembles polycythemia vera in that cells of the megakaryocytic series have a diminished requirement for growth factors. Dysfunctions of platelets derived from the neoplastic clone probably contribute to the major clinical features of bleeding and thrombosis.

Morphology

Marrow cellularity is usually mildly to moderately increased; megakaryocytes are often markedly increased in number and include abnormally large forms. Peripheral smears reveal thrombocytosis (usually >600,000 cells/mm^3) and abnormally large platelets, frequently accompanied by mild leukocytosis. Neoplastic extramedullary hematopoiesis can produce mild organomegaly (50% of cases). Uncommonly, essential thrombocytosis can evolve to a spent phase of marrow fibrosis or transform to AML.

Clinical Features

Essential thrombocytosis is the rarest of the chronic MPDs; it usually occurs after age 60 but is also seen in young adults. Qualitative and quantitative abnormalities in platelets underlie the major clinical manifestations of thrombosis and hemorrhage. *Erythromelalgia,* the throbbing and burning of hands and feet caused by occlusion of small arterioles by platelet aggregates, is a characteristic symptom.

Prognosis

Essential thrombocytosis has an indolent course; long asymptomatic periods are punctuated by thrombotic or hemorrhagic crises. Median survival time is 12 to 15 years.

Primary Myelofibrosis (p. 700)

Primary marrow fibrosis (myelofibrosis) with myeloid metaplasia also arises from a transformed multipotent myeloid stem cell but differs in that progression to myelofibrosis (identical to the spent phase of other chronic MPDs) occurs early in the course.

Pathophysiology

The pathologic features stem from extensive collagen deposition in the marrow by non-neoplastic fibroblasts, inexorably displacing hematopoietic elements, including stem cells. Marrow obliteration leads to extensive extramedullary hematopoiesis in spleen, liver, and sometimes lymph nodes. Fibrosis may be caused by inappropriate release of two fibroblast mitogens from neoplastic megakaryocytes, platelet-derived growth factor, and TGF-β.

Morphology

- Early, the marrow is often hypercellular and contains large, dysplastic, and abnormally clustered megakaryocytes. With progression, diffuse fibrosis displaces hematopoietic elements. Late in the course, the fibrotic marrow space can be largely converted to bone (osteosclerosis).
- Fibrotic obliteration of the marrow space leads to extensive extramedullary hematopoiesis, principally in the spleen (to a lesser degree in liver and lymph nodes), with splenic enlargement to weights above 4000 gm.
- Nucleated erythroid progenitors and early granulocytes are inappropriately released from the fibrotic marrow and sites of extramedullary hematopoiesis; their appearance in the circulation is termed *leukoerythroblastosis*. Other frequent peripheral blood findings include tear-drop erythrocytes, increased basophils, and abnormally large platelets.

Laboratory Findings

Moderate to severe normochromic, normocytic anemia is common. The white blood cell count is usually normal or reduced but can be markedly elevated (80,000–100,000 cells/mm³) during the early cellular marrow phase. Thrombocytopenia, often severe, appears with disease progression.

Clinical Features

Primary myelofibrosis is uncommon in individuals younger than 60 years of age. The disorder comes to attention because of progressive anemia or marked splenic enlargement. Nonspecific symptoms (e.g., fatigue, weight loss, and night sweats) result from increased metabolism associated with the expanded mass of hematopoietic cells. Owing to high cell turnover, hyperuricemia and secondary gout can complicate the picture.

Prognosis

Prognosis is variable, with median survival periods of 1 to 5 years. Threats to life include intercurrent infections, thrombotic episodes or bleeding related to platelet abnormalities, and transformation to AML (5%–20% of cases).

Langerhans Cell Histiocytosis (p. 701)

There are three types of *histiocytoses* (an archaic term for proliferations of dendritic cells and macrophages):

- True histiocytic lymphomas (rare)
- Benign, reactive histiocytoses
- Langerhans cell histiocytoses

The Langerhans cell histiocytoses (also referred to as *histiocytosis X*) represent clonal proliferations of a subtype of antigen-presenting dendritic cells.

Morphology and Immunophenotype

Tumor cells have abundant, often vacuolated cytoplasm, with vesicular oval or indented nuclei; expression of HLA-DR, S100, and CD1a is characteristic. Electron microscopy reveals cytoplasmic structures called *HX bodies (Birbeck granules)*; they resemble a tennis racquet. A prominent reactive infiltrate of plasma cells, macrophages, and eosinophils (scant or numerous) is admixed with the neoplastic dendritic cells.

Clinical Features and Prognosis

Three patterns of disease occur, each with a different course and prognosis:

- *Multifocal multisystem Langerhans cell histiocytosis (Letterer-Siwe disease)* is an aggressive systemic disorder in which Langerhans cells infiltrate and proliferate within skin, spleen, liver, lung, and bone marrow; anemia and destructive bony lesions are also seen. Usually occurring before age 2, Letterer-Siwe disease is rapidly fatal if untreated. Intensive chemotherapy yields 5-year survival rates of about 50%.
- *Unifocal Langerhans cell histiocytosis (eosinophilic granuloma)* usually affects the skeleton as an erosive, expanding accumulation of Langerhans cells within calvarium, ribs, or femur; it may also occur in skin, lungs, or stomach. Lesions can be asymptomatic or painful; pathologic fractures may occur. This is an indolent disorder of children and young adults, usually male. Unifocal lesions can remit spontaneously or may be cured by local excision or irradiation.
- *Multifocal unisystem Langerhans cell histiocytosis* usually affects children, who present with fever and diffuse eruptions, particularly on the scalp and in the ear canals. There is also frequent otitis media, mastoiditis, upper respiratory tract infections, bone lesions, mild lymphadenopathy, hepatomegaly, and splenomegaly. In 50%, the posterior pituitary stalk of the hypothalamus is involved, leading to diabetes insipidus. The combination of calvarial bone defects, diabetes insipidus, and exophthalmos is referred to as the *Hand-Schüller-Christian triad*. Spontaneous regression may be seen; persistent disease is treated with chemotherapy.

SPLENOMEGALY (p. 703)

The spleen can be enlarged in a variety of conditions (Table 14–5). Splenic enlargement is often a feature of hematolymphoid disorders. *Hypersplenism* is observed in a minority of patients with splenic enlargement; it is characterized by splenomegaly, reduction of one or more cellular elements of the blood (due to increased sequestration and splenic macrophage lysis), and correction of cytopenias after splenectomy.

TABLE 14–5   **Disorders Associated with Splenomegaly**

I. Infections

Nonspecific splenitis of various blood-borne infections (particularly
infective endocarditis)
Infectious mononucleosis
Tuberculosis
Typhoid fever
Brucellosis
Cytomegalovirus
Syphilis
Malaria
Histoplasmosis
Toxoplasmosis
Kala-azar
Trypanosomiasis
Schistosomiasis
Leishmaniasis
Echinococcosis

II. Congestive States Related to Portal Hypertension

Cirrhosis of the liver
Portal or splenic vein thrombosis
Cardiac failure

III. Lymphohematogenous Disorders

Hodgkin lymphoma
Non-Hodgkin lymphomas and lymphocytic leukemias
Multiple myeloma
Myeloproliferative disorders
Hemolytic anemias
Thrombocytopenic purpura

IV. Immunologic-Inflammatory Conditions

Rheumatoid arthritis
Systemic lupus erythematosus

V. Storage Diseases

Gaucher disease
Niemann-Pick disease
Mucopolysaccharidoses

VI. Miscellaneous

Amyloidosis
Primary neoplasms and cysts
Secondary neoplasms

Nonspecific Acute Splenitis (p. 704)

Nonspecific acute splenitis is associated with splenic enlargement, and can occur with any blood-borne infection. Grossly,
the spleen is red and extremely soft. Microscopically, there is
acute red pulp congestion with lymphoid follicle effacement
and reticuloendothelial hyperplasia.

Congestive Splenomegaly (p. 704)

Passive chronic venous congestion and enlargement can
result from

- Systemic congestion, encountered in right-sided cardiac
  failure
- Intrahepatic derangement of portal venous drainage (e.g.,
  due to cirrhosis)
- Extrahepatic portal vein obstruction (e.g., spontaneous
  portal vein thrombosis); inflammatory involvement of the

portal vein *(pylephlebitis)*, with intraperitoneal infections; and thrombosis of the splenic vein

In all these settings, there is moderate to marked splenic enlargement (500–1000 gm). Microscopically, the red pulp is suffused with erythrocytes during the early phases but becomes increasingly more fibrous and cellular with time. Organization of focal hemorrhages gives rise to areas of fibrosis containing deposits of iron and calcium salts encrusted on connective tissue and elastic fibers *(Gandy-Gamna nodules)*.

Splenic Infarcts (p. 705)

The spleen is prone to infarction in a wide variety of conditions. Embolic infarcts occur in endocarditis and in severe atherosclerosis. Infarction due to enlargement and compromise of intrasplenic blood flow can occur in virtually any condition that causes significant splenomegaly (see Table 14–5). Grossly, infarcts are wedge-shaped and subcapsular. Fresh infarcts are hemorrhagic and red; older infarcts are yellow-gray and fibotic.

SPLENIC NEOPLASMS (p. 705)

Benign splenic tumors include fibromas, osteomas, chondromas, lymphangiomas, and hemangiomas. Malignant hematolymphoid neoplasms (e.g., lymphoid leukemias, Hodgkin and non-Hodgkin lymphomas, myeloproliferative disorders) often involve the spleen secondarily and much less commonly originate at this site. Rarely, hemangiosarcomas can arise primarily within the spleen. Metastasis of solid tumors to the spleen is not common and is usually observed only in advanced malignancies.

THYMIC DEVELOPMENTAL DISORDERS (p. 706)

Thymic developmental disorders are classified as follows:

- *Thymic hypoplasia or aplasia* is accompanied by parathyroid aplasia and variable defects involving the heart and great vessels; these changes occur in *DiGeorge syndrome.*
- *Thymic cysts* are uncommon lesions lined by stratified or columnar epithelium; they are probably developmental in origin and of little clinical significance.

THYMIC HYPERPLASIA (p. 706)

Thymic hyperplasia refers to the appearance of reactive B-cell lymphoid follicles within the thymus. It is seen in chronic inflammatory and immunologic states, particularly myasthenia gravis (65%–75% of cases).

THYMOMAS (p. 707)

Thymomas are neoplasms derived from cortical or medullary thymic epithelial cells.

Morphology

Macroscopically, thymomas are usually lobulated, firm, gray-white masses up to 15 to 20 cm in greatest dimension; they can have areas of cystic necrosis and calcification. In malignant tumors (20%–25% of cases), there is invasion of adjacent structures; benign tumors are well encapsulated.

Microscopically, thymomas are composed of a mixture of neoplastic epithelial cells and variable numbers of reactive thymocytes. They are classified according to their appearance and pattern of growth:

- *Benign medullary thymoma:* This type is composed of proliferating elongated or spindle-shaped cells, often with few admixed thymocytes.
- *Benign cortical thymoma:* The neoplastic epithelial cells are plump, have abundant cytoplasm and rounded vesicular nuclei, and are often mixed with large numbers of reactive thymocytes.
- *Benign mixed thymoma:* These masses exhibit both medullary and cortical patterns.
- *Malignant thymoma type I:* This type is cytologically benign and morphologically resembles a cortical thymoma; however, it invades local structures.
- *Malignant thymoma type II:* Better thought of as *thymic carcinoma,* these are uncommon (5% of thymomas), cytologically malignant tumors. Grossly, they are usually fleshy and obviously invasive. Microscopically, they either resemble *squamous cell carcinoma* or are composed of anaplastic cortical-type epithelial cells scattered against a dense background of non-neoplastic thymocytes (so-called *lymphoepithelioma*). The lymphoepithelioma type is more common in Asia and often contains clonal EBV genomes.

Clinical Course

These are tumors of adults; about 40% present with local pressure symptoms, and an additional 30% to 45% present with *myasthenia gravis.* Thymomas are associated with other paraneoplastic syndromes (e.g., acquired hypogammaglobulinemia, pure red blood cell aplasia, Graves disease, pernicious anemia, dermatomyositis-polymyositis, and Cushing syndrome).

Prognosis

When minimally invasive or noninvasive, simple excision yields greater than 90% 5-year survival rate. Extensive invasion is often accompanied by local metastasis and is associated with a 5-year survival rate of less than 50%.

CHAPTER 15

The Lung

CONGENITAL ANOMALIES (p. 713)

Pulmonary hypoplasia (p. 713) indicates defective development resulting in small lungs (weight, volume, and acinar number). Causes include oligohydramnios, congenital diaphragmatic hernia, renal cystic diseases, and anencephaly.

Foregut cysts (p. 713) are formed by abnormal detachment of primitive foregut. The most common are bronchogenic cysts, lined by bronchial-type epithelium found in the mediastinum or hilum. Usually incidental, they can present as a mass lesion or become apparent after infection or rupture.

Congenital pulmonary airway malformation (p. 713) is a hamartomatous lesion; type 1 (of five subtypes)—with large cysts and good prognosis—is most common.

Pulmonary sequestration (p. 713) is lung tissue (lobes or segments) *without* a normal connection to the airway system and *with* a vascular supply derived from the aorta or its branches (rather than the pulmonary artery).

- *Extralobar sequestrations* are found most often in infants as abnormal mediastinal masses and in association with other congenital anomalies.
- *Intralobar sequestrations* are found *within the lung parenchyma* in older children and adults. They are often acquired lesions, associated with recurrent infections.

ATELECTASIS (COLLAPSE) (p. 713)

Atelectasis refers to incomplete expansion or collapse of parts of a lung. In adults, there are *three* basic types:

- *Resorption atelectasis* follows complete airway obstruction (e.g., from bronchial secretions in chronic bronchitis, foreign body aspiration, or bronchial neoplasms). It is reversible if the obstruction is removed.
- *Compressive atelectasis* occurs when the pleural space is expanded by fluid (e.g., effusions from cardiac failure or neo-

plasms, blood from rupture of a thoracic aneurysm) or by air (pneumothorax). It is reversible if the air or fluid is removed.
- *Contraction atelectasis* occurs when local or generalized fibrotic changes in the lung or pleura prevent full expansion. This is *not* reversible.

ACUTE LUNG INJURY (p. 714)

Acute lung injury can produce a spectrum of pulmonary lesions including congestion, edema, surfactant disruption, and atelectasis; all can progress to acute respiratory distress syndrome or acute interstitial pneumonia.

Pulmonary Edema (p. 714)

Hemodynamic disturbances or changes in microvascular permeability cause pulmonary edema (Table 15–1). In addition to impairing normal respiratory function, chronic edema predisposes to infection.

Morphology

Regardless of cause, lungs become heavy, wet, and subcrepitant. Fluid accumulates, especially in dependent, basal regions of the lower lobes. *Histologic findings* include engorged capillaries and airspace filling by granular pink precipitate. In chronic congestion and edema (e.g., with mitral stenosis), interstitial fibrosis may supervene, associated with numerous hemosiderin-laden macrophages *(brown induration)*.

TABLE 15–1 **Classification and Causes of Pulmonary Edema**

Hemodynamic Edema
Increased hydrostatic pressure (increased pulmonary venous pressure)
    Left-sided heart failure (common)
    Volume overload
    Pulmonary vein obstruction
Decreased oncotic pressure (less common)
    Hypoalbuminemia
    Nephrotic syndrome
    Liver disease
    Protein-losing enteropathies
Lymphatic obstruction (rare)

Edema Due to Microvascular Injury (Alveolar Injury)
Infections: pneumonia, septicemia
Inhaled gases: oxygen, smoke
Liquid aspiration: gastric contents, near-drowning
Drugs and chemicals: chemotherapeutic agents (bleomycin), other
    medications (amphotericin B), heroin, kerosene, paraquat
Shock, trauma
Radiation
Transfusion related

Edema of Undetermined Origin
High altitude
Neurogenic (central nervous system trauma)

Acute Respiratory Distress Syndrome (Diffuse Alveolar Damage) (p. 715)

Acute respiratory distress syndrome (ARDS) is characterized by diffuse alveolar capillary damage, leading to severe pulmonary edema, respiratory failure, and arterial hypoxemia refractory to oxygen therapy. Causes are listed under "Microvascular Injury" in Table 15–1. X-rays show diffuse bilateral infiltrates; there are frequent superimposed infections and the overall mortality rate is about 60%.

Pathogenesis

The basic lesion is diffuse alveolar wall damage, initially involving capillary endothelium but also eventually involving the epithelium. Early ARDS is characterized by increased capillary permeability and edema, fibrin exudation, formation of hyaline membranes (composed of necrotic epithelial debris and exuded proteins), and septal inflammation (*diffuse alveolar damage*, or *DAD*).

- *Activated neutrophils* aggregate in the pulmonary vasculature and damage the epithelium by secreting oxygen-derived free radicals and lysosomal enzymes (proteases), as well as arachidonic acid metabolites that further augment neutrophil aggregation.
- *Activated pulmonary macrophages* release oxidants, proteases, and proinflammatory cytokines.
- *Surfactant is lost or damaged,* contributing to atelectasis; in combination with pulmonary edema, atelectasis causes the stiff lungs characteristic of ARDS.

Morphology

- *Acute stage:* lungs are diffusely firm, red, boggy, and heavy with DAD (edema, hyaline membranes, acute inflammation).
- *Proliferative/organizing stage:* interstitial fibrosis and type II pneumocyte proliferation develop; bacterial infections are frequently superimposed in fatal cases.

Acute Interstitial Pneumonia (p. 716)

Acute interstitial pneumonia is similar to ARDS, except that its etiology is unknown. Mortality rate is 50% in the first 1 to 2 months; survivors often develop chronic disease.

OBSTRUCTIVE VERSUS RESTRICTIVE PULMONARY DISEASES (p. 716)

Diffuse pulmonary disease is classified physiologically as:

- *Obstructive disease:* increased resistance to airflow
- *Restrictive disease:* reduced expansion of lung parenchyma, with decreased total lung capacity

OBSTRUCTIVE PULMONARY DISEASE (p. 717)

The individual disorders—emphysema, chronic bronchitis, asthma, and bronchiectasis—have distinct characteristics

(Table 15–2). Emphysema and chronic bronchitis are often grouped together as *chronic obstructive pulmonary disease* (COPD); many patients have overlapping features due to the pathogenic common denominator, cigarette smoking.

Emphysema (p. 717)

Emphysema is defined morphologically as the abnormal permanent enlargement of airspaces distal to the terminal bronchioles with alveolar wall destruction and minimal fibrosis. Emphysema is further classified according to the anatomic distribution of the lesions (Fig. 15–1).

Centriacinar (Centrilobular) Emphysema (p. 718)

- Destruction and enlargement of the central or proximal parts of the respiratory unit—the acinus—sparing distal alveoli
- Predominant involvement of upper lobes and apices
- Severe lesions, seen primarily in male smokers, often associated with chronic bronchitis

Panacinar (Panlobular) Emphysema (p. 718)

- Uniform destruction and enlargement of the acinus
- Predominance in lower basal zones
- Strong association with α_1-antitrypsin deficiency

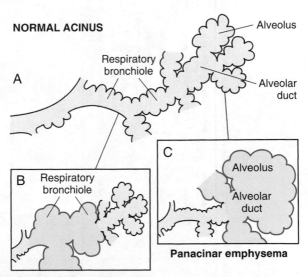

FIGURE 15–1 *A,* Diagram of normal structures within the acinus, the fundamental unit of the lung. A terminal bronchiole (not shown) is immediately proximal to the respiratory bronchiole. *B, Centriacinar emphysema* with dilation that initially affects the respiratory bronchioles. *C, Panacinar emphysema* with initial distention of the peripheral structures (alveolus and alveolar duct); the disease later extends to affect the respiratory broinchioles.

TABLE 15-2 Disorders Associated with Airflow Obstruction: The Spectrum of Chronic Obstructive Pulmonary Disease

Clinical Term	Anatomic Site	Major Pathologic Changes	Etiology	Signs/Symptoms
Chronic bronchitis	Bronchus	Mucous gland hyperplasia, hypersecretion	Tobacco smoke, air pollutants	Cough, sputum production
Bronchiectasis	Bronchus	Airway dilation and scarring	Persistent or severe infections	Cough, purulent sputum, fever
Asthma	Bronchus	Smooth muscle hyperplasia, excess mucus, inflammation	Immunologic or undefined causes	Episodic wheezing cough, dyspnea
Emphysema	Acinus	Airspace enlargement; wall destruction	Tobacco smoke	Dyspnea
Small airway disease,* bronchiolitis	Bronchiole	Inflammatory scarring/obliteration	Tobacco smoke, air pollutants, miscellaneous	Cough, dyspnea

*A feature of chronic bronchitis (see text).

Distal Acinar (Paraseptal) Emphysema (p. 719)

- Involves mostly the distal acinus
- Typically near the pleura and adjacent to fibrosis or scars
- Frequently the underlying lesion in spontaneous pneumothorax

Airspace Enlargement with Fibrosis (Irregular Emphysema) (p. 719)

Airspace enlargement with fibrosis refers to irregular acinar involvement and is associated with scarring. It is usually asymptomatic. Other related entities are *bullous emphysema* (blebs or bullae >1 cm) and *interstitial emphysema* (entrance of air into lung connective tissue, mediastinum, or subcutaneous tissue).

Pathogenesis

The *protease-antiprotease hypothesis* holds that alveolar wall destruction in emphysema results from imbalances between pulmonary proteases and their inhibitors:

- Individuals with hereditary deficiency of the major protease inhibitor, α_1-antitrypsin, invariably develop emphysema, and it develops at a younger age if they smoke.
- Experimental pulmonary instillation of proteolytic enzymes, including neutrophil elastase, causes emphysema.

Tobacco smoking contributes to emphysema by:

- Activating alveolar macrophages that, in turn, recruit neutrophils into the lung
- Enhancing neutrophil and macrophage elastase activity
- Inactivating α_1-antitrypsin (via oxidants in tobacco smoke or free radicals released by activated neutrophils)

Smoke particle impaction in small bronchioles leads to inflammatory cell recruitment, increased elastase, and decreased α_1-antitrypsin, resulting in the centriacinar pattern of emphysema seen in smokers.

Morphology

With diffuse disease, lungs can become voluminous and overlap the heart. Microscopically, alveolar spaces are enlarged, separated by thin septa; septal capillaries are compressed and bloodless. Alveolar wall rupture can produce very large airspaces (*blebs* and *bullae*).

Chronic Bronchitis (p. 722)

Chronic bronchitis is clinically defined as persistent cough with sputum production for at least 3 months in at least 2 consecutive years.

Pathogenesis

Chronic irritation of the airways by inhaled substances—especially tobacco smoke—is the dominant pathogenic mechanism. The irritants cause:

- Mucus hypersecretion with mucous gland hypertrophy
- Goblet cell metaplasia in bronchiolar epithelium
- Bronchiolitis

- Secondary infections maintain and promote the smoking-initiated injury

Morphology

- Hyperemia and edema of lung mucous membranes
- Mucinous secretions or casts filling airways
- Increased mucous gland size
- Bronchial or bronchiolar mucus plugging, inflammation, and fibrosis
- Squamous metaplasia or dysplasia of bronchial epithelium

Asthma (p. 723)

This chronic relapsing inflammatory disorder is characterized by paroxysmal reversible bronchospasm of tracheobronchial airways due to smooth muscle hyper-reactivity. Its incidence has increased significantly in the past 3 decades in the Western world. Asthma can be classified according to clinical severity, response to therapy, and triggering agents. Pathophysiologically, two major types are recognized:

- *Atopic (allergic, reagin-mediated) asthma* is the most common type; it is triggered by environmental antigens (e.g., dust, pollen, food), often with a family history of atopy. T-cell differentiation in these patients appears to be skewed to overproduce T_H2-type cells (see Chapter 6) with subsequent immunoglobulin E (IgE)- and eosinophil-dominated immune responses; in presensitized patients, repeat antigen exposure causes a classic type I (IgE)-mediated hypersensitivity reaction:

  In the acute phase, antigen binding to IgE-coated mast cells causes primary (e.g., leukotriene) and secondary (e.g., cytokine, neuropeptide) mediator release. The acute-phase mediators cause bronchospasm, edema, mucus secretion, and leukocyte recruitment.

  A late-phase reaction is mediated by recruited leukocytes (e.g., eosinophils, lymphocytes, neutrophils, monocytes); it is characterized by persistent bronchospasm and edema, leukocytic infiltration, and epithelial damage and loss.

- *Nonatopic asthma* (nonreaginic, nonimmune) is often triggered by respiratory tract infections, chemical irritants, or drugs, usually without a family history, and with no apparent IgE involvement. The cause of increased airway reactivity is unknown.

Morphology

Lungs are overinflated with patchy atelectasis and airway occlusion by mucus plugs. *Microscopically,* the lungs exhibit edema, bronchiolar inflammatory infiltrates with numerous eosinophils, sub-basement membrane fibrosis, and bronchial wall smooth muscle and submucosal gland hypertrophy. Whorled mucus plugs (Curschmann spirals) and crystalloid eosinophil granule debris (Charcot-Leyden crystals) deposit in airways.

Bronchiectasis (p. 727)

Bronchiectasis represents a chronic necrotizing infection of bronchi and bronchioles leading to abnormal permanent dilation of these airways. Clinical features include cough, fever, and abundant purulent sputum. In severe cases, obstructive respiratory insufficiency may be seen. Complications include cor pulmonale, metastatic abscesses, and systemic amyloidosis.

Bronchiectasis is associated with:

- Congenital or hereditary conditions (e.g., cystic fibrosis, immunodeficiency states)
- Postinfectious conditions (necrotizing bacterial, viral, or fungal pneumonia)
- Bronchial obstruction (e.g., by tumor or foreign body)
- Other conditions (e.g., rheumatoid arthritis, or chronic graft-versus-host disease)

Obstructions and infection are the major causes of bronchiectasis. With obstruction, secretions pool and become infected, leading to inflammation, necrosis, fibrosis, and irreversible airway dilation. *Allergic bronchopulmonary aspergillosis* (a hypersensitivity reaction to *Aspergillus fumigatus* with intense eosinophil-rich airway inflammation) can complicate cystic fibrosis and asthma and can cause bronchiectasis.

Morphology

The most severe changes occur in lower lobe distal airways; dilations have different shapes (*cylindrical, fusiform, or saccular*). Histology shows a spectrum of mild to necrotizing acute and chronic inflammation of the larger airways with bronchiolar fibrosis.

DIFFUSE INTERSTITIAL (INFILTRATIVE, RESTRICTIVE) DISEASES (p. 728)

These are a heterogeneous group of disorders, many of unknown etiology. There is characteristic involvement of pulmonary connective tissue, principally the alveolar interstitium, with characteristic clinical, radiologic, and pathologic changes.

- *Clinically:* Restrictive lung disease, including dyspnea, decreased lung volumes, and decreased compliance
- *Radiologically:* Diffuse infiltrates, ground-glass shadows
- *Pathologically:* Diffuse, chronic inflammation and fibrosis of alveolar interstitium, occasionally with pathognomonic findings (e.g., asbestos bodies)

Pathogenesis

- The *initial event* is epithelial or endothelial injury by inhaled or blood-borne toxins or agents.
- *Early acute* changes of alveolitis follow, consisting of chemokine-mediated recruitment of activated inflammatory cells. These cells release injurious (oxidants, cytokines) and fibrogenic (platelet-derived growth factor, fibroblast growth factor, interleukin-1) mediators.
- *Late stages* progress to interstitial fibrosis.

Fibrosing Diseases (p. 729)

Idiopathic Pulmonary Fibrosis (p. 729)

This disorder of unknown cause is *characterized by progressive pulmonary interstitial fibrosis resulting in hypoxemia.*

Repeated cycles of acute lung injury (alveolitis) are postulated to cause abnormal "wound healing" resulting in excessive fibroblast proliferation. The disease is most common between ages 40 and 70, and is typically progressive, causing pulmonary insufficiency, cor pulmonale, and cardiac failure.

Morphology

The pathologic pattern is denoted *usual interstitial pneumonia (UIP):*

- There is *patchy interstitial fibrosis,* with characteristic subpleural and interlobular septal distribution and a lower lobe predominance.
- New *fibroblastic foci,* typically in bronchiolar walls, occur within older fibrotic areas.
- Ongoing lung destruction leads to *honeycomb lung* with dense fibrosis and cystic spaces lined by hyperplastic type II pneumocytes or bronchiolar epithelium.

Nonspecific Interstitial Pneumonia (p. 731)

Nonspecific interstitial pneumonia (NSIP) is of unknown etiology. There is patchy or diffuse interstitial involvement; the histologic patterns may be either inflammatory or fibrosing. These patients have a better prognosis than those with UIP.

Cryptogenic Organizing Pneumonia (p. 731)

Formerly called *bronchiolitis obliterans organizing pneumonia (BOOP),* it may be idiopathic (cryptogenic) or may be a response to infection or inflammation.

- *Clinically,* there is cough, dyspnea, and often a recent respiratory tract infection; other etiologic associations include inhaled toxins, drugs, collagen vascular disease, or graft-versus-host disease. Many patients improve gradually or with steroid therapy.
- *Pathologically,* there are loose fibrous tissue plugs within bronchioles, alveolar ducts, and alveoli. The underlying lung is normal, although atelectatic.

Pulmonary Involvement in Collagen Vascular Diseases (p. 731)

Many collagen vascular diseases (e.g., systemic lupus erythematosus, rheumatoid arthritis, and scleroderma) can involve the lung; patterns include NSIP, UIP, vascular sclerosis, organizing pneumonia, and bronchiolitis.

Pneumoconioses (p. 732)

These disorders are caused by aerosols, including mineral dusts, organic dusts, fumes, and vapors. The following factors determine the outcome of inhalation:

- *The amount of dust retained:* This is a function of the original concentration, duration of exposure, and effectiveness of clearance mechanisms.
- *The size, shape, and buoyancy of particles:* Particles larger than 5 μm are filtered in upper airways; those smaller than 1 μm typically remain suspended and are exhaled; particles between 1 and 5 μm tend to settle in the alveoli and will be the most pathologically significant.

- *The physicochemical reactivity and solubility of particles:*
  For example, quartz can directly injure cells via free radicals on the particle surface. Highly soluble particles may
  rapidly cause toxicity; other particles may resist dissolution
  and by persisting can potentially induce a chronic fibrotic
  reaction.

Coal Workers' Pneumoconiosis (p. 733)

The range of pulmonary effects of carbon dust includes:

- *Anthracosis:* small, harmless accumulations in the lungs of
  urban dwellers and smokers.
- *Simple coal workers' pneumoconiosis* (CWP): more prominent, numerous aggregates of coal dust–laden macrophages
  forming coal *macules.* Clinical features include cough and
  blackish sputum, but no significant dysfunction is seen in
  uncomplicated cases.
- *Progressive massive fibrosis or complicated CWP:* manifested by severe fibrosis and scarring in areas of dust accumulation. This pattern reflects a much heavier dust burden
  and results in disabling respiratory insufficiency.

Factors involved in determining the progression of simple
CWP to progressive massive fibrosis include duration and magnitude of exposure and secretion of fibrogenic factors by coal
dust–laden macrophages.

Morphology
- In *simple* CWP, 1- to 5-mm black coal macules, composed of
  dust-filled macrophages are diffusely present, especially in
  the lobar upper zones.
- In *complicated* CWP, large, blackened scars replace substantial portions of the lung *(black lung disease),* especially in the
  upper zones.

Silicosis *(p. 734)*

*Prolonged inhalation of silica particles produces a chronic,
nodular, dense pulmonary fibrosis.* Sources of exposure include
mining (gold, tin, copper, coal) and quarrying, sandblasting,
metal grinding, and ceramics manufacture.
Pathogenesis. Macrophage ingestion of silica leads to activation, with release of oxidants, cytokines, and growth factors
that ultimately cause fibroblast proliferation and collagen deposition. Direct toxic effects on the macrophage can also result
in cell death with subsequent silica release—restarting the
injury cycle.
Morphology. Distinct collagenous nodules start as small
lesions in the upper lung becoming larger and more diffuse
with disease progression. Lesion coalescence forms large areas
of dense scar. Calcification or concomitant blackening by coal
dust often occurs. Microscopically, there are hyalinized whorls
of collagen with scant inflammation. Polarized light often
shows birefringent silica particles within nodules.

Asbestos-Related Diseases (p. 735)

Asbestos is a family of fibrous silicates including curled, flex-
ible *serpentines* (e.g., chrysotile) and brittle straight *amphiboles*
(e.g., crocidolite). Heavy occupational exposure causes:

- *Interstitial fibrosis (asbestosis)* that is morphologically similar
  to UIP except for the presence of numerous asbestos bodies
  (see following section) within fibrotic areas.

- *Pleural reactions,* manifested by benign effusions, fibrous pleural adhesions, and dense fibrous plaques, found on the pleura or diaphragm. The plaques can be calcified; they do not contain asbestos bodies.
- Increased risk of lung carcinoma and malignant mesothelioma.

Pathogenesis. Amphiboles (straight, stiff) reach the deep lung more than serpentine fibers, accounting for their greater pathogenicity. Inhaled fibers that reach the alveoli are ingested by alveolar macrophages, stimulating release of complement C5a and other chemoattractants. Most of the inhaled asbestos is cleared by the macrophages; the rest reaches the interstitium and lymphatics. Some ingested fibers are coated by hemosiderin and glycoproteins to form characteristic, beaded, dumbbell-shaped *asbestos bodies.*

Possible mechanisms for lung injury and progressive fibrosis include:

- Enzyme or toxic free radical release by macrophages and neutrophils recruited to sites of asbestos deposition
- Fibrogenic cytokines and growth factors released by alveolar macrophages after fiber phagocytosis
- Direct stimulation of fibroblast collagen synthesis by asbestos

Complications of Therapies (p. 737)

- *Drug-induced lung disease,* ranging from acute bronchospasm to pneumonitis to fibrosis.
- *Radiation-induced lung disease,* in which acute pneumonitis occurs 1 to 6 months after therapy (usually for thoracic tumors). The initial pathology is that of DAD; fibrosis may follow.

Granulomatous Diseases (p. 737)

Sarcoidosis (p. 737)

Sarcoidosis is a relatively common disease of unknown etiology, characterized by noncaseating granulomas in virtually any tissue. Women are affected more frequently than men, and American blacks are affected 10 times more often than whites.

Sarcoidosis may be entirely asymptomatic and discovered only incidentally at autopsy, or as bilateral hilar adenopathy on a chest radiograph. Alternatively, it can present as isolated cutaneous or ocular lesions, peripheral lymphadenopathy, or hepatosplenomegaly; with the insidious onset of respiratory difficulties or constitutional symptoms (fever, night sweats, weight loss); or with an aggressive onset accompanied by fever, erythema nodosum, and polyarthritis.

Although elevated serum IgG and calcium, characteristic chest x-ray changes, and a typical clinical history may strongly suggest the diagnosis, *sarcoidosis can be definitively established only by biopsy (often lung, liver, or lymph node) to document noncaseating granulomas.* Since other diseases (e.g., tuberculosis and fungal infections) can exhibit the same histologic features, they must be ruled out by culture or special stains; sarcoidosis is then a diagnosis of exclusion.

Pathogenesis

Genetic factors may also contribute, and the distinctive granulomatous response suggests an immune-mediated phenomenon; several immune abnormalities may be seen:

- Lymphocytic alveolitis, with numerous activated CD4+ T cells (MHC expression), with increased T_H1 cytokine production (interleukin-2 and interferon-γ) cause macrophage activation.
- Cutaneous anergy may be caused by multiple agents that normally induce a local delayed hypersensitivity reaction (e.g., tuberculin).
- Polyclonal hypergammaglobulinemia may be seen.
- Activated helper T cells and their secreted cytokines account for the influx of monocytes, as well as the subsequent granulomas and cell-mediated injury.
- Elevated circulating γ-δ T cells (associated with mycobacterial disease) and (occasionally) positive polymerase chain reaction assays for mycobacterial DNA in sarcoidal tissue have revived interest in an underlying infectious cause; nevertheless, the etiology remains unknown.

Morphology

Other than organomegaly (liver, spleen, lymph nodes), no distinctive macroscopic change is apparent in sarcoidosis. The granulomas are characteristically composed of tightly clustered epithelioid histiocytes, often including multinucleated giant cells; there is rarely central necrosis. In 60% of granulomas *Schaumann bodies* (laminated, calcified proteinaceous concretions) and *asteroid bodies* (stellate inclusions within giant cells) occur.

- *Lung* is a common site of involvement. Diffuse, scattered granulomas (forming a reticulonodular pattern on x-rays) are not grossly apparent except for foci where they coalesce. Pulmonary lesions tend to heal, so only residual hyalinized scars may be seen.
- *Lymph nodes* are virtually always involved, most commonly in the hilar and mediastinal regions. Tonsils are affected 25% to 33% of the time.
- *Spleen and liver* are microscopically affected in 75% of patients. Splenomegaly occurs in only 20% and hepatomegaly is rarer.
- *Skin* is involved in 33% to 50% of patients, as discrete subcutaneous nodules, erythematous scaling plaques, and mucous membrane lesions.
- *Eyes* are affected in 20% to 50% of cases, as iritis, iridocyclitis, or choroid retinitis.
- *Skeletal muscle* involvement is often underdiagnosed since it may be asymptomatic.

Clinical Features

Sarcoidosis follows an unpredictable course:

- It can be slowly progressive.
- It may pursue a remitting and resolving course (with or without steroid therapy).
- It can spontaneously resolve.
- In 65% to 70% of patients, there are no or only minimal residual manifestations; 20% have permanent lung or ocular dysfunction; and 10% of patients die, primarily from progressive pulmonary fibrosis.

Hypersensitivity (Allergic) Pneumonitis
(p. 739)

This immunologically mediated disorder is caused by inhaled dusts or antigens:

- *Farmer's lung:* spores of thermophilic actinomycetes in hay
- *Pigeon breeder's lung:* proteins from bird feathers or excreta
- Humidifier or air-conditioner lung: thermophilic bacteria

Histologic changes include bronchiolocentric interstitial pneumonitis and fibrosis and a variable number of noncaseating, loosely formed granulomas. Early cessation of exposure to the injurious agent prevents progression to serious chronic fibrosis. The clinical manifestations are varied and include cough, dyspnea, fever, diffuse and nodular radiographic densities, and a restrictive pattern of pulmonary dysfunction.

Pulmonary Eosinophilia (p. 740)

Pulmonary eosinophilia refers to diverse clinicopathologic conditions characterized by eosinophil infiltrates in pulmonary interstitial or alveolar spaces:

- *Acute eosinophilic pneumonia* with respiratory failure: etiology unknown
- *Simple pulmonary eosinophilia (Loeffler syndrome):* etiology uncertain; transient, benign infiltrates with prominent eosinophilia in blood and lung
- *Tropical eosinophilia:* caused by microfilariae
- *Secondary eosinophilia:* induced by infections, hypersensitivity, asthma, and allergic bronchopulmonary aspergillosis
- *Idiopathic chronic eosinophilic pneumonia:* unknown etiology; manifested by focal lung consolidation with extensive lymphocyte and eosinophil infiltration

Acute and idiopathic chronic eosinophilic pneumonias are generally steroid responsive.

Smoking-Related Interstitial Diseases (p. 740)

Desquamative Interstitial Pneumonia (p. 740)

Desquamative interstitial pneumonia is characterized by large intra-alveolar collections of dusty brown (smokers') macrophages with mild interstitial inflammation and minimal fibrosis. Emphysema is often present. Steroid therapy or smoking cessation yields improvement.

Respiratory Bronchiolitis-Associated Interstitial Lung Disease (p. 740)

This disease causes a gradual development of mild but significant pulmonary symptoms, with abnormal pulmonary function and imaging. Cessation of smoking results in improvement.

Pulmonary Alveolar Proteinosis (p. 741)

Pulmonary alveolar proteinosis (PAP) is a rare entity occurring in three forms:

- *Acquired PAP* accounts for 90% of cases. Autoimmune anti-GM-CSF (granulocyte-macrophage colony-stimulating

factor) antibodies may be pathogenic, leading ultimately to impaired surfactant clearance by pulmonary macrophages.
- *Congenital PAP* occurs in newborns and is rapidly fatal.
- *Secondary PAP* follows exposure to irritating dusts or chemicals, or occurs in immunosuppressed individuals.

PAP is characterized *clinically* by respiratory difficulty, cough, and sputum containing gelatinous material; *radiologically* by diffuse pulmonary opacification; and *histologically* by accumulation of dense, amorphous, periodic acid–Schiff (PAS)-positive, lipid-laden material in intra-alveolar spaces. The alveolar protein exudate consists largely of granular acellular surfactant and cholesterol clefts.

DISEASES OF VASCULAR ORIGIN (p. 742)

Pulmonary Embolism, Hemorrhage, and Infarction (p. 742; see also Chapter 4)

Pulmonary artery occlusions are almost always embolic; *in situ* thromboses are rare, but can occur in DAD, pulmonary hypertension, and pulmonary atherosclerosis. Deep leg veins are the source of over 95% of pulmonary emboli (PE) and the prevalence of PE correlates with predisposition to leg thrombosis. The autopsy incidence of PE ranges from 1% in the general population to 30% in hospitalized patients with severe burns, trauma, fractures, or cancer.
- Large emboli (about 5% of PE) impact in the major pulmonary arteries or astride the pulmonary artery bifurcation *(saddle embolus):*
  Large emboli frequently cause instantaneous death.
  They can cause cardiovascular collapse (e.g., acute *cor pulmonale* [right-sided heart failure]). Multiple or recurrent small emboli can have the same effect.
  Hemodynamic compromise is due not only to vascular obstruction, but also to reflex vasoconstriction caused by agents such as thromboxane A_2.
- Small emboli are involved in 60% to 80% of cases of PE:
  Small emboli can be clinically silent in patients without cardiovascular failure.
  They can cause transient chest pain and sometimes hemoptysis from pulmonary hemorrhage.
  In patients with compromised pulmonary circulation (cardiac failure), PE can cause pulmonary infarctions, manifest as peripheral, wedge-shaped hemorrhagic areas of necrosis.
- Middle-sized emboli (about 20%–35% of PE) occlude moderate-sized peripheral pulmonary arteries and usually induce hemorrhage or infarction.
- Uncommonly, multiple small PE (overt or covert) produce right-sided heart strain (chronic cor pulmonale) and eventually pulmonary hypertension and vascular sclerosis.

Clinical Significance

Diagnosis of PE is often difficult; many are silent. Roughly 65% (even those causing pulmonary infarction or death) are diagnosed only postmortem. Even without treatment (provided the patient lives), perfusion typically improves within 24 hours owing to fibrinolysis and thrombus contraction. The embolus can completely resolve or be reduced to a fibrous mural plaque within weeks or months; infarcts will be converted to a fibrous scar. With diagnosis and fibrinolytic agents, improvement is greatly speeded, and mortality rates may be reduced to 5% to 10%.

Pulmonary Hypertension (p. 743)

Elevated pulmonary artery pressure is caused by increased pulmonary vascular resistance. Most commonly, pulmonary hypertension is secondary to:

- Chronic obstructive or interstitial lung disease
- Congenital or acquired heart disease with left-sided heart failure
- Recurrent PE
- Autoimmune disorders

Primary (or idiopathic) pulmonary hypertension is uncommon, typically occurring in women 20 to 40 years old; it generally progresses to severe respiratory insufficiency, cor pulmonale, and death over several years. Therapies include vasodilators and occasionally lung transplantation. The cause is unknown in the majority; however, in 50% of familial cases and 25% of sporadic disease, mutations in the bone morphogenetic protein receptor type 2 are pathogenic. In *secondary pulmonary hypertension*, endothelial dysfunction and injury (triggered by chemical or dietary agents) lead to persistent vasoconstriction, with subsequent intimal and medial hypertrophy and increased vascular resistance.

Morphology

Vascular lesions include:

- Atheromas in large elastic arteries
- Intimal fibrosis or medial hypertrophy in medium-sized muscular arteries and smaller arterioles
- So-called *plexogenic arteriopathy* (tufts within capillary channels creating a vascular plexus), seen in primary pulmonary hypertension and with some congenital cardiovascular anomalies
- Numerous organized thrombi, suggesting recurrent pulmonary thromboembolism as an etiology

Diffuse Pulmonary Hemorrhage Syndromes (p. 745)

Pulmonary hemorrhage is a serious complication of some interstitial lung diseases, particularly the so-called *pulmonary hemorrhage syndromes:*

- *Goodpasture syndrome:* This necrotizing, hemorrhagic interstitial pneumonitis with progressive glomerulonephritis is caused by circulating autoantibodies against basement membrane antigens in lungs and kidneys. It is more common in men and in smokers.
- *Idiopathic pulmonary hemosiderosis:* This rare disease of children, of unknown cause, with intermittent diffuse alveolar hemorrhage, responds to immunosuppression, leaving residual prominent hemosiderin deposition and variable fibrosis.

- *Vasculitis-associated hemorrhage:* This form is seen with *Wegener granulomatosis,* systemic lupus erythematosus, and hypersensitivity angiitis.

PULMONARY INFECTIONS (p. 747)

Pulmonary infections occur when lung or systemic defenses are impaired. Pulmonary defenses include nasal, tracheo-bronchial, and alveolar mechanisms to filter, neutralize, and clear inhaled organisms and particles:

- Decreased cough reflex leading to aspiration (seen in coma, anesthesia, drug effects)
- Injury to mucociliary apparatus (as with cigarette or other inhalations)
- Decreased phagocytic or bactericidal function of the alveolar macrophage (owing to alcohol, tobacco, oxygen toxicity)
- Edema or congestion (congestive heart failure)
- Secretion accumulation
- Defects in innate or specific immunity

Pneumonias are classified by the specific etiologic agent or the clinical setting (Table 15–3). In the latter, the implicated pathogens are specific to each category.

Community-Acquired Acute Pneumonias
(p. 748)

These pneumonias may be bacterial or viral (viral are considered under *atypical pneumonias,* discussed later). Bacterial infections occur in two frequently overlapping morphologic patterns *(bronchopneumonia* and *lobar pneumonia)* and are caused by various gram-positive or gram-negative organisms. Depending on bacterial virulence and host resistance, the same organism can cause bronchopneumonia, lobar pneumonia, or something intermediate.

- *Streptococcus pneumoniae,* or *pneumococcus,* is the most common organism; gram-positive, lancet-shaped diplococci within neutrophils.
- *Haemophilus influenzae* are pleomorphic, gram-negative, encapsulated (six serotypes) or unencapsulated (untypable) bacteria; they cause life-threatening lower respiratory tract infections and meningitis in children and are a common cause of pneumonia in adults, especially those with COPD. An effective vaccine is widely available.
- *Moraxella catarrhalis* causes bacterial pneumonia, especially in the elderly; this infection exacerbates COPD and is a common cause of otitis media in children.
- *Staphylococcus aureus* pneumonia often complicates viral illnesses and infects intravenous drug abusers; infection results in abscess and empyema.
- *Klebsiella pneumoniae* is the most common cause of gram-negative pneumonia; it afflicts debilitated individuals, especially chronic alcoholics.
- *Pseudomonas aeruginosa* is common in cystic fibrosis and neutropenic patients.
- *Legionella pneumophilia* spreads through aerosolization; infection causes severe pneumonia in the immunocompromised patient.

TABLE 15-3 **The Pneumonia Syndromes**

Community-Acquired Acute Pneumonia

Streptococcus pneumoniae
Haemophilus influenzae
Moraxella catarrhalis
Staphylococcus aureus
Legionella pneumophilia
Enterobacteriaceae *(Klebsiella pneumoniae)* and *Pseudomonas* spp.

Community-Acquired Atypical Pneumonia

Mycoplasma pneumoniae
Chlamydia spp. *(C. pneumoniae, C. psittaci, C. trachomatis)*
Coxiella burnetti (Q fever)
Viruses: respiratory syncytial virus, parainfluenzavirus (children); influenzavirus A and B (adults); adenovirus (military recruits); SARS* virus

Nosocomial Pneumonia

Gram-negative rods belonging to Enterobacteriaceae *(Klebsiella* spp., *Serratia marcescens, Escherichia coli)* and Pseudomonas spp.
Staphylococcus aureus (usually penicillin-resistant)

Aspiration Pneumonia

Anaerobic oral flora *(Bacteroides, Prevotella, Fusobacterium, Peptostreptococcus),* admixed with aerobic bacteria *(Streptococcus pneumoniae, Staphylococcus aureus, Haemophilas influenzae,* and *Pseudomonas aeruginosa)*

Chronic Pneumonia

Nocardia
Actinomyces
Granulomatous: *Mycobacterium tuberculosis* and atypical mycobacteria, *Histoplasma capsulatum, Coccidioides immitis, Blastomyces dermatitidis*

Necrotizing Pneumonia and Lung Abscess

Anaerobic bacteria (extremely common), with or without mixed aerobic infection
Staphylococcus aureus, Klebsiella pneumoniae, Streptococcus pyogenes, and type 3 pneumococcus (uncommon)

Pneumonia in the Immunocompromised Host

Cytomegalovirus
Pneumocystis jiroveci (carinii)
Mycobacterium avium-intracellulare
Invasive aspergillosis
Invasive candidiasis
"Usual" baterial, viral, and fungal organisms (listed above)

*SARS, severe acute respiratory syndrome.

Morphology

- *Bronchopneumonia is marked by patchy exudative consolidation of lung parenchyma:* staphylococci, pneumococci, *Haemophilus influenzae, Pseudomonas aeruginosa,* and coliform bacteria are the most common agents. Grossly, the lungs show dispersed, elevated, focal areas of palpable consolidation and suppuration. Histologically, there is acute (neutrophilic) suppurative exudation filling airways and airspaces, usually around bronchi and bronchioles. Resolution of the exudate usually restores normal lung structure, but organization with fibrous scarring can occur, or aggressive disease can produce abscesses.
- *Lobar pneumonia involves a large portion of or an entire lobe of lung.* Most lobar pneumonias are caused by pneumococci

entering the lungs via the airways. Occasionally, they are caused by other organisms (*K. pneumoniae,* staphylococci, streptococci, *H. influenzae*).

Stages of Disease. The following sequence of stages portray the natural history of uncomplicated lobar pneumonia; such *classic* pneumonia is now seen infrequently due to antibiotic therapy:

- *Congestion* predominates in the first 24 hours.
- *Red hepatization* (consolidation) describes lung tissue with confluent exudates of neutrophils and red blood cells, giving a red, firm, liverlike gross appearance.
- *Gray hepatization* follows, as the red blood cells disintegrate and the remaining fibrinosuppurative exudate persists, giving a gray-brown gross appearance.
- *Resolution* is the favorable final stage in which consolidated exudate undergoes enzymatic and cellular degradation and clearance. Normal structure is restored.

Complications

Complications of lobar pneumonia, and sometimes bronchopneumonia, are:

- Abscess formation
- Empyema (spread of infection to pleural cavity)
- Organization of exudate into fibrotic scar tissue
- Bacteremia and sepsis, with infection of other organs

Community-Acquired Atypical (Viral and Mycoplasmal) Pneumonias (p. 751)

Infections by viruses (e.g., *influenza A* or *B, respiratory syncytial virus, adenovirus, rhinovirus, herpes simplex, cytomegalovirus*) or *Mycoplasma pneumoniae* range from relatively mild upper respiratory tract involvements (e.g., the common cold) to severe lower respiratory tract disease.

Morphology

Patchy or lobar areas of congestion are seen *without* the consolidation of bacterial pneumonias (hence the term *atypical pneumonia*). Other findings are as follows:

- Predominant interstitial pneumonitis with widened, edematous alveolar walls containing mononuclear inflammatory cell infiltrates may be seen.
- *Hyaline membranes* reflect diffuse alveolar damage.
- Frequent, superimposed bacterial infection is seen.
- Certain viruses cause necrosis of bronchial or alveolar epithelium in severe infections (herpes simplex, adenovirus, varicella); in some, characteristic cytopathic changes occur (e.g., cytomegaly and nuclear inclusions in cytomegalovirus infection).

Influenza Infections (p. 751)

Type A influenzaviruses infect humans and are the major cause of influenza epidemics through viral mutations. Types B and C do not mutate; consequently, childhood infections result in largely life-long antibody-mediated protection against future disease.

Severe Acute Respiratory Syndrome (p. 752)

Severe acute respiratory syndrome (SARS) first appeared in China in November 2002 before spreading to other countries. One-third of patients recover; the remainder progress to severe respiratory disease and nearly 10% die. It is caused by a previously unknown coronavirus, spread mainly through infected respiratory secretions. The lungs show DAD with multinucleated giant cells; virus can be visualized by electron microscopy.

Nosocomial Pneumonia (p. 752)

Nosocomial pneumonia is defined as infection acquired during hospitalization. These pneumonias occur in patients with severe underlying disease or invasive access devices, and are serious life-threatening complications.

Aspiration Pneumonia (p. 752)

Aspiration pneumonia occurs in markedly debilitated or unconscious patients; it results in partly chemical (gastric acid) and partly bacterial (mixed oral flora) pneumonia.

Lung Abscess (p. 753)

Lung abscess is an infection marked by localized suppurative necrosis of lung tissue. Commonly involved are staphylococci, streptococci, numerous gram-negative species, and anaerobes. Mixed infections are frequent, reflecting aspiration of oral contents as a common etiology. Abscesses can be due to:

- Aspiration of infective material, as in oropharyngeal surgical procedures or aspiration secondary to diminished consciousness from coma, drugs, anesthesia, or seizures. Aspiration abscesses are more common on the right, reflecting the more vertical right bronchus.
- Antecedent primary bacterial infection.
- Septic emboli from infected thrombi or right-sided cardiac valve vegetations.
- Obstructive tumors.
- Direct traumatic punctures.
- Spread of infection from adjacent organs.

Complications include extension into the pleural cavity, hemorrhage, septic embolization, and secondary amyloidosis.

Morphology

Abscesses vary in number (single or multiple) and size (microscopic to many centimeters). They contain variable mixtures of pus and air, depending on available drainage through airways. Chronic abscesses are often surrounded by a reactive fibrous wall.

Chronic Pneumonia (p. 753)

Chronic pneumonia is typically a localized granulomatous inflammation in immunocompetent patients, with or without regional lymph node involvement. In the immunocompromised, the infection may become disseminated. Tuberculosis is described in Chapter 8.

Histoplasmosis (p. 754)

Acquired by inhalation, histoplasmosis is endemic along the Ohio and Mississippi Rivers and in the Caribbean. Infection by *Histoplasma capsulatum* produces granulomas with coagulative necrosis that subsequently undergo fibrosis and concentric calcification. Silver stain identifies the 3- to 5-μm thin-walled cyst of the fungus, which can persist for years.

Blastomycosis (p. 755)

Blastomycosis occurs in the central and southeastern United States, Canada, Mexico, the Middle East, Africa, and India. *Blastomyces dermatidis* is a 5- to 15-μm thick-walled yeast that divides by broad-based budding; it causes suppurative granulomas.

Coccidioidomycosis (p. 755)

Coccidioidomycosis is endemic in the Southwest and western United States and Mexico. *Coccidioides immitis* causes lesions varying from pyogenic to granulomatous; silver stains demonstrate a 20- to 60-μm thick-walled spherule containing small endospores.

Pneumonia in the Immunocompromised Host (p. 755)

Opportunistic infections (bacteria, viruses, and fungi) rarely cause infection in normal hosts, but can cause life-threatening pneumonias in the immunocompromised host. Often, more than one agent is involved.

Pulmonary Disease in Human Immunodeficiency Virus Infection (p. 756)

In these patients pulmonary disease may be due to more than one cause and symptoms may be atypical; the CD4+ T-cell count can define the risk of infection with specific organisms.
* In addition to opportunistic infections, the usual bacterial pathogens cause severe disease.
* Malignancies (Kaposi sarcoma, lymphoma, lung cancer) also cause pulmonary disease.

LUNG TRANSPLANTATION (p. 756)

Lung transplantation is typically performed in otherwise healthy patients for emphysema, idiopathic pulmonary fibrosis, cystic fibrosis, and primary pulmonary hypertension. Complications include infections (similar to those in other immunocompromised patients), acute rejection (vascular and airway inflammatory infiltrates), and chronic rejection *(bronchiolitis obliterans)*. One- and 6-year survival rates are 90% and 54%, respectively.

TUMORS (p. 757)

Carcinomas (p. 757)

Carcinomas constitute 90% to 95% of lung tumors; they are the most common cause of cancer death in both men and women.

Pathogenesis

Tobacco smoking is well established as the most important etiologic factor in lung cancer development.

- *Statistically,* there is an unequivocal link between lung cancer frequency and number of smoking pack-years.
- *Clinically,* hyperplastic and atypical changes occur in the bronchial epithelium of smokers and in the vicinity of bronchial cancer.
- *Experimentally,* numerous cigarette smoke carcinogens (e.g., polycyclic aromatic hydrocarbons) are known, although bronchogenic cancers are not readily induced by inhalation in experimental animals.
- *Environmental exposures* include radiation (e.g., radon), asbestos (especially combined with smoking), air pollution (particulates), and occupational inhaled substances (e.g., nickel, chromates, arsenic).
- *Genetic mechanisms* include dominant oncogenes (*c-MYC, K-RAS, EGFR,* and *HER-2/neu*) and loss of tumor-suppressor genes (e.g., *p53, RB, p16^{INK4a}*).

Precursor Lesions

Three types of precursor lesions are recognized: squamous dysplasia and carcinoma *in situ,* atypical adenomatous hyperplasia, and diffuse idiopathic pulmonary neuroendocrine cell hyperplasia.

Classification

Lung carcinomas are classified by their predominant histologic appearance (Table 15–4), although the most relevant clinical grouping is *small cell* versus *non–small cell carcinoma.*

- *Adenocarcinoma* is the most common lung cancer. It typically presents as a peripheral mass, with characteristic micro-

TABLE 15–4 **Histologic Classification of Malignant Epithelial Lung Tumors**

Squamous cell carcinoma
Small cell carcinoma
　Combined small cell carcinoma
Adenocarcinoma
　Acinar, papillary, bronchioloalveolar, solid, mixed subtypes
Large cell carcinoma
　Large cell neuroendocrine carcinoma
Adenosquamous carcinoma
Carcinomas with pleomorphic, sarcomatoid, or sarcomatous elements
Carcinoid tumor
　Typical, atypical
Carcinomas of salivary gland type
Unclassified carcinoma

scopic features including gland formation—usually producing mucin—and an adjacent desmoplastic response.

- *Bronchioloalveolar carcinoma* is an uncommon form of adenocarcinoma arising in the terminal bronchioloalveolar regions. Grossly, there may be single or multiple nodules or a diffuse, pneumonia-like tumor consolidation. Histologically, there are distinctive tall, columnar, often mucin-producing tumor cells arrayed along preserved alveolar septa, and forming papillary projections. Clinically, these occur equally in men and women and are not usually associated with smoking. Prognosis is relatively favorable after solitary nodule resection, but dismal in diffuse disease.
- *Squamous cell carcinoma* has the closest correlation with smoking. Most arise in or near the lung hilus. Microscopically, they vary from well-differentiated keratinizing neoplasms to anaplastic tumors with only focal squamous differentiation.
- *Small cell carcinoma* is the most malignant of lung cancers and usually presents as a central or hilar tumor. It is strongly associated with cigarette smoking. The characteristic microscopic features include nests or clusters of small, *oatlike* cells with little cytoplasm, and without squamous or glandular differentiation. Ultrastructurally the cancer cells can exhibit neurosecretory granules and immunohistochemical stains usually demonstrate neuroendocrine markers. These tumors most often produce *paraneoplastic syndromes* (described later).
- *Large cell carcinoma* probably represents poorly differentiated squamous cell carcinomas or adenocarcinomas. There may be peculiar histologic variants (e.g., with giant cells, clear cells, or spindle cells).

Clinical Features

Lung carcinomas usually present with cough, weight loss, chest pain, and dyspnea. Outcome depends on stage at presentation. Overall 5-year survival rate is 15%; surgical resection of solitary (non–small cell) tumors (a minority of patients) has better survival rate (48%). Small cell carcinoma has almost always metastasized by the time of diagnosis, precluding surgical intervention. It is responsive to chemotherapy but ultimately recurs. Other types show disappointing responses to chemotherapy.

Paraneoplastic syndromes associated with lung carcinoma result from tumor release of:

- Antidiuretic hormone (syndrome of inappropriate antidiuretic hormone)
- Corticotropin (Cushing syndrome)
- Parathormone or prostaglandin E (hypercalcemia)
- Calcitonin (hypocalcemia)
- Gonadotropins (gynecomastia)
- Serotonin (carcinoid syndrome)

Other paraneoplastic syndromes include myopathy, peripheral neuropathy, acanthosis nigricans, and hypertrophic pulmonary osteoarthropathy (finger clubbing).

Neuroendocrine Proliferations and Tumors
(p. 764)

Carcinoid Tumors (p. 764)

Carcinoid tumors (1%–5% of all lung tumors) have neuroendocrine differentiation. The tumors are subclassified into *typical* (low-grade, 87% 10-year survival rate) and *atypical* (more mitoses and necrosis, 56% 5-year and 35% 10-year survival rates) tumors.

Grossly the tumors are usually intrabronchial, highly vascular, polypoid masses less than 3 or 4 cm. Microscopically, there are nests and cords of uniform, small, round cells resembling intestinal carcinoids. Occasional tumors show atypia, mitoses, or pleomorphism. Neurosecretory granules are seen ultrastructurally, and neuroendocrine differentiation is confirmed by immunostaining for neuron-specific enolase, serotonin, calcitonin, or bombesin.

Miscellaneous Tumors (p. 765)

Hamartomas are relatively common, benign, nodular neoplasms composed of cartilage and other mesenchymal tissues (e.g., fat, blood vessels, fibrous tissue). *Mediastinal tumors* arise from local structures or may represent metastatic disease (Table 15–5).

Metastatic Tumors (p. 765)

Secondary involvement of the lung by metastatic tumor is common and can occur via direct extension from contiguous organs, or lymphatics or hematogenous routes. Patterns of disease include discrete masses or nodules, growth within peribronchial lymphatics *(lymphangitis carcinomatosa),* and (rarely) multiple tumor microemboli.

TABLE 15–5 **Mediastinal Tumors and Other Masses**

Superior Mediastinum
Lymphoma
Thymoma
Thyroid lesions
Metastatic carcinoma
Parathyroid tumors

Anterior Mediastinum
Thymoma
Teratoma
Lymphoma
Thyroid lesions
Parathyroid tumors

Posterior Mediastinum
Neurogenic tumors (schwannoma, neurofibroma)
Lymphoma
Gastroenteric hernia

Middle Mediastinum
Bronchogenic cyst
Pericardial cyst
Lymphoma

PLEURA (p. 766)

Most pleural lesions are secondary to underlying lung disease.

Pleural Effusions (p. 766)

Accumulations of transudate (hydrothorax) or serous exudate occur with:

- Increased hydrostatic pressure (e.g., heart failure)
- Increased vascular permeability (e.g., pneumonia)
- Decreased oncotic pressure (e.g., nephrotic syndrome)
- Increased negative intrapleural pressure (e.g., atelectasis)
- Decreased lymphatic drainage (e.g., carcinomatosis)

Inflammatory Pleural Effusions (p. 766)

Various patterns may be seen:

- *Serofibrinous pleuritis* reflects pulmonary inflammation (e.g., tuberculosis, pneumonia, infarcts, abscesses, or systemic diseases [e.g., rheumatoid arthritis, uremia]).
- *Suppurative pleuritis* or empyema usually reflects pleural space infection leading to pus accumulation.
- *Hemorrhagic pleuritis* occurs with bleeding disorders, neoplastic involvement, and certain rickettsial diseases.

Organization of these exudates with dense fibrous adhesions can affect lung expansion.

Noninflammatory Pleural Effusions (p. 767)

Other pleural fluid accumulations include hemothorax (a fatal complication of a ruptured aortic aneurysm) and chylothorax (a collection of milky lymph fluid, usually with neoplastic lymphatic obstruction).

Pneumothorax (p. 767)

Pneumothorax refers to air or gas in the pleural cavity. Pneumothorax can be traumatic (e.g., after rib fractures that puncture the lung) or spontaneous, occurring after peripheral apical bleb rupture. *Tension pneumothorax* occurs when lung and mediastinal structures are compressed by the collected air and represents a serious, potentially fatal complication.

Pleural Tumors (p. 768)

Most common pleural tumors are metastases from lung, breast, ovaries, or other organs. Metastases often cause malignant effusions containing cytologically detectable tumor cells.

Solitary (Localized) Fibrous Tumors (p. 768)

These noninvasive, fibrosing, rarely malignant tumors are composed of pleural fibroblasts; they also occur in other sites and are not related to asbestos exposure. Resection is usually curative.

Malignant Mesothelioma (p. 768)

This uncommon tumor of mesothelial cells occurs most often in the pleura (less frequently in the peritoneum or other sites). It is associated with occupational exposure to asbestos in 90% of cases; only 20% of these patients have pulmonary asbestosis. The lifetime risk (not affected by smoking) in heavily exposed individuals is 7% to 10%, with a latency period between exposure and tumor development of 25 to 45 years. Among asbestos workers, *carcinoma remains the most common lung tumor;* the risk of lung carcinoma is markedly increased by concomitant smoking.

Clinical Features

Patients present with chest pain, dyspnea, and recurrent pleural effusion. Mesotheliomas are highly malignant tumors that invade the lung and can metastasize widely. Few patients survive longer than 2 years.

Morphology

Tumor spreads diffusely over the lung surface and fissures, forming an encasing sheath. Microscopic patterns are *epithelioid* (70%), *sarcomatoid* (20%), and mixed *(biphasic)* (10%) tumors.

- *Epithelioid pattern* shows epithelium-like cells forming tubules and papillary projections resembling adenocarcinomas. Antigenic (calretinin, WT-1 and CK5/6 positivity) and ultrastructural (long, slender microvilli) features allow distinction from adenocarcinomas (MOC31 and BG8 positivity and short, plump microvilli).
- *Sarcomatoid pattern* shows malignant, spindle-shaped cells resembling fibrosarcoma.

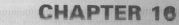
Head and Neck

ORAL CAVITY (p. 774)

Teeth and Supporting Structures (p. 774)

Caries (tooth decay) (p. 774) is focal tooth degradation due to mineral dissolution; it occurs through acids released by oral bacteria during sugar fermentation. Caries is a common worldwide disease and the most common reason for tooth loss before age 35.

Gingivitis (p. 775) is inflammation of the soft tissues around teeth typically resulting from inadequate oral hygiene (causing dental plaque and calculus accumulation). Therapy involves reducing etiologic factors to allow gingival healing.

Periodontitis (p. 775) is an inflammation affecting tooth-supporting structures (e.g., periodontal ligaments, alveolar bone, and cementum). Periodontitis can progress to complete destruction of the periodontal ligament and alveolar bone, with tooth loss.

- While typically presenting in isolation, periodontal disease can also occur in several systemic diseases, including AIDS (acquired immunodeficiency syndrome), Crohn's disease, diabetes mellitus, hemochromatosis, sarcoidosis, and syndromes associated with neutrophil defects.
- Conversely, periodontal infections can be causal in systemic diseases (e.g., infective endocarditis, pulmonary and brain abscesses, and adverse pregnancy outcomes).

Inflammatory/Reactive Lesions (p. 775)

Reactive Lesions (p. 775)

For the following benign reactive lesions, surgical excisions are usually curative:

401

- *Irritation fibroma* is the most common (61% of all the reactive lesions); it can occur throughout the oral cavity, but is most common along the "bite line." It is essentially fibrous tissue covered by squamous mucosa.
- *Pyogenic granulomas* (12%) are highly vascular lesions similar to granulation tissue.
- *Peripheral ossifying fibroma* (22%) can arise through maturation of pyogenic granulomas, although most have unknown etiologies. They are red, ulcerated nodular gingival lesions; even with surgical excision to the periosteum, there is 15% to 20% recurrence.
- *Peripheral giant cell granuloma (giant cell epulis)* (5%) is a striking aggregation of multinucleated foreign body–like giant cells separated by fibroangiomatous stroma.

Apthous Ulcers (Canker Sores) (p. 776)

Apthous ulcers are extremely common lesions (40% of the U.S. population); they are painful and tend to be recurrent with a familial predilection, although the etiology is unknown. Lesions are shallow, hyperemic ulcerations initially infiltrated by mononuclear inflammatory cells; secondary bacterial infection recruits neutrophils.

Glossitis (p. 776)

Glossitis implies tongue inflammation, but is more commonly applied to the "beefy-red" tongues of certain deficiency states. The latter appearance is due to papillae atrophy with mucosal thinning and therefore more apparent vasculature; it occurs in sprue and in vitamin B_{12}, riboflavin, niacin, iron, and pyridoxine deficiencies.

Infections (p. 776)

Normal oral mucosa resists infections due to competitive suppression from low-virulence commensal organisms, high levels of immunoglobulin A, the antibacterial properties of saliva, and dilution from ingested food and liquids. Imbalance of these protective mechanisms (e.g., due to antibiotics) contributes to infections.

Herpes Simplex Virus Infections (p. 776)

Herpes simplex virus (HSV) type 1 (and sometimes HSV2) infections cause "cold sores"; they also cause a severe infection called *acute herpetic gingivostomatitis,* seen in children. Lesions consist of vesicles, large bullae, or shallow ulcerations. Histologically, there is intra- and intercellular edema *(acantholysis),* eosinophilic intranuclear inclusions, and giant cells. Vesicles heal spontaneously in 3 to 4 weeks; reactivation frequently occurs with crops of small vesicles that clear in 4 to 6 days.

Oral Candidiasis (Thrush) (p. 777)

Oral candidiasis presents as superficial gray-white inflammatory membranes comprising fungus in a fibrinosuppurative exudate. It occurs with diabetes, neutropenia, or immunodeficiency.

Oral Manifestations of Systemic Disease
(p. 777)

Characteristic oral lesions occur in:
* Infections (e.g., scarlet fever, measles, and infectious mononucleosis)
* Dermatologic conditions (e.g., lichen planus and erythema multiforme)
* Hematologic disorders (e.g., pancytopenias and leukemias, especially monocytic leukemia)
* Miscellaneous conditions

    Melanotic pigmentations of Addison disease and pregnancy

    Fibrous gingival enlargement of chronic phenytoin (Dilantin) ingestion

    Telangiectasias of Rendu-Osler-Weber syndrome

Hairy Leukoplakia (p. 777)

Hairy leukoplakia is a distinctive oral lesion seen in immunocompromised patients (80% have human immunodeficiency virus [HIV] infection); caused by Epstein-Barr virus (EBV), the lesions are white patches of fluffy ("hairy") hyperkeratosis on tongue lateral borders. Occasionally, superimposed candidal infections augment the "hairiness."

Tumors and Precancerous Lesions (p. 778)

Leukoplakia and Erythroplakia (p. 778)

Both are associated with chronic tobacco use.

* *Leukoplakia* is the clinical term for a white plaque on the oral mucous membranes that cannot be removed by scraping and cannot be classified as another disease entity. Thus defined, lesions vary from benign epithelial thickenings to highly atypical dysplasia that merges into carcinoma *in situ*. Leukoplakic lesions occur in 3% of individuals; 5% to 25% are premalignant. Thus, until proved otherwise, leukoplakia should be considered precancerous.
* *Erythroplakia* is a red, velvety, relatively flat lesion; it is less common than leukoplakia but more ominous because the epithelium is markedly atypical and has greater risk of malignant transformation.

Squamous Cell Carcinoma (p. 780)

Squamous cell carcinoma constitutes 95% of oral cancers; these are typically diagnosed between ages 50 and 70, most commonly in the mouth floor, tongue, soft palate, and tongue base. Lesions can be raised, firm, ulcerated, or verrucous; histologically, they are typical squamous carcinomas of variable differentiation. They tend to infiltrate locally before metastasizing, particularly to cervical lymph nodes, lungs, liver, and bones. Prognosis is best with lip lesions, and poorest with mouth floor and tongue base lesions (20%–30% 5-year survival rate).

Pathogenesis

* Tobacco and alcohol are the most common associations; smokers can have 15-fold greater risk (than nonsmokers) of malignancy.

- Human papillomavirus (HPV) types 6, 16, and 18 are implicated in 10% to 15% of cases.
- Betel nut and paan chewing are important causes in India and parts of Asia.
- Genetic factors may also play a role (deletions in chromosomes 18q, 10p, 8p, and 3p are implicated).

Odontogenic Cysts (p. 782)

These epithelium-lined cysts in the mandible and maxilla are derived from odontogenic epithelium remnants; they may be either inflammatory or developmental.

- *Dentigerous cysts* originate near crowns of unerupted teeth and may result from dental follicle separation. They are unilocular lesions and are most often associated with impacted third molars. Complete removal is curative.
- *Odontogenic keratocyst (OKC)* is important to distinguish owing to its aggressive potential. Treatment requires complete resection (recurrence rates of 60%). Patients with multiple OKCs merit evaluation for nevoid basal cell carcinoma syndrome *(Gorlin syndrome),* related to *PATCHED* tumor-suppressor gene mutations (Chapter 25).
- *Periapical cysts* are extremely common lesions found at tooth apices; these develop from long-standing pulpitis caused either by advanced caries or tooth trauma; persistent bacteria or necrotic debris leads to chronic inflammation, granulation tissue, and proliferation of quiescent rests of odontogenic epithelium.

Odontogenic Tumors (p. 782)

These lesions demonstrate diverse histology and clinical behavior. Some are true neoplasms (both benign and malignant); others are hamartomas. They are composed of either odontogenic epithelium or ectomesenchyme.

- *Ameloblastoma* is a true neoplasm arising from odontogenic epithelium and showing *no* ectomesenchymal differentiation. It is commonly cystic, slow growing, and locally invasive, but typically has a benign course.
- *Odontoma* is the most common odontogenic tumor. It is likely a hamartoma, arising from epithelium with extensive enamel and dentin deposition.

UPPER AIRWAYS (p. 783)

Nose (p. 783)

Inflammations (p. 783)

- *Infectious rhinitis* ("common cold"), caused by adeno-, echo-, and rhinoviruses, produces erythematous and edematous nasal mucosa with profuse catarrhal discharge; bacterial superinfection can induce mucopurulent exudates.
- *Allergic rhinitis* ("hay fever") affects 20% of individuals; it is an IgE-mediated immune reaction (see Chapter 6) with mucosal edema and erythema, and eosinophil-rich infiltrates.
- *Nasal polyps* occur after recurrent rhinitis attacks; they are edematous mucosa infiltrated by neutrophils, eosinophils, and plasma cells. When multiple or large, they obstruct the airway and impair sinus drainage, necessitating removal.

- *Sinusitis* is commonly preceded by acute or chronic rhinitis; maxillary sinusitis can occur by extension of a periapical tooth infection through the sinus floor. Offending organisms are normal oral commensals (commonly mixed microbial flora), although diabetics can develop severe chronic sinusitis due to fungi (e.g., *mucormycosis*). In *Kartagener syndrome*, congenitally defective cilia cause a triad of *sinusitis*, *bronchiectasis*, and *situs inversus*.

Necrotizing Lesions of the Nose and Upper Airways (p. 784)

- Spreading fungal infections
- Wegener granulomatosis (Chapter 11)
- Lethal midline granulomas; actually an angiocentric non-Hodgkin lymphoma (natural killer cell neoplasm [Chapter 14])

Nasopharynx Inflammation (p. 784)

Pharyngitis and *tonsillitis* are frequent concomitants of viral upper respiratory infections; there is mucosal edema and erythema with reactive lymphoid hyperpalasia. Bacterial superinfection exacerbates the process, particularly in immunocompromised individuals or children without protective immunity.

Tumors of the Nose, Sinuses, and Nasopharynx (p. 784)

- *Nasopharyngeal angiofibroma* is a highly vascularized benign tumor occurring in adolescent boys; serious bleeding can complicate surgical resection.
- *Inverted papilloma* is a benign but locally aggressive neoplasm of squamous epithelium.
- *Olfactory neuroblastomas (esthesioneuroblastomas)* are uncommon, highly malignant tumors composed of neuroendocrine cells.
- *Nasopharyngeal carcinomas* have characteristic geographic distributions, have a close anatomic relationship to lymphoid tissue, and are associated with epithelial EBV infection. They classically occur in Africa (in children) and southern China (in adults). Tumors may be nonkeratinizing squamous cell carcinomas or undifferentiated carcinomas with abundant lymphocytic infiltrate *(lymphoepithelioma)*. At initial diagnosis, they are often unresectable with nodal metastases. Most are sensitive to radiotherapy: 3-year survival rates are 50% to 70%.

Larynx (p. 786)

Inflammations (p. 786)

Laryngitis can be caused by allergic, viral, bacterial, or chemical injury; most common causes are nonspecific infection or heavy tobacco smoke exposure. In children, *Haemophilus influenzae* laryngitis can be life-threatening due to airway obstruction from rapid-onset severe mucosal edema; the inspiratory stridor it produces is called *croup*.

Reactive Nodules (Vocal Cord Polyps) (p. 786)

Reactive nodules occur most often in heavy smokers or singers *(singer's nodules)* and are small (millimeters), smooth, rounded excrescences on true vocal cords. These are myxoid, occasionally vascular, connective tissue covered by (occasionally hyperplastic) squamous epithelium. Although they often cause progressive hoarseness, malignant transformation is rare.

Carcinoma of the Larynx (p. 786)

Tobacco smoke is the major cause, although alcohol is also a risk factor; up to the point of frank malignancy, changes typically regress after smoking cessation. Epithelial changes range from *hyperplasia* and *atypical hyperplasia* to *dysplasia, carcinoma in situ,* and invasive cancer. The likelihood of developing overt carcinoma is proportional to the atypia seen at first diagnosis.

Typical squamous cell carcinoma accounts for 95% of laryngeal cancers; usually occurring on the vocal cords, these can also develop on the epiglottis or pyriform sinuses. They present as persistent hoarseness, but later can produce pain, dysphagia, and hemoptysis. With surgery and radiation, more than 65% of patients are cured.

Squamous Papilloma and Papillomatosis (p. 786)

Squamous papillomas are benign lesions, usually on the true vocal cords; in children, they may be multiple *(juvenile laryngeal papillomatosis)* and can spontaneously regress at puberty. Lesions are caused by HPV (human papillomavirus) types 6 and 11; they frequently recur, but cancerous transformation is rare.

EARS (p. 787)

Inflammatory Lesions (p. 788)

- *Otitis media* occurs mostly in infants and children; typical organisms are *Streptococcus pneumoniae, H. influenzae,* and β-hemolytic streptococci. *Chronic disease* is usually caused by *Pseudomonas* and *Staphylococcus.*
- *Cholesteatomas* are associated with chronic otitis media; they are 1- to 4-cm cystic lesions, lined by keratinizing squamous epithelium and filled with amorphous debris, sometimes containing cholesterol spicules.

Otosclerosis (p. 788)

Otosclerosis is *abnormal bone deposition* in the middle ear, hampering stapes footplate mobility. The cause of osseous overgrowth is obscure, although there is a familial autosomal dominant predilection with variable penetrance. The process is slowly progressive, eventually causing marked hearing loss.

NECK (p. 788)

Branchial Cysts (Lymphoepithelial Cysts)
(p. 788)

Branchial cysts are 2- to 5-cm benign lesions with fibrous walls lined by stratified squamous or pseudostratified columnar epithelium accompanied by lymphocytic infiltrates or reactive lymphoid tissue. They arise on the anterolateral neck either from branchial arch remnants or as salivary gland inclusions within cervical nodes.

Thyroglossal Duct Cysts (p. 789)

These cysts arise from embryonic residua of the thyroid gland (see Chapter 24).

Paraganglioma (Carotid Body Tumor) (p. 789)

Paraganglioma is a tumor arising in extra-adrenal paraganglia—either paravertebral, or more commonly, around the great vessels, including the *carotid bodies*. It consists of nests *(zellballen)* of polygonal neuroendocrine cells enclosed by fibrous trabeculae and elongated sustentacular cells. Sporadic forms typically occur singly; familial forms (i.e., part of the multiple endocrine neoplasia 2 syndrome [Chapter 24]) are usually multiple and bilateral. Paragangliomas may recur after excision in half of cases, and may prove fatal due to infiltrative growth.

SALIVARY GLANDS (p. 790)

Xerostomia (p. 790)

Xerostomia, or dry mouth, is due to lack of salivary secretions; it may occur as a major feature of the autoimmune *Sjögren syndrome* (Chapter 6), due to salivary gland inflammation and fibrosis, or may be a complication of radiation therapy.

Inflammation (Sialadenitis) (p. 790)

Sialadenitis may be traumatic, viral, bacterial, or autoimmune.

- *Mucoceles* are the most common salivary gland lesions; they result from ductal blockage or rupture with saliva leakage into surrounding stroma. Most often on the lower lip, they typically result from trauma; lesions fluctuate in size, particularly in association with meals. Incomplete excision can result in recurrence.
- *Nonspecific* (bacterial) *sialoadenitis* usually follows ductal obstructions by stones, *(sialolithiasis),* with *S. aureus* or *Streptococcus viridans* overgrowth inducing painful enlargement and purulent discharge.

Neoplasms (p. 790)

Some 30 benign and malignant tumors of salivary glands have been described (Table 16–1 lists the more common tumors). Parotids account for 65% to 80% (of which 15%–30% are malignant); 10% occur in the submandibular glands (30%–40% malignant), with the remainder being in the minor salivary glands (70%–90% malignant).

Pleomorphic Adenoma (p. 791)

The most common salivary gland neoplasm (60% of all parotid tumors); these tumors exhibit mixed epithelial and mesenchymal differentiation, with epithelial nests dispersed in a variable matrix of myxoid, hyaline, chondroid, or osseous differentiation.

Tumors are painless, slow-growing, mobile, discrete masses. Recurrence rates approach 25% if not well excised. Malignant transformation (usually as adenocarcinoma or undifferentiated carcinoma) occurs in 10% of tumors after more than 15 years.

Warthin Tumor (Papillary Cystadenoma Lymphomatosum) (p. 792)

A benign tumor of unknown histogenesis typically found in the parotid, 10% are multifocal and bilateral. The tumor is most common in smokers. It is well-encapsulated, consisting of glandular spaces lined by a double layer of epithelial cells atop a dense lymphoid stroma.

Mucoepidermoid Carcinoma (p. 793)

Mucoepidermoid carcinoma is the most common primary malignant salivary tumor, constituting 15% of all salivary gland neoplasms. Up to 8 cm in size, these lack well-defined capsules. Histologically, there are cords, sheets, or cystic arrangements of squamous, mucous, or intermediate cells with mucus-filled vacuoles. Low-grade tumors can invade locally with 15% recurrence rates; high-grade tumors have 25% recurrence rates and 50% 5-year survival rates.

TABLE 16–1 **Histologic Classification and Approximate Incidence of Benign and Malignant Tumors of the Salivary Glands**

Benign	Malignant
Pleomorphic adenoma (50%) (mixed tumor)	Mucoepidermoid carcinoma (15%)
Warthin tumor (5%–10%)	Adenocarcinoma (NOS) (10%)
Oncocytoma (1%)	Acinic cell carcinoma (5%)
Other adenomas (5%–10%)	Adenoid cystic carcinoma (5%)
Basal cell adenoma	Malignant mixed tumor (3%–5%)
Canalicular adenoma	Squamous cell carcinoma (1%)
Ductal papillomas	Other carcinomas (2%)

NOS, not otherwise specified.
Data from Ellis GL, Auclair PL: Tumors of the Salivary Glands. Atlas of Tumor Pathology, Third Series. Washington, DC, Armed Forces Institute of Pathology, 1996.

Other Salivary Gland Tumors (p. 793)

- *Adenoid cystic carcinoma* (p. 793) is relatively uncommon; half occur in minor salivary glands. Histologically, tumor cells are small with scant cytoplasm; they are arrayed in tubular or cribriform patterns with intercellular spaces filled with excess basement membrane–like material. Although slow-growing, they are stubbornly recurrent and invasive, eventually becoming metastatic. Five-year survival rates of 60% to 70% drop to 15% at 15 years.
- *Acinic cell tumor* (p. 794) constitute 2% to 3% of all salivary gland tumors and arise most commonly in the parotid glands; tumor cells resemble normal salivary serous acinar cells. Clinical behavior is dependent on cellular pleomorphism; 10% to 15% metastasize to lymph nodes, and 5-year survival rate is 90%.

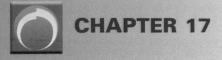

CHAPTER 17

The Gastrointestinal Tract

ESOPHAGUS (p. 798)

The esophagus is 10 to 11 cm long in newborns; it is 25 cm in adults, with a distance of 40 cm from incisors to the gastroesophageal junction. The upper and lower esophageal sphincters are functional, not anatomic, and there is no serosa, allowing rapid mediastinal spread of invasive lesions.

Symptoms of esophageal disorders include:

- *Dysphagia:* Subjective swallowing difficulty, seen in mechanical and functional disorders
- *Heartburn:* Retrosternal burning pain, usually reflecting gastric reflux into lower esophagus
- *Hematemesis:* Vomiting blood; due to inflammation, ulceration, or blood vessel rupture
- *Pain:* Retrosternal, nonspecific

Anatomic Anomalies (p. 799)

Atresia and Fistulas (p. 800)

These anomalies are uncommon; they are usually discovered shortly after birth. Many are incompatible with life, and may be associated with congenital heart disease or other gastrointestinal tract malformations.

- *Atresia:* A portion of the esophagus is replaced by a thin, noncanalized cord, with blind pouches above and below the atretic segment.
- *Fistula:* A connection between the esophagus and the trachea or a mainstem bronchus; swallowed material or gastric fluids enter the respiratory tract.

Webs, Rings, and Stenosis (p. 800)

These anomalies describe esophageal narrowings heralded by progressive dysphagia (difficulty swallowing), especially with solid foods.

- *Stenosis,* due to esophageal wall fibrous thickening; may be congenital or acquired (gastroesophageal reflux, radiation, scleroderma, or caustic injury).
- *Mucosal webs* are ledgelike mucosal protrusions, usually in the upper esophagus. The constellation of webs, iron deficiency anemia, glossitis, and cheilosis is called the *Plummer-Vinson syndrome.*
- *Esophageal rings* are concentric tissue plates protruding into the distal esophageal lumen. If above the gastroesophageal junction, a ring is designated "A" ring; if at the gastroesophageal junction, it is designated "B" or *Schatzki ring.*

Lesions Associated With Motor Dysfunction (p. 800)

Achalasia (p. 800)

Achalasia (literally "failure to relax") presents with dysphagia in young adulthood (or earlier). Patients have diminished myenteric ganglia leading to esophageal *aperistalsis* (lack of peristalsis), incomplete relaxation of the lower esophageal sphincter (LES) with swallowing, and increased LES resting tone. Secondary features are proximal esophageal dilation, thickened (muscular hypertrophy) or thinned muscular walls, and regurgitation with mucosal damage. Complications include candidal esophagitis, diverticula, and aspiration pneumonia. The risk of esophageal carcinoma is 2% to 7%.

Secondary achalasia occurs with Chagas disease *(Trypanosoma cruzi),* disorders of the vagal dorsal motor nuclei (polio, surgical ablation), diabetic autonomic neuropathy, and infiltrative disorders (malignancy, amyloidosis, sarcoidosis).

Hiatal Hernia (p. 801)

In this saclike dilation of stomach with protrusion above the diaphragm, there is separation of the diaphragmatic crura and widening of the esophageal foramen.

- *Sliding* (axial) *hiatal hernia* (95% of cases): Shortened esophagus, traction of upper stomach into thorax, bell-like dilation of stomach within the thoracic cavity are typical.
- *Paraesophageal hiatal hernia* (rolling hernia) (<5% of cases): Cardia of stomach dissects into the thorax adjacent to the esophagus; vulnerable to strangulation and infarction.

Clinical Findings. Hiatal hernia occurs in 1% to 20% of normal adults, and can affect infants and children. Only 9% have symptoms (retrosternal chest pain, gastric reflux). A paraesophageal hiatal hernia may ulcerate or strangulate, with bleeding or perforation.

Diverticula (p. 802)

Diverticula are outpouchings of the alimentary tract containing one or more wall layers. Typical symptoms of esophageal diverticulum are food regurgitation, dysphasia, and a mass in the neck. In the esophagus, diverticula are classified as:

- *Pharyngeal (Zenker) diverticulum:* Occurs in the upper esophagus, presumably due to motor dysfunction
- *Traction diverticulum:* More distal location; attributed to fibrosing mediastinal processes or abnormal motility
- *Epiphrenic diverticulum:* Immediately above esophageal sphincter; unclear cause

Lacerations (Mallory-Weiss Syndrome) (p. 802)

These lacerations are longitudinal tears in the esophagus at the esophagogastric junction. They are due to episodes of excessive vomiting with failure of LES relaxation and are commonly seen in alcoholics. They may lead to potentially massive hematemesis, inflammation, residual ulcer, mediastinitis, or peritonitis.

Morphology. Irregular longitudinal tears (millimeters to centimeters in length) span the esophagogastric junction. Lacerations typically involve only the mucosa but may be full-thickness.

Clinical Findings. Lacerations account for 5% to 10% of upper gastrointestinal bleeding events. Lacerations are not usually fatal; healing tends to be prompt.

Esophageal Varices (p. 802)

Prolonged and severe portal hypertension from liver cirrhosis induces formation of collateral bypass channels through the coronary veins of the stomach into esophageal subepithelial and submucosal veins *(varices),* eventually emptying into the azygous veins and systemic circulation. Varices occur in 90% of cirrhotic patients; hepatic schistosomiasis is a common cause worldwide. Other portosystemic shunts include the rectal canal *(hemorrhoids)* and falciform ligament *(caput medusa).*

Morphology. Tortuous dilated veins are within the distal esophageal and proximal gastric submucosa; there is irregular luminal protrusion of overlying mucosa, with superficial ulceration, inflammation, or adherent blood clots.

Clinical Findings. Varices are clinically silent until they rupture with catastrophic hematemesis. The fatality rate is 40% for each episode of bleeding; in survivors, there is a 90% chance of recurrence within a year.

Esophagitis (p. 803)

Reflux Esophagitis (p. 804)

Reflux of gastric contents is the foremost cause of esophagitis. Contributing factors include:

- Decreased efficacy of esophageal antireflux mechanisms
- Sliding hiatal hernias

- Delayed gastric emptying and increased gastric volume
- Reduced reparative capability of the esophageal mucosa

Morphology
- Hyperemia and edema
- Thickened basal zone (exceeding 20% of the epithelium) and thinning of superficial epithelial layers
- Neutrophil or eosinophil infiltration
- Superficial necrosis and ulceration with adherent inflammatory exudate

Clinical Findings
Reflux esophagitis most commonly affects adults. Symptoms include dysphagia, heartburn, regurgitation of gastric contents into the mouth, hematemesis, and melena. Stricture or Barrett esophagus can develop as a result of long-standing reflux.

Barrett Esophagus (p. 804)

Barrett esophagus refers to *replacement of the distal esophageal squamous epithelium by a metaplastic columnar epithelium,* typically after long-standing gastroesophageal reflux with ulceration and inflammation of the squamous mucosa. Re-epithelialization by pluripotent stem cells in a low pH setting induces differentiation into gastric- or intestinal-type epithelium. It is most common in adults. There is substantial risk of ulceration and stricture.

Morphology
- *Gross:* Irregular circumferential band of red, velvety mucosa at the gastroesophageal junction, with linear streaks or patches of similar mucosa in the distal esophagus.
- *Microscopic:* Intestinal-type columnar epithelium (both absorptive epithelial cells and mucin-secreting goblet cells) interspersed with glandular gastric columnar mucosa. Epithelial cell dysplasia can arise in Barrett esophagus. Adenocarcinoma risk is increased 30- to 40-fold.

Infectious and Chemical Esophagitis (p. 805)

Unusual causes of esophageal mucosal inflammation include:

- Prolonged gastric intubation
- Ingestion of irritants: alcohol, corrosive acids or alkalis, excessively hot fluids, smoking
- Uremia
- Bacterial, viral (e.g., herpesvirus, cytomegalovirus), or fungal (candidiasis, mucormycosis, aspergillosis) infection
- Chemo- or radiotherapy

Systemic desquamative disorders (pemphigoid, epidermolysis bullosa), graft-versus-host disease, autoimmune diseases, or Crohn disease can also cause esophagitis.

Tumors (p. 806)

Benign Tumors (p. 806)

- *Intramural or submucosal:* leiomyoma, fibroma, lipoma, hemangioma, neurofibroma, lymphangioma
- *Mucosal,* rarely larger than 3 cm: squamous papilloma, fibrovascular polyp (with overlying epithelium), inflamma-

tory polyp (severely inflamed mesenchyme with overlying epithelium)

Malignant Tumors (p. 806)

Esophageal carcinomas constitute 6% of all GI tract cancers but have a disproportionately high death rate. Malignant stromal tumors (smooth muscle or fibroblast origin) are rare.

Squamous Cell Carcinoma (p. 806)

The most common malignant tumor in the esophagus. Squamous cell carcinoma typically occurs in adults older than 50 years, in men more often than women, in blacks more often than whites. There is considerable geographic variability, with highest incidences in Northern China, Iran, Russia, and South Africa.

Pathogenesis. The pathogenesis is multifactorial; environment and diet contribute synergistically, modified by genetic factors (Table 17–1). Achalasia, Plummer-Vinson syndrome, and long-standing celiac disease increase risk.

Morphology. The upper third of the esophagus has 20% of these tumors, the middle and lower thirds, 50% and 30%, respectively. Squamous cell carcinomas begin as *in situ* gray-white, plaquelike mucosal thickenings. Lesions subsequently extend longitudinally, and circumferentially, and invade deeply. Tumors spread via rich submucosal lymphatic networks to nearby lymph nodes, and extend deeply into adjacent mediastinal structures.

- Grossly, lesions may be polypoid (60%), exhibit necrotizing excavation (25%), or be diffusely infiltrative (15%).
- Histologically, tumors are usually moderately to well differentiated, with or without keratinization.

Clinical Findings. Onset is insidious; symptoms typically develop late and include dysphagia, obstruction, weight loss,

TABLE 17–1 **Factors Associated With the Development of Squamous Cell Carcinoma of the Esophagus**

Dietary
Deficiency of vitamins (A, C, riboflavin, thiamine, pyridoxine)
Deficiency of trace elements (zinc, molybdenum)
Fungal contamination of foodstuffs
High content of nitrites/nitrosamines
Betel chewing

Lifestyle
Burning-hot beverages or food
Alcohol consumption
Tobacco use
Urban environment

Esophageal Disorders
Long-standing esophagitis
Achalasia
Plummer-Vinson syndrome

Genetic Predisposition
Long-standing celiac disease
Ectodermal dysplasia
Epidermolysis bullosa
Racial disposition

hemorrhage, sepsis secondary to ulceration, or respiratory tree fistulas with aspiration. Resection is possible in 80% of cases; although 5-year survival rates for *all* esophageal cancers is 9%, superficial carcinomas have a 5-year survival rate of 75%.

Adenocarcinoma (p. 808)

Adenocarcinoma constitutes approximately 50% of esophageal cancers in the United States. Adenocarcinomas largely evolve from dysplastic changes in Barrett mucosa; risk factors are the same for both, and most are in the distal third of esophagus.

Pathogenesis. Genetic alterations from Barrett esophagus to adenocarcinoma are well documented (e.g., p53 overexpression and 17p allelic losses, with loss of cell cycle control at the G_1 to S transition).

Morphology
- *Grossly,* findings range from exophytic nodules to excavated and deeply infiltrative masses.
- *Microscopically,* typically mucin-producing glandular tumors with intestinal features, or diffusely infiltrative signet ring cells are seen; rarely, there is adenosquamous or small cell type (poorly differentiated) appearance.

Clinical Findings. Tumors typically arise in patients older than age 40, men more often than women, with symptoms as for squamous cell carcinoma. Interestingly, previous symptoms of gastroesophageal reflux are present in fewer than 50%. Overall 5-year survival rate is less than 20%; screening programs detect disease earlier.

STOMACH (p. 810)

Congenital Anomalies (p. 812)

Uncommon anomalies include *pancreatic heterotopia* in the gastric muscle wall and *in utero* displacement of the stomach cephalad through a *diaphragmatic hernia*. Such hernias are due to a weakness or a defect in the diaphragm (usually on left) and do not involve the hiatal orifice. If herniation of abdominal viscera is substantial, respiratory impairment with pulmonary hypoplasia is life threatening.

Pyloric Stenosis (p. 812)

Congenital hypertrophic pyloric stenosis (p. 812) refers to hypertrophy or hyperplasia of the pyloric muscularis propria. Occurring in 1:300 to 1:900 live births, the male-female ratio is 4:1; regurgitation and projectile vomiting occur in the first 3 weeks of life. Other findings include externally visible peristalsis and a palpable firm ovoid mass. Inheritance is multifactorial with high twin concordance.

- Mucosal edema and inflammation aggravate narrowing.
- Full-thickness, muscle-splitting incision *(pyloromyotomy)* is curative.

Acquired pyloric stenosis (p. 812) is a complication of chronic antral gastritis, peptic ulcers close to the pylorus, and malignancy (e.g., carcinoma, lymphoma, pancreatic carcinoma).

Gastritis (p. 812)

Gastritis is inflammation of the gastric mucosa.

Acute Gastritis (p. 812)

Acute gastritis is an acute, usually transient, mucosal inflammatory process. The most common associations are chronic, heavy use of nonsteroidal anti-inflammatory drugs (particularly aspirin), excessive alcohol consumption, and heavy smoking. Severe stress (burns, surgery), ischemia, and shock also cause acute gastritis, as can chemotherapy, uremia, systemic infections, ingestion of acid or alkali, gastric irradiation, mechanical trauma, and distal gastrectomy.

Pathogenesis. General etiologic mechanisms include increased acid production with back-diffusion, decreased bicarbonate production, and direct mucosal damage.

Morphology
- *Grossly,* there is moderate edema and hyperemia, occasionally with hemorrhage *(acute hemorrhagic erosive gastritis).*
- *Microscopically,* neutrophils invade the epithelium, with superficial epithelial sloughing *(erosion).*

Clinical Findings. Findings range from asymptomatic, to minor abdominal pain, to acute abdominal pain with hematemesis.

Chronic Gastritis (p. 813)

Chronic gastritis is defined as the presence of chronic mucosal inflammatory changes leading eventually to mucosal atrophy and epithelial metaplasia. This condition constitutes a background for dysplasia, hence carcinoma.

Pathogenesis. Chronic infection with *Helicobacter pylori* is the leading cause (see following list). Diseases associated with chronic *H. pylori* infection are listed in Table 17–2. Other causes include:
- Immunologic (autoimmune)

  Antibodies to parietal cells (including the H^+/K^+-ATPase) or vitamin B_{12}-binding intrinsic factor
  Gland destruction and atrophy
  Decreased intrinsic factor secretion by parietal cells, leading to pernicious anemia

TABLE 17–2 **Diseases Associated With *Helicobacter pylori* Infection**

Disease	Association
Chronic gastritis	Strong causal association
Peptic ulcer disease	Strong causal association
Gastric carcinoma	Strong causal association
Gastric MALT lymphoma*	Definitive etiologic role

*MALT, mucosa-associated lymphoid tissue.

- Toxic: alcohol and tobacco usage
- Postsurgical: postantrectomy bile reflux
- Motor/mechanical: obstruction, atony
- Radiation
- Granulomatous conditions: Crohn disease
- Graft-*versus*-host disease, uremia, amyloidosis

Helicobacter pylori (p. 813) colonizes more than 50% of Americans over age 50. It is an S-shaped gram-negative rod present in 90% of patients with chronic antral gastritis. *H. pylori* can be diagnosed by antibody serologic test, breath test, bacterial culture, direct bacterial visualization in gastric biopsy, or DNA-based tests. *H. pylori* infection is a risk factor for peptic ulcer disease, gastric adenocarcinoma, and gastric lymphoma. Traits that allow it to flourish in the stomach include:

- *Motility* via flagella
- *Urease production* buffering gastric acid
- Bacterial *adhesins* to bind surface epithelial cells
- Proinflammatory peptides (e.g., cagA and vacA cytotoxins)

Autoimmune gastritis (p. 814) causes less than 10% of chronic gastritis; it is due to autoantibodies to gastric parietal cells and intrinsic factor, and is associated with other autoimmune diseases, including Hashimoto thyroiditis and Addison disease.

Morphology
- Grossly, chronic gastritis exhibits a reddened, boggy, coarse-textured mucosa. The distribution depends on the etiology:

  Environmental causes (including *H. pylori*) yield a variable and patchy distribution in the antrum or corpus.
  Autoimmune causes produce diffuse involvement of the body and fundus.
- Histologically:

  Lymphocyte and plasma cell infiltrate in lamina propria
  Intraepithelial neutrophilic infiltrates
  Regenerative change of surface columnar cells
  Variable mucosal gland atrophy
  Metaplasia of surface columnar epithelium to intestinal-type epithelium
  Dysplasia in some cases of long-standing chronic gastritis

Clinical Findings. Chronic gastritis is usually asymptomatic, although nausea, vomiting, or upper abdominal discomfort can occur; rarely, overt pernicious anemia occurs. Laboratory findings include gastric hypochlorhydria and serum hypergastrinemia. Long-term cancer risk is 2% to 4%.

Peptic Ulcer Disease (p. 816)

An ulcer is *a breach of the mucosa extending through the muscularis mucosa into deeper layers*. The first portion of the duodenum is most commonly affected (>80% of cases).

Peptic Ulcers (p. 816)

Chronic, typically solitary ulcers arise from exposure to acid-peptic secretion. The lifetime incidence is 10% for American men and 4% for women, typically middle-aged and older; tend to recur. There are no apparent genetic tendencies.

Pathogenesis. The ulcers are attributed to imbalanced gastroduodenal mucosal defense mechanisms and damage from gastric acid and pepsin, combined with superimposed environmental or immunologic injury. Mucosal defenses are impaired by ischemia and shock, delayed gastric emptying, or duodenal-gastric reflux. Normal defenses include:

- Surface mucus and bicarbonate secretion
- Apical epithelial cell transport systems
- Mucosal blood flow sustaining mucosal integrity and epithelial regeneration
- Prostaglandins

Most peptic ulcers are associated with *H. pylori* infection; it is present in 70% of gastric ulcers, and virtually all patients with duodenal ulcers. *H. pylori* causes injury by several mechanisms:

- *H. pylori* secrete urease, proteases, and phospholipases that are directly toxic to the mucosa.
- Bacterial lipopolysaccharide stimulates mucosal production of proinflammatory cytokines (e.g., interleukin 8 and tumor necrosis factor [TNF]) that recruit and activate inflammatory cells; these, in turn, release proteases and oxygen-derived free radicals.
- Bacterial platelet-activating factor promotes capillary thrombosis.
- Mucosal damage permits nutrient leakage onto the surface microenvironment, thus sustaining the bacillus in the mucus layer.

Other promoters of gastric mucosal ulceration include:

- Gastric hyperacidity: increased parietal cell mass from excess gastrin production (e.g., a gastrinoma), causing multiple peptic ulcerations *(Zollinger-Ellison syndrome)*
- Chronic NSAID (nonsteroidal anti-inflammatory drug) use, suppressing mucosal prostaglandin synthesis
- Cigarette smoking, alcoholic cirrhosis, corticosteroids, and hypercalcemia (e.g., chronic renal failure or hyperparathyroidism)

Morphology. About 98% of ulcers occur in duodenum and stomach (ratio of 4:1). Gross findings include a sharply punched-out defect with overhanging mucosal borders and smooth, clean ulcer bases. Microscopically, there are thin superficial layers of necrotic debris with underlying inflammation merging into granulation tissue and deep scarring. The surrounding mucosa usually exhibits chronic gastritis.

Clinical Findings. Epigastric gnawing, burning, or aching pain, worse at night and 1 to 3 hours after meals. Nausea, vomiting, bloating, belching, and weight loss occur. Complications include anemia, hemorrhage, perforation, and obstruction. Malignant transformation is rare and related to underlying gastritis.

Acute Gastric Ulceration (p. 819)

Acute gastric ulceration refers to focal, acute mucosal defects in the setting of severe stress *(stress ulcer)*. These occur after shock, extensive burns, or severe trauma (Curling ulcers), or with elevated intracranial pressure, as in trauma or surgery (Cushing ulcers). NSAIDs may also cause acute ulceration. The pathogenesis is unclear, but may be related to impaired oxygenation, vagal stimulation (leading to gastric acid hypersecretion), or systemic acidosis.

Morphology. Ulcers are usually less than 1 cm in diameter, multiple, and shallow. Ulcer base is brown (blood); adjacent mucosa is normal.

Clinical Findings. Acute gastric erosions or ulcers occur in 5% to 10% of intensive care unit patients. The single most important determinant of outcome is the *ability to correct the underlying conditions.*

Miscellaneous Conditions (p. 820)

Gastric Dilation and Bezoars

Gastric dilation can arise from gastric outlet obstruction (pyloric stenosis, tumors) or from gastric and intestinal atony (ileus). Rarely, gastric rupture may occur.

Bezoars are luminal concretions of indigestible ingested material: A phytobezoar is derived from plant material; a trichobezoar is a *hairball. Eosinophilic gastritis* is caused by heavy eosinophilic infiltration of the mucosa or submucosa; it can be idiopathic or due to allergy for ingested material.

Hypertrophic Gastropathy (p. 820)

Hypertrophic gastropathy refers to uncommon conditions featuring giant cerebriform enlargement of gastric rugal folds, caused by hyperplasia of mucosal epithelial cells.

* *Ménétrier disease:* hyperplasia of surface mucous (foveolar) cells, often accompanied by fundic gland atrophy, and hence *hypochlorhydria.* It also causes clinical hypoproteinemia. Transforming growth factor-α (TGF-α) overexpression is implicated.
* *Hypertrophic-hypersecretory gastropathy:* hyperplasia of parietal and chief cells (fundic glands). Patients are often *hyperchlorhydric.*
* *Gastric gland hyperplasia:* mainly parietal cell hyperplasia secondary to excessive gastrin secretion by a (usually pancreatic) gastrinoma (Zollinger-Ellison syndrome). Patients are typically *hyperchlorhydric.*

Clinical Findings. Hypertrophic gastropathy can mimic diffuse gastric cancer or lymphoma on radiographic studies. Patients are at risk for peptic ulceration. Excess secreted protein may cause hypoalbuminemia and *protein-losing gastroenteropathy.* The hyperplastic mucosa may become dysplastic, with risk of adenocarcinoma.

Gastric Varices (p. 821)

Gastric varices develop in the setting of portal hypertension, near the gastroesophageal junction. These are less common than esophageal varices.

Tumors (p. 821)

Benign Tumors (p. 821)

In the alimentary tract, *polyp* refers to any nodule or mass that projects above the level of the surrounding mucosa; it generally refers to lesions arising from the mucosa.

Non-Neoplastic Polyps

- *Hyperplastic* or *inflammatory polyps* constitute 90% of gastric polyps. They are smooth, and sessile (without a stalk) or pedunculated (with a stalk), with epithelial tubules and cysts interspersed with an inflamed stroma. They are common in chronic gastritis, frequently multiple, and have no malignant potential per se.
- *Fundic gland polyps* involve innocuous fundic gland dilation. They occur sporadically or in the setting of familial adenomatous polyposis (FAP).
- *Inflammatory fibroid polyps* arise from the submucosa, and involve fibroblast proliferation with inflammatory cell infiltrate (especially eosinophils).
- Hamartomatous polyps usually occur in the setting of Peutz-Jeghers syndrome or juvenile polyposis syndrome.

Neoplastic Polyps

Gastric adenomas (5%–10% of gastric polyps) are true neoplasms with *proliferative dysplastic epithelium* (i.e., with malignant potential). Usually single, they can be sessile or pedunculated. Incidence increases with age, and 40% can harbor carcinoma. They arise on a background of chronic gastritis or genetic polyposis syndromes.

Gastric Carcinoma (p. 822)

Of gastric malignancies, 90% to 95% are carcinoma (versus lymphomas, carcinoids, or spindle cell tumors). Worldwide distribution is widely variable; U.S. incidence has decreased fourfold over the last 60 years. Prognosis is dismal, with 5-year survival rates of 20%; it represents 2.5% of U.S. cancer deaths.

Pathogenesis. Gastric carcinoma occurs as either *intestinal* or *diffuse* types (see below). Risk factors for diffuse cancer are poorly defined; contributing factors for intestinal-type tumors include:

- Environment
  Diet: lack of refrigeration, use of preservatives, lack of fresh fruit and vegetables
  Cigarette smoking (increases risk 1.5- to 3-fold)
- Host
  Infection by *H. pylori* with chronic gastritis
  Autoimmune gastritis
  Partial gastrectomy permitting gastroduodenal reflux

Gastric mucosa *dysplasia* is a common result with genetic instability in DNA repair genes, telomerase expression, and c-*met*, K-*sam*, and c-*ERB-B2* abnormalities (growth factor receptor pathways).

Morphology. The lesser curvature is involved in 40% of cases, and the greater curvature in 12%; 50% to 60% of cancers occur in the pylorus and antrum, 25% in the cardia, and 15% to 25% in the body and fundus. Tumors are classified by:

- *Depth of invasion: Early gastric carcinoma* is confined to the mucosa and submucosa, regardless of presence or absence of lymph node metastases. *Advanced gastric carcinoma* extends beyond the submucosa.
- *Macroscopic growth pattern:* Tumors are exophytic, flat or depressed, or excavated. Uncommonly, diffuse invasion throughout the wall creates a rigid thickened stomach, so-called *linitis plastica.*
- Histologic subtype (Lauren classification)

    Intestinal: Gland-forming columnar epithelium; usually mucin producing; usually polypoid expansile growth pattern; almost always associated with mucosal intestinal metaplasia; mean age, 55 years; male-female ratio of 2:1; decreasing incidence.

    Diffuse: Poorly differentiated, single signet-ring cells; mucin producing; infiltrative growth pattern; mean age, 48 years; male-female ratio, 1:1; does not appear to be related to environmental factors. Familial gastric cancer exhibits this histologic type.

- *Dissemination:* Ovarian involvement generates *Krukenberg tumors.*

Clinical Findings. Gastric carcinoma is an insidious disease, initially asymptomatic, although patients exhibit weight loss, abdominal pain, anorexia, vomiting, altered bowel habits, dysphagia, anemia, and hemorrhage. Prognosis after resection depends only on *depth of invasion:*

- *Early gastric cancer:* 90% to 95% 5-year survival rate
- *Advanced disease:* less than 15% 5-year survival rate

Less Common Gastric Tumors (p. 826)

- *Lymphomas* (also referred to as MALT lymphoma—*m*ucosa-*a*ssociated *l*ymphoid *t*issue) represent 5% of gastric malignancies. They are associated with *H. pylori* infection; antibiotic treatment can induce tumor regression. Antibiotic-resistant tumors often harbor a t(11:18) translocation.
- *Gastrointestinal stromal tumor (GIST)* is a solid tumor of the gastric submucosa or wall with unpredictable malignant potential. Tumor cells exhibit either epithelioid (plump and cohesive cells) or spindle cell features. The majority harbor c-*kit* gene mutations (c-KIT is the stem cell factor receptor), while a minority exhibit *platelet-derived growth factor receptor-α* mutations; both receptors have cytoplasmic tyrosine kinases that activate downstream signaling pathways. The tumors are responsive to the tyrosine kinase inhibitor STI571 (also called *Gleevec* or *Imatinib*).
- Other rare tumors include *carcinoid tumors* (enterochromaffin-like cell tumor), *schwannomas,* and *lipomas.* Diffusely invasive metastatic tumors (as from breast) may produce a linitis plastica-like picture.

SMALL AND LARGE INTESTINES (p. 828)

Congenital Anomalies (p. 830)

These anomalies are fairly rare. The first two may be silent for decades; the latter two present in the newborn and are severe to catastrophic:

- *Duplication* of a portion of bowel
- *Malrotation* of the entire bowel
- *Omphalocele* (abdominal musculature fails to form)
- *Gastroschisis* (a portion of the abdominal wall fails to develop altogether)

Atresia and stenosis (p. 830) are due to developmental failure (e.g., intrauterine vascular events) or intussusception; the duodenum is most commonly affected. Failure of cloacal diaphragm rupture causes *imperforate anus.*

Meckel Diverticulum (p. 830)

A *diverticulum* is a blind pouch leading off the alimentary tract, lined by mucosa and communicating with the gut lumen. Meckel diverticula occur in 2% of the population, and result from persistence of the vitelline duct (connects yolk sac with gut lumen) leaving a solitary outpouching within approximately 85 cm of the ileocecal valve. These are *true* diverticula, consisting of all three bowel wall layers, *mucosa, submucosa, and muscularis propria. In roughly half the diverticula, heterotopic gastric mucosa (or pancreatic tissue) is present and can cause peptic ulceration in the adjacent small intestinal mucosa.* Diverticula may also intussuscept, incarcerate, or perforate, although most are asymptomatic.

Congenital Aganglionic Megacolon— Hirschsprung Disease (p. 830)

Arrested (proximal to distal) migration of neural crest cells into the gut results in an aganglionic segment with functional obstruction and proximal dilation. The rectum is always affected; proximal involvement is more variable.

Morphology. Absence of ganglion cells and ganglia in muscle wall (Auerbach plexus) and submucosa (Meissner plexus) of the affected segment. There is progressive dilation and hypertrophy of unaffected proximal colon.

Clinical Findings. Hirschsprung disease occurs in 1:5000 to 1:8000 live births; male-female ratio is 4:1. There is an association with Down syndrome and neurologic abnormalities. Hirschsprung disease presents with neonatal failure to pass meconium or abdominal distention; patients risk perforation, sepsis, or enterocolitis with fluid derangement.

Acquired megacolon may occur in Chagas disease, bowel obstruction, inflammatory bowel disease, and psychosomatic disorders.

Enterocolitis (p. 831)

Diarrhea and Dysentery (p. 831)

Diarrhea is roughly defined as greater than *250 gm daily stool production, containing 70% to 95% water;* patients perceive it as *increased stool volume, fluidity,* or *frequency.* Low-volume, painful diarrhea is called *dysentery.* Table 17–3 lists major causes of diarrhea; mechanisms may overlap.

- *Secretory diarrhea:* Net intestinal fluid secretion is greater than 500 mL/day, isotonic with plasma, and persists during fasting.

TABLE 17–3 Major Causes of Diarrheal Illnesses

Secretory Diarrhea
Infectious: viral damage to mucosal epithelium
   Rotavirus
   Caliciviruses
   Enteric adenoviruses
   Astroviruses
Infectious: enterotoxin mediated
   Vibrio cholerae
   Escherichia coli
   Bacillus cereus
   Clostridium perfringens
Neoplastic
   Tumor elaboration of peptides, serotonin, prostaglandins
   Villous adenoma in distal colon (nonhormone mediated)
Excess laxative use

Osmotic Diarrhea
Disaccharidase (lactase) deficiencies
Lactulose therapy (for hepatic encephalopathy, constipation)
Prescribed gut lavage for diagnostic procedures
Antacids ($MgSO_4$ and other magnesium salts)
Primary bile acid malabsorption

Exudative Diseases
Infectious: bacterial damage to mucosal epithelium
   Shigella
   Salmonella
   Campylobacter
   Entamoeba histolytica
Idiopathic inflammatory bowel disease
Typhlitis (neutropenic colitis in the immunosuppressed)

Malabsorption
Defective intraluminal digestion
Primary mucosal cell abnormalities
Reduced small intestinal surface area
Lymphatic obstruction
Infectious: impaired mucosal cell absorption
   Giardia lamblia infection

Deranged Motility
Decreased intestinal transit time
   Surgical reduction of gut length
   Neural dysfunction, including irritable bowel syndrome
   Hyperthyroidism
   Diabetic neuropathy
   Carcinoid syndrome
Decreased motility (increased intestinal transit time)
   Small intestinal diverticula
   Surgical creation of a "blind" intestinal loop
   Bacterial overgrowth in the small intestine

- *Osmotic diarrhea:* Osmotic forces exerted by luminal solutes lead to greater than 500 mL stool/day; diarrhea abates during fasting and exhibits osmotic gap (stool osmolality exceeds plasma electrolyte concentration by >50 mOsm).
- *Malabsorption:* Voluminous, bulky stools have excess fat and high osmolarity; diarrhea abates on fasting.
- *Exudative diseases:* Purulent, bloody stools persist during fasting; stools are frequent but of variable volume.
- *Deranged motility:* Features are variable; other causes must be excluded.

Infectious Enterocolitis (p. 832)

- Half of all deaths before age 5 worldwide are due to infectious enterocolitis; it causes more than 12,000 deaths *per day* in children in developing countries.
- In industrialized nations, individuals experience on average one or two episodes of vomiting or diarrhea per year; 40% of U.S. population is affected annually.
- Parasitic and protozoal disease affects more than 50% of the world's population on a chronic or recurrent basis.

Viral Gastroenterocolitis (p. 832)

Incubation periods range from hours to days; acute illness lasts from 1 to 7 (or more) days. Besides diarrhea, anorexia, headache, and fever can develop.

- *Rotavirus (group A):* 70-nm dsRNA virus; person-to-person transmission via food and water; mainly affects infants 6 to 24 months old. Virus selectively infects and destroys mature small intestinal enterocytes; accounts for 25% to 65% of severe childhood diarrhea (worldwide, 140 million cases and 1 million deaths annually). Minimal infective inoculum is 10 particles, and infected hosts shed 10^{12} particles/mL of stool. Consequently, outbreaks are characteristic.
- *Caliciviruses* (includes *Norwalk virus, Norwalk-like viruses,* and *Sapporo-like viruses*): ssRNA virus; person-to-person transmission via cold food, water, and raw shellfish. It accounts for the majority of cases of nonbacterial food-borne epidemic gastroenteritis in all age groups.
- *Enteric adenoviruses:* 80-nm dsDNA virus, person-to-person transmission mostly in children.
- *Astroviruses:* ssRNA viruses affecting children; person-to-person transmission via water, cold foods, and raw shellfish.

Morphology. Infected small intestine exhibits modestly shortened villi, lamina propria inflammation, enterocyte damage (brush border loss and cytoplasmic vacuolization), and crypt hyperplasia.

Bacterial Enterocolitis (p. 833)

Mechanisms of Injury

- *Ingestion of preformed toxin* in contaminated food (food poisoning), for example, *Staphylococcus aureus, Vibrio species, Clostridium perfringens.* Botulinum toxin is neurotoxic, not diarrheogenic.
- Infection by toxigenic organisms (*Vibrio cholerae,* toxigenic *Escherichia coli*), which proliferate in the gut lumen and elaborate toxins.
- Infection by enteroinvasive organisms (*Shigella, Salmonella, Yersinia, Campylobacter,* enteroinvasive *E. coli*) that proliferate, invade, and destroy mucosal epithelial cells.

Key pathogenic bacterial virulence factors:

- *Bacterial adhesion and replication:* Ingested organisms must adhere to the mucosal epithelial cells (to avoid elimination by peristalsis); requires plasmid-encoded *adhesin* proteins expressed on the bacterial surface.
- *Bacterial enterotoxins:* Polypeptides cause diarrhea. Two mechanisms are involved (*E. coli* can produce both toxin forms):

   Secretagogues (e.g., cholera toxin from *Vibrio cholerae*) stimulate fluid secretion by activating endogenous secretion pathways.

   Cytotoxins (e.g., Shiga toxin) cause direct tissue damage via epithelial cell necrosis.

- *Bacterial invasion:* Microbe-stimulated endocytosis permits intracellular proliferation, cell lysis, cell-to-cell spread, and entry into the circulation (e.g., enteroinvasive *E. coli, Shigella, Salmonella,* and *Yersinia enterocolitica*).

Morphology. Morphologic features are extremely variable. Nonspecific features include surface epithelium damage, increased mitotic rate, lamina propria hyperemia and edema, and neutrophilic infiltration.

- *Salmonella:* Ileum and colon are inflamed, with Peyer patches involved. *S. typhimurium* causes *typhoid fever* (bacteremia with biliary, joint, bone, and meningeal dissemination) with generalized lymphoid hyperplasia.
- *Shigella:* Colonic inflammation, shallow ulcerations, and exudates *(bacillary dysentery)* are seen.
- *Campylobacter jejuni* and other species: Small intestine, appendix, and colon are involved, with ulcers, inflammation, and exudate.
- *Y. enterocolitica* and *Y. pseudotuberculosis:* Ileum Peyer patches, appendix, colon, and mesenteric lymph nodes exhibit necrotizing granulomas; systemic spread is characteristic.
- *V. cholerae:* No histologic abnormality in the small intestine.
- *Clostridium perfringens:* Usually changes are minimal; some strains cause severe necrotizing enterocolitis with perforation *(pigbel).*
- *E. coli: Enterotoxigenic E. coli* produce cholera-like toxin; *enterohemorrhagic E. coli* produce shiga-like toxin (the prototype strain *E. coli* O157:H7 causes hemolytic uremic syndrome [HUS]). *Enteropathogenic* strains attach and efface epithelium but do not invade; *enteroinvasive* strains are like shigellosis. All cause "traveler's diarrhea."

Clinical Findings

- *Ingestion of preformed toxins:* Explosive diarrhea and abdominal pain within hours.
- *Infection with enteric pathogens:* Hours to days incubation period, followed by diarrhea and dehydration or dysentery.
- *Insidious infection:* Yersinial and mycobacterial infections. All enteroinvasive organisms can mimic (or coexist with) acute onset of inflammatory bowel disease.

Antibiotic-Associated Colitis—Pseudomembranous Colitis (p. 836)

This acute colitis is characterized by *formation of adherent inflammatory pseudomembranes overlying sites of mucosal injury.* Classically, it is caused by toxins produced by *Clostrid-*

ium difficile that has overgrown after competing bowel organisms were eliminated by broad-spectrum antibiotic therapy.

Morphology. Disease most commonly involves the right colon. There is plaquelike adhesion of fibrinopurulent-necrotic, gray-yellow debris and mucus to the damaged colonic mucosa. *The pseudomembrane is not specific for this colitis; it also may form with any severe mucosal injury, such as ischemia, volvulus, or infection.* Toxin detection in stool yields the definitive diagnosis.

Parasitic Enterocolitis (p. 838)

Parasitic enterocolitis collectively affects more than 50% of the world's population on a chronic or recurrent basis. Key organisms include:

- *Nematodes* (roundworms)

  Ascaris: This is the most common nematode. Fecal-oral transmission occurs with intestine-liver-lung-intestine life cycle. They can cause physical obstruction of intestine or biliary tract, hepatic abscesses, or *Ascaris* pneumonitis.

  Strongyloides: Life cycle begins with penetration of skin or intestinal mucosa progressing sequentially to lung and intestine. They typically incite strong tissue eosinophil reactions. Autoinfection (intestinal luminal larvae penetrate the mucosa and directly invade into the body) can be fatal in immunocompromised individuals.

  Hookworms: Life cycle begins with larvae penetration through skin-lung-duodenum. Worms attach to mucosa and extract blood, causing mucosal damage and iron deficiency anemia.

  Pinworms (Enterbius vermicularis): Transmission is fecal-oral; entire life cycle occurs in the intestinal lumen. No direct tissue invasion occurs; adult worms migrate to anal orifice where eggs are deposited, causing irritation and pruritus.

  Whipworms (Trichuris trichiura): Infection primarily affects children. No direct tissue invasion occurs; heavy infections cause diarrhea and rectal prolapse.

- *Cestodes:* Infection occurs by ingesting raw or undercooked meat. Parasites reside within the lumen without tissue invasion; scolex attaches to the mucosa, proglottids contain eggs.

- *Protozoa*

  Entamoeba histolytica: Human infection occurs by ingesting cysts; cysts release trophozoites that colonize the mucosal surface (cecum and ascending colon). Amoebae cause epithelial damage with gland invasion and formation of flask-shaped ulcers (narrow neck and broad base). Amoebae can also cause liver abscess, but rarely systemic infection. Metronidazole therapy targets the organism-specific enzyme ferridoxin-dependent pyruvate oxidoreductase.

  Giardia lamblia: This common human parasitic infection is spread typically from contaminated water and food. Duodenal trophozoites exhibit characteristic morphology (pear-shaped and binucleate); *Giardia* does not invade the tissue, but protein products damage the microvillus brush border and cause malabsorption.

  In acquired immunodeficiency syndrome (AIDS) patients, *microsporidia, cryptosporidia,* and *Isospora belli* are frequent causes of diarrheal illness.

Necrotizing Enterocolitis (p. 840)

This acute, necrotizing small bowel and colon inflammation occurs in low-birth-weight or premature neonates. It presents as mild diarrhea to fulminant illness with gangrene, perforation, sepsis, and shock. Extensive bowel resection may be required. It results from:

- Immature gut immunity
- Onset of oral feeding, initiating mucosal proinflammatory cytokine release
- Bacterial colonization exposing the mucosa to endotoxin
- Mucosal injury
- Impaired intestinal blood flow followed by rapidly progressive injury

Morphology. Mucosal edema, hemorrhage, and necrosis involve the terminal ileum and proximal colon or entire gut.

Collagenous and Lymphocytic Colitis (p. 840)

Both types present as chronic watery diarrhea with abdominal pain in middle-aged patients; female-male ratio is 6:1. Endoscopic findings are grossly normal, hence the designation "microscopic colitis." Both forms tend to follow a benign course.

- *Collagenous colitis* exhibits patches of bandlike collagen under the surface epithelium.
- *Lymphocytic colitis* exhibits a prominent intraepithelial infiltrate of lymphocytes; it is associated with autoimmune diseases and sprue.

Miscellaneous Intestinal Inflammatory Disorders (p. 841)

- *AIDS-associated diarrheal illness* (p. 841) occurs in 50% of U.S. patients and in 100% of AIDS patients in developing countries. Besides other known infectious organisms, HIV is thought to directly affect mucosal epithelium.
- *Transplantation* (bone marrow transplantation especially; p. 841) can result in graft-*versus*-host disease involving the gut mucosa; it can be fatal. Characteristic histologic findings include a mild lymphocytic infiltrate and associated crypt epithelial cell apoptosis.
- *Drug-induced intestinal injury* (p. 841) most commonly is manifest as focal ulceration or mucosal inflammation from NSAID use.
- *Radiation enterocolitis* (p. 841) may be indolent or cause an inflammatory diarrhea.
- *Neutropenic colitis (typhlitis)* (p. 841) is a life-threatening acute inflammatory destruction of the cecal region occurring in neutropenic patients (e.g., after bone marrow transplant); it is attributed to impaired mucosal immunity in conjunction with compromised blood flow.
- *Diversion colitis* (p. 841) is an iatrogenic inflammatory colitis occurring after surgical diversion of the fecal stream (as with an enterostomy). It is proposed that the lack of short-chain fatty acid delivery to the mucosa (i.e., inadequate nutrition) is responsible for this disorder. Microscopically, there is a chronic lymphoplasmacytic inflammation, and a characteristic lymphoid follicular hyperplasia.
- *Colitis cystica profunda* (the localized form is also referred as *"solitary rectal ulcer syndrome"*; p. 842) is attributed to

dysregulation of the anorectal sphincter, causing acute angulation of the anterior rectal shelf and overlying mechanical abrasion. Patients present with rectal bleeding and mucus discharge. Microscopically, there is distorted, cystically dilated glands surrounded by proliferating smooth muscle cells.

Malabsorption Syndromes (p. 842)

Malabsorption syndromes are characterized by inadequate absorption of fats, fat-soluble and other vitamins, proteins, carbohydrates, electrolytes, minerals, and water (Table 17–4). Clinical consequences include effects on several areas of the body:

- *Alimentary tract:* Diarrhea; flatus; pain; weight loss; passage of bulky, frothy, greasy stools. Excessive diarrhea can be life threatening.
- *Hematopoietic system:* Anemia, bleeding.
- *Musculoskeletal system:* Osteopenia, tetany.
- *Endocrine system:* Amenorrhea, impotence, infertility, hyperparathyroidism.
- *Skin:* Purpura and petechiae, edema, dermatitis.
- *Nervous system:* Peripheral neuropathy.

TABLE 17–4 **Major Malabsorption Syndromes**

Defective Intraluminal Digestion

Digestion of fats and proteins
    Pancreatic insufficiency, owing to pancreatitis or cystic fibrosis
    Zollinger-Ellison syndrome, with inactivation of pancreatic enzymes by excess gastric acid secretion
Solubilization of fat, owing to defective bile secretion
    Ileal dysfunction or resection, with decreased bile salt uptake
    Cessation of bile flow from obstruction, hepatic dysfunction
Nutrient preabsorption or modification by bacterial overgrowth

Primary Mucosal Cell Abnormalities

Defective terminal digestion
    Disaccharidase deficiency (lactose intolerance)
    Bacterial overgrowth, with brush border damage
Defective epithelial transport
    Abetalipoproteinemia
    Primary bile acid malabsorption owing to mutations in the ileal bile acid transporter

Reduced Small Intestinal Surface Area

Gluten-sensitive enteropathy (celiac disease)
Crohn disease

Lymphatic Obstruction

Lymphoma
Tuberculosis and tuberculous lymphadenitis

Infection

Acute infectious enteritis
Parasitic infestation
Tropical sprue
Whipple disease (*Tropheryma whippelii*)

Iatrogenic

Subtotal or total gastrectomy
Short-gut syndrome, following extensive surgical resection
Distal ileal resection or bypass

The most common causes of malabsorption syndromes in the United States are celiac disease, chronic pancreatitis with pancreatic insufficiency, and Crohn disease. Mechanistically, malabsorption results from defects in:

* *Intraluminal digestion,* including secreted enzymes and emulsification
* *Terminal digestion* (i.e., enzyme catabolism at enterocyte membranes)
* *Transepithelial transport* through enterocytes

Celiac Disease (p. 843)

This T cell–mediated inflammatory disorder leads to impaired nutrient absorption; the disorder improves with withdrawal of gluten gliadins and related grain proteins from the diet. Also called *gluten-sensitive enteropathy, nontropical sprue,* and *celiac sprue,* it is generally a disease of whites; the prevalence ranges from 1 in 200 to 1 in 2000.

Pathogenesis. Celiac disease results from a sensitivity to gluten (specifically the *gliadin* protein component) found in wheat, oat, barley, and rye. The antigenic epitopes recognized by T cells are found in residues 57 to 75 of the gliadin.

* From 90% to 95% of patients express the DQ2 (and HLA B8) histocompatibility molecules suggesting a genetic (immunologic) susceptibility.
* Immune-mediated injury likely underlies the disease; patients express antibody to gliadin that potentially cross-reacts with type 12 adenovirus.

Morphology. Diffuse enteritis with flattened (atrophic) villi, elongated regenerative crypts, surface epithelial damage with intraepithelial lymphocytes, and exuberant lamina propria chronic inflammation are seen. Severity is greatest in the more proximal intestine. Histologic appearance reverts to normal with gluten withdrawal.

Clinical Findings. Celiac disease presents in infants up to mid-adult life with diarrhea, flatulence, weight loss, and fatigue. Other causes must be excluded. Serologic tests include detecting antibodies to tissue transglutaminase and gliadin. The disease responds to gluten withdrawal.

* Celiac disease is often associated with *dermatitis herpetiformis.*
* Complications include iron and vitamin deficiencies and a 10% to 15% risk of gastrointestinal lymphoma, usually T-cell lymphoma.

Tropical (Postinfectious) Sprue (p. 844)

Tropical sprue occurs after appropriate travel or habitation exposure (e.g., in tropical climes). Although the cause is unknown, infectious etiologies (e.g., enterotoxigenic *E. coli*) are suspected. It responds to broad-spectrum antibiotic therapy; folate and vitamin B_{12} are also used for treatment.

Morphology. Variable histologic features are seen, ranging from normal to villous blunting resembling celiac disease; the lamina propria has abundant lymphocytes and more eosinophils than in celiac disease. The majority of the injury involves the distal small intestine.

Whipple Disease (p. 844)

This rare, systemic condition principally involves intestine, central nervous system, and joints. It is attributed to infection by *Tropheryma whippelii,* a gram-positive actinomycete that invades macrophages.

Morphology. Lamina propria of small intestine is laden with distended macrophages, each containing abundant bacilli (demonstrable by electron microscopy or highlighted by diastase-resistant periodic acid–Schiff [PAS] stain). Similarly laden macrophages are present in lymphatics, lymph nodes, joints, and brain. Active inflammation is largely absent, consistent with the absence of bacterial-induced immune responses.

Clinical Findings. Patients have diarrhea, steatorrhea, malabsorption, abdominal cramps, distention, fever, and weight loss; migratory arthritis and heart disease may also occur.

Whites in their 30s to 40s are affected, with a male-female ratio of 10:1. Although this condition is potentially fatal, Whipple disease usually responds to antibiotic therapy.

Lactase Deficiency

Disaccharidase (lactase) is an apical membrane enzyme of surface absorptive cells; with *lactase deficiency* (p. 844), lactose remains in the bowel lumen exerting an osmotic pull, and causing diarrhea and malabsorption.

- Rare congenital form: explosive, frothy stools and abdominal distention in infants exposed to milk/milk products
- Acquired form: common among North American blacks, with milder symptoms; worsens with enteric infections, owing to superimposed mucosal injury
- No abnormalities of mucosa or mucosal cells

Abetalipoproteinemia (p. 846)

Abetalipoproteinemia has an autosomal recessive inheritance; patients cannot synthesize apolipoprotein B required for lipoprotein export from mucosal cells. Presents in infancy with failure to thrive, diarrhea, and steatorrhea; there is severe hypolipoproteinemia related to depressed levels of chylomicrons, pre-β-lipoproteins (very-low-density lipoproteins), and β-lipoproteins (low-density lipoproteins). Patients can have neurologic and liver disorders, and retinitis pigmentosa.

- Abnormal intraepithelial triglyceride stores manifest as *lipid vacuolation* visualized on routine hematoxylin and eosin (H&E) sections.
- Altered erythrocyte lipid membrane constituents result in peripheral blood acanthocytes (*burr cell*s).

Idiopathic Inflammatory Bowel Disease
(p. 846)

Idiopathic inflammatory bowel disease (IBD) refers to chronic, relapsing idiopathic inflammatory disorders of the gastrointestinal tract likely resulting from unregulated and exaggerated local immune responses to normal gut flora in genetically susceptible individuals. There are two major forms; salient differences are listed in Table 17–5. In both forms of IBD, epithelial dysplasia may progress to carcinoma. The risk increases with extent of mucosal involvement and duration of disease. Thus, surveillance for dysplasia constitutes an importance step in patient management.

* *Crohn disease* (CD): Granulomatous IBD affecting any portion of gut, but most often small intestine and colon
* *Ulcerative colitis* (UC): IBD without granuloma formation affecting only the colon

Pathogenesis (p. 846). IBD ultimately results from *activation of inflammatory cells* whose products cause tissue injury. The following factors contribute:

* *Genetic:* familial clustering without particular HLA associations. Mutations of the *NOD2* gene are implicated in some cases of CD; NOD2 regulates proinflammatory cytokine production and innate defense against microbial pathogens.
* *Infectious:* no specific pathogen. Many agents are associated with IBD.

TABLE 17–5 **Distinctive Features of Crohn Disease and Ulcerative Colitis***

Feature	Crohn Disease—SI	Crohn Disease—C	Ulcerative Colitis
Macroscopic			
Bowel region	Ileum ± colon	Colon ± ileum	Colon only
Distribution	Skip lesions	Skip lesions	Diffuse
Stricture	Early	Variable	Late/rare
Wall appearance	Thickened	Thin	Thin
Dilation	No	Yes	Yes
Microscopic			
Inflammation	Transmural	Transmural	Limited in mucosa
Pseudopolyps	No to slight	Marked	Marked
Ulcers	Deep, linear	Deep, linear	Superficial
Lymphoid reaction	Marked	Marked	Mild
Fibrosis	Marked	Moderate	Mild
Serositis	Marked	Variable	Mild to none
Granulomas	Yes (50%)	Yes (50%)	No
Fistulae/sinuses	Yes	Yes	No
Clinical			
Fat/vitamin malabsorption	Yes	Yes, if ileum involved	No
Malignant potential	Yes	Yes	Yes
Response to surgery	Poor	Fair	Good

*SI, Crohn disease of the small intestine; C, Crohn disease of the colon. Features are often not all present in a single case.

- *Mucosal integrity:* Increased intestinal permeability and altered mucoproteins may affect ability of microbes to breach the epithelium and trigger inflammatory responses.
- *Abnormal host immunoreactivity:* exaggerated host responses to otherwise innocuous antigenic stimuli.

Crohn Disease (p. 847)

CD has an annual incidence in the United States of 3 per 100,000; it presents at any age, with a peak incidence in the teens to the 20s, females are more often affected than males, and whites more often than nonwhites. It is characterized by:

- Regional involvement *(skip lesions)*
- Sharply delimited, typically transmural lesions with inflammation and mucosal damage
- Fissuring and fistula formation due to transmural inflammation
- Noncaseating granulomas (50% of cases)
- Systemic manifestations

Morphology. CD involves the small intestine alone in 40% of cases, the small intestine and colon in 30%, and colon alone in 39%. The duodenum, stomach, esophagus, and mouth are uncommonly involved.

- Gross findings:

  Skip lesions with granular and inflamed serosa and adherent *"creeping"* mesenteric fat

  Rubbery thick bowel wall with edema, inflammation, fibrosis, muscular hypertrophy, and often stricture

  Punched-out mucosal *aphthous* ulcers and linear ulcers

- Microscopic findings:

  Mucosal inflammation and ulceration with intraepithelial neutrophils and *crypt abscesses,* lamina propria with mononuclear inflammation

  Chronic mucosal damage with villus blunting, atrophy, metaplasia, and architectural disarray

  Transmural inflammation with *lymphoid aggregates* in submucosa, muscle wall, and subserosal fat

  Noncaseating granulomas present throughout the gut, even in uninvolved segments

  Fibrosis with muscle and neural hypertrophy and vasculitis

  Dysplasia in the mucosa

Clinical Findings

- Intermittent attacks of diarrhea, fever, abdominal pain, anorexia, weight loss; intervening asymptomatic periods
- *Complications* from fibrotic strictures; fistulas to adjacent viscera, abdominal and perineal skin, bladder, or vagina; malabsorption and malnutrition; loss of albumin (protein-losing enteropathy)
- With extensive terminal ileal involvement vitamin B_{12} deficiency with pernicious anemia and malabsorption of bile salts with steatorrhea.
- Increased risk of bowel cancer
- Extraintestinal manifestations: migratory polyarthritis, sacroiliitis, ankylosing spondylitis, erythema nodosum, uveitis, cholangitis, amyloidosis

Ulcerative Colitis (p. 849)

This ulcerating inflammatory disease is limited to the colon, and affects only the mucosa and submucosa (except in the most severe cases). In contrast to CD, UC extends in a continuous fashion beginning in the rectum, and granulomas are absent. The annual U.S. incidence is 4 per 100,000 to 12 per 100,000, typically occurring in young to older adulthood with a peak incidence in ages 20 to 25 years, females more than males and whites more than nonwhites.

Morphology. UC is a disease of continuity with no *skip* lesions, involving the rectum and extending proximally in retrograde fashion to involve the entire colon (pancolitis); the distal ileum may also show some inflammation.

- Gross findings:

  Mucosa may be reddened, granular, or friable with inflammatory *pseudopolyps,* and easy bleeding; extensive ulceration or may be atrophic and flattened.
  Mural thickening and stricture do not occur.
  Dysplasia may develop in the mucosa.

- Microscopic findings:

  Mucosal inflammation is similar to CD with crypt abscesses, ulceration, chronic mucosal damage, glandular architectural distortion, and atrophy.
  Fissures, aphthous ulcers, and granulomas are absent.
  In treated or inactive disease, the mucosa may revert to near normal.

Clinical Findings
- Intermittent attacks of bloody mucoid diarrhea and abdominal pain
- Rarely presents as explosive illness with severe electrolyte disturbances and *toxic megacolon* (a massively dilated, nonfunctional colon)
- *Extraintestinal manifestations:* migratory polyarthritis, sacroiliitis, ankylosing spondylitis, uveitis, cholangitis and primary sclerosing cholangitis (up to 5% of patients), and skin lesions
- *Risk of carcinoma arising from dysplasia:* highest risk in patients with pancolitis of greater than 10 years' duration

Vascular Disorders (p. 851)

Ischemic Bowel Disease (p. 851)

Predisposing conditions:

- *Arterial thrombosis* due to atherosclerosis, vasculitis, dissecting aneurysm, angiography, surgery, hypercoagulable states
- *Arterial embolism* due to cardiac vegetations, angiography, aortic atheroembolism
- *Venous thrombosis* due to hypercoagulable states, cirrhosis, sepsis, surgery and abdominal trauma, neoplasms
- *Nonocclusive ischemia:* cardiac failure, shock, dehydration, vasoconstrictive drugs
- *Miscellaneous:* radiation, volvulus, stricture, herniation

Morphology

- *Mucosal infarction:* patchy mucosal hemorrhage, but with normal serosa. Extent of inflammation depends on duration of injury. Infarction may be due to any of the causes listed previously.
- *Mural infarction:* complete mucosal necrosis, with variable necrosis of submucosa and muscularis propria. Generally, this infarction is due to major vascular compromise (vascular occlusion, volvulus, herniation). Distribution may be patchy, but is typically segmental.
- *Transmural infarction:* sudden and total occlusion of major vasculature (thrombosis, volvulus, herniation) with infarction of all bowel layers. Bowel segment is usually hemorrhagic due to blood suffusion into damaged area. Bacterial overgrowth produces gangrene, and perforation develops within days.
- *Venous thrombosis:* Acute mesenteric venous occlusion (e.g., due to portal vein thrombosis) produces massive small bowel congestion with infarction.
- *Chronic ischemia:* Chronic vascular insufficiency causes mucosal inflammation, ulceration, fibrosis, and stricture. Ischemia has a segmental patchy distribution. Transmural infarction is more common in the small bowel (completely dependent on mesenteric blood supply); large bowel has posterior abdominal wall collaterals.

Clinical Findings. Total bowel infarction has a 50% to 75% mortality rate. Typically occurring in severely ill patients, it presents as severe abdominal pain, bloody diarrhea or gross melena, nausea, vomiting, bloating, and abdominal wall rigidity. With incomplete infarction, there are nonspecific abdominal complaints.

Angiodysplasia (p. 854)

Angiodysplasia features tortuous, abnormal dilations (small and focal, to large and dilated) of submucosal veins extending into the lamina propria of the cecum or ascending colon; these areas may bleed intermittently.

Pathogenesis. Acquired ectasias are attributed to partial, intermittent occlusion of submucosal veins. These occur largely in the cecum because the maximal wall tension is greatest there owing to its larger diameter (LaPlace law).

Hemorrhoids (p. 854)

Hemorrhoids are variceal dilations of anal and perianal submucosal venous plexi; they affect 5% of adults. Hemorrhoids are causally associated with constipation (straining at stool), venous stasis during pregnancy, and cirrhosis (portal hypertension). *External hemorrhoids* occur with ectasia of the inferior hemorrhoidal plexus below the anorectal line; *internal hemorrhoids* are due to ectasia of the superior hemorrhoidal plexus above the anorectal line. Secondary thrombosis (with recanalization), strangulation, or ulceration with fissure formation can occur.

Diverticular Disease (p. 854)

Acquired diverticula may occur in the esophagus, stomach, small intestine, or colon. Acquired *colonic diverticula (diverticulosis)* are uncommon in patients younger than age 30, but occur in 50% of Western populations in those after age 60.

Morphology. Multiple flask-like outpouchings, 0.5 to 1 cm in diameter, are found typically in the distal colon. They occur where the vasculature penetrates the inner circular layer of the muscularis propria (at the taeniae coli), and dissect into the subjacent appendices epiploicae. The thin diverticulum wall is lined by mucosa and submucosa without significant muscularis propria, although the muscularis between diverticuli is hypertrophic. *Diverticulitis*—inflammation of diverticulum after obstruction or perforation—is a complication.

Pathogenesis. *Focal bowel wall weakness* (at sites of penetrating blood vessels) allows mucosal outpouching when there is *increased intraluminal pressure* due to exaggerated peristaltic contractions (e.g., due to decreased dietary bulk).

Clinical Findings. Diverticular disease is usually asymptomatic, but may be associated with cramping, abdominal discomfort, and constipation. Diverticulitis can result in pericolic abscesses, sinus tracts, and peritonitis.

Intestinal Obstruction (p. 855)

Tumors and infarctions account for 10% to 15% of obstructions; 80% are attributable to the following four entities:

Hernias (p. 855)

Peritoneal wall weakness or defect permits protrusion of a peritoneal sac *(hernia sac)* in which bowel segments can be trapped *(external herniation)*. Subsequent vascular stasis and edema lead to *incarceration;* vascular compromise leads to *strangulation.* Locations include the femoral and inguinal canals (internal and external), umbilicus, retroperitoneum, and surgical scars.

Adhesions (p. 856)

Adhesions are residua of localized peritoneal inflammation *(peritonitis)* following surgery, infection, endometriosis, or radiation; healing leads to fibrous bridging between viscera; they may also be congenital. *Complications* include *internal herniation* (within peritoneal cavity), obstruction, and strangulation.

Intussusception (p. 856)

Intussusception refers to telescoping of one intestinal segment (usually small bowel) into the immediately distal segment. In *infants and children,* intussusception is spontaneous and reversible; rotaviral vaccination or infection can cause intussusception in some children. In *adults,* the point of traction is usually a tumor.

Volvulus (p. 856)

Volvulus is complete twisting of a bowel loop about its mesenteric vascular base, leading to obstruction and infarction. Volvulus occurs most often in small bowel or redundant loops of sigmoid colon.

Tumors of the Small and Large Intestine (p. 856)

The colon (including the rectum) is the gastrointestinal tract segment most commonly affected by tumors (Table 17–6). Benign tumors are primarily epithelial and occur in 25% to 50% of older adults.

Tumors of the Small Intestine (p. 856)

The small intestine represents 75% of the length of the gastrointestinal tract, yet contributes only 3% to 6% of tumors (malignant-benign ratio, 1.5 : 1). *Benign lesions* include leiomyomas, adenomas, lipomas, neuromas, vascular malformations, and hamartomatous lesions. *Adenomas* frequently occur in the region of the ampulla of Vater, especially in patients with familial polyposis syndromes. *Adenocarcinomas* and *carcinoids* occur with roughly equal incidence.

Clinical Findings. Adenomas are clinically silent unless they obstruct the intestinal lumen or common bile duct. Adenocarcinomas typically present with obstruction (cramping pain,

TABLE 17–6   **Tumors of the Small Intestine and Colon**

Non-Neoplastic (Benign) Polyps
Hyperplastic polyps
Hamartomatous polyps
   Juvenile polyps
   Peutz-Jeghers polyps
Inflammatory polyps
Lymphoid polyps

Neoplastic Epithelial Lesions
Benign
   Adenoma*
Malignant
   Adenocarcinoma*
   Carcinoid tumor
   Anal zone carcinoma

Mesenchymal Lesions
Gastrointestinal stromal tumor (GIST) (gradation from benign to malignant)
Other benign lesions
   Lipoma
   Neuroma
   Angioma
Kaposi sarcoma

Lymphoma

*Benign and malignant counterparts of the most common neoplasms in the intestines; virtually all lesions are in the colon.

nausea, vomiting), weight loss, and bleeding. Metastatic spread is to mesentery, regional lymph nodes, and liver. Five-year survival rate is 70% with wide en bloc excisions.

Tumors of the Colon and Rectum (p. 857)

Benign Tumors

Polyps are tumorous masses that protrude into the gut lumen; they may be *pedunculated* (with a stalk) or *sessile* (without a stalk). They may be *non-neoplastic* or *neoplastic*.

Non-neoplastic Polyps (p. 858). These polyps result from abnormal mucosal maturation, inflammation, or architecture. They usually have no malignant potential and represent 90% of colonic epithelial polyps.

- *Hyperplastic polyp:* found in over 50% of persons older than 60 years. These nipple-like hemispheric protrusions are usually less than 5 mm in diameter. Polyps are composed of well-formed mature glands exhibiting crowding; they result from delayed surface epithelial cell shedding. Although formerly considered entirely benign, a subset of hyperplastic polyps (identified as *"serrated adenomas"*) may reflect microsatellite instability (MSI) along the pathway to colonic cancer.
- *Juvenile polyp:* focal, usually sporadic hamartomatous malformations of small intestine and colon mucosa. Polyps are typically large (1–3 cm), rounded, and pedunculated with cystically dilated glands and abundant lamina propria. Most occur in children younger than 5 years old, and involve the rectum. The rare *juvenile polyposis syndrome* is autosomal dominant, with numerous polyps, and increased risk of adenomas and adenocarcinoma.
- *Peutz-Jeghers polyp:* sporadic, hamartomatous mucosal polyps of small intestine and colon. These polyps are large, pedunculated, and lobulated with arborizing smooth muscle surrounding normal abundant glands. The rare *Peutz-Jeghers syndrome* is autosomal dominant, with melanotic pigmentation of mucosal and skin surfaces, and increased risk of carcinomas (pancreas, breast, lung, ovary, uterus).
- *Other polyps: lymphoid aggregates* (normal); *inflammatory polyps* in IBD; small isolated hamartomatous polyps *(retention polyps)* found in adult colons.

Adenomas (Neoplastic Polyps) (p. 859). These polyps arise from dysplastic epithelium; adenocarcinoma generally arises from adenomas. Prevalence of adenomas approaches 50% after age 60; they are frequently multiple. All adenomas arise as the result of epithelial proliferative dysplasia. Four histologic appearances are recognized:

- *Tubular adenoma:* tubular glands, smooth surface
- *Villous adenoma:* villous frondlike projections of epithelial surface
- *Tubulovillous adenoma:* mixture of the first two
- *Serrated adenoma:* features of both hyperplastic polyp and adenoma, often associated with MSI

Most tubular adenomas are small, but become pedunculated as they grow; most villous adenomas are large but remain sessile. Adenomas are slow growing; doubling time is approximately 10 years. *Risk of coexistent malignancy is correlated to:*

- Polyp size.
- Histologic architecture.
- Severity of dysplasia: Larger villous adenomas typically show more severe dysplasia.

Morphology. Most (90%) adenomas are in the colon, but they may occur in stomach or small intestine; they may be single or multiple. *By definition, all adenomas exhibit dysplastic epithelium* (tall, hyperchromatic disorderly cells with increased nuclear-cytoplasmic ratio, cigar-shaped nuclei) that may be mild (nuclei still basally oriented) to severe (stratified nuclei over full thickness of epithelium). Dysplastic cells line the entire colonic crypt and mucosal surface. Any adenoma can harbor *intramucosal carcinoma* (overt malignancy confined to mucosa) or *invasive carcinoma* (extending beyond the mucosa), regardless of size or histology.

- *Tubular adenomas* begin as smooth mucosal bumps involving only a few adjacent crypts; with growth, they become bulky neoplasms (up to 4 cm diameter) protruding into the lumen; branching dysplastic glands are embedded in the lamina propria. Traction creates a submucosal stalk lined by normal mucosa.
- *Villous adenomas* tend to be larger when discovered and may carpet up to 10 cm of colonic mucosa. Finger-like projections with a lamina propria core are lined by dysplastic epithelium.
- *Tubulovillous adenomas* are intermediate in size, usually with a stalk and mixed architecture.
- *Serrated adenomas* exhibit a transitional mixture of glands with "hyperplastic" scalloped contours and "adenomatous" dysplastic nuclei.

Adenomas with *severe dysplasia (carcinoma in situ)* cannot yet metastasize and are not yet malignant. Polyps with *intramucosal carcinoma* confined to mucosa have little to no metastatic potential since lymphatic channels are mostly absent in mucosa (in colon). Polyps with *invasive adenocarcinoma* are malignant and have metastatic potential because they have crossed into submucosa and can access lymphatics.

Clinical Findings. Adenomas may be asymptomatic or may cause occult bleeding with anemia. Small intestine adenomas can cause obstruction and intussusception. Rarely, large villous adenomas in colon hypersecrete copious amounts of protein- and potassium-rich mucus.

- *Endoscopic removal of pedunculated malignant polyps is adequate provided that* the invasive component is superficial and does not approach the margin, there is no evident vascular or lymphatic invasion, and the invasive component is not poorly differentiated.
- Invasive adenocarcinoma arising in a sessile polyp cannot be adequately resected by polypectomy; further surgery is required.
- *The only adequate treatment for any adenoma is resection,* regardless of whether carcinoma is present. Any residual adenomatous tissue is still a premalignant lesion, and could even harbor invasive adenocarcinoma.

Familial Syndromes (p. 861)

Many familial syndromes exhibit gastrointestinal tract polyps; the genetic basis for some of these syndromes is listed in Table 17–7.

TABLE 17–7   **Hereditary Syndromes Involving the Gastrointestinal Tract**

Syndromes	Altered Gene	Pathology in GI Tract
Familial adenomatous polyposis (FAP) Classic FAP Attenuated FAP Gardner syndrome Turcot syndrome	*APC*	Multiple adenomatous polyps
Peutz-Jeghers syndrome	*STK11*	Hamartomatous polyps
Juvenile polyposis syndrome	*SMAD4* *BMPRIA*	Juvenile polyps
Hereditary nonpolyposis colorectal carcinoma	Defects in DNA mismatch repair genes	Colon cancer
Tuberous sclerosis	*TSC1* *TSC2*	Inflammatory polyps
Cowden disease	*PTEN*	Hamartomatous polyps

Familial adenomatous polyposis (FAP) is the prototypical autosomal dominant polyposis syndrome.

- Innumerable adenomatous polyps in colon (and other GI sites); a minimum of 100 colonic adenomas is required for diagnosis.
- Average age of onset is 20s to 30s. Progression to cancer starts within 10 to 15 years of onset, and there is a 100% risk of colon adenocarcinoma by mid-adulthood; prophylactic colectomy is curative.

There are multiple variants to this syndrome: *classic FAP; attenuated FAP; Gardner syndrome; and Turcot syndrome.* In addition to GI polyps, *Gardner syndrome* exhibits multiple osteomas (mandible, skull, long bones), epidermal cysts, fibromatosis (desmoid tumors), abnormal dentition (impacted teeth), and increased incidence of duodenal and thyroid cancers. *Turcot syndrome* is rarer; besides adenomas, there are central nervous system tumors (gliomas). Only two thirds of Turcot syndrome patients are formally considered as FAP variants; in these, the brain tumor is typically medulloblastoma. The remainder of Turcot patients have DNA mismatch repair gene mutations (*hereditary nonpolyposis colorectal cancer syndrome, or HNPCC*), and the brain tumors are usually glioblastomas.

Colorectal Carcinogenesis (p. 862)

Evidence for an adenoma-to-carcinoma progression:

- *Epidemiology:* Populations at risk are similar.
- *Topology:* Colorectal distributions are similar.
- *Chronology:* Peak incidence years are offset slightly.
- *Histology:* Adenomas commonly harbor adenocarcinoma.
- *Quantity:* Cancer risk is related to number of polyps.
- *Intervention:* Screening programs for adenomas reduce incidence of colorectal carcinoma.

Genetic alterations in the progression from colon adenomas to carcinomas have been characterized (Fig. 17–1):

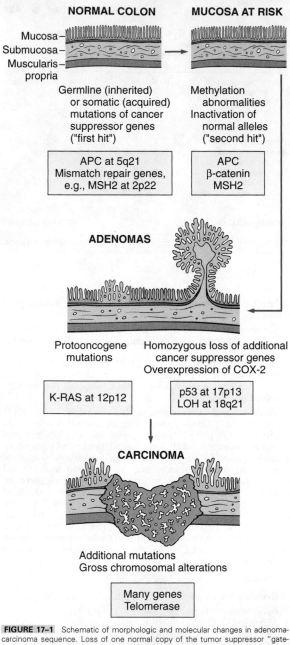

NORMAL COLON

Mucosa
Submucosa
Muscularis propria

MUCOSA AT RISK

Germline (inherited) or somatic (acquired) mutations of cancer suppressor genes ("first hit")

APC at 5q21
Mismatch repair genes, e.g., MSH2 at 2p22

Methylation abnormalities
Inactivation of normal alleles ("second hit")

APC
β-catenin
MSH2

ADENOMAS

Protooncogene mutations

K-RAS at 12p12

Homozygous loss of additional cancer suppressor genes
Overexpression of COX-2

p53 at 17p13
LOH at 18q21

CARCINOMA

Additional mutations
Gross chromosomal alterations

Many genes
Telomerase

FIGURE 17–1 Schematic of morphologic and molecular changes in adenoma-carcinoma sequence. Loss of one normal copy of the tumor suppressor "gate-keeper" gene *APC* occurs early, representing the "first hit" in Knudson's hypothesis (individuals may be born with mutant *APC* alleles); loss of the remaining normal *APC* copy is a "second hit." *K-RAS* oncogene mutations occur next, followed by mutations or losses of heterozygosity that inactivate *p53* and *SMAD 2* and *4*. As the carcinoma emerges, it accrues additional mutations. Although presented sequentially, *it is the accumulation of mutations rather than their specific order that is most important.*

- FAP patients have mutations in the tumor-suppressor *APC* gene (*a*denomatous *p*olyposis *c*oli); mutations occur in sporadic cancers as well.
- *DNA methylation:* Loss of DNA methyl groups occurs early in colonic adenomas.
- *K-RAS gene* and other oncogenes are mutated with increasing frequency as adenomas increase in size and develop into carcinomas.
- SMADs are involved in the tumor growth factor-β (TGF-β) signaling pathway; mutations are associated with cancer formation.
- Losses at 17p (site of *p53 gene*) are common in cancers.
- *Telomerase* is an enzyme that maintains chromosome telomere length and cell replicative ability; it is expressed in cancers but not in adenomas.

Cumulative alterations in the genome appear to lead to progressive increases in dysplasia and invasive potential of neoplastic lesions. No single event or sequence of events is requisite, but a multihit genetic mechanism appears to be operative.

DNA mismatch repair gene mutations occur in *HNPCC*, and cause faulty DNA *proofreading*, widespread alterations in the genome, and predisposition to cancer. Sporadic cancers can exhibit the same defect. This pathway for carcinogenesis is considered a separate pathway for colorectal cancer, *versus* the classic adenoma-carcinoma sequence described earlier.

Colorectal carcinoma (p. 864) causes 56,600 deaths per year in the United States, second only to lung cancer. Peak incidence is between ages 60 and 79 except in polyposis syndromes. The male-female ratio is 1:1, except for rectal cancer, in which men are favored. Worldwide distribution is higher in industrialized countries; 98% are adenocarcinomas.

Pathogenesis. Hereditary polyp syndromes, HNPCC, and IBD significantly increase the risk of developing carcinoma. However, most colonic cancers arise sporadically in polypoid adenomas. *Diet* likely contributes to risk in these sporadic cancers, although causality is not proved; such diets may promote increased mucosal exposure to bile acids and bacterial degradative byproducts:

- Energy intake greater than requirement
- Low vegetable fiber intake
- High content of refined carbohydrates
- High intake of red meat
- Decreased intake of *protective micronutrients* (vitamins A, C, E)

Morphology. Roughly a quarter of colon cancers occur in the cecum and ascending colon, with 11% in the transverse colon, 6% in the descending colon, and 55% in the rectosigmoid; 1% of colon cancers will be multifocal at presentation. *Grossly* there may be a *polypoid, exophytic mass* (especially in capacious cecum and right colon) or an *annular mass* with "*napkin-ring*" obstruction (characteristic of distal colon). Both forms penetrate the bowel wall over the course of many years.

Histologically, these tumors are typically composed of tall, columnar cells resembling adenomatous neoplastic epithelium but with invasion into the submucosa, muscularis propria, or beyond; a minority produce copious extracellular mucin. Carcinomas may also be poorly differentiated, solid tumors without gland formation. Less commonly, foci of neuroendocrine differentiation, signet-ring features, or squamous differentiation occur. Tumors characteristically incite *desmoplastic stromal responses,* with mesenchymal inflammation and fibrosis.

Clinical Findings. Colorectal carcinoma is usually asymptomatic at first. Fatigue, weakness, iron deficiency anemia, abdominal discomfort, progressive bowel obstruction, and liver enlargement (metastases) eventually occur. *Prognosis varies with the stage of disease at diagnosis;* 5-year survival rates are related to the depth of tumor penetration and lymph node involvement, and range from 100% for lesions limited to the mucosa to 25% for extensively invasive tumors. Currently, only surgery can be curative.

Carcinoid Tumors (p. 866)

Carcinoid tumors are tumors of gut endocrine cells *(carcinoid = cancer-like)*. Although most arise in the gut, they can also occur in the pancreas, lungs, biliary tree, and liver. Carcinoid tumors represent 50% of small intestine cancers. Peak incidence is in the sixth decade.

- Appendiceal and rectal carcinoids rarely metastasize.
- Ileal, gastric, and colonic carcinoids are frequently aggressive. Because of their endocrine cell origin, many elaborate bioactive products (e.g., amines or peptides).

Morphology. Typically, these tumors are small, firm, yellow-tan intramural or submucosal masses. They are usually solitary in the appendix and rectum but tend to be multiple elsewhere. Fibrosis ensuing from invasion of the muscularis may cause kinking and intestinal obstruction. Metastases are usually small and dispersed. *Microscopically,* the tumors range from islands to sheets of uniform cohesive cells with scant, granular cytoplasm and oval, stippled nuclei; cell clusters are separated by dense fibrous stroma. The cells usually stain positive for neuroendocrine markers, such as chromogranin and synaptophysin.

Clinical Findings. Carcinoid tumors are generally asymptomatic, although local symptoms can occur from obstruction or bleeding. Symptoms can also be caused by tumor secretory products:

- Gastrin causing *Zollinger-Ellison syndrome* with peptic ulceration
- Corticotropin causing Cushing syndrome
- Insulin causing hyperinsulinism
- Serotonin and other bioactive amines causing *carcinoid syndrome*

Carcinoid syndrome is seen only with extraintestinal carcinoid or with extensive hepatic metastases (allowing bioactive amines to reach the systemic circulation without being metabolized). Symptoms include:

- *Vasomotor disturbances:* flushing, cyanosis.
- *Intestinal hypermotility:* diarrhea, cramps, nausea, vomiting.
- *Asthmatic bronchoconstriction:* cough, wheezing, dyspnea.
- *Hepatomegaly* from hepatic metastases
- *Systemic fibrosis:* pulmonary and tricuspid valve thickening and stenosis, endocardial fibrosis, retroperitoneal and pelvic fibrosis, collagenous pleural and aortic intimal plaques.

Carcinoid syndrome is diagnosed by documenting excess urinary 5-hydroxyindoleacetic acid (5-HIAA; a breakdown product of serotonin). Appendiceal and rectal carcinoids are almost always innocuous. Five-year survival rate for other carcinoids is 90%; with hepatic metastases, 5-year survival rate is 50%.

Gastrointestinal Lymphoma (p. 868)

The gut is the most common location for the 40% of lymphomas arising in extranodal sites. Although they usually arise as sporadic neoplasms (1%–3% of GI malignancies), *primary GI lymphomas occur more frequently in chronic sprue-like malabsorption syndromes, natives of Mediterranean region, congenital immunodeficiency states, human immunodeficiency virus (HIV) infection, and after organ transplantation with immunosuppression.*

Sporadic B-cell lymphomas are the most common form of GI lymphoma in the Western hemisphere; these derive from *m*ucosa-*a*ssociated *l*ymphoid *t*issue *(MALT)* with 55% to 60% arising in the stomach, 25% to 30% in the small intestine, and 20% to 25% in the colon. They may be related to chronic mucosal lymphoid activation (e.g., chronic gastric inflammation with *H. pylori* infection).

Morphology. *Early lesions* are plaquelike mucosal or submucosal expansions. *Advanced lesions* are of full mural thickness or are polypoid, exophytic masses protruding to lumen. *Microscopically,* atypical lymphocytes infiltrate and replace normal structures. Extreme numbers of lymphocytes may populate the mucosal epithelium *(lymphoepithelial lesion)*. B-cell lesions (95%) may be low or high grade; T-cell lesions (5%) are all high grade.

Clinical Findings. Sporadic lymphomas are amenable to surgical resection and are chemoresponsive. Outcome depends on size, grade, and tumor invasiveness at resection. Low-grade lymphomas associated with *H. pylori* infection may be treatable by eradicating the *Helicobacter* organism.

Mesenchymal Tumors (p. 869)

- *Lipomas* are the most common GI mesenchymal tumor, generally found in the small intestine or colon submucosa.
- *Gastrointestinal stromal tumors* exhibit spindle or epitheloid morphology; cells are c-KIT positive.
- *Smooth muscle tumors:* Spindle-cell lesions exhibit a smooth muscle phenotype; benign *(leiomyoma)* and malignant forms *(leiomyosarcoma)* occur.
- *Kaposi sarcoma:* Visceral involvement is common.

Clinical Findings. Most mesenchymal tumors are asymptomatic. Larger lesions may cause mucosal ulceration with bleeding (especially in stomach), obstruction, or intussusception.

APPENDIX (p. 870)

Acute Appendicitis (p. 870)

Acute appendicitis is the most common acute abdominal condition requiring surgery. The differential diagnosis includes virtually every acute process that can occur in the abdomen as well as some acute thorax conditions.

Pathogenesis. Obstruction of the appendiceal lumen by a fecalith, calculus, tumor, or worms (*Oxyuriasis vermicularis* or *pinworm*) causes increased intraluminal pressure, followed by ischemia (exacerbated by edema and exudate), and bacterial invasion.

Morphology

- *Early acute appendicitis* involves scant appendiceal wall neutrophil exudate with congestion of subserosal vessels and perivascular neutrophil emigration. Serosa is dull, granular, and red.
- *Advanced acute appendicitis (acute suppurative appendicitis)* involves more severe neutrophilic infiltration with fibrinopurulent serosal exudate, luminal abscess formation, ulceration, and suppurative necrosis. This stage can progress to gangrenous necrosis *(acute gangrenous appendicitis)*, followed by perforation.

Clinical Findings. Acute appendicitis can occur at any age, but mainly affects adolescents and young adults. Classically, there is periumbilical pain migrating to the right lower quadrant; nausea or vomiting; abdominal tenderness; mild fever; and leukocytosis greater than 15,000 cells per mm^3. Symptoms may be variably present in very young and elderly patients making clinical diagnosis more difficult. Other entities that mimic appendicitis include enterocolitis, mesenteric lymphadenitis, systemic viral infection, acute salpingitis, ectopic pregnancy, mittelschmerz, and Meckel diverticulitis. Since untreated appendiceal perforation has a 2% mortality rate, a false-positive clinical diagnosis rate of 20% to 25% (with a histologically normal appendix) is considered quite acceptable. Pyelophlebitis and thrombosis of portal venous drainage, liver abscess, and bacteremia are other important complications of appendicitis.

Tumors of the Appendix (p. 871)

Mucocele and Pseudomyxoma Peritonei (p. 871)

Mucocele simply means dilation of the appendiceal lumen by mucinous secretions; it can be due to innocuous obstruction with inspissated mucus, to mucin-secreting adenomas, or to adenocarcinoma.

- Non-neoplastic *mucosal hyperplasia* can produce copious amounts of mucin.
- Neoplastic mucin-producing *mucinous cystadenoma* can lead to mechanical distention, with appendiceal rupture and spillage of neoplastic cells into the abdomen; this is not malignant dissemination but rather local rupture.
- *Mucinous cystadenocarcinoma* is indistinguishable from cystadenomas except for *appendiceal wall invasion by neoplastic cells and peritoneal implants*. The peritoneum becomes distended with tenacious, semisolid, mucin-producing anaplastic adenocarcinoma cells—*pseudomyxoma peritonei;* it is ultimately fatal.

PERITONEUM (p. 872)

Inflammation (p. 872)

Sterile peritonitis can result from bile or pancreatic enzyme spillage. *Surgical procedures* can cause foreign body reaction and adhesions. *Endometriosis* (ectopic endometrial implants) will periodically bleed causing peritoneal inflammation.

Peritoneal Infection (p. 872)

Bacterial infections can result from appendicitis, peptic ulcer, cholecystitis, diverticulitis, bowel strangulation, acute salpingitis, abdominal trauma, or peritoneal dialysis. Spontaneous bacterial peritonitis can develop in the setting of ascites of other causes (e.g., nephrotic syndrome or cirrhosis).

Morphology. Peritoneal membranes become dull and gray, followed by exudation and frank suppuration; localized abscesses can develop (subhepatic, subdiaphragmatic), although the inflammation tends to remain superficial. In *tuberculous peritonitis,* the exudate is studded with minute, pale granulomas.

Clinical Findings. Infections can resolve spontaneously or with therapy. Exudates may organize, leaving fibrous adhesions, and residual, walled-off abscesses may persist, serving as new infectious foci.

Sclerosing Retroperitonitis (p. 873)

Sclerosing retroperitonitis is a dense infiltrative fibrosing overgrowth of retroperitoneal tissues; the accompanying lymphocyte, plasma cell, and neutrophil infiltrate suggests an inflammatory rather than a neoplastic process. The fibrosis may encircle ureters (causing hydronephrosis) or bowel segments. Although usually sporadic, sclerosing retroperitonitis can occur with methysergide use (for migraine headaches) or in fibrosing disorders (e.g., carcinoid tumors, sclerosing cholangitis, Riedel fibrosing thyroiditis).

Mesenteric Cysts (p. 873)

These cysts arise from sequestered lymphatic channels, pinched-off enteric diverticula of developing foregut or hindgut, developmental cysts of urogenital origin, pancreatic pseudocysts, or walled-off infections. Occasionally, these cysts are malignant, arising from other primary sites.

Tumors (p. 873)

Tumors may be primary or secondary; virtually all are malignant.

- *Primary* tumors are rare and include *mesothelioma* (similar to pleural or pericardial mesotheliomas) and *desmoplastic small round cell tumor.* The latter resembles other such tumors and has a characteristic t(11;22)(p13;q12) translocation yielding *EWS-WT1* fusion.
- *Secondary* tumors are common and may be any form of advanced cancer. These tumors tend to diffusely seed peritoneal surfaces.

CHAPTER 18

Liver and Biliary Tract

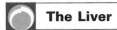

The Liver

GENERAL FEATURES OF HEPATIC DISEASE
(p. 879)

The adult human liver weighs 1400 to 1600 gm. It has a dual blood supply—portal vein and hepatic artery. Histologically, the key anatomic features are portal tracts (hepatic artery, portal vein, and bile duct), the hepatocellular parenchyma, and hepatic veins. The parenchyma is perfused by blood within sinusoids lined by a fenestrated endothelium permitting free exchange of plasma solutes with hepatocytes. Scattered macrophages *(Kupffer cells)* adhere to the sinusoidal endothelium. Hepatic *stellate cells* reside in the subendothelial *space of Disse;* these cells normally contain vitamin A–rich fat vacuoles but can transform into *myofibroblasts* during liver injury. Subendothelial lymphocytes are also normally present.

The enormous functional hepatic reserve masks the clinical impact of early liver damage. Although the liver is vulnerable to a host of metabolic, toxic, microbial, circulatory, and neoplastic insults, the most common liver diseases in the United States are hepatitis B and C viral infections, alcohol-related liver disease, and nonalcoholic fatty liver disease.

Patterns of Hepatic Injury (p. 880)

- *Inflammation (hepatitis):* influx of acute or chronic inflammatory cells into portal tracts or the parenchyma. Granulomas can be induced by foreign bodies, organisms, or drugs. Abscesses may also occur.
- *Degeneration:* characterized by hepatocyte swelling either with fat or with water and solute. Certain materials can also

accumulate, such as retained bile pigments, iron, copper, or viral particles.

- *Cell death:* coagulative necrosis due to ischemia. *Apoptosis is due to toxic, viral, or immunologic injury; ballooning degeneration is due to almost any form of injury.* Lesions may be focal (scattered through the parenchyma), zonal (periportal or perivenous), submassive, or massive.
- *Regeneration:* occurs in all but the most fulminant diseases. Hepatocyte proliferation produces thickened hepatocyte cords or swirls of immature tubular and acinar structures.
- *Fibrosis:* develops after inflammation or direct toxic insult. Ongoing fibrosis divides the liver into nodules of regenerating hepatocytes surrounded by scar tissue, termed *cirrhosis.*

Hepatic Failure (p. 881)

The major clinical consequences of liver disease are listed in Table 18–1. *Hepatic failure* is at the most severe end of this spectrum; it occurs only when greater than 80% to 90% of hepatic function is lost, and has an overall mortality rate of 70% to 95%. Frequently, patients with marginal hepatic function can be tipped toward decompensation (failure) when intercurrent disease places a greater demand on hepatic function (e.g., gastrointestinal hemorrhage, systemic infection, electrolyte disturbances, severe physiologic stress, drug dosages that would be nontoxic for a normal liver). Some patients survive with supportive measures only; others require liver transplantation. The following conditions can cause hepatic failure:

- *Massive hepatic necrosis,* such as that due to fulminant viral hepatitis or exposure to hepatotoxic drugs and chemicals

TABLE 18–1 **Clinical Consequences of Liver Disease**

Characteristic Signs
Hepatic dysfunction
Jaundice and cholestasis
Hypoalbuminemia
Hyperammonemia
Hypoglycemia
Fetor hepaticus
Palmar erythema
Spider angiomas
Hypogonadism
Gynecomastia
Weight loss
Muscle wasting
Portal hypertension from cirrhosis
Ascites
Splenomegaly
Hemorrhoids
Caput medusae—abdominal skin
Life-Threatening Complications
Hepatic failure
Multiple organ failure
Coagulopathy
Hepatic encephalopathy
Hepatorenal syndrome
Portal hypertension from cirrhosis
Esophageal varices, risk of rupture
Malignancy with chronic disease
Hepatocellular carcinoma

(e.g., acetaminophen, halothane, mushroom poisoning), can lead to hepatic failure.

- *Chronic liver disease* is the most common route to hepatic failure; causes include relentless chronic hepatitis (including inherited metabolic disorders) ending in cirrhosis.
- *Hepatic dysfunction without overt necrosis* can occur with tetracycline toxicity, acute fatty liver of pregnancy, or the mitochondrial dysfunction caused by some HIV (human immunodeficiency virus) therapies.

Clinical Features

Clinical features include jaundice; hypoalbuminemia; hyperammonemia; *fetor hepaticus* (a peculiar body odor related to mercaptan formation); and hyperestrogenemia with palmar erythema, spider angiomas of the skin, hypogonadism, and gynecomastia. Complications include coagulopathy (inadequate hepatic synthesis of clotting factors), multiple organ failure, *hepatic encephalopathy,* and *hepatorenal syndrome.*

Hepatic encephalopathy is a life-threatening disorder of central nervous system and neuromuscular transmission; it is reversible if the underlying liver conditions are corrected. It is caused by loss of hepatocellular function and blood shunting around the liver, leading to an altered metabolic milieu bathing the CNS; excess ammonia levels appear to be important. Only minor morphologic changes are actually seen in the brain (e.g., edema, astrocytic reaction). Clinical features include:

- Disturbances in consciousness (e.g., behavioral abnormalities, confusion, stupor, coma)
- Electroencephalogram changes
- Limb rigidity and hyperreflexia
- Seizures
- Asterixis (a flapping tremor of outstretched hands)

Hepatorenal syndrome is life-threatening renal failure (without intrinsic renal pathology) in the setting of severe liver disease. The cause is decreased renal perfusion pressure, followed by renal vasoconstriction. Although the patients are oliguric, the concentrating ability of the kidney is maintained; the resulting urine is hyperosmolar, devoid of proteins, and surprisingly *low in sodium.* Kidney function promptly improves if hepatic failure is reversed.

Cirrhosis (p. 882)

Cirrhosis is among the top 10 leading causes of death in the Western world. It is defined by three characteristics:

- *Fibrosis*—Bridging septa in the form of delicate bands or broad scars
- *Nodules* created by regeneration of hepatocytes encircled by fibrosis
- Disruption of hepatic parenchymal architecture

The fibrosis is accompanied by vascular reorganization, with abnormal interconnections between vascular inflow and outflow: arterioportal venous shunts, arteriohepatic venous shunts, and portal venous–hepatic venous shunts. As a result, the liver may be seriously underperfused. Although the bridging fibrous septa were previously believed to be irreversible, with cessation of injury, the severity of hepatic fibrosis may diminish; the abnormal vascular channels tend to persist.

Cirrhosis is generally classified according to cause, with the caveat that once cirrhosis develops, the etiology may be impossible to establish. Major causes in Western nations are as follows:

Alcoholic liver disease	60–70%
Viral hepatitis	10%
Biliary diseases	5–10%
Primary hemochromatosis	5%
Wilson disease	rare
α_1-antitrypsin (α_1-AT) deficiency	rare
Cryptogenic cirrhosis	10%–15%

Many cases of cryptogenic cirrhosis may be the consequence of nonalcoholic fatty liver disease or autoimmune hepatitis.

Pathogenesis

Cirrhosis is characterized by *progressive fibrosis and reorganization of the vascular microarchitecture.* Interstitial collagen (types I and III) is found normally in portal tracts and around central veins, with occasional bundles in the space of Disse associated with a delicate reticulin (collagen type IV). In cirrhosis, types I and III collagen are extensively deposited in all parts of the liver, thin bands of subendothelial collagen divide the parenchyma, and portal tract fibrosis creates broad portal-portal bridges. Sinusoidal endothelium lose their fenestrations. Pre-existing myofibroblasts within portal tracts are the major source of fibrosis there. The major source of excess sinusoidal collagen is the perisinusoidal hepatic stellate cell *(Ito cell);* normally involved in vitamin A and fat-storage, with injury, stellate cells transform into myofibroblast-like cells. Stellate cells and portal myofibroblasts are activated by:

- Proinflammatory cytokines (e.g., tumor necrosis factor-α [TNF-α] and interleukin 1 [IL1]) from chronic inflammation
- Cytokines released by endogenous cells (Kupffer cells, endothelial cells, hepatocytes, bile duct epithelial cells)
- Disruption of the normal extracellular matrix
- Direct toxin stimulation of stellate cells or portal tract myofibroblasts

Clinical Features

Cirrhosis can be clinically silent for years; it ultimately presents with anorexia, weight loss, weakness, osteoporosis, and debilitation. Death is caused by:

- Hepatic failure (discussed earlier)
- Complications of portal hypertension (see following section)
- Hepatocellular carcinoma (see later discussion)

Portal Hypertension (p. 883)

Defined as increased resistance to portal blood flow, portal hypertension has the following causes:

- *Prehepatic:* obstructive thrombosis and narrowing of the portal vein or massive splenomegaly with shunting of blood into the splanchnic circulation
- *Intrahepatic: cirrhosis,* schistosomiasis, veno-occlusive disease, massive fatty change, diffuse fibrosing granulomatous disease, or nodular regenerative hyperplasia

- *Posthepatic:* severe right-sided heart failure, constrictive pericarditis, or hepatic vein outflow obstruction *(Budd-Chiari syndrome)*

Major clinical consequences of portal hypertension are:

- Ascites, especially in cirrhosis
- Formation of portosystemic venous shunts
- Congestive splenomegaly
- Hepatic encephalopathy

Ascites (p. 884) is defined as the collection of excess serous fluid in the peritoneal cavity. Pathogenesis involves:

- Hepatic sinusoidal hypertension
- Percolation of hepatic lymph into the peritoneal cavity
- Intestinal fluid leakage into the peritoneal cavity
- Renal retention of sodium and water

Portosystemic shunts (p. 884) develop because the principal sites for portal-systemic venous bypasses are the following:

- Cardioesophageal junction *(esophagogastric varices).* These varices rupture and bleed to cause massive hematemesis and death in one half of cirrhotic patients.
- Rectum (hemorrhoids).
- Retroperitoneum.
- Falciform ligament and umbilicus *(caput medusa).*

Splenomegaly (p. 885) is caused by long-standing congestion; it can cause hematologic abnormalities due to hypersplenism.

Jaundice and Cholestasis (p. 885)

Jaundice and *icterus* denote yellow skin and sclera discoloration, respectively; they both reflect systemic bilirubin retention. *Cholestasis* denotes systemic retention of bilirubin, bile salts, and cholesterol due to inadequate biliary elimination of these solutes.

Jaundice

Jaundice occurs when bilirubin production exceeds hepatic clearance capacity; there can be *unconjugated* or *conjugated hyperbilirubinemia.*

Unconjugated Hyperbilirubinemia

- *Bilirubin overproduction:* excessive erythrocyte hemolysis, resorption of major hemorrhages, or ineffective erythropoiesis
- *Reduced hepatic uptake of bilirubin* formed peripherally: Gilbert syndrome, some drugs (rifampin)
- *Impaired hepatic conjugation of bilirubin:* transient deficiency of bilirubin uridine diphosphate-glucuronosyltransferase (UGT1A1) in newborns *(neonatal jaundice)* or hereditary hyperbilirubinemias

Crigler-Najjar syndrome type I (autosomal recessive): total absence of bilirubin UGT1A1, severe jaundice and high serum levels of unconjugated bilirubin, histologically normal liver. Without liver transplantation, fatal kernicterus will ensue.

Crigler-Najjar syndrome type II (autosomal dominant): less severe UGT1A1 deficiency, nonfatal. Kernicterus with neurologic damage can occur.

Gilbert syndrome: mild, fluctuating unconjugated hyper-bilirubinemia. It is a heterogeneous inherited condition that affects 6% of the population, and is usually detected during intercurrent illness or fasting. Heterozygous missense mutations or promoter region mutations cause reduced UGT1A1 activity or expression. There are no clinical consequences of this condition.

Conjugated Hyperbilirubinemia

Conjugated hyperbilirubinemia is designated when greater than 50% of an elevated serum bilirubin is conjugated. It is typically associated with cholestasis. There are two common hereditary causes:

- *Dubin-Johnson syndrome* (autosomal recessive): defective hepatocyte secretion of bilirubin conjugates due to absent transport protein (multidrug resistance-associated protein 2, MRP2) for bilirubin glucuronides in the canalicular plasma membrane. The liver is brown, with accumulated pigment granules (polymers of epinephrine metabolites, *not* bilirubin pigment). Most patients are asymptomatic but chronically jaundiced; life expectancy is normal.
- *Rotor syndrome* (autosomal recessive): asymptomatic conjugated hyperbilirubinemia with multiple defects in hepatocellular uptake and excretion of bilirubin pigments. The liver is not pigmented; most patients have chronic jaundice with normal life span.

Cholestasis

Cholestasis results from hepatocellular dysfunction or biliary obstruction. Consequences include jaundice, *pruritus* from bile salt retention, and *xanthomas* (skin accumulations of cholesterol). Serum alkaline phosphatase is characteristically elevated because this enzyme is present in bile duct epithelium and hepatocyte canalicular membranes.

Morphology

- Bile pigment accumulates within the hepatic parenchyma, leading to dilated bile canaliculi and hepatocyte degeneration.
- Biliary obstruction leads to distended, proliferating bile ducts in the portal tracts, with edema and periductular neutrophils.
- Necrotic parenchymal foci may coalesce to form *bile lakes.*
- Prolonged obstruction causes *portal tract fibrosis* and eventually cirrhosis.

Clinical Features

- *Intrahepatic cholestasis* (hepatocellular dysfunction or intrahepatic bile duct disease) cannot be surgically treated, short of liver transplantation for life-threatening disease.
- *Extrahepatic cholestasis (obstruction)* may be amenable to surgical correction.

Familial intrahepatic cholestasis is a heterogeneous group of autosomal recessive disorders, usually presenting with cholestasis in infancy.

- Benign recurrent intrahepatic cholestasis (BRIC): intermittent attacks of cholestasis without progression to chronic liver disease.

- Progressive familial intrahepatic cholestasis (PFIC): mutations in one of three ATP-dependent transporter proteins:

  PFIC-1 *(Byler disease):* mutations in *ATP8B1* gene (an aminophospholipid translocase in canalicular membranes); progresses to liver failure before adulthood. Gene defect is the same as for BRIC, but is more severe clinically. There is no damage to the canalicular membranes or biliary tree; thus, serum γ-glutamyl transpeptidase (GGT) levels are low.

  PFIC-2: mutation in *ABCB11* gene (transports bile salts across canalicular membranes); cholestasis, pruritus, growth failure, and progression to cirrhosis in the first decade. Serum GGT levels are low.

  PFIC-3: mutations in *ABCB4* gene (encodes MDR3 protein responsible for phosphatidylcholine secretion into bile). Damage to the biliary tree results in high serum GGT levels.

INFECTIOUS DISORDERS (p. 890)

Viral Hepatitis (p. 890)

Any blood-borne bacterial, fungal, or parasitic infection can involve the liver. A number of systemic viral infections can also involve the liver, including infectious mononucleosis (Epstein-Barr virus), cytomegalovirus, and herpesvirus. More rarely, rubella, adenovirus, enterovirus, and yellow fever *(flavivirus)* can affect the liver. *Unless otherwise specified, viral hepatitis refers to infection of the liver by a small group of hepatotropic viruses.* All produce similar patterns of clinical and morphologic acute hepatitis but vary in their potential to induce carrier states, or chronic or fulminant disease (Table 18–2).

Hepatitis A Virus (p. 890)

Hepatitis A virus (HAV) was originally called *infectious hepatitis.* HAV is a single-stranded RNA virus (*picornavirus* family) causing a benign, self-limited disease; fulminant HAV is rare (fatality rate <0.1%) (see Table 18–2). HAV accounts for 20% to 25% of acute hepatitis in the developing world. Acute infection is marked by anti-HAV immunoglobulin M (IgM) in serum; IgG appears as IgM declines (within a few months) and persists for years, conferring long-term immunity. An effective vaccine is available.

Hepatitis B Virus (p. 891)

Hepatitis B virus (HBV) was originally called *serum hepatitis.* HBV chronically infects 350 million people worldwide with great geographic variations; there are 1.2 million carriers in the United States. Besides chronic and carrier states, HBV can cause fulminant hepatitis with massive liver necrosis (<1%). HBV can also lead to the development of hepatocellular carcinoma (chronic HBV carriers have 100 times greater risk for liver cancer). HBV is spread mainly by perinatal, parenteral routes (transfusion, blood products, needle-stick accidents, or shared needles), or via body fluids (saliva, semen, and vaginal fluid), hence the risk of sexual transmission (see Table 18–2). Treatment includes interferon-α (IFN-α) and antiviral reagents. Effective vaccines are available.

TABLE 18-2 The Hepatitis Viruses

Features	Hepatitis A Virus	Hepatitis B Virus	Hepatitis C Virus	Hepatitis D Virus	Hepatitis E Virus	Hepatitis G Virus*
Agent	Icosahedral capsid, ssRNA	Enveloped dsDNA	Enveloped ssRNA	Enveloped ssRNA	Unenveloped ssRNA	ssRNA virus
Transmission	Fecal-oral	Parenteral; close contact	Parenteral; close contact	Parenteral; close contact	Waterborne	Parenteral
Incubation period	2–6 wk	4–26 wk	2–26 wk	4–7 wk	2–8 wk	Unknown
Carrier state	None	0.1%–1.0% of blood donors in U.S. and Western world	0.2%–1.0% of blood donors in U.S. and Western world	1%–10% in drug addicts and hemophiliacs	Unknown	1%–2% of blood donors in U.S.
Chronic hepatitis	None	5%–10% of acute infections	>60%	<5% co-infection, 80% upon superinfection	None	None
Hepatocellular carcinoma	No	Yes	Yes	No increase above HBV	Unkonwn, but unlikely	None

*At present, hepatitis G virus is not considered pathogenic.

Molecular Biology

HBV is a circular, partially double-stranded DNA virus member of the *hepadnavirus* family. It exists as a spherical, 42-nm diameter *Dane particle* with many viral genotypes. The viral coat contains three surface proteins (PreS1, PreS2, and S protein/HBsAg); the nucleocapsid has HBV DNA, DNA polymerase (with reverse transcriptase activity), hepatitis B core antigen (HBcAg), and X protein (required for viral replication and infectivity, it modulates host cell signal transduction). Viral replication occurs through reverse transcription from the pregenomic RNA template.

Pathogenesis

HBV itself does not cause cell death. Hepatocyte killing is mediated by cytotoxic CD8+ T lymphocytes directed against virus-infected cells. Viral DNA sequences can also integrate into host genomes, constituting a pathway for cancer development.

Serum Markers

HBsAg appears before symptoms, peaks during overt disease, and declines over months. HBeAg (a longer polypeptide containing core protein and precore protein) is detectable in serum during viral replication; HBeAg and HBV DNA appear soon after HBsAg, before onset of acute disease. HBV mutants may lack the ability to form HBeAg. HBeAg usually declines within weeks; persistence indicates probable progression to chronic disease. IgM anti-HBc is usually the first antibody to appear, followed shortly by anti-HBe (seroconversion) and IgG anti-HBc. Anti-HBs signifies the end of acute disease and persists for years, conferring immunity. A chronic carrier is defined by the presence of HBsAg in serum for 6 months. Using sensitive PCR based testing, low levels of viral DNA are detectable even in the presence of the anti-HBe antibody.

Hepatitis C Virus (p. 894)

In the United States, 3.9 million individuals are infected; the incidence is declining as a result of blood supply screening. *Persistent infection and chronic hepatitis are the hallmarks of HCV infection;* 60% to 85% of infected patients develop chronic infection, and a subset progress eventually to cirrhosis, with risk of hepatocellular carcinoma (see Table 18–2). Primary risk groups are intravenous drug abusers, hemophiliacs, hemodialysis patients, and homosexuals. Sexual transmission is lower than for HBV. Like HBV, hepatocellular damage is immune-mediated. Therapy includes combinations of interferon and ribavirin, with only partial efficacy. No vaccine is available.

Molecular Biology

HCV is a single-stranded RNA enveloped virus (*flaviviridae* family), with six major genotypes in different geographic distribution; genotype 1 accounts for 75% of all U.S. HCV infections. Genomic variability constitutes a major obstacle to vaccine development. A single 3010–amino acid polypeptide is processed into nucleocapsid protein, envelope proteins, and seven nonstructural proteins.

Serum Markers

HCV RNA is detectable in blood for 1 to 3 weeks during active infection; it frequently persists despite neutralizing antibodies. Episodic elevations in serum transaminases are seen in chronic disease states. *Elevated titers of anti-HCV IgG after active infection do not confer effective immunity, either against reactivation of endogenous HCV or by infection with a new HCV strain.* Patients are initially screened for anti-HCV antibody, followed by qualitative or quantitative HCV RNA tests (viral load assay).

Hepatitis D Virus (p. 895)

This defective RNA virus can replicate and cause infection only when encapsulated by HBsAg. Hence, *HDV infection can develop only when there is concomitant HBV infection. Acute co-infection* by HDV and HBV leads to hepatitis that can vary from mild to fulminant, but chronicity rarely develops. *Superinfection* of chronic HBV by HDV leads to eruption of acute hepatitis, conversion of mild chronic disease into fulminant disease, or exacerbation of chronic disease terminating in cirrhosis (see Table 18–2). HDV is endemic in Africa, the Middle East, Italy, and elsewhere; in the United States, it is primarily seen in drug addicts and male homosexuals.

Molecular Biology

HDV is composed of a *Dane particle* with HBV envelope; there is an internal, 24-kD polypeptide (δ *antigen,* HDV Ag) and circular single-stranded RNA.

Serum Markers

HDV RNA appears in blood and liver just before and during early acute symptomatic infection. IgM anti-HDV indicates recent HDV exposure. Differentiating acute co-infection from superinfection requires correlation with HBV markers.

Hepatitis E Virus (p. 896)

Hepatitis E virus (HEV) is an enterically transmitted, waterborne infection, with endemics in Asia and the Indian subcontinent. *There is a high rate of fulminant hepatitis in pregnant women* (20%); otherwise, HEV is a self-limiting disease, with no tendency to chronic disease (see Table 18–2).

Molecular Biology

HEV is an nonenveloped single-stranded RNA *calicivirus.* HEV antigen is found in hepatocytes during active infection.

Other Hepatitis Viruses (p. 897)

Hepatitis G is a nonpathogenic RNA virus (similar to HCV), with serologic evidence of exposure in 1% to 2% of U.S. blood donors.

Clinicopathologic Syndromes (p. 897)

Acute Infection With Recovery (p. 897)

Acute infection is similar for all hepatitis viruses, with a variable incubation period, asymptomatic preicteric phase, symptomatic icteric phase, and convalescence. A fulminant course with high mortality rate occurs in fewer than 1% of cases. Acute infection can also be subclinical without overt syptomatology. Drug reactions can mimic acute hepatitis.

Chronic Hepatitis (p. 898)

Chronic hepatitis refers to symptomatic, biochemical, or serologic evidence of ongoing hepatic inflammation for more than 6 months without steady improvement. Major causes are viral hepatitis, Wilson disease, α_1-AT deficiency, alcohol, drugs, and autoimmunity. Cause—rather than histology—is the single most important factor that determines whether progressive chronic hepatitis will occur. Drug reactions can also mimic chronic hepatitis. Likelihood of developing chronic hepatitis after viral infection (see also Table 18–2) is as follows:

- HAV: none
- HBV: over 90% in infected neonates; 10% of adults
- HCV: over 60% (half will then progress to cirrhosis)
- HDV: rarely in acute HBV/HDV co-infection but is the most frequent outcome of HDV superinfection of HBV-infected patient
- HEV: none

Carrier State

A *carrier* is an individual without manifest symptoms who harbors and therefore can transmit an organism. There are two types: those with little or no adverse effects *(healthy carriers)* and those with chronic disease but few or no symptoms (see also Table 18–2).

- HAV and HEV do not produce a carrier state.
- HBV: From 90% to 95% of infants infected at birth become carriers; 1% to 10% of individuals infected as adults (especially with impaired immunity) are carriers.
- HCV: Less than 1% become healthy carriers.
- HDV: Low (but real) potential of becoming carrier.

Fulminant Hepatitis (p. 899)

Fulminant hepatitis is recognized when hepatic insufficiency with hepatic encephalopathy occurs within 2 to 3 weeks after symptom onset; subfulminant hepatic failure denotes a course of up to 3 months. The presentation is as described earlier for hepatic failure. Overall, fulminant hepatic failure has a viral etiology in 12% of cases, and over 50% of fulminant hepatic failures are due to drug or chemical toxicity; 18% have unknown causes. Mortality rate is 25% to 90% without transplantation.

Morphology

- In *acute viral hepatitis,* the liver is slightly enlarged and green. There is hepatocyte necrosis ranging from scattered hepatocytes, to clumps, to an entire lobule; necrotic hepatocytes are eosinophilic and rounded (undergoing *apoptosis*), or swollen *(ballooning degeneration)*. Lymphocytes are present and macrophages engulf necrotic hepatocytes. Lobular architecture is disrupted by necrosis *(lobular disarray); portal-to-central (bridging)* necrosis portends more severe disease. Kupffer cells and sinusoidal lining cells exhibit hypertrophy and hyperplasia, and there is portal tract inflammation (mainly lymphocytes and macrophages), hepatocellular regeneration, and occasional cholestasis.

- *Chronic hepatitis* ranges from exceedingly mild, to severe, to cirrhosis. In mild disease, the chronic inflammatory infiltrate is limited to portal tracts. Progressive disease is marked by extension of chronic inflammation from portal tracts into parenchyma with hepatocyte necrosis *(interface hepatitis);* linking of portal-portal and portal-central regions constitutes *bridging necrosis. Continued loss of hepatocytes results in fibrous septum formation; associated hepatocyte regeneration results in cirrhosis.*

- The *carrier state* for HBV may exhibit normal liver architecture and hepatocytes. Isolated cells or clusters show a finely granular, eosinophilic cytoplasm *(ground glass)* and stain positive for HBsAg. Tubules and spheres of HBsAg in the cytoplasm are seen by electron microscopy. HCV-infected patients typically exhibit chronic hepatitis.

- In *fulminant hepatitis,* the entire liver, or just portions, may be involved; the liver is shrunken. Affected areas are soft, muddy-red or bile-stained. Entire lobules are destroyed, leaving cellular debris and a collapsed reticulin network; inflammation may be minimal. With massive destruction, regeneration is disorderly, and scar may form, producing a coarsely lobulated pattern of cirrhosis.

Clinical Features

Viral hepatitis may be a subclinical event, may run a self-limited course, may persist as indolent chronic disease without progression for many years, or may progress to cirrhosis. Symptoms of acute and chronic hepatitis are similar: fatigue, malaise, anorexia, and bouts of jaundice. With chronic hepatitis, symptoms may persist or be intermittent. Associated findings with chronic liver disease are spider angiomas, palmar erythema, mild hepatosplenomegaly, and hepatic tenderness. Laboratory findings include persistently or intermittently elevated serum liver enzymes, prolonged prothrombin time, hyperglobulinemia, and hyperbilirubinemia. Major causes of death are cirrhosis with liver failure and hepatic encephalopathy, massive hematemesis from esophageal varices, and hepatocellular carcinoma.

Bacterial, Parasitic, and Helminthic Infections (p. 902)

Parasitic infections (e.g., amebic, echinococcal, other protozoal, or helminthic organisms) are common causes of hepatic abscesses in developing countries. Abscesses occurring in developed countries are rare and are usually bacterial or candidal, resulting from complications of infection elsewhere in the body. Abscesses are associated with fever, right upper quadrant pain, tender hepatomegaly, and possibly jaundice. Mortality rate ranges from 30% to 90%; survival is improved by early recognition.

- Sources of infection are intra-abdominal (via portal vein), systemic (via arterial supply), biliary tree *(ascending cholangitis),* direct extension, and penetrating injuries.
- Histologic features are those seen in any abscess; parasitic fragments or fungal organisms may be identifiable.

AUTOIMMUNE HEPATITIS (p. 903)

Autoimmune hepatitis (AIH) refers to hepatitis of a primary immunologic basis; these typically respond dramatically to immunosuppressive therapy. There is a female predominance, an increased frequency of HLA B8 or DRw3 alleles, absence of viral serologic markers, elevated serum IgG levels, and high titers of autoantibodies in 80% of cases (antinuclear antibody [ANA] or anti–smooth muscle antibody [SMA]); subsets exhibit antiliver and kidney microsome antibodies (LKM). Antimitochondrial antibody (elevated in primary biliary cirrhosis) is usually negative in AIH. AIH is sometimes associated with other autoimmune diseases (e.g., rheumatoid arthritis, thyroiditis, Sjögren syndrome, and ulcerative colitis). The morphology is similar to chronic viral hepatitis, with robust portal and lobular infiltrates of lymphocytes and prominent plasma cells.

DRUG- AND TOXIN-INDUCED LIVER DISEASE
(p. 903)

Reaction to a toxin or therapeutic agent should be included in the differential diagnosis of any form of liver disease. Injury is caused by direct drug toxicity, hepatic conversion of an agent to an active toxin, or injury via immune mechanisms. Injury may be immediate or develop over weeks to months. Injury may take the form of *hepatocyte necrosis, hepatitis, cholestasis, fibrosis,* or *insidious onset of liver dysfunction.* Examples of drug- and toxin-induced hepatic injury are given in Table 18–3.

Alcoholic Liver Disease (p. 904)

Alcohol abuse constitutes the major form of liver disease in most Western countries. More than 10 million Americans are affected, with 200,000 deaths per year in the United States related to alcohol abuse (including automobile accidents).

TABLE 18–3 **Drug- and Toxin-Induced Hepatic Injury**

Hepatocellular Damage	Examples
Microvesicular fatty change	Tetracycline, salicylates, yellow phosphorus, ethanol
Macrovesicular fatty change	Ethanol, methotrexate, amiodarone
Centrilobular necrosis	Bromobenzene, CCl₄, acetaminophen, halothane, rifampin
Diffuse or massive necrosis	Halothane, isoniazid, acetaminophen, methyldopa, trinitrotoluene, *Amanita phalloides* (mushroom) toxin
Hepatitis, acute and chronic	Methyldopa, isoniazid, nitrofurantoin, phenytoin, oxyphenisatin
Fibrosis-cirrhosis	Ethanol, methotrexate, amiodarone, most drugs that cause chronic hepatitis
Granuloma formation	Sulfonamides, methyldopa, quinidine, phenylbutazone, hydralazine, allopurinol
Cholestasis (with or without hepatocellular injury)	Chlorpromazine, anabolic steroids, erythromycin estolate, oral contraceptives, organic arsenicals

There are three distinctive, albeit overlapping, forms of alcohol-related liver disease, characterized by morphology.

- *Hepatic steatosis (fatty liver)* is marked initially by small *(microvesicular)* lipid droplets accumulating within hepatocytes with even moderate alcohol intake. With chronic alcohol intake, lipid accumulates in *macrovesicular* droplets, displacing the nucleus. At first centrilobular, lipid accumulation can expand to involve the entire lobule. The liver becomes enlarged, soft, greasy, and yellow. There is little to no fibrosis at the outset and the condition is reversible.
- *Alcoholic hepatitis* is characterized by *liver cell necrosis* (both in the form of ballooning degeneration and apoptosis), particularly in the centrilobular region. There is also *Mallory body* formation (intracellular eosinophilic aggregates of intermediate filaments), *neutrophilic reaction* to degenerating hepatocytes, portal inflammation that spills into lobules, and *fibrosis* (sinusoidal, pericentral, and periportal).
- *Alcoholic cirrhosis* is the final and largely irreversible outcome of alcoholic liver disease. The liver is transformed from fatty and enlarged to brown, shrunken, and nonfatty. Regenerative nodules may be prominent or buried in dense fibrous scar. End-stage alcoholic cirrhosis resembles postnecrotic cirrhosis.

Pathogenesis (p. 906)

- *Steatosis* results from shunting of substrates toward lipid biosynthesis, impaired lipoprotein assembly and secretion, and increased peripheral catabolism of fat.
- Cellular injury results from:

  Induction of cytochrome P-450 augmenting catabolism of other drugs to potentially toxic metabolites
  Free radicals generated by the microsomal ethanol oxidizing system that react with proteins and membranes
  Acetaldehyde generated from alcohol to induce lipid peroxidation and acetaldehyde-protein adduct formation
- Alcohol induces an *immunologic attack* on hepatic neoantigens, possibly due to alterations in native proteins.
- Alcohol is a *caloric food source,* displacing nutrients.
- *Fibrosis* is the result of collagen deposition by perisinusoidal stellate cells, eventuating in cirrhosis. Stimuli include:

  Kupffer cell activation with proinflammatory cytokine release
  Amplification of cytokine stimuli by *platelet-activating factor,* a lipid released by endothelial and Kupffer cells
  Influx of neutrophils into the parenchyma, with release of free radicals, proteases, and other inflammatory mediators
- *Deranged hepatic blood flow* is the result of progressive fibrosis and alcohol-induced release of vasoconstrictive *endothelins* from sinusoidal endothelial cells.

Clinical Features (p. 907)

- *Hepatic steatosis:* Asymptomatic and reversible mild elevation of serum bilirubin and alkaline phosphatase.
- *Alcoholic hepatitis:* Acute, mild to fulminant hepatic failure; may be transient or fatal.

- *Alcoholic cirrhosis:* Manifestation similar to any other form of cirrhosis; irreversible.

  Proximate causes of death are hepatic coma, massive gastrointestinal hemorrhage, intercurrent infection, hepatorenal syndrome, and hepatocellular carcinoma.

METABOLIC LIVER DISEASE (p. 907)

Nonalcoholic Fatty Liver Disease and Steatohepatitis (p. 907)

Nonalcoholic fatty liver disease (NAFL) is a clinicopathological condition characterized by elevated serum transaminase levels and hepatic steatosis in the absence of heavy alcohol consumption. Nonalcoholic steatohepatitis (NASH) is defined as steatosis plus liver inflammation, characterized by the presence of neutrophil infiltrates. The rising incidence of NAFL is attributed to the increasing prevalence of obesity in developed countries. NAFL has strong associations with obesity, and may be accompanied by a metabolic syndrome of dyslipidemia, hyperinsulinemia, insulin resistance, and type 2 diabetes. It is estimated that 31% of men and 16% of women have NAFL, representing 31 million Americans.

Pathogenesis

Although the mechanisms of NAFL are not completely understood, a net retention of lipids (mostly triglycerides) within hepatocytes is a prerequisite for its development. This can occur through changes in hepatocyte lipid uptake, synthesis, or secretion. Insulin resistance also appears to be an important factor in pathogenesis, as are cytokines, particularly TNF-α.

Morphology

Hepatocytes are filled with fat vacuoles in the absence of inflammatory infiltration (steatosis), or with inflammatory infiltrates (steatohepatitis). Varying degrees of fibrosis are present. There are no distinctive features to separate alcoholic versus nonalcoholic steatosis based on histologic findings.

Clinical Features

Most patients with NAFL have no symptoms or signs of liver disease at diagnosis, although many report fatigue or malaise and a sensation of fullness or right upper quadrant discomfort. Most cases are detected by elevated serum transaminase levels. Hepatomegaly is the only physical finding in most patients, although acanthosis nigricans may be found in children with NAFL. Findings of chronic liver disease and low platelets suggest onset of cirrhosis. Some patients with cryptogenic cirrhosis share many of the clinical and demographic features of patients with NAFL, suggesting NAFL as an etiology.

Hemochromatosis (p. 908)

Hemochromatosis is excessive iron accumulation deposited in the parenchymal cells of various organs, particularly liver and pancreas. Hereditary hemochromatosis (also called *primary hemochromatosis*) is a homozygous recessive heritable disorder. Secondary hemochromatosis denotes disorders with identifiable sources of excess iron (e.g., repetitive transfusions, ineffective erythropoiesis, increased iron intake, or chronic liver disease).

The frequency of the hereditary hemochromatosis allele is 6% in white populations of Northern European descent; homozygosity occurs in 0.45% and heterozygosity in 11%. The male-female ratio of the disease is 6:1, most likely owing to physiologic iron loss in women (e.g., menstruation, pregnancy).

Pathogenesis

The hemochromatosis gene *HFE* is on the short arm of chromosome 6, close to the HLA locus. It encodes an HLA class I–like molecule that regulates intestinal absorption of dietary iron; the fundamental defect appears to be unregulated intestinal absorption. The most common mutation (>70% of patients) is a cysteine-to-tyrosine substitution at amino acid 282 (C282Y). However, disease penetrance is low even with homozygous C282Y (about 20%), so that the genetic condition alone does not invariably lead to hemochromatosis. Tissue damage is attributed to direct iron toxicity presumably by free radical formation with lipid peroxidation, stimulation of collagen formation, and iron-DNA interactions.

Morphology

Iron accumulates as ferritin and hemosiderin in parenchymal tissues (liver, pancreas, myocardium, endocrine glands) and in synovial joint linings. *Prussian blue reaction (potassium ferrocyanide and hydrochloric acid) highlights tissue hemosiderin. Biochemical determination of hepatic iron content can be performed; normal level is less than 1000 µg/gm dry weight of liver. Adult patients with hereditary hemochromatosis have hepatic iron content exceeding 10,000 µg/gm.*

Clinical Features

Hereditary hemochromatosis presents at age 20 to 30 with hepatomegaly, abdominal pain, skin pigmentation, diabetes mellitus, cardiac dysfunction, arthritis, and hypogonadism. Potentially fatal complications occur from cirrhosis (including hepatocellular carcinoma) and cardiac involvement. Regular phlebotomy is sufficient treatment; early diagnosis can therefore enable normal life expectancy. Genetic screening for *HFE* gene mutations in family members of probands is important.

Wilson Disease (p. 910)

This autosomal recessive disorder is marked by toxic accumulation of copper in liver, brain, and eye (*hepatolenticular degeneration*).

Pathogenesis

The genetic defect is in the *ATP7B* gene on chromosome 13, encoding a hepatocyte canalicular membrane transmembrane copper-transporting adenosine triphosphatase (ATPase). Copper absorption and delivery to the liver is normal, but there is increased hepatic export into the circulation most likely due to defective secretion of copper into bile. More than 30 mutations have been identified; most affected patients are compound heterozygotes with different mutations. Abnormal allele frequency is 1 : 200; disease incidence is 1:30,000. Proposed mechanisms for copper-related injury include poisoning of hepatic enzymes, abnormal binding of copper to serum proteins, and free radical formation.

Morphology

Liver damage ranges from minor to severe, and is manifested by *fatty change, acute* and *chronic hepatitis* (with Mallory bodies), *cirrhosis,* and (rarely) *massive liver necrosis.* Toxicity in the brain predominantly affects the basal ganglia, which become atrophied and even cavitated. Nearly all patients with neurologic involvement also develop eye lesions called *Kayser-Fleischer rings;* these are green-brown copper deposits in the Desçemet membrane of the corneal limbus.

Clinical Features

Age at onset and clinical presentation are extremely variable; typically there will be some liver disease in the first couple of decades of life. Neuropsychiatric disorders are also possible, including mild behavioral changes, frank psychosis, and Parkinson disease–like symptoms. Diagnosis is suggested by *decreased serum ceruloplasmin* (a copper-binding serum protein), *increased hepatic copper content, and increased urinary copper excretion. Serum copper levels are of no diagnostic value.* Copper chelation can ameliorate problems; liver transplantation may be necessary.

α_1-Antitrypsin (α_1-AT) Deficiency (p. 911)

α_1-Antitrypsin (α_1-AT) deficiency is an autosomal co-dominant disorder resulting in abnormally low serum levels of this protease inhibitor; deficiency leads to emphysema and hepatic disease (cholestasis or cirrhosis).

Pathogenesis

α_1-AT is a 394–amino acid serum protease inhibitor (Pi) synthesized primarily in liver. The gene on chromosome 14 has extensive polymorphism with more than 75 protein isoforms. The most common isoform (>90% of people) is designated PiM. Homozygotes for the PiZ allele (the most common disease genotype; homozygote frequency = 1 : 7000) have circulating α_1-AT levels below 10% of normal. PiZ has a Glu_{342} to Lys_{342} substitution: the resulting polypeptide misfolds and forms polymers that cannot be secreted normally by hepatocytes. Impaired hepatic α_1-AT secretion leads to protein accumulation within hepatocyte endoplasmic reticulum, although the mechanism of liver damage is unclear. Lung damage results from inadequate levels of protease inhibitor.

Morphology

Hepatic lesions include *neonatal hepatitis* (inflammation with cholestasis) and *childhood* and *adult cirrhosis.* α_1-AT deficiency is diagnosed by identifying periodic acid–Schiff (PAS)-positive (diastase-resistant) cytoplasmic globules in periportal hepatocytes.

Clinical Features

Neonatal hepatitis with cholestatic jaundice occurs in 10% to 20% of newborns with α_1-AT deficiency; later presentation may be attributable to acute hepatitis or complications of cirrhosis. Hepatocellular carcinoma develops in 2% to 3% of PiZZ homozygous adults. Treatment is liver transplantation. Avoiding smoking is extremely important in patients with α_1-AT deficiency, since smoking accentuates their lung emphysematous damage.

Neonatal Cholestasis (p. 912)

Neonatal cholestasis is a nonspecific term for hepatic disorders of many possible etiologies in the neonate (Table 18–4). In 50% of cases no cause is identified. Patients present with prolonged conjugated hyperbilirubinemia *(neonatal cholestasis)*, hepatomegaly, and variable degrees of hepatic dysfunction (e.g., hypoprothrombinemia).

Morphology

There is hepatocyte necrosis and lobular disarray, panlobular giant cell transformation (multinucleate hepatocytes), prominent cholestasis, inflammation of portal tracts, Kupffer cell activation, and extramedullary hematopoiesis. Neonatal hepatitis should be distinguished from the bile duct proliferation seen in obstructive bile duct disease.

TABLE 18–4　**Major Causes of Neonatal Cholestasis**

Bile duct obstruction
　Extrahepatic biliary atresia
Neonatal infection
　Cytomegalovirus
　Bacterial sepsis
　Urinary tract infection
　Syphilis
Toxic
　Drugs
　Parenteral nutrition
Metabolic disease
　Tyrosinemia
　Niemann-Pick disease
　Galactosemia
　Defective bile acid synthetic pathways
　α_1-Antitrypsin deficiency
　Cystic fibrosis
Miscellaneous
　Shock/hypoperfusion
　Indian childhood cirrhosis
　Alagille syndrome (paucity of bile ducts)
Idiopathic neonatal hepatitis

INTRAHEPATIC BILIARY TRACT DISEASE (p. 913)

Secondary Biliary Cirrhosis (p. 913)

Etiology

- Obstruction from extrahepatic cholelithiasis (stones)
- Biliary atresia
- Malignancies of biliary tree or pancreatic head
- Strictures from previous surgical procedures

Morphology

Cholestasis may be severe but is reversible. *Periportal fibrosis* eventually leads to *cirrhosis,* which is irreversible. The end-stage liver is yellow-green and finely divided by fibrous tissue bile ducts that are distended and contain inspissated bile. Ascending bacterial infection incites bile duct neutrophilic infiltration with abscess formation.

Primary Biliary Cirrhosis (p. 914)

Primary biliary cirrhosis is a chronic, progressive cholestatic liver disease characterized by intrahepatic bile duct destruction, and portal inflammation and scarring, with progression to cirrhosis and liver failure. The presymptomatic phase may span 2 decades. It is primarily a disease of middle-aged women, and has an autoimmune pathogenesis. Onset is insidious, with pruritus and hepatomegaly; jaundice and xanthomas (from retained cholesterol) develop later, with progression to hepatic failure after a prolonged clinical course. Liver transplantation is required for end-stage disease.

Laboratory findings include elevated serum alkaline phosphatase and cholesterol, with serum antimitochondrial antibodies (especially to the mitochondrial pyruvate dehydrogenase E-2 subunit) positive in 90% of patients. Associated conditions include Sjögren syndrome, scleroderma, thyroiditis, rheumatoid arthritis, Raynaud phenomenon, membranous glomerulonephritis, and celiac disease.

Morphology

- *Portal tract lesion:* destruction of interlobular and septal bile ducts by lymphocytic inflammation (florid bile duct lesion) and chronic portal tract inflammation
- *Granulomas* in portal tracts and parenchyma
- *Progressive lesion:* global involvement of hepatic portal tracts; secondary obstructive changes with eventual cirrhosis
- *End-stage:* indistinguishable from other forms of cirrhosis

Primary Sclerosing Cholangitis (p. 915)

Primary sclerosing cholangitis is a chronic, progressive cholestatic liver disease most common in middle-aged men; it is characterized by inflammation, obliterative fibrosis, and segmental dilation of intrahepatic and extrahepatic bile ducts. It occurs in association with inflammatory bowel disease (70% of cases), particularly ulcerative colitis. The cause is unknown and autoantibodies are usually absent; it runs a chronic course over many years; end-stage disease requires transplantation.

Morphology

Morphologic features include inflammation and concentric (onion-skin) fibrosis around bile ducts, with progressive atrophy and eventual bile duct luminal obliteration; ductal obstruction culminates in biliary cirrhosis and hepatic failure.

Anomalies of the Biliary Tree (p. 915)

- *Von Meyenberg complexes (bile duct hamartomas)* are small clusters of dilated bile ducts or cysts within a fibrous stroma; they are portal tract lesions of probable embryologic origin.
- *Polycystic liver disease:* Few to hundreds of biliary epithelium-lined 0.5- to 4-cm cystic lesions are found. Familial polycystic liver disease is associated with polycystic kidney disease and is caused by an autosomal dominant mutation in the gene encoding the protein hepatocystin, a substrate for protein kinase C.
- *Congenital hepatic fibrosis* involves incomplete involution of embryonic ductal structures. The liver is subdivided by dense fibrous septa with embedded irregular biliary structures. Portal hypertension can develop.
- *Caroli disease:* Segmental dilation of larger ducts of intrahepatic biliary tree is complicated by cholelithiasis, hepatic abscesses, and cholangiocarcinoma. *Caroli syndrome* is the combination of Caroli disease with congenital hepatic fibrosis.
- Alagille syndrome is an uncommon autosomal dominant condition characterized by almost complete absence of intrahepatic bile ducts. It is caused by mutations in the Jagged 1 cell surface protein that normally binds Notch. The Jagged:Notch signaling pathway is critical in the development of many organ systems. Consequently, patients with Alagille syndrome often also have extrahepatic anomalies including peculiar facies, and vertebral and cardiovascular defects.

CIRCULATORY DISORDERS (p. 917)

Impaired Blood Flow Into the Liver (p. 917)

- *Extrahepatic:* portal vein thrombosis (e.g., due to peritoneal sepsis or pancreatitis), postsurgical compromise of hepatic artery, idiopathic portal hypertension (histologically manifested as *hepatoportal* sclerosis without cirrhosis)
- *Intrahepatic:* thrombosis with infarction (rare), idiopathic fibrosing obliterative portal vein lesions

Impaired Blood Flow Through the Liver (p. 918)

Cirrhosis is the most important cause. Sinusoidal occlusion can also be caused by disseminated intravascular coagulation (e.g., eclampsia), sickle cell disease, metastatic tumors, and sarcoidosis.

Systemic hypoperfusion (e.g., shock) leads to hepatocyte necrosis around the central vein *(centrilobular necrosis)*. With superimposed passive congestion (e.g., right-sided heart failure or constrictive pericarditis), there is hemorrhage as well, producing *centrilobular hemorrhagic necrosis.* Protracted right-sided heart failure causes chronic passive congestion and peri-central fibrosis *(cardiac sclerosis),* eventually culminating in cirrhosis.

Peliosis hepatitis is hepatic sinusoid dilation associated with exposure to anabolic steroids (rarely oral contraceptives and danazol). The liver is mottled and blotchy with irregular blood-filled lakes. Microscopically, there are irregular blood-filled cystic spaces, with or without an endothelial lining.

Hepatic Venous Outflow Obstruction (p. 919)

Budd-Chiari syndrome occurs when two or more major hepatic veins are obstructed. It typically occurs in thrombotic conditions, such as polycythemia vera, pregnancy and the post-partum state, oral contraceptive use, paroxysmal nocturnal hemoglobinuria, and intra-abdominal cancers (e.g., hepatocel-lular carcinoma). A membranous inferior vena cava valve can also cause hepatic venous obstruction. Budd-Chiari syndrome is characterized by hepatomegaly, weight gain, ascites, and abdominal pain, and can be acute or chronic. In acute cases, the liver is swollen and red-purple and the parenchyma has profound centrilobular congestion and necrosis. Subacute or chronic cases may develop superimposed fibrosis.

Veno-occlusive disease (VOD) was originally described in Jamaican drinkers of pyrrolizidine alkaloid-containing bush tea; it now occurs primarily in the bone marrow transplant pop-ulation as a toxic complication of chemotherapy. VOD is char-acterized by patchy obliteration of smaller hepatic vein radicles by endothelial swelling and collagen. Clinical features are the same as for Budd-Chiari syndrome.

HEPATIC DISEASE ASSOCIATED WITH PREGNANCY (p. 920)

Preeclampsia and Eclampsia (p. 920)

Preeclampsia affects 7% to 10% of pregnancies; it is char-acterized by hypertension, proteinuria, peripheral edema, coagulation abnormalities, and varying degrees of dissemi-nated intravascular coagulation. When hyperreflexia and con-vulsions occur, the condition is called *eclampsia.* The *HELLP* syndrome (*h*emolysis, *e*levated *l*iver enzymes, and *l*ow *p*latelets) is common in preeclampsia. Definitive treatment is termination of pregnancy.

Morphology

Gross morphologic findings are small, red, hemorrhagic patches, with occasional yellow-white patches of infarction. Fibrin deposits in periportal sinusoids, periportal necrosis, and hemorrhage occur. Hemorrhage coalescence forms hepatic hematomas with potential for fatal rupture into the abdomen.

Acute Fatty Liver of Pregnancy (p. 920)

This disorder is histologically characterized by *hepatocyte microvesicular fatty transformation.* The pathogenesis is unknown, although *maternal* heterozygous deficiency in long-chain 3-hydroxyacyl coenzyme A dehydrogenase and *fetal* homozygous deficiency (the other deficient allele is *paternal*) has been implicated. Incipient hepatic failure in the third trimester of pregnancy leads to bleeding, nausea and vomiting, jaundice, coma, and potentially death. Definitive treatment is termination of pregnancy.

Intrahepatic Cholestasis of Pregnancy (p. 921)

Intrahepatic cholestasis of pregnancy is characterized by onset of pruritus and jaundice in the third trimester of pregnancy. The liver shows cholestasis, attributed to estrogenic hormones. The condition is generally benign, but pruritus may be severe.

HEPATIC COMPLICATIONS OF ORGAN OR BONE MARROW TRANSPLANTATION (p. 921)

Drug Toxicity After Bone Marrow Transplantation (p. 921)

Administration of cytotoxic drugs prior to marrow transplantation causes hepatic dysfunction in up to 50% of patients, heralded by weight gain, tender hepatomegaly, edema, ascites, hyperbilirubinemia, and a fall in urinary sodium excretion. *Clinical features are indistinguishable from venoocclusive disease;* the morphologic features are nonspecific (hepatocyte necrosis and cholestasis). Outcome depends on severity of hepatic injury.

Graft-Versus-Host Disease and Liver Rejection (p. 921)

Graft-versus-host disease (GVHD) is characterized by *direct lymphocyte attack on liver cells, particularly bile duct epithelium.* Most GVHD occurs in the setting of bone marrow or stem cell transplantation, although it occasionally occurs in solid organ transplants. *Acute GVHD* is characterized by hepatitis (parenchymal inflammation and hepatocyte necrosis), vascular lymphocytic inflammation and intimal proliferation *(endothelialitis),* and *bile duct destruction. Chronic GVHD* exhibits portal tract inflammation, bile duct destruction (or complete bile duct loss), and fibrosis.

Acute rejection of liver allografts exhibits portal tract inflammation (frequently including eosinophils), bile duct damage, and endothelialitis. Typically occurring within weeks of transplantation, acute rejection can also occur at later points, especially if immunosuppression is interrupted. *Chronic rejection* occurs months or years after the transplantation and is characterized by bile duct loss and arteriopathy, with eventual graft failure. *Hyperacute rejection* (due to preformed circulating antibodies against graft antigens) is rare.

Nonimmunologic Damage to Liver Allografts (p. 921)

- Preservation injury occurs from oxygen-derived radical damage in hypoxic organ with insufficient reserves of oxygen scavengers.
- Technical complications include hepatic artery or portal vein occlusion and bile duct obstruction (e.g., stricture).

NODULES AND TUMORS (p. 922)

Hemangiomas and non-neoplastic biliary cysts are common benign lesions.

Nodular Hyperplasias (p. 922)

Nodular hyperplasias are solitary or multiple benign hepatocellular nodules in the absence of cirrhosis; the putative cause is focal hepatic vascular obliteration, with compensatory hypertrophy of well-vascularized lobules. *Focal nodular hyperplasia* occurs in young to middle-aged adults and is an irregular, unencapsulated tumor containing a central stellate fibrous scar. *Nodular regenerative hyperplasia* is a diffuse nodular transformation of the liver *without fibrosis,* occurring rarely with virtually any systemic inflammatory condition.

Benign Neoplasms (p. 922)

Liver cell adenomas are benign hepatocyte neoplasms up to 30 cm in diameter; they typically occur in younger women, usually when taking oral contraceptives. Adenomas are composed of sheets of hepatocytes, and include arteries and veins; *portal tracts with bile ducts are absent.* Adenomas may be confused with malignancy, may rupture with massive hemorrhage, and rarely may harbor hepatocellular carcinoma.

Malignant Tumors (p. 923)

In the United States, most tumors involving the liver are metastatic. Most *primary* liver cancers are hepatocellular carcinomas. Rare variants include:

- *Hepatoblastoma:* This tumor of young childhood exhibits *epithelial* features of fetal liver or *mixed* features with epithelial and mesenchymal differentiation. The Wnt/β-catenin signaling pathway appears to play a role in tumorigenesis, since more than 80% of hepatoblastomas harbor β-catenin mutations.
- *Angiosarcoma:* Similar to angiosarcomas occurring elsewhere, this tumor can be associated with exposure to vinyl chloride, arsenic, or Thorotrast (a contrast agent used in the 1950s).

Hepatocellular Carcinomas (p. 924)

Hepatocellular carcinomas (HCC) constitute 90% of primary liver cancers; they arise in the middle to late decades. The male-female ratio is 3:1 to 4:1. There is a strong causal relationship between hepatotropic viral infection (especially HBV and HCV) and hepatocellular carcinoma.

Epidemiology

Global distribution is closely linked to HBV infection rates, with higher incidence in men and black populations in any geographic area. HCC represents 40% of all cancers in high-incidence locales (Africa, Southeast Asia); in comparison, only 2% to 3% of cancers in the United States and Europe are HCC. HCC is strongly associated with protracted HBV infection, particularly when acquired early in life, presumably due to HBV integration into the hepatocellular genome. Individuals infected at birth may develop HCC at age 20 to 40; other risk populations develop it later in life. *Universal vaccination against HBV in endemic areas has dramatically decreased the incidence of HCC.* Chronic HCV infection is also strongly implicated. Other associated environmental influences are cirrhosis (alcoholism, primary hemochromatosis, tyrosinemia) and iatrogenic carcinogens (Thorotrast). The environmental hepatic carcinogen *aflatoxin* is produced by the fungus *Aspergillus flavus,* which grows on peanuts and grains.

Pathogenesis

HCC usually arises in the background of chronic liver disease (e.g., chronic hepatitis and cirrhosis). Chronic inflammation is associated with genotoxic products, cytokine production, and hepatocyte regeneration; such changes—along with an underlying genetic susceptibility—presumably underlie tumorigenesis. In addition, the high incidence of HCC with HBV and HCV infections suggests that viral factors also contribute.

- For *HBV-related malignancy,* key events appear to be integration of HBV DNA into the host genome (inducing oncogene activation) and binding viral proteins (e.g., X protein) to activate various proto-oncogenes and disrupt normal cell cycle regulation.
- For *HCV-related malignancy,* viral proteins such as core protein may modulate normal cell signaling pathways to affect cell growth control and apoptosis.
- For *aflatoxin-related malignancy,* the toxin covalently binds cellular DNA and causes gene mutations, particularly *p53.*

Morphology

There may be a solitary mass, multifocal nodules, or a diffusely infiltrative cancer with massive liver enlargement, frequently in a background of cirrhosis. Tumors are pale pink-yellow or bile-stained; intrahepatic spread and vascular invasion are common. Histologically, lesions may range from well differentiated to highly anaplastic and undifferentiated.

- *Well-differentiated to moderately differentiated HCC:* Hepatocytes are arranged in trabecular (sinusoidal) or acinar (tubular) pseudoglandular patterns.
- *Poorly differentiated HCC:* HCC characterized by markedly pleomorphic giant cells; small, completely undifferentiated cells; spindle cells; or completely anaplastic cells.
- Tumor cells form bile (by light microscopy) or bile canaliculi (by electron microscopy); cytoplasmic inclusions resemble Mallory bodies; there is positive staining for α-fetoprotein and α_1-antitrypsin.

Clinical Features

Features include hepatomegaly, right upper quadrant pain, weight loss, and elevated serum α-fetoprotein. Prognosis depends on the resectability of the tumor; usually death occurs within 6 months of diagnosis.

Fibrolamellar Variant of Hepatocellular Carcinoma (p. 925)

This carcinoma arises in the absence of identifiable risk factors or underlying liver disease in children, adolescents, and young adults. This variant is more often resectable; at 5 years, survival rate is 60%. Usually, a single, sometimes encapsulated, multinodular mass is present. The mass contains prominent fibrous bands separating trabeculae of large, eosinophilic polygonal hepatocytes. Cytoplasmic hyalin globules and PAS-positive inclusions may be present.

Cholangiocarcinoma (p. 926)

Cholangiocarcinoma arises from elements of the intrahepatic biliary tree. Although most cases arise without antecedent risk conditions, it can be associated with Thorotrast administration, protracted parasitic infection of the biliary tree with *Clonorchis (Opisthorchis sinensis)*, and Caroli disease. Cholangiocarcinoma may appear as a single large mass or as multifocal nodules, or may be diffusely infiltrative. In contrast to HCC, it is typically pale (because biliary epithelium does not secrete bilirubin pigment) and firm. Microscopically, there are variably differentiated bile duct elements that resemble adenocarcinomas elsewhere in the alimentary tract. Clinical outlook is dismal because they are rarely resectable. Mixed variants of *hepatocellular-cholangiocarcinoma* can also rarely occur.

Metastatic Tumors (p. 927)

The liver and lung are the visceral organs most often involved by metastatic cancer. Any cancer in any site of the body may spread to the liver, including those of the blood-forming elements. The overwhelming majority of hepatic malignancy is therefore metastatic; breast, lung, and colonic primary sites are most common. Malignant melanoma in the eye (choroidal melanoma) also has a propensity to metastasize to the liver. Typically, multiple implants are present, with massive hepatic enlargement. Large implants tend to have defective vascular supplies and become centrally necrotic. Massive involvement of the liver is usually present before hepatic failure develops.

🖰 The Biliary Tract (p. 927)

CONGENITAL ANOMALIES (p. 928)

In normal biliary tree anatomy, the pancreatic and common bile ducts either join to form a common intrapancreatic channel, or enter the duodenum separately. Variants of the normal gallbladder anatomy are folded fundus *(phrygian cap)*, congenitally absent, duplicated, bilobed, or aberrant location.

DISORDERS OF THE GALLBLADDER (p. 928)

Cholelithiasis (Gallstones) (p. 928)

Bile secretion allows hepatic elimination of bilirubin, xenobiotics, and cholesterol (as free cholesterol and as bile salts). Detergent bile salts are necessary to disperse and hydrolyze dietary lipids and facilitate their intestinal absorption. Cholesterol is solubilized by bile salts and co-secreted lecithin; supersaturation of bile with cholesterol or bilirubin salts promotes stone formation. Besides such *cholesterol* stones (>50% crystalline cholesterol monohydrate), *pigmented* cholesterol stones may also form (predominantly bilirubin calcium salts).

Prevalence and Risk Factors

Gallstones afflict 10% to 20% of adult populations in developed countries. Risk factors for *cholesterol gallstones* include:

- Native Americans, adults in industrialized countries
- Increasing age, with a male-female ratio of 1:2
- Estrogenic influences, clofibrate, obesity, or rapid weight loss
- Gallbladder stasis, as in spinal cord injury or pregnancy
- Hypercholesterolemic syndromes

Risk factors for *pigmented gallstones* include:

- Asian more than Western, rural more than urban
- Chronic hemolytic syndromes (sickle cell disease)
- Biliary tract infection
- Ileal disease (resection or bypass)
- Cystic fibrosis with pancreatic insufficiency

Pathogenesis

Four conditions are necessary to form *cholesterol stones:*

- Bile must be supersaturated with cholesterol.
- Gallbladder hypomotility promotes crystal nucleation.
- Cholesterol nucleation in bile is accelerated. Nucleation is promoted by microprecipitates of calcium salts (inorganic or bilirubin salts).
- Mucus hypersecretion in the gallbladder traps the crystals, permitting their agglomeration into stones.

The pathogenesis of *pigmented stones* is based on the presence in the biliary tree of unconjugated bilirubin and precipitation of calcium bilirubin salts. *Chronic hemolytic conditions promote formation of unconjugated bilirubin in the biliary tree. Infection of the biliary tract with Escherichia coli, Ascaris lumbricoides, or the liver fluke Opisthorchis sinensis promotes bilirubin glucuronide deconjugation.*

Morphology

Cholesterol stones arise exclusively in the gallbladder and are hard and pale yellow, although bilirubin salts may impart a black color. Single stones are ovoid; multiple stones tend to be faceted. *Pigmented stones* are classified as *black* or *brown;* black stones occur in sterile gallbladders, while brown stones occur in infected intra- or extrahepatic bile ducts. Both are soft and usually multiple; brown stones are greasy. Based on calcium content, cholesterol stones are typically radiolucent, and pigment stones are frequently radiopaque.

Clinical Features

From 70% to 80% of gallstone patients remain asymptomatic throughout life. *Asymptomatic patients become symptomatic at the rate of 1% to 3% per year, and risk diminishes with time.* Symptoms include spasmodic, *colicky* pain, owing to obstruction of bile ducts by passing stones. Gallbladder obstruction per se generates right upper abdominal pain. *Complications* are gallbladder inflammation *(cholecystitis),* empyema, perforation, fistulas, biliary tree inflammation *(cholangitis),* obstructive cholestasis or pancreatitis, and erosion of a gallstone into adjacent bowel *(gallstone ileus).* Clear mucinous secretions in an obstructed gallbladder distend the gallbladder *(mucocele).*

Cholecystitis (p. 931)

Acute Cholecystitis (p. 931)

Acute cholecystitis is an acute inflammation of the gallbladder, precipitated most frequently by gallstone obstruction. The 10% of cases without gallstone obstruction usually occur in severely ill patients: postoperative state, severe trauma, severe burns, multisystem organ failure, sepsis, prolonged hyperalimentation, or postpartum state. *Symptoms* include right upper quadrant or epigastric pain, mild fever, anorexia, tachycardia, diaphoresis, and nausea and vomiting. Jaundice suggests common bile duct obstruction.

Pathogenesis

Acute inflammation due to gallstone obstruction is initiated by chemical irritation of the gallbladder by bile acids, with release of inflammatory mediators (lysolecithin, prostaglandins), gallbladder dysmotility, distention, and ischemia; bacterial contamination is a later complication. With severe illness, cholecystitis is likely a direct consequence of ischemic compromise.

Morphology

An enlarged, tense gallbladder is observed, bright red to blotchy green-black with a serosal fibrin covering. Luminal contents range from turbid to purulent.

Clinical Features

Acute cholecystitis may be mild and intermittent or may be a surgical emergency. Self-limited attacks subside over several days; overall mortality rate is less than 1%. In severely ill patients symptoms may not be evident, and mortality rate is higher. Complications include:

• Bacterial superinfection with cholangitis and sepsis
• Gallbladder perforation or rupture
• Enteric fistula formation
• Aggravation of preexisting illness

Chronic Cholecystitis (p. 932)

Chronic cholecystitis can occur through repeated bouts of symptomatic acute cholecystitis or without antecedent attacks. Although gallstones are usually present, they may not play a direct role in initiating inflammation. Rather, chronic supersaturation of bile with cholesterol permits cholesterol suffusion of the gallbladder wall and initiation of inflammation and gallbladder dysmotility. Patient populations and symptoms are the same as for the acute form.

Morphology

Gallbladders can be contracted (from fibrosis), normal in size, or enlarged (from obstruction). The wall is variably thickened and gray-white. Mucosa is generally preserved but may be atrophied. Cholesterol-laden macrophages in the lamina propria are frequently seen *(cholesterolosis)* and gallstones are frequent. Inflammation in the mucosa and wall is variable; mucosal outpouchings through the wall *(Rokitansky-Aschoff sinuses)* may be present. Rare findings are mural dystrophic calcification *(porcelain gallbladder)* and a fibrosed, nodular gallbladder with marked histiocytic inflammation *(xanthogranulomatous cholecystitis)*.

Clinical Features

Recurrent attacks of steady or colicky epigastric or right upper quadrant pain occur. Complications are the same as for acute cholecystitis.

DISORDERS OF THE EXTRAHEPATIC BILE DUCTS (p. 933)

Choledocholithiasis and Ascending Cholangitis (p. 933)

Choledocholithiasis refers to stones within the biliary tree; it occurs in 10% of patients with cholelithiasis. In Western nations, almost all stones are gallbladder-derived and are cholesterol; in Asia, they usually arise in the biliary tree and are pigmented. *Symptoms* are due to obstruction, pancreatitis, cholangitis, hepatic abscess, secondary biliary cirrhosis, and acute calculous cholecystitis.

Ascending cholangitis refers to bile duct bacterial infection; it usually occurs in the setting of choledocholithiasis. Uncommon causes include indwelling stents or catheters, tumors, acute pancreatitis, and benign strictures. Infections are typically due to bacteria entering the biliary tract through the sphincter of Oddi (e.g., *E. coli, Klebsiella,* other enteroforms).

Biliary Atresia (p. 933)

Extrahepatic biliary atresia is complete obstruction of bile flow due to destruction or absence of some part of the extrahepatic bile ducts; it occurs in 1:10,000 live births. It is the single most frequent cause of death from liver disease in early childhood (due to rapidly progressive biliary cirrhosis), and accounts for 50% to 60% of children referred for liver transplantation.

Pathogenesis

There are fetal forms and perinatal forms. The early, severe *fetal form* (20% of cases) is due to aberrant intrauterine development of the biliary tree; it is frequently associated with other anomalies. The perinatal form is more common, but the exact cause is unknown; viral infections and genetic susceptibilities may contribute.

Morphology

In both forms of biliary atresia, there is inflammation and fibrosing stricture of the extrahepatic biliary tree, progressing into the intrahepatic biliary system. The liver shows florid features of duct obstruction:

- Marked bile ductular proliferation
- Portal tract edema
- Fibrosis progressing to cirrhosis within 3 to 6 months

In the early severe form, aberrant intrahepatic biliary morphology is evident at the time of initial diagnosis, with severe paucity of intrahepatic bile ducts.

Clinical Features

Neonatal cholestasis is seen in an infant of normal birth weight and postnatal weight gain. If untreated (liver transplantation), death occurs within 2 years of birth.

Choledochal Cysts (p. 934)

These cysts are congenital dilations of the common bile duct, presenting most often in children younger than 10 years old with nonspecific symptoms of jaundice and recurrent abdominal pain; cysts may coexist with Caroli's disease (intrahepatic bile duct dilation). The cysts predispose to stone formation, stenosis and stricture, pancreatitis, obstructive biliary complications, and bile duct carcinoma in the adult.

TUMORS (p. 934)

The primary neoplasms of the gallbladder are epithelial. Benign neoplasms are adenomas, including tubular, papillary, and tubulopapillary configurations.

Carcinoma of the Gallbladder (p. 934)

Carcinoma of the gallbladder is the fifth most common cancer of the digestive tract. It is slightly more common in women, typically presenting over the age of 60. Gallstones coexist in 60% to 90% of U.S. patients, but it is unclear whether there is a causal relationship. Chronic gallbladder inflammation (with or without stones) may be a more critical risk factor. Gallstones are less common in Asian populations, in which pyogenic and parasitic disease dominate as causes.

Morphology

Tumors may be *infiltrating,* with diffuse gallbladder thickening and induration, or *exophytic*—tumor growing into the lumen as an irregular, cauliflower-like mass. Most gallbladder carcinomas are adenocarcinomas; the histologic appearance can be papillary; infiltrating; moderately to poorly differentiated or undifferentiated; and, rarely, squamous or adenosquamous, carcinoid, or mesenchymal. Tumors spread by local invasion of liver; extension to cystic duct and portohepatic lymph nodes; and seeding of peritoneum, viscera, and lungs.

Clinical Features

Symptoms are insidious and indistinguishable from those caused by cholelithiasis. Tumors are usually unresectable when discovered. Prognosis is rarely good.

Carcinoma of the Extrahepatic Bile Ducts
(p. 935)

Carcinoma of the extrahepatic bile ducts refers to uncommon malignancies of the extrahepatic biliary tree down to the ampulla of Vater. There is an increased risk in patients with choledochal cysts, ulcerative colitis, and chronic infections with *C. sinensis* and *Giardia lamblia*.

Morphology

Most are adenocarcinomas; uncommonly, squamous metaplasia gives rise to squamous cell carcinomas or adenosquamous carcinomas. Carcinoma may take the form of papillary exophytic masses, intraductal nodules, or diffuse infiltrative lesions of the duct walls. Histologically, the tumor exhibits irregular glandular structures with prominent desmoplastic reaction. Tumors arising at the confluence of the right and left hepatic bile ducts are called *Klatskin tumors,* notable for slow growth, sclerosing behavior, and infrequency of distant metastasis.

Clinical Features

Symptoms are similar to those of cholelithiasis. There is progressive obstruction, which may wax and wane as tumor necrosis periodically reestablishes ductal patency. Most have invaded adjacent structures at the time of diagnosis, and the prognosis is only fair.

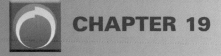
The Pancreas

CONGENITAL ANOMALIES (p. 941)

Definitions

Aberrant (or ectopic) pancreas   Pancreatic parenchyma in an abnormal location occurs in 2% of all routine postmortem examinations. Common sites include stomach, duodenum, jejunum, Meckel diverticulum, and ileum. Single or multiple firm, yellow-gray nodules in the gut wall (typically submucosal) measure from several millimeters to 4 cm. May cause pain, or rarely can incite mucosal bleeding.

Agenesis   The complete congenital absence of the pancreas is associated with other severe congenital malformations; it is usually incompatible with life.

Annular pancreas   A bandlike ring of normal pancreatic tissue completely encircles the second portion of the duodenum; can cause duodenal obstruction.

Pancreas divisum   Failure of fusion of the fetal duct system of the dorsal and ventral pancreatic primordia; this causes most pancreatic secretions to drain through the smaller minor papilla and predisposes to recurrent pancreatitis.

PANCREATITIS (p. 941)

By definition, in *acute pancreatitis*, the condition is reversible if the inciting stimulus is withdrawn; *chronic pancreatitis* is defined by irreversible destruction of exocrine pancreatic parenchyma.

Acute Pancreatitis (p. 942)

This group of disorders is characterized by pancreatic inflammation. Patients typically present with abdominal pain, associated with increased pancreatic enzymes (amylase and lipase) in blood or urine. Mild forms feature interstitial edema and

TABLE 19–1   **Etiologic Factors in Acute Pancreatitis**

Metabolic
Alcoholism
Hyperlipoproteinemia
Hypercalcemia
Drugs (e.g., thiazide diuretics)
Genetic

Mechanical
Trauma
Gallstones
Iatrogenic injury
  Perioperative injury
  Endoscopic procedures with dye injection

Vascular
Shock
Atheroembolism
Polyarteritis nodosa

Infectious
Mumps
Coxsackievirus
Mycoplasma pneumoniae

inflammation of the pancreas *(acute interstitial pancreatitis)*. In more severe cases, tissue necrosis develops *(acute necrotizing pancreatitis)*. The most severe form, *acute hemorrhagic pancreatitis*, exhibits extensive hemorrhage into the pancreatic parenchyma. About 80% of cases are associated with cholelithiasis or alcoholism (Table 19–1).

Pathogenesis

The pancreas secretes a number of enzymes; amylase and lipase are secreted in their active form, while proteases, elastases, and phospholipase are secreted as proenzymes that normally require activation by trypsin in the duodenum. Trypsin itself is normally activated by duodenal enteropeptidase. The pathogenesis of acute pancreatitis centers on inappropriate activation of trypsin in the pancreas; activated trypsin will convert (i) various proenzymes to active enzymes and (ii) prekallikrein to kallikrein, activating the kinin system and clotting. The net result is pancreatic inflammation and thrombosis. Features of pancreatitis include *tissue proteolysis, lipolysis, and hemorrhage,* resulting from the destructive effect of pancreatic enzymes released from acinar cells.

Proposed mechanisms for pancreatic enzyme activation include the following:

- *Pancreatic duct obstruction.* Gallstones can impact in the ampulla of Vater; behind the obstruction, enzyme-rich fluid accumulates and injures the pancreatic parenchyma. Resident tissue leukocytes release proinflammatory cytokines, promoting local inflammation and edema.
- *Primary acinar cell injury.* May be due to damage by viruses (mumps), drugs, trauma, or ischemia.
- *Defective intracellular transport of proenzymes.* Exocrine enzymes are misdirected toward lysosomes rather than toward secretion; lysosomal hydrolysis of the proenzymes causes enzyme activation and release.

- *Alcohol* may promote acinar cell injury by misdirecting intracellular proenzyme traffic and by promoting deposition of inspissated protein plugs within pancreatic ducts, leading to local obstruction and inflammation.
- Hereditary pancreatitis is characterized by recurrent attacks of severe pancreatitis usually beginning in childhood. This disorder is caused by germ line mutations in:

  Cationic trypsinogen gene *(PRSS1)*, leading to a loss of a site on trypsin that is essential for its own inactivation (an important failsafe mechanism for regulating trypsin enzymatic activity)

  Serine protease inhibitor, Kazal type 1 (SPINK1) gene, leading to a defective protein that can no longer inhibit trypsin activity

Morphology

The basic pancreatic alterations in acute pancreatitis are:

- Vascular leakage causing edema
- Necrosis of regional fat by lipolytic enzymes
- Acute inflammation
- Proteolytic destruction of the pancreatic substance
- Vascular injury with subsequent interstitial hemorrhage

Mild pancreatitis (acute interstitial pancreatitis) features only the first three of these. Acute necrotizing pancreatitis exhibits gray-white parenchymal necrosis and chalky white fat necrosis. In acute hemorrhagic pancreatitis, there is patchy red-black hemorrhage interspersed with focal yellow-white, chalky fat necrosis.

Clinical Features

Full-blown, acute pancreatitis is a medical emergency with acute abdomen, constant and intense abdominal pain radiating to the upper back, peripheral vascular collapse, and shock from explosive activation of the systemic inflammatory response. Death can occur from shock, acute respiratory distress syndrome, or acute renal failure. Laboratory findings include marked serum amylase elevations during the first 24 hours, followed within 72 to 96 hours by a rising serum lipase. Glycosuria occurs in 10% of cases. Hypocalcemia may result from precipitation of calcium soaps in the fat necrosis; if persistent, it is a poor prognostic sign. In less severe cases, common sequelae include sterile *pancreatic abscesses* from tissue liquefaction and *pancreatic pseudocysts,* localized collections of necrotic, hemorrhagic material rich in pancreatic enzymes. The pancreas can return to normal function if the acute pancreatitis resolves.

Chronic Pancreatitis (p. 945)

Chronic pancreatitis is characterized by pancreatic inflammation with destruction of exocrine parenchyma and fibrosis; in late stages, there is destruction of the endocrine parenchyma. The chief distinction between acute and chronic pancreatitis is the irreversible impairment in pancreatic function characteristic of chronic pancreatitis; chronic pancreatitis can be severely debilitating due to loss of pancreatic function.

Pathogenesis

The most common associated condition is alcoholism. Less commonly, hypercalcemia, hyperlipidemia, pancreas divisum, hereditary pancreatitis (see previous section), and protein-deficient malnutrition can be causes. Postulated inciting events include:

- Ductal obstruction by concretions (as with alcohol).
- Toxic-metabolic effects. Toxins, including alcohol and its metabolites, can exert a direct toxic effect on acinar cells.
- Oxidative stress from alcohol-induced oxygen-derived radical generation.
- Interstitial fibrosis initiated by acute pancreatitis.

Morphology

There is replacement of pancreatic acinar tissue by dense fibrous connective tissue, with relative sparing of the islets of Langerhans, and variable dilation of the pancreatic ducts. The pancreas is hard with focal calcification; fully developed calculi may be present *(chronic calcifying pancreatitis),* particularly in alcoholics. *Chronic obstructive pancreatitis* with impacted ampullary stones is characteristically centered around ducts and is irregular in its glandular distribution. Pseudocyst formation is common, especially in alcoholics.

Clinical Features

Chronic pancreatitis can be silent, or recurrent attacks of pain may occur at scattered intervals. Attacks are precipitated by alcohol abuse, overeating, and drug use. Late complications relate primarily to the loss of exocrine and endocrine function, and include:

- Diarrhea (malabsorption)
- Steatorrhea
- Diabetes mellitus
- Pseudocysts

The long-term outlook for patients with chronic pancreatitis is poor, with a mortality rate of 50% within 20 to 25 years.

TUMORS (p. 946)

Non-Neoplastic Cysts (p. 946)

- *Congenital cysts* (p. 946) are caused by anomalous development of the pancreatic ducts, and frequently exist concurrently with kidney and liver cysts in *congenital polycystic disease.* In *von Hippel–Lindau disease,* pancreatic cysts and angiomas of the central nervous system are seen.
- *Pseudocysts* (p. 947) are localized, usually unilocular collections of necrotic-hemorrhagic material rich in pancreatic enzymes. They almost always occur after bouts of acute or chronic pancreatitis. They may become infected or hemorrhagic. They do not possess an epithelial lining but instead are lined by fibrosed granulation tissue. Symptoms include abdominal pain.

Neoplasms (p. 947)

Neoplasms of the pancreas can be broadly grouped into cystic and solid neoplasms.

Cystic Tumors (p. 947)

Cystic tumors constitute fewer than 5% of pancreatic neoplasms; they typically present as painless, slow-growing masses.

- *Serous cystadenoma:* Predominantly occurring in women older than age 65, these neoplasms are usually solitary, 6 to 10 cm, well-circumscribed nodules with a central stellate scar. They are composed of numerous tiny cysts lined by a uniform cuboidal epithelium; a few larger cysts are filled with straw-colored, watery fluid. The epithelium contains abundant glycogen. Prognosis is excellent, with minimal risk of malignant transformation.
- *Mucinous cystic neoplasm:* These unilocular or multiloculated cystic neoplasms, up to 10 cm in diameter, are filled with thick mucinous material and lined by mucin-producing tall columnar cells. The majority occur in women (90%) and most arise in the tail of the gland. Noninvasive mucinous cystic neoplasms are classified as cystadenoma, borderline, or in situ carcinoma on the basis of epithelial pleomorphism. One third of mucinous cystic neoplasms are associated with an invasive adenocarcinoma. Prognosis depends on the presence or absence of an invasive cancer and on adequacy of surgical resection.
- *Intraductal papillary mucinous neoplasm:* These extensively involve the larger pancreatic ducts and produce copious amounts of mucin. The neoplastic epithelium is columnar, mucin-producing, and usually papillary. A characteristic feature is mucin oozing from a patulous ampulla of Vater. Most arise in the head of the gland, and one third have an associated invasive carcinoma. Prognosis depends on the presence or absence of invasive cancer and on adequacy of surgical resection.
- *Solid-pseudopapillary tumor:* These round, well-circumscribed neoplasms have solid and cystic regions; the latter are primarily due to hemorrhage and cystic degeneration. Neoplastic cells are small and uniform, growing in solid sheets or papillary projections. Most of these are seen in adolescent girls and women younger than age 35; surgical resection is the treatment of choice. Although some solid-pseudopapillary tumors are locally aggressive, most pursue a benign course if completely resected.

Solid Neoplasms (p. 948)

Solid neoplasms are more common than cystic, and are more often malignant.

Pancreatic Carcinoma (p. 948)

Infiltrating carcinoma of the exocrine pancreas almost always shows ductal epithelial differentiation and is therefore an adenocarcinoma.

Epidemiology. Carcinoma of the pancreas accounts for 5% of all cancer deaths in the United States. Each year, approximately 31,000 new patients are identified in the United States and 31,000 die from the disease. Incidence rates are twice as high in smokers compared to nonsmokers. Chronic pancreatitis, consumption of a high-energy diet rich in fats, a family history of pancreatic cancer, and diabetes mellitus impose a modestly increased risk. Peak incidence is between ages 60 and 80. Five-year survival rate is less than 4%.

Pathogenesis. Invasive adenocarcinomas of the pancreas arise from morphologically defined noninvasive precursor lesions called *pancreatic intraepithelial neoplasia.* Inherited (germline) mutations in the *BRCA2, STK11, p16,* and *PRSS1* genes predispose to pancreatic cancer. Mutational activation of the *KRAS* oncogene occurs in more than 90% of all pancreatic cancers. The *p16/CDKN2A* tumor suppressor gene is inactivated in more than 90%, *TP53* in 50% to 70%, and *SMAD4/DPC4* in 55% (Table 19–2). Other genetic alterations include hypermethylation of tumor-suppressor gene promoters, and amplification of other genes, including the *AKT2* gene. The reasons for this striking pattern of genetic alterations are not yet known.

Morphology. Distribution of pancreatic adenocarcinoma is as follows:

- Head, 60%
- Body, 15%
- Tail, 5%
- Diffuse or widely spread, 20%

Carcinomas may be small or large (8–10 cm), but are almost always ill-defined. Local invasion into the bile duct is common and results in jaundice. Metastases to regional lymph nodes and distant metastasis to the liver are present at diagnosis in most cases. *Microscopically,* the neoplastic cells form more or less differentiated glandular patterns *(adenocarcinoma)* resembling ductal epithelium. Extensive perineural and vascular invasion are common. Less common histologic variants include:

- *Adenosquamous carcinoma* with both squamous and glandular differentiation
- *Undifferentiated carcinoma* containing prominent reactive multinucleated osteoclast-like giant cells
- *Acinar cell carcinoma* producing exocrine enzymes and with granular eosinophilic cytoplasm

Clinical Features. Weight loss and pain are typical presenting symptoms; obstructive jaundice develops with tumors in the head of the gland. Metastases are common, and 85% of pancreatic adenocarcinomas are unresectable at presentation;

TABLE 19–2 **Molecular Alterations in Invasive Pancreatic Adenocarcinoma**

Gene (Chromosomal Region)	Percent of Tumors With Genetic Alteration
KRAS (12p)	>90%
p16/CDKN2A (9p)	>95%
TP53 (17p)	50%–70%
SMAD4 (18q)	55%
AKT2 (19q)	10%–20%
MYB (6q)	10%
AIB1 (20q)	10%
BRCA2 (13q)	7%–10%
LKB1/STK11 (19p)	<5%
MKK4 (17p)	<5%
TGFβ-R1 (9q) or *TGFβ-R2* (3p)	<5%
RB1 (13q)	<5%

massive liver metastasis frequently develops. The outlook is dismal: first-year mortality rate exceeds 80%. Migratory thrombophlebitis *(Trousseau syndrome)* may occur with pancreatic neoplasms (as well as other adenocarcinomas).

Other Solid Pancreatic Neoplasms

- *Periampullary carcinomas* refer to invasive carcinomas in the immediate vicinity of the ampulla of Vater. These include carcinomas of the pancreas, of the most distal common bile duct, the periampullary duodenum, and of the ampulla itself.
- *Pancreatoblastoma* is a rare tumor primarily of childhood with both acinar differentiation and squamoid nests.

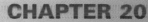

CHAPTER 20

The Kidney

Renal diseases are traditionally divided into four categories, based on the four basic anatomic compartments principally affected:

- Glomeruli
- Tubules
- Interstitium
- Blood vessels

Many disorders affect more than one structure; the anatomic interdependence of these compartments typically means that damage to one secondarily affects the others. Whatever the initial insult, there is a tendency for all forms of *chronic* renal disease to ultimately destroy all four kidney elements, culminating in end-stage kidneys and chronic renal failure.

CLINICAL MANIFESTATIONS OF RENAL DISEASES (p. 960)

Renal diseases clinically manifest themselves within reasonably well-defined syndromes (Table 20–1).

- *Acute nephritic syndrome* is seen with certain glomerular diseases (e.g., poststreptococcal glomerulonephritis). It is characterized by the acute onset of usually grossly visible hematuria, mild to moderate proteinuria, and hypertension.
- *Nephrotic syndrome* is characterized by heavy proteinuria (>3.5 gm/day), hypoalbuminemia, severe edema, hyperlipidemia, and lipiduria.
- *Asymptomatic hematuria or proteinuria* is usually a manifestation of mild glomerular abnormalities.
- *Acute renal failure* is dominated by acute onset of azotemia with oliguria or anuria resulting from severe injury to either glomeruli, tubules, interstitium, or blood vessels.
- *Chronic renal failure* is characterized by prolonged uremia. It is the end result of all chronic renal diseases.
- *Renal tubular defects* are dominated by polyuria, nocturia, and electrolyte disorders (e.g., metabolic acidosis). These

483

TABLE 20–1 **The Glomerular Syndromes**

Syndrome	Clinical Features
Acute nephritic syndrome	Hematuria, azotemia, variable proteinuria, oliguria, edema, and hypertension
Rapidly progressive glomerulonephritis	Acute nephritis, proteinuria, and acute renal failure
Nephrotic syndrome	>3.5 gm proteinuria, hypoalbuminemia, hyperlipidemia, lipiduria
Chronic renal failure	Azotemia → uremia progressing for years
Asymptomatic hematuria or proteinuria	Glomerular hematuria; subnephrotic proteinuria

defects are seen in acquired or genetic diseases affecting the tubules and/or interstitium.

- *Urinary tract infections* affect the kidney *(pyelonephritis)* or bladder *(cystitis)*, with bacteriuria and pyuria.
- *Nephrolithiasis* is manifested by renal colic, hematuria, and recurrent stone formation.

Renal Failure (p. 960)

- *Azotemia* refers to an elevation of the blood urea nitrogen (BUN) and creatinine levels; it is largely related to decreased glomerular filtration rate (GFR).
- *Prerenal azotemia* occurs with hypoperfusion of the kidneys (e.g., with congestive heart failure, shock, volume depletion, or hemorrhage).
- *Postrenal azotemia* occurs with urinary outflow obstruction below the level of the kidney.
- *Uremia* is azotemia associated with a constellation of clinical signs and symptoms (Table 20–2); it is the *sine qua non* of chronic renal failure.

Stages of renal disease progression:

1. Diminished renal reserve (approximately 50% of normal GFR)
2. Renal insufficiency (20%–50% of normal GFR)
3. Renal failure (<20% of normal GFR)
4. End-stage renal disease (<5% of normal GFR)

CONGENITAL ANOMALIES (p. 961)

Approximately 10% of newborns have potentially significant malformations of the urinary system. Renal dysplasias and hypoplasias account for 20% of pediatric chronic renal failure. Most arise from developmental defects rather than inherited genes.

- *Renal agenesis* may be bilateral or unilateral.

  Bilateral absence of renal development is incompatible with life.

  Unilateral agenesis is associated with compensatory hypertrophy of the remaining kidney; in later life the hypertrophied kidney may develop progressive glomerulosclerosis and renal failure.

- *Hypoplasia* describes failure to develop to normal size, usually unilateral. A truly hypoplastic kidney shows no scars

TABLE 20–2 **Principal Systemic Manifestations of Chronic Renal Failure and Uremia**

Fluid and Electrolytes
Dehydration
Edema
Hyperkalemia
Metabolic acidosis

Calcium Phosphate and Bone
Hyperphosphatemia
Hypocalcemia
Secondary hyperparathyroidism
Renal osteodystrophy

Hematologic
Anemia
Bleeding diathesis

Cardiopulmonary
Hypertension
Congestive heart failure
Pulmonary edema
Uremic pericarditis

Gastrointestinal
Nausea and vomiting
Bleeding
Esophagitis, gastritis, colitis

Neuromuscular
Myopathy
Peripheral neuropathy
Encephalopathy

Dermatologic
Sallow color
Pruritus
Dermatitis

and possesses a reduced number (≤6) of renal lobes and pyramids.
- *Ectopic kidneys* lie either just above the pelvic brim or sometimes within the pelvis. Kinking or tortuosity of the ureters may cause urinary obstruction, predisposing to bacterial infection.
- *Horseshoe kidney:* Fusion of the upper (10%) or lower (90%) poles produces a horseshoe-shaped structure continuous across the midline anterior to the aorta and inferior vena cava.

CYSTIC DISEASES OF THE KIDNEY (p. 962)

Table 20–3 lists the genetics, pathologic findings, and clinical presentations of the various cystic diseases.

Cystic Renal Dysplasia (p. 962)

Cystic renal dysplasia refers to sporadic, nonfamilial disease resulting from abnormal metanephric differentiation. It is frequently associated with obstructive abnormalities of the ureter and lower urinary tract and may be uni- or bilateral. Affected kidneys are enlarged and multicystic; histologically, there are

TABLE 20-3　Summary of Renal Cystic Diseases

	Inheritance	Pathologic Features	Clinical Features or Complications	Typical Outcome
Adult polycystic kidney disease	Autosomal dominant	Large multicystic kidneys, liver cysts, berry aneurysms	Hematuria, flank pain, urinary tract infection, renal stones, hypertension	Chronic renal failure beginning at age 40–60 yr
Childhood polycystic kidney disease	Autosomal recessive	Enlarged, cystic kidneys at birth	Hepatic fibrosis	Variable, death in infancy or childhood
Medullary sponge kidney	None	Medullary cysts on excretory urography	Hematuria, urinary tract infection, recurrent renal stones	Benign
Familial juvenile nephronophthisis	Autosomal recessive	Corticomedullary cysts, shrunken kidneys	Salt wasting, polyuria, growth retardation, anemia	Progressive renal failure beginning in childhood
Adult-onset medullary cystic disease	Autosomal dominant	Corticomedullary cysts, shrunken kidneys	Salt wasting, polyuria	Chronic renal failure beginning in adulthood
Simple cysts	None	Single or multiple cysts in normal-sized kidneys	Microscopic hematuria	Benign
Acquired renal cystic disease	None	Cystic degeneration in end-stage kidney disease	Hemorrhage, erythrocytosis, neoplasia	Dependence on dialysis

immature ducts surrounded by undifferentiated mesenchyme, often with focal cartilage formation.

Autosomal Dominant (Adult) Polycystic Kidney Disease (p. 962)

This disease affects 1:400 to 1:1000 persons and accounts for about 5% to 10% of cases of chronic renal failure. The genetic defect has high penetrance; 95% of individuals with a *PKD1* gene abnormality develop overt disease by age 75.

Genetics and Pathogenesis

The disease is caused by mutations primarily in one of two genes:

- *PKD1,* located on chromosome 16p13.3, accounts for about 85% of cases. It encodes a large (460 kD) protein named *polycystin 1.* Although the precise function is unknown, polycystin I normally localizes to tubular epithelial cells and has homology to proteins involved in cell-cell and cell-matrix interactions.
- *PKD2,* located on chromosome 4q21, accounts for most of the remaining cases. It encodes *polycystin 2,* an integral membrane protein with homology to certain calcium- and sodium-channel proteins, as well as to polycystin 1.

Although the specific mechanisms are unclear, these mutations are thought to alter cell-cell and cell-matrix interactions that are important for tubular epithelial growth and differentiation.

Morphology

Polycystic changes are always bilateral and can present from early childhood to as late as 80 years of age. The kidneys are enlarged, achieving massive size, and are composed virtually entirely of cysts up to 3 to 4 cm in diameter. Cysts arise anywhere along the nephron and compress adjacent parenchyma. In late disease, there is interstitial inflammation and fibrosis.

Clinical Features

Patients have flank pain from hemorrhage into cysts, hematuria, hypertension, proteinuria, progressive renal failure, and bilateral abdominal masses inducing a dragging sensation. Progression is accentuated in the presence of hypertension. About 40% of patients have scattered *liver cysts* (polycystic liver disease), and 5% to 10% have *cerebral berry aneurysms;* mitral valve prolapse occurs in 20% to 25%. About 40% of patients die of hypertensive or coronary heart disease, 25% of infections, 15% from ruptured berry aneurysm (causing subarachnoid hemorrhages) or hypertensive brain hemorrhage, and the rest of other causes.

Autosomal Recessive (Childhood) Polycystic Kidney Disease (p. 964)

This is a rare bilateral anomaly presenting from the perinatal through juvenile periods. Infants often succumb rapidly to renal failure. Kidneys are enlarged by multiple, cylindrically dilated collecting ducts, oriented at right angles to the cortex and filling both the cortex and medulla. The liver almost always has cysts and proliferating bile ducts; in the infantile and juvenile forms these cysts give rise to *congenital hepatic fibrosis.*

Cystic Diseases of Renal Medulla (p. 965)

Medullary Sponge Kidney (p. 965)

This entity consists of multiple cystic dilations in the collecting ducts of the medulla, usually presenting in adults. Although it is typically an innocuous lesion discovered incidentally by radiographic studies, it can predispose to renal calculi.

Nephronophthisis-Medullary Cystic Disease Complex (p. 965)

This complex is actually a family of progressive renal disorders, usually with onset in childhood. They are characterized by small medullary cysts (especially in the corticomedullary area) associated with cortical tubular atrophy and interstitial fibrosis. There are four variants:

- Sporadic, nonfamilial (20%)
- Familial juvenile nephronophthisis (50%); autosomal recessive
- Renal-retinal dysplasia (15%); autosomal recessive
- Adult-onset medullary cystic disease (15%); autosomal dominant

Children present with polyuria, sodium wasting, and tubular acidosis, followed by progression to renal failure. At least five gene loci have been identified for this complex. *NPH1 (nephrocystin), NPH2,* and *NPH3* underlie the juvenile form of nephronophthisis and cause autosomal recessive disease. These disorders should be strongly considered in children with otherwise unexplained chronic renal failure, a positive family history, and chronic tubulointerstitial nephritis on biopsy.

Acquired (Dialysis-Associated) Cystic Disease (p. 966)

End-stage kidneys of patients undergoing prolonged renal dialysis can develop multiple cortical and medullary cysts. They are often lined by atypical, hyperplastic epithelium that can undergo malignant transformation to renal cell carcinoma.

Simple Cysts (p. 966)

Commonly encountered, single or multiple cysts of the cortex (rarely medulla) are lined by low cuboidal epithelium and usually are 2 to 5 cm in diameter, but can measure up to 10 cm. They have smooth walls and are filled with clear serous fluid; occasionally, hemorrhage and stromal reaction can cause flank pain and irregular contours, thus mimicking renal carcinoma.

GLOMERULAR DISEASES (p. 966)

Glomerular injury is a major cause of renal disease.

- In *primary glomerulonephritis* (GN), the kidney is the principal organ involved.

TABLE 20–4 **Glomerular Diseases**

Primary Glomerulopathies
Acute diffuse proliferative golmerulonephritis
　Poststreptococcal
　Non-poststreptococcal
Rapidly progressive (crescentic) glomerulonephritis
Membranous glomerulopathy
Minimal change disease
Focal segmental glomerulosclerosis
Membranoproliferative glomerulonephritis
IgA nephropathy
Chronic glomerulonephritis

Systemic Diseases With Glomerular Involvement
Systemic lupus erythematosus
Diabetes mellitus
Amyloidosis
Goodpasture syndrome
Microscopic polyarteritis/polyangiitis
Wegener granulomatosis
Henoch-Schönlein purpura
Bacterial endocarditis

Hereditary Disorders
Alport syndrome
Thin basement membrane disease
Fabry disease

- In *secondary glomerular disease,* the kidney is one of many organ systems damaged by a systemic disease (Table 20–4).
- *Chronic GN* is one of the most common causes of chronic renal failure.

Some glomerular diseases present mainly as *nephritic syndrome,* others cause *nephrotic syndrome,* and still others present as a mixture.

Pathogenesis of Glomerular Injury (p. 968)

Immune mechanisms predominate in glomerular injury, although various nonimmune factors can initiate GN or cause its progression.

Immune Mechanisms

Glomerular deposition of antigen-antibody complexes is a major mechanism of glomerular injury; these can be formed in situ with glomerular antigens or can be trapped circulating complexes (Table 20–5). With *in situ* immune complex formation, antibodies can be directed against:

- Fixed intrinsic antigens

  Anti-glomerular basement membrane (GBM) nephritis is an autoimmune disease in which antibodies bind to the noncollagenous domain of the α3 chain of GBM type IV collagen; this yields a *linear* immunofluorescence staining pattern. Anti-GBM GN accounts for less than 5% of primary GN.

  Heymann nephritis of rats: Antibodies react with a large 330-kD *megalin* protein antigen expressed on visceral epithelial cells; megalin is complexed to a smaller 44-kD *receptor-associated protein* (RAP). The resultant lesions exhibit *subepithelial deposits* of antigen-antibody com-

TABLE 20–5 **Immune Mechanisms of Glomerular Injury**

Antibody-Mediated Injury

In Situ **Immune Complex Deposition**
Fixed intrinsic tissue antigens
  NC1 domain of collagen type IV antigen (anti-GBM nephritis)
  Heymann antigen (membranous glomerulopathy)
  Mesangial antigens
  Others
Planted antigens
  Exogenous (infectious agents, drugs)
  Endogenous (DNA, nuclear proteins, immunoglobulins, immune
    complexes, IgA)

Circulating Immune Complex Deposition
Endogenous antigens (e.g., DNA, tumor antigens)
Exogenous antigens (e.g., infectious products)

Cytotoxic Antibodies

Cell-Mediated Immune Injury

Activation of Alternative Complement Pathway

plexes resembling those in human *membranous GN*. The deposits give a *granular* pattern of immunofluorescence staining for immunoglobulin G (IgG) and complement. The pathogenesis of the rat injury closely models human membranous glomerulopathy, although the human equivalent of the Heymann antigen has not yet been identified.

- Planted circulating exogenous (e.g., infectious agents) or endogenous (e.g., DNA) antigens can occur.

- *Circulating immune complexes:* Antigens may be endogenous (e.g., thyroglobulin) or exogenous (e.g., infectious agents) but in most cases are not known. Complexes are usually deposited subendothelially or in the mesangium, and yield a granular immunofluorescence pattern. Once deposited, immune complexes cause injury by both cellular and soluble mediators, including the following:

  Neutrophils release proteases, oxygen-derived free radicals, and arachidonic acid metabolites, often following complement activation.

  Monocytes, macrophages, lymphocytes, and natural killer (NK) cells release cytokines, cytotoxic cell mediators, growth factors, and other biologically active molecules.

  Platelets aggregate and release eicosanoids and growth factors.

  Resident glomerular cells, particularly mesangial cells can initiate inflammatory responses by releasing cytokines, growth factors, chemokines, oxygen free radicals, eicosanoids, and endothelin.

  C5b-C9, the terminal membrane attack complex of complement cause cell lysis and also induce cellular activation.

  Coagulation proteins, especially fibrin, can stimulate crescent formation in crescentic GN.

  Hemodynamic regulators (e.g., eicosanoids, nitric oxide, endothelin) may be involved.

  Cytokines may include interleukin 1, tumor necrosis factor, and *chemokines* (e.g., MCP-1).

  Growth factors may include platelet-derived growth factor, transforming growth factor-β (the latter being important for extracellular matrix deposition in glomerulosclerosis) and vascular endothelial growth factor.

Mechanisms of Progression in Glomerular Diseases (p. 972)

Once any renal disease (glomerular or otherwise) destroys functioning nephrons and reduces the GFR to 30% to 50% of normal, progression to end-stage renal failure proceeds at a relatively constant rate, independent of the original stimulus or activity of the underlying disease. The two major histologic characteristics of such progressive renal damage are *glomerulosclerosis* (both focal and segmental glomerulosclerosis) and *tubulointerstitial inflammation* and *fibrosis*.

Glomerulosclerosis is initiated by *adaptive change* occurring in the relatively unaffected glomeruli of diseased kidneys. Similar changes occur in rats following loss of renal mass by subtotal nephrectomy. *Compensatory hypertrophy* of the remaining glomeruli maintains renal function in these animals, but proteinuria and glomerulosclerosis soon develop, leading eventually to glomerular sclerosis and uremia. Glomerular hypertrophy is associated with *hemodynamic changes,* including increases in single-nephron GFR, blood flow, and transcapillary pressure *(capillary hypertension),* often with systemic hypertension.

Tubulointerstitial injury is a component of many acute and chronic glomerulonephritides. Typically, decline in renal function correlates better with the extent of tubulointerstitial damage than with the severity of glomerular injury. Many factors contribute to tubulointerstitial injury, including ischemia distal to sclerotic glomeruli, concomitant immune reactions to shared tubular and glomerular antigens, phosphate or ammonia retention leading to interstitial fibrosis, and the effects of proteinuria on tubular cell structure and function. Proteinuria, in particular, causes direct injury to and activation of tubular cells. In turn, activated tubular cells elaborate proinflammatory cytokines and growth factors that drive interstitial fibrosis.

Acute Glomerulonephritis (p. 973)

Acute Proliferative (Poststreptococcal, Postinfectious) Glomerulonephritis (p. 974)

Acute proliferative GN is characterized by *acute nephritic syndrome (hematuria, red blood cell casts, and moderate proteinuria and edema),* presenting 1 to 4 weeks after a pharyngeal streptococcal infection (less commonly in the United States, after a skin infection). Other bacterial, viral, and parasitic infections can produce the same disease picture. Poststreptococcal GN is an antibody-mediated disease, although the precise causal streptococcal antigen is unknown; only certain strains (types 12, 4, 1) of group A β-hemolytic streptococci are nephritogenic.

- Biopsy specimens show *diffuse* GN (all glomeruli involved) with *global* hypercellularity due to proliferation of endothelial, mesangial, and epithelial cells, and neutrophil and monocyte infiltration.

- Immunofluorescence shows a granular IgG, IgM, and C3 deposition, and electron microscopy shows subepithelial, *humplike* deposits, supporting the contention that the pathogenesis is due to immune complex deposition.
- Serum antistreptococcal antibody levels are elevated and serum complement C3 concentrations are decreased.
- Clinically, more than 95% of children recover. A few develop a rapidly progressive disease, with the remainder progressing to chronic renal failure. In adults, the epidemic form has a good prognosis, although only 60% recover after the sporadic form; the remainder develop rapidly progressive disease, chronic renal failure, or delayed (but eventual) resolution.

Rapidly Progressive (Crescentic) Glomerulonephritis (p. 976)

This clinicopathologic syndrome is characterized by cellular accumulation in Bowman space in the form of crescents accompanied by a rapid, progressive decline in renal function. The common denominator in all types of rapidly progressive GN (RPGN) is severe glomerular injury. RPGN is divided into three broad groups; in each, the disease may be associated with another systemic disorder, or may be idiopathic (Table 20–6).

- *Type I RPGN is an anti-GBM disease* characterized by linear IgG (and in many cases C3) deposits in the GBM. In some, the anti-GBM antibodies cross-react with pulmonary alveolar basement membranes to produce pulmonary hemorrhages *(Goodpasture syndrome)*. The Goodpasture antigen is a peptide within the noncollagenous domain of the $\alpha 3$ chain of type IV collagen. What triggers these antibodies is unclear, although there is a high prevalence of certain HLA haplotypes, a finding suggesting genetic predisposition to autoimmunity.
- *Type II RPGN* is an *immune complex–mediated disease.* It can be a complication of any of the immune complex nephritides, including postinfectious GN, but in some cases, the underlying cause is undetermined. In all these cases, immunofluorescence shows characteristic *("lumpy bumpy")* granular staining.

TABLE 20–6 **Rapidly Progressive Glomerulonephritis (RPGN)**

Type I RPGN (Anti-GBM Antibody)
Idiopathic
Goodpasture syndrome

Type II RPGN (Immune Complex)
Idiopathic
Postinfectious
Systemic lupus erythematosus
Henoch-Schönlein purpura (IgA)
Others

Type III RPGN (Pauci-Immune)
ANCA associated
Idiopathic
Wegener granulomatosis
Microscopic polyarteritis nodosa/microscopic polyangiitis

ANCA, antineutrophil cytoplasmic antibodies.

- *Type III RPGN,* also called *pauci-immune type,* is defined by the lack of either anti-GBM antibodies or immune complexes. Most of these patients have *antineutrophil cytoplasmic antibody (ANCA)* in the serum, which plays a role in some vasculitides. In some cases, type III RPGN is part of a systemic vasculitis (e.g., Wegener granulomatosis or microscopic polyarteritis). In many cases, however, pauci-immune crescentic glomerulonephritis is isolated and hence *idiopathic.* In idiopathic cases, over 90% have serologic c-ANCA (cytoplasmic-ANCA) or p-ANCA (perinuclear-ANCA).

RPGN cases are distributed as follows:

- Approximately 20% have anti-GBM disease (RPGN type I).
- 25% are type II RPGN.
- Over 50% are pauci-immune (type III RPGN).

Morphology

The *histologic picture* of RPGN is dominated by distinctive *crescents* formed by parietal cell proliferation and monocyte and macrophage migration into Bowman space. Neutrophils and lymphocytes may also be present. Electron microscopy discloses subepithelial deposits in some cases, but in many cases shows distinct *ruptures in the GBM.* In time, many crescents undergo sclerosis.

Clinical Features

All forms include hematuria with urinary red blood cell casts, moderate proteinuria, and variable hypertension and edema. In Goodpasture syndrome, the course may be dominated by recurrent hemoptysis. Serum analyses for anti-GBM, antinuclear antibodies, and ANCA are helpful in diagnostic subtyping. Renal involvement is usually progressive over the course of a few weeks, culminating in severe oliguria. Functional recovery may occur with intensive plasmapheresis (plasma exchange to remove antibodies) combined with steroids and cytotoxic agents (e.g., in Goodpasture syndrome).

Nephrotic Syndrome (p. 978)

Nephrotic syndrome is characterized by excessive permeability of the glomerular capillary wall to plasma proteins, with proteinuria above 3.5 gm per day. Depending on the lesions, the proteinuria may be highly selective, such as low molecular weight proteins (chiefly albumin). With more severe injury, relatively nonselective proteinuria leads to loss of higher molecular weight proteins in addition to albumin. Heavy proteinuria leads to hypoalbuminemia, decreased colloid osmotic pressure, and systemic edema. There are also *sodium and water retention, hyperlipidemia, lipiduria, vulnerability to infection, and thrombotic complications.* The diseases causing the nephrotic syndrome in children and adults are listed in Table 20–7.

Membranous Glomerulopathy (p. 979)

Membranous GN is a major cause of nephrotic syndrome in adults; it is manifested by diffuse glomerular capillary wall thickening due to deposition of immunoglobulin-containing, electron-dense material along the *subepithelial* side of the GBM. The disease is idiopathic in 85% of patients; it may be caused by autoantibodies to visceral epithelial antigens yet

TABLE 20–7 **Causes of Nephrotic Syndrome**

	Prevalence (%)*	
Disease	Children	Adults
Primary Glomerular Disease		
Membranous glomerulopathy	5	30
Minimal change disease	65	10
Focal segmental glomerulosclerosis	10	35
Membranoproliferative glomerulonephritides	10	10
Other proliferative glomerulonephritis (focal, "pure mesangial," IgA nephropathy)	10	15
Systemic Diseases		
Diabetes mellitus		
Amyloidosis		
Systemic lupus erythematosus		
Drugs (nonsteroidal anti-inflammatory, penicillamine, "street heroin")		
Infections (malaria, syphilis, hepatitis B and C, acquired immunodeficiency syndrome)		
Malignant disease (carcinoma, lymphoma)		
Miscellaneous (bee-sting allergy, hereditary nephritis)		

*Approximate prevalence of primary disease = 95% in children, 60% in adults. Approximate prevalence of systemic disease = 5% in children, 40% in adults.

to be identified. The remaining 15% of membranous GN is associated with underlying malignant tumors (lung, colon, melanoma), systemic lupus erythematosus, exposure to gold or mercury, drugs (penicillamine, captopril), infections (hepatitis B and C, syphilis, schistosomiasis, malaria), or metabolic disorders (thyroiditis).

Morphology

By light microscopy, there is diffuse thickening of the capillary wall, hence the term *membranous.* By immunofluorescence, there is a diffuse granular staining pattern of immunoglobulin and complement along the GBM. By electron microscopy, there are subepithelial GBM deposits, which eventually incorporate into the GBM and assume an intramembranous location.

Clinical Features

The condition usually starts with the insidious onset of nephrotic syndrome or subnephrotic-range proteinuria. Some 40% of cases progress to renal insufficiency over an unpredictable time span of 2 to 20 years. Secondary causes of membranous GN (cited earlier) should be excluded in any new case.

Minimal Change Disease (Lipoid Nephrosis)
(p. 981)

This disease is the major cause of nephrotic syndrome in children. It is characterized by normal glomeruli on light microscopy but uniform and diffuse effacement of the foot processes of visceral epithelial cells on electron microscopy. Immunofluorescence shows no immune deposits. The most characteristic feature of this condition is the dramatic response to corticosteroid therapy.

The cause and pathogenesis are unknown, but several features suggest an immune defect of T cells resulting in the elaboration of a circulating cytokine that affects visceral epithelial cells and increases glomerular permeability. Despite the heavy proteinuria, the long-term prognosis is excellent.

Focal Segmental Glomerulosclerosis (p. 982)

A cause of nephrotic syndrome or heavy proteinuria, focal segmental glomerulosclerosis (FSG) is characterized by *sclerosis* of some, but not all, glomeruli (thus, it is *focal*); in affected glomeruli, only a portion of the capillary tuft is involved, and thus it is *segmental*. FSG can be:

* Idiopathic
* A secondary event, reflecting glomerular scarring, consequent to another primary glomerular disease (e.g., IgA nephropathy)
* Associated with loss of renal mass (renal ablation FSG) as the result of chronic reflux, analgesic abuse, or unilateral renal agenesis
* Secondary to other known disorders (e.g., heroin abuse, HIV infection, obesity)
* The result of inherited mutations of proteins present in podocytes *(podocin, α-actinin)* or in the slit diaphragm between podocytes *(nephrin)*

It is controversial whether idiopathic FSG is part of a pathologic continuum with minimal change disease at one end of the spectrum. The primary glomerular lesion in all cases is *visceral epithelial damage* (effacement or detachment) in affected glomerular segments. Segmental IgM and C3 depositions in glomeruli are also frequently present in FSG, often in areas of sclerosis, as is segmental hyalinosis involving capillary walls and lumens. In contrast to minimal change disease, the proteinuria in FSG is relatively nonselective. Moreover, FSG patients more likely exhibit hematuria, reduced GFR, and hypertension. Idiopathic FSG responds poorly to steroids, and progression to chronic renal failure is common. FSG recurs in 25% to 50% of patients receiving allografts, with proteinuria occurring rapidly after transplantation. A circulating factor (perhaps a cytokine) is suspected as the underlying cause.

In FSG associated with HIV, there is *collapse* and *sclerosis* of the entire glomerular tuft, as well as *endothelial tuboreticular inclusions* seen by electron microscopy.

Membranoproliferative Glomerulonephritis (p. 984)

The name *membranoproliferative* (MP) reflects both thickened capillary loops and glomerular cell proliferation. It accounts for up to 20% of nephrotic syndrome in children and adults. Some patients have hematuria or proteinuria, while others demonstrate a combined *nephritic-nephrotic* picture. Glomeruli have a *lobular* appearance because of mesangial proliferation, and the capillary walls often have a *double-contour* or *tram-track* appearance. The latter is caused by interposition of cellular elements (usually mesangial, endothelial, or leukocyte) between split or reduplicated capillary basement membranes; hence, the alternative name *mesangiocapillary GN*.

There are two major types of MPGN:

* *Type I* has *subendothelial* electron-dense deposits and occasional granular subepithelial and mesangial immunoglogulin and C3, C1q, and C4 deposits. Type I MPGN occurs in

patients with systemic lupus erythematosus, hepatitis B, hepatitis C with cryoglobulinemia, infected ventriculoatrial shunts, schistosomiasis, α_1-antitrypsin deficiency, chronic liver disease, and certain malignancies; it can also be idiopathic.

- *Type II (dense-deposit disease)* has electron-dense GBM deposition in a confluent ribbon-like fashion; subepithelial *humplike* deposits are also occasionally found. C3 is present, but there are no early complement components.

Type I disease is related to immune complex deposition, whereas type II is due to activation of the alternate complement pathway. Most type II patients have *C3 nephritic factor* in the serum, an autoantibody against C3 convertase that stabilizes C3 convertase activity. Although steroids may slow the progression of MPGN, about 50% of patients develop chronic renal failure within 10 years. There is a high recurrence rate in transplant recipients, particularly in patients with type II disease.

IgA Nephropathy (Berger Disease) (p. 986)

IgA nephropathy is probably the most common type of glomerulonephritis worldwide and is a major cause of recurrent glomerular hematuria. It is characterized by mesangial proliferation and IgA deposition detectable by immunofluorescence. By light microscopy, the glomeruli can appear nearly normal, showing only subtle mesangial hypercellularity, or can reveal focal proliferative or sclerotic lesions.

Pathogenesis

The pathogenesis is unclear, although a genetic or acquired defect in immune regulation leading to increased mucosal IgA secretion in response to ingested or inhaled antigens is postulated. There is also decreased clearance of IgA complexes by the liver. Increased systemic IgA or qualitative alterations in the IgA molecule leads to augmented IgA deposition in the mesangium, but it is unclear how this leads to disease. Similar IgA deposits are seen in *Henoch-Schönlein purpura* in children.

Clinical Features

The hematuria typically lasts for several days, then subsides, only to recur. Although most patients have an initially benign course, chronic renal failure develops in 50% over a period of 20 years. Recurrence occurs in 20% to 60% of grafts. Onset in old age, heavy proteinuria, hypertension, crescents, and vascular sclerosis portend a poorer prognosis.

Hereditary Syndromes of Isolated Hematuria (p. 988)

Hereditary nephritides comprise a heterogeneous group manifesting primarily as glomerulopathies, usually presenting with hematuria, and sometimes progressing to renal failure.

Alport Syndrome

The best characterized—Alport syndrome—(p. 988) *is a glomerulopathy associated with nerve deafness, lens dislocation, cataracts, and corneal dystrophy.* In most patients, electron microscopy demonstrates irregular GBM thickening, with pronounced splitting of the lamina densa, often with a basketweave appearance. The X-linked form of the disease (males are most severely affected) is due to gene mutations in the α5 chain of collagen type IV, a component of the GBM. As a result of this defect, there is decreased α3 chain synthesis, and kidneys from Alport patients do not express the Goodpasture antigen.

Thin Membrane Disease (p. 989)

Thin membrane disease is associated with the fairly common entity of benign (asymptomatic) familial hematuria. Renal function is normal, and the prognosis is excellent. The GBM is approximately 150 to 250 nm thick (normal, 300–400 nm). The genetic basis is still unclear.

Chronic Glomerulonephritis (p. 989)

Chronic GN is a common end-stage of a number of different glomerulonephritides; the following percentiles indicate the risk that a particular entity will progress to chronic GN:

- Poststreptococcal GN (1%–2%)
- RPGN (90%)
- Membranous GN (up to 40%)
- Focal glomerulosclerosis (50%–80%)
- MPGN (50%)
- IgA nephropathy (30%–50%)

Some chronic GNs arise mysteriously with no history of any well-recognized precursor. Glomeruli in chronic GN are completely effaced by hyalinized connective tissue, making it impossible to identify the cause of the antecedent lesion. An overview of the various forms of primary GN is presented in Table 20–8.

Glomerular Lesions Associated With Systemic Disease (p. 990)

- *Systemic lupus erythematosus* (SLE) (p. 990): SLE is covered in detail in Chapter 6.
- *Henoch-Schönlein purpura* (p. 990): Systemic lesions include purpuric skin lesions (leukocytoclastic vasculitis), abdominal symptoms (pain, vomiting, bleeding), arthralgia, and GN. GN lesions vary from focal mesangial proliferation to crescentic GN but are always associated with *mesangial IgA deposition*. This condition usually occurs in children, and the course is variable; resolution of the lesions is the rule. Chronic renal failure may ensue, especially in those with diffuse lesions, crescents, or the nephrotic syndrome.
- *Bacterial endocarditis* (p. 990): Variably severe, immune complex–mediated GN is found, showing a morphologic continuum from focal necrotizing GN to diffuse GN, sometimes with crescents.
- *Diabetic glomerulosclerosis* (p. 990): The disease produces proteinuria (sometimes in the nephrotic range) in about 50% of type I and type II diabetics. It is usually discovered 1 to 2 decades after onset (in type I) and heralds the beginning of end-stage renal disease within 4 to 5 years in about 30% of juvenile diabetics. Glomerular morphologic changes include:

Capillary basement membrane thickening
Diffuse mesangial sclerosis

TABLE 20–8 Summary of Major Primary Glomerulonephrides

Disease	Most Frequent Clinical Presentation	Pathogenesis	Glomerular Pathology		
			Light Microscopy	Fluorescence Microscopy	Electron Microscopy
Poststreptococcal glomerulonephritis	Acute nephritis	Antibody mediated; circulating or planted antigen	Diffuse proliferation; leukocytic infiltration	Granular IgG and C3 in GBM and mesangium	Subepithelial humps
Goodpasture syndrome	Rapidly progressive glomerulonephritis	Anti-GBM COL4-A3 antigen	Proliferation; crescents	Linear IgG and C3; fibrin in crescents	No deposits; GBM disruptions; fibrin
Idiopathic RPGN	Rapidly progressive glomerulonephritis	Anti-GBM antibody immune complex ANCA-associated	Proliferation; focal necrosis; crescents	Linear IgG and C3 / Granular IgG or IgA or IgM / Negative or equivocal	No deposits / Deposits may occur / No deposits
Membranous glomerulopathy	Nephrotic syndrome	In situ antibody-mediated; antigen unknown	Diffuse capillary wall thickening	Granular IgG and C3; diffuse	Subepithelial deposits
Minimal change disease	Nephrotic syndrome	Unknown, loss of glomerular polyanion; podocyte injury	Normal; lipid in tubules	Negative	Loss of foot processes; no deposits
Focal segmental glomerulosclerosis	Nephrotic syndrome; non-nephrotic proteinuria	Unknown, ablation nephropathy plasma factor(?); podocyte injury	Focal and segmental sclerosis and hyalinosis	Focal; IgM and C3	Loss of foot processes; epithelial denudation
Membranoproliferative glomerulonephritis (MPGN) type I	Nephrotic syndrome	(I) Immune complex	Mesangial proliferation; basement membrane thickening; splitting	(I) IgG + C3; C1q + C4	(I) Subendothelial deposits
Dense deposit disease (MPGN type II)	Hematuria Chronic renal failure	(II) Autoantibody: alternative complement pathway		(III) C3 ± IgG; no C1q or C4	(II) Dense deposits
IgA nephropathy	Recurrent hematuria or proteinuria	Unknown; see text	Focal proliferative glomerulonephritis; mesangial widening	IgA +/– IgG, IgM, and C3 in mesangium	Mesangial and paramesangial dense deposits
Chronic glomerulonephritis	Chronic renal failure	Variable	Hyalinized glomeruli	Granular or negative	

ANCA, antineutrophil cytoplasmic antibody; GBM, glomerular basement membrane; RPGN, rapidly progressive glomerulonephritis.

Nodular glomerulosclerosis (also known as *Kimmelstiel-Wilson disease*)

- Diabetics also develop hyaline arteriosclerosis and pyelonephritis, sometimes associated with papillary necrosis. Diabetes and renal changes are further discussed in Chapter 24.
- *Amyloidosis* (p. 992): Amyloid deposited in glomeruli and in vessel walls (either primary or secondary form of the disease) produces heavy proteinuria. Eventually, end-stage renal disease occurs, although the kidneys tend to be either normal-sized or slightly enlarged.
- *Miscellaneous:* Goodpasture syndrome, polyarteritis nodosa, allergic vasculitis, and Wegener granulomatosis all produce similar forms of GN ranging from focal segmental necrotizing GN to crescentic GN. Essential mixed cryoglobulinemia can induce cutaneous vasculitis, synovitis, and GN. Plasma cell dyscrasias can be associated with amyloidosis, monoclonal cryoglobulinemia, and a peculiar nodular GN (granular dense deposits) ascribed to the deposition of nonfibrillar light chains usually of the κ type, known as *light-chain glomerulopathy* (p. 993).

DISEASES AFFECTING TUBULES AND INTERSTITIUM (p. 993)

Acute Tubular Necrosis (p. 993)

Acute tubular necrosis (ATN) is the most common cause of acute renal failure; it is characterized by renal tubular epithelial cell destruction due to either *ischemia* or *nephrotoxins.*

- *Ischemic ATN* is a reversible lesion that arises in a variety of clinical settings (e.g., shock, circulatory collapse, dehydration); all such settings are characterized by period of inadequate blood flow to the kidney, causing hypoxia.
- *Nephrotoxic ATN* is caused by a wide variety of drugs (e.g., gentamicin, cephalosporin, methoxyflurane, cyclosporine, contrast media) and toxins (e.g., mercury; lead; arsenic; methyl alcohol; ethylene glycol; and certain mushrooms, insecticides, and herbicides). ATN can also follow massive hemoglobinuria or myoglobinuria (from rhabdomyolysis), usually associated with dehydration and hypoxia.

Pathogenesis

Reversible and irreversible tubular damage are thought to be primary events leading to diminished renal function (Fig. 20–1):

- Arteriolar vasoconstriction (with tubuloglomerular feedback involving the renin-angiotensin system and endothelial dysfunction) leading to increased endothelin and decreased nitric oxide and prostaglandin I_2
- Tubular obstruction by casts derived from necrotic and apoptotic epithelial cells and proteinaceous material
- Back-leak of tubular fluids
- Altered glomerular ultrafiltration

Morphology

Findings may be microscopically subtle, but careful evaluation usually reveals the following changes:

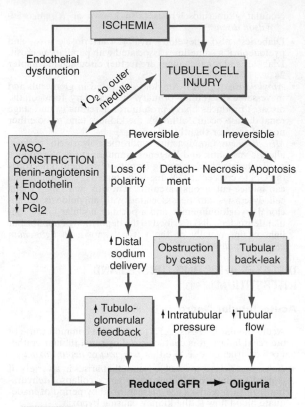

FIGURE 20–1 Pathogenetic mechanisms in ischemic acute renal failure.

- *Ischemic ATN:* Patchy tubular necrosis with lesser degrees of tubular cell injury typically involve the proximal tubule straight segments and thick ascending loop of Henle.
- *Nephrotoxic ATN:* Variable degrees of tubular injury and necrosis, mostly in proximal tubules, occur, although other tubular segments can be affected.
- In both types, the distal tubules and collecting ducts contain cellular and protein casts. The recovery phase shows epithelial regeneration (i.e., tubular cells with hyperchromatic nuclei and mitotic figures).

Clinical Features

The clinical course of ATN is highly variable, but it classically proceeds through these stages:

- *An initiating stage* is dominated by the inciting event.
- *A maintenance stage* is dominated by persistent renal failure, diminished urine production, and hyperkalemia.
- *A recovery stage* is dominated by rising urine volumes and perhaps hypokalemia.
- Prognosis depends in part on the cause; it is *good* in most cases of nephrotoxic ATN, but is poor for ATN secondary to overwhelming sepsis

Pyelonephritis and Urinary Tract Infection
(p. 996)

Urinary tract infection (UTI) denotes infection of the bladder *(cystitis),* the urethra or ureter, the kidneys *(pyelonephritis),* or all of the above. UTI may be clinically silent (asymptomatic bacteriuria) but more often causes dysuria and frequency, and—in pyelonephritis—flank pain and fever. UTI is much more common in women, perhaps because of the shorter urethra and hormonal changes affecting mucosal bacterial adherence. Other UTI risk factors include long-term catheterization, vesicoureteral reflux, pregnancy, diabetes mellitus, immunosuppression, and lower urinary tract obstructions due to congenital defects, benign prostatic hypertrophy, tumors, or calculi.

Pathogenesis

Pyelonephritis in either gender is most commonly the result of *ascending infection* from the bladder. In women, this may occur as a consequence of *bacterial colonization* of the distal urethra and introitus. The typical sequence of events is:

- Multiplication of bacteria in the bladder (cystitis).
- Vesicoureteral reflux through an incompetent vesicoureteral orifice. Vesicoureteral reflux is most often due to congenital defects in the intravesicular portion of the ureter and may be accentuated by cystitis, allowing retrograde seeding of the renal pelvis and renal papillae.
- Intrarenal reflux through open papillae to renal tissue.

Escherichia coli, Proteus, Klebsiella, and *Enterobacter* are the most frequent bacterial pathogens.

Hematogenous seeding of kidneys occurs most often in the setting of septicemia or infective endocarditis and is frequently due to *Staphylococcus* or *E. coli.*

Acute Pyelonephritis (p. 998)

Acute infection of the kidney is marked by patchy, suppurative inflammation, tubular necrosis, and intratubular neutrophilic casts. More advanced changes include abscesses, necrotizing papillitis (especially in diabetics and in those with obstruction), pyonephrosis (pelvis filled with pus), perinephric abscesses, and eventually renal scars with fibrotic deformation of the cortex and underlying calyx and pelvis (see chronic pyelonephritis, discussed next).

Clinically, acute pyelonephritis is associated with flank pain, fever, dysuria, pyuria (with pus casts in the urine), and bacteriuria. Uncomplicated acute pyelonephritis follows a benign course with antibiotic therapy but may recur or progress in the presence of vesicoureteral reflux, obstruction, immunocompromise, diabetes, and other conditions.

Chronic Pyelonephritis and Reflux Nephropathy (p. 1000)

Chronic pyelonephritis (CPN) is a disorder in which *tubulointerstitial inflammation causes discrete, corticomedullary scars overlying dilated, blunted, and deformed calyces.* Previously, CPN was the cause of 10% to 20% of cases of chronic renal failure, but this prevalence has decreased with better diagnosis of predisposing conditions. It can be divided into two forms: *obstructive CPN* and *reflux nephropathy-associated CPN*.

- In *obstructive CPN*, chronic obstruction predisposes the kidney to infections, and multiple recurrences over time produce CPN. It is usually caused by enteric bacteria.
- *Reflux nephropathy-associated CPN* is the most common cause of CPN. It begins in childhood, as a result of infections superimposed on congenital vesicoureteral reflux and intrarenal reflux. Reflux nephropathy may have a silent, insidious onset, sometimes presenting with hypertension or evidence of renal dysfunction in the absence of persisting infection.
- *Xanthogranulomatous pyelonephritis* is an uncommon form of CPN associated with gram-negative infections; there is a mixed inflammatory infiltrate with abundant foamy macrophages producing large, yellow-orange nodules that can clinically and radiologically mimic renal cell carcinoma.

Morphology

Both major types of CPN are associated with broad scars, deformed calyces, and significant tubulointerstitial inflammation and fibrosis. Secondary FGS and hypertensive changes can also be present.

Tubulointerstitial Nephritis Induced by Drugs and Toxins (p. 1002)

Acute drug-induced interstitial nephritis is an adverse hypersensitivity reaction to a variety of drugs. It begins 2 to 40 days after exposure. The disorder is immune-mediated; the offending agents act as immunizing haptens. During tubular secretion, the drugs covalently bind to cytoplasmic or extracellular matrix components, become immunogenic, and induce antibody (IgE) and T cell–mediated immune reactions.

Clinical Features

Fever, eosinophilia, skin rash, hematuria, mild proteinuria, sterile pyuria, azotemia, and acute renal failure can all be variably present. Drug withdrawal usually leads to full recovery. Biopsy will show edema, patchy tubular necrosis, and tubulointerstitial infiltrates, with variable combinations of lymphocytes, histiocytes, eosinophils, neutrophils, plasma cells, and occasionally well-formed granulomas.

Analgesic Abuse Nephropathy (p. 1003)

Analgesic abuse nephropathy is caused by excessive intake of analgesic mixtures. It is characterized by chronic tubulointerstitial nephritis with papillary necrosis. Most affected patients consume phenacetin-containing mixtures, and cases ascribed to aspirin, phenacetin, or acetaminophen alone are uncommon. The drugs act synergistically to cause papillary necrosis; tubulointerstitial nephritis is a secondary phenomenon.

Clinical Features

Patients may have polyuria, headaches, anemia, gastrointestinal symptoms, pyuria, UTIs, and hypertension. These patients have an increased incidence of transitional cell carcinoma of the renal pelvis. Chronic renal failure can result, but drug withdrawal often stabilizes renal function. Renal papillary necrosis can be diagnosed radiologically, although it is not specific for analgesic nephropathy (e.g., it also occurs in diabetes mellitus, sickle cell disease, and urinary tract obstruction).

Other Tubulointerstitial Diseases (p. 1004)

- *Urate nephropathy* can cause acute renal failure or chronic renal failure, depending on the time course of uric acid deposition. Acute renal failure is more likely in patients with hematolymphoid malignancies undergoing chemotherapy; chronic renal failure is more common in patients with gout. Patients with increased lead exposure can develop gout and a chronic interstitial disease.
- *Hypercalcemia* of any cause can cause stones *(nephrolithiasis)* or deposition within the kidney *(nephrocalcinosis)*; both can cause renal insufficiency.
- *Multiple myeloma* can cause proteinuria, as well as acute or chronic renal failure; renal insufficiency occurs in 50% of patients. Several factors contribute to renal damage:

  Bence Jones proteinuria and cast nephropathy: Some light chains are directly toxic to epithelial cells. In addition, Bence Jones proteins combine with the urinary glycoprotein *(Tamm-Horsfall protein)* under acidic conditions to form large, histologically distinct tubular casts that obstruct the tubular lumens and induce a peritubular inflammatory reaction (cast nephropathy).

  Amyloidosis occurs in 6% to 24% of patients with myeloma.

  Light-chain deposition disease: Light chains can deposit in glomeruli in nonfibrillar forms, causing a glomerulopathy, or in tubular basement membranes, causing a tubulointerstitial nephritis.

  Hypercalcemia and hyperuricemia are often present in patients with myeloma.

  Vascular disease commonly occurs in the elderly population, which is typically most frequently afflicted by myeloma.

  Urinary tract obstruction from stones or casts can lead to secondary pyelonephritis.

DISEASES OF BLOOD VESSELS (p. 1006)

Nearly all diseases of the kidney and many systemic diseases secondarily affect the blood vessels of the kidney. In particular, hypertension markedly affects renal vessels; conversely, any vascular changes augment the hypertension.

Benign Nephrosclerosis (p. 1006)

Benign nephrosclerosis is the term used to describe renal changes associated with sclerosis of renal arterioles and small arteries. The vascular lesions are characterized by narrowing of arteriolar lumens, caused by wall thickening and hyalinization.

Larger muscular arteries show *fibroelastic hyperplasia,* with both medial and intimal thickening. The changes are more severe in patients with essential hypertension, diabetes mellitus, or both. *The vascular lesions cause diffuse ischemic atrophy of nephrons; as a result, the kidneys are relatively small and exhibit diffuse granular surfaces due to scarring and contraction of individual glomeruli.* Benign nephrosclerosis rarely causes renal failure, but can cause mild proteinuria. Three groups of patients are at risk of developing renal failure: blacks, those with more severe blood pressure elevations, and those with underlying diseases, particularly diabetes.

Malignant Hypertension and Accelerated Nephrosclerosis (p. 1007)

Malignant nephrosclerosis is the kidney disease associated with an accelerated phase of hypertension. Although occasionally developing in previously normotensive people, most cases are superimposed on preexisting benign essential hypertension, chronic renal disease (particularly GN or reflux nephropathy), or scleroderma.

The condition occurs in 1% to 5% of patients with hypertension. Its pathogenesis involves injury with fibrinoid necrosis of the vessel walls caused by severe hypertension, intravascular thrombosis, and arteritis. These cause renal ischemia, with stimulation of the renin-angiotensin and other vasoconstrictive systems, perpetuating an ever-increasing cycle of escalating blood pressures.

Morphology

Pathologic changes include fibrinoid necrosis of arterioles; hyperplastic arteriolopathy (onion-skinning); and necrotizing glomerulitis, and a glomerular thrombotic microangiopathy. Patients have a diastolic blood pressure greater than 130 mm Hg, marked proteinuria, hematuria, papilledema, encephalopathy, cardiovascular abnormalities, and eventually renal failure. There are marked increases in plasma renin, angiotensin, and aldosterone.

Renal Artery Stenosis (p. 1008)

Unilateral renal artery stenosis accounts for 2% to 5% of cases of renal hypertension, resulting from excessive renin secretion by the involved kidney. Of stenoses, 70% are caused by obstructive *atheromatous plaque* at the origin of the renal artery and the remainder by *fibromuscular dysplasia.* The latter is a heterogeneous group of disorders, usually occurring at a younger age (20s to 30s), characterized by nonarteriosclerotic *intimal, medial, or adventitial* thickening. Before arteriosclerosis develops in the opposite kidney, surgery cures about 80% with fibromuscular dysplasia and 60% with atherosclerotic stenosis.

Thrombotic Microangiopathies (p. 1009)

This group of diseases has overlapping clinical manifestations (e.g., microangiopathic hemolytic anemia, thrombocytopenia, renal failure, and manifestations of intravascular coagulation). The diseases include:

- Classic (childhood) hemolytic-uremic syndrome (HUS)
- Adult HUS associated with infection, antiphospholipid antibodies, contraceptives, complications of pregnancy, certain drugs, radiation, and scleroderma
- Familial HUS
- Idiopathic HUS and thrombotic thrombocytopenic purpura (TTP)

Although these diseases can have diverse causes, endothelial injury and intravascular platelet aggregation and coagulation appear to be shared pathogenetic mechanisms. They are characterized morphologically by thromboses in the interlobular arteries, afferent arterioles, and glomeruli, together with necrosis and thickening of the vessel walls. The morphologic changes are similar to those in malignant hypertension, but the changes can precede the development of hypertension or be seen in its absence.

Classic (Childhood) HUS (p. 1010)

Classic HUS usually occurs after a gastrointestinal or flulike prodrome; it is manifested by acute renal failure with oliguria, hematuria, microangiopathic hemolytic anemia, hypertension, and (in some patients) neurologic signs. Up to 75% of patients are infected with *verocytotoxin-producing E. coli.*

Pathogenesis

Pathogenesis is related to the endothelial effects of the shigella toxin-like verocytotoxin:

- Increased leukocyte adhesion
- Increased endothelin and decreased nitric oxide production (both favoring vasoconstriction)
- Endothelial lysis

Morphology

Kidneys show patchy renal cortical necrosis, glomerular capillary wall thickening (due to deposition of fibrin-related materials and subendothelial swelling), mesangiolysis, and arteriolar changes (fibrinoid necrosis, intimal hyperplasia, and thrombi).

Adult HUS/TTP (p. 1010)

This form occurs in a variety of settings:

- *In association with infection,* such as typhoid fever, *E. coli* septicemia, viral infections, and shigellosis.
- In the *antiphospholipid syndrome,* either primary or secondary to systemic lupus erythematosus (lupus anticoagulant) (Chapter 4).
- Related to complications of pregnancy (placental hemorrhage) or the postpartum period. *Postpartum renal failure* usually occurs after an uneventful pregnancy, 1 day to several months after delivery, and is characterized by microangiopathic hemolytic anemia, oliguria, anuria, and initially mild hypertension.
- Associated with *vascular renal diseases,* such as scleroderma, and malignant hypertension.
- In patients treated with chemotherapeutic and immunosuppressive drugs, such as mitomycin and cyclosporine.

Idiopathic TTP (p. 1011)

Idiopathic TTP and various forms of HUS overlap considerably both clinically and morphologically. *Classic idiopathic TTP* is manifested by fever, neurologic symptoms, hemolytic anemia, thrombocytopenic purpura, and thrombi in glomerular capillaries and afferent arterioles. The disease is more common in women, mostly in those younger than 40 years. The thrombi are composed largely of platelets and are found in arterioles of many organs throughout the body. Untreated, the disease was once highly fatal, but exchange transfusions and corticosteroid therapy have reduced mortality rate to below 50%. Idiopathic TTP is caused by an acquired or genetic defect of ADAMTS-13, a protease that normally cleaves large von Willebrand factor (vWF) multimers; the abnormal, noncleaved forms of vWF lead to enhanced platelet aggregation.

Other Vascular Disorders (p. 1011)

Atheroembolic Renal Disease (p. 1011)

Cholesterol crystals and debris embolize from atheromatous plaques after manipulation of severely diseased aortas, usually for repair of aortic aneurysms or during intra-aortic cannulation. They lodge in intrarenal vessels, causing arterial narrowing and focal ischemic injury. Rarely, renal function becomes compromised.

Renal Infarcts (p. 1012)

Kidneys are favored sites of infarction because they receive 25% of cardiac output and because of their "end organ" arterial blood supply with only a very limited collateral circulation. Infarcts usually develop in a clinical setting of atrial fibrillation or myocardial infarction complicated by mural thrombosis, with subsequent renal embolization. Most renal infarcts are asymptomatic but may cause pain and hematuria. Large infarcts of one kidney can cause hypertension.

URINARY TRACT OBSTRUCTION (OBSTRUCTIVE UROPATHY) (p. 1012)

Obstruction increases susceptibility to infection and to stone formation. Unrelieved obstruction almost always leads to permanent renal atrophy. *Hydronephrosis is the term used to describe dilation of the renal pelvis and calyces associated with progressive atrophy of the kidney following urinary outflow obstruction.* Causes of urinary tract obstruction include:

- Congenital anomalies (urethral valves, urethral strictures, meatal stenosis, bladder neck obstruction, ureteropelvic junction narrowing or obstruction, severe vesicoureteral reflux)
- Urinary calculi
- Prostatic hypertrophy or carcinoma
- Tumors
- Inflammation (prostatitis, ureteritis, urethritis, retroperitoneal fibrosis)
- Sloughed papillae or blood clots
- Normal pregnancy
- Functional disorders (neurogenic bladder)

When obstruction is sudden and complete, the reduction of GFR usually leads to only mild dilation of the pelvis and calyces but only sometimes cause renal parenchymal atrophy. When the obstruction is subtotal or intermittent, GFR is not suppressed, and progressive dilation ensues. Unilateral (complete or partial) obstruction may remain silent for long periods because the unaffected kidney can usually compensate to maintain adequate renal function. In bilateral partial obstruction, the earliest manifestations are inability to concentrate the urine; this is reflected by polyuria and occasionally acquired distal tubular acidosis, salt wasting, renal calculi, tubulointerstitial nephritis, atrophy, and hypertension.

UROLITHIASIS (RENAL CALCULI, STONES)
(p. 1014)

Calculi can arise at any level in the urinary tract, frequently causing clinical symptoms, including obstruction, ulceration, bleeding, and pain *(renal colic)*; they also predispose to renal infection. There are four types of calculi (Table 20–9); an organic matrix of mucoprotein (1%–5% by weight) is present in all four types:

- About 70% of stones are *calcium containing,* composed of calcium oxalate plus/minus calcium phosphate. *Calcium-containing stones* are usually associated with hypercalcemia or hypercalciuria (about 60%); hyperoxaluria and hyperuricosuria are associated in others. In about 15% to 20%, there is no demonstrable metabolic abnormality.
- About 15% to 20% are so-called *triple phosphate* or *struvite* stones composed of magnesium ammonium phosphate. Struvite stones are associated with infection by urea-splitting bacteria that convert urea to ammonia. So-called *staghorn* calculi are struvite stones and are almost always associated with infection.
- From 5% to 10% are *uric acid stones;* these may or may not form in the presence of hyperuricemia or hyperuricosuria.
- Between 1% and 2% of calculi are made up of cystine.

TABLE 20–9   **Prevalence of Various Types of Renal Stones**

Types of Stones	Percentage of All Stones
Calcium Oxalate and Phosphate	70
Idiopathic hypercalciuria (50%)	
Hypercalciuria and hypercalcemia (10%)	
Hyperoxaluria (5%)	
Enteric (4.5%)	
Primary (0.5%)	
Hyperuricosuria (20%)	
Hypocitraturia	
No known metabolic abnormality (15%–20%)	
Magnesium Ammonium Phosphate (Struvite)	15–20
Uric Acid	5–10
Associated with hyperuricemia	
Associated with hyperuricosuria	
Idiopathic (50% of uric acid stones)	
Cystine	1–2
Others or Unknown	±5

Increased concentrations of stone constituents, changes in urinary pH, decreased urine volume, and bacteria all play a role in stone formation, but many calculi occur in the absence of these factors. Thus, *loss of inhibitors* of crystal formation (e.g., citrate, pyrophosphate, glycosaminoglycans, osteopontin, and an α-glycoprotein called *nephrocalcin*) may play a pathogenic role in such cases.

TUMORS OF THE KIDNEY (p. 1015)

Benign Tumors (p. 1015)

- *Renal papillary adenoma:* Small, discrete (usually yellow) tumors are seen in 7% to 22% of autopsies. Histologically, most consist of vacuolated epithelial cells forming tubules and complex branching papillary structures. The cells may be histologically indistinguishable from those of low-grade papillary renal cell carcinoma, and they share some of their cytogenetic features. Most are small (0.5 mm in diameter).
- *Renal fibroma or hamartoma:* These small (<1 cm) nodules of fibroblast-like cells and collagen are found in the medulla; they are completely benign.
- *Angiomyolipoma:* Often associated with tuberous sclerosis (25%–50% of patients), these tumors are considered to be hamartomas.
- *Oncocytomas:* These epithelial tumors are composed of eosinophilic cells, arising from the intercalated cells of collecting ducts; on electron microscopy, the cells are packed with mitochondria. They may be large (up to 12 cm) but almost never metastasize.

Malignant Tumors (p. 1016)

Renal Cell Carcinoma (Hypernephroma or Adenocarcinoma of Kidney) (p. 1016)

These carcinomas represent about 1% to 3% of all visceral cancers and 85% of renal cancers in adults. They usually occur in patients 50 to 70 years old and show a male preponderance; tobacco use is the most prominent risk factor. Most renal cancer is sporadic, but autosomal dominant familial cancers account for 4% of cases.

- *von Hippel–Lindau (VHL) syndrome:* In VHL, 50% to 70% of patients develop renal cysts, as well as bilateral, frequently multicentric renal cell carcinomas. The *VHL* gene is implicated in carcinogenesis of both familial and sporadic clear cell tumors.
- *Hereditary (familial) clear cell carcinoma:* This type occurs without the other VHL manifestations.
- *Hereditary papillary carcinoma:* This autosomal dominant entity manifests with multiple bilateral tumors with papillary histologic appearance; the syndrome is ascribed to mutations in the *MET* proto-oncogene.

The major types of *renal cell carcinomas* are as follows:

- *Clear cell (nonpapillary) carcinoma* is the most common type, accounting for 70% to 80% of primary renal cancers. Tumors are composed of cells with clear to granular cytoplasm. In 98% of these tumors, *whether familial, sporadic, or associated with VHL,* there is a loss of sequences on the short arm of chromosome 3 at a locus that harbors *VHL,* a tumor-suppressor gene.

- *Papillary carcinoma* accounts for 10% to 15% of renal cell cancers, and occurs in both familial and sporadic forms. The gene for the familial form is on chromosome 7; it encompasses the locus for *MET,* a proto-oncogene that exhibits both germ line and somatic mutations. A second gene called *PRCC* (for papillary renal cell carcinoma) on chromosome 1 is implicated in sporadic tumors, largely in children.
- *Chromophobe renal carcinoma* represents 5% of renal cell cancers. These tumors have cells with prominent membranes and pale eosinophilic cytoplasm, usually with a halo around the nucleus; they are thought to derive from intercalated cells of collecting ducts. Although they exhibit multiple chromosome losses and extreme hypodiploidy, they have an excellent prognosis.

Morphology

Clear cell carcinomas are spherical masses, 3 to 15 cm in diameter, composed of bright yellow-gray-white tissue that distorts the renal outline. There are large areas of ischemic opaque, gray-white necrosis, foci of hemorrhagic discoloration, and areas of softening. Tumors may bulge into the calyces and pelvis, and invade the renal vein to grow as a solid column of cells within this vessel.

Clinical Features

Patients may show hematuria (90%), fever, constitutional symptoms, or a paraneoplastic syndrome (polycythemia, hypercalcemia, hypertension, feminization or masculinization, Cushing syndrome, eosinophilia, leukemoid reaction, and amyloidosis). *Prognosis* depends on tumor size and the extent of spread (either local or distant) at diagnosis. Renal cell carcinoma has a tendency to metastasize widely before giving rise to any local symptoms; in 25% of new patients, there is radiographic evidence of metastases at presentation. The time course of disease is variable, but on average 45% survive 5 years and—in the absence of distant metastasis at diagnosis—up to 70% survive 5 years.

Urothelial Carcinomas of Renal Pelvis (p. 1018)

About 5% to 10% of renal tumors occur in the pelvis, where they manifest relatively early either due to hematuria or obstruction. Their histologic type is the same as for urothelial tumors in the bladder, ranging from well-differentiated papillary lesions to anaplastic, invasive carcinomas. They are often multifocal, and in 50% of cases there is a synchronous or metachronous bladder tumor. Despite such observations, evidence suggests they are clonal in origin. Five-year survival rate varies from 70% for low-grade superficial tumors to 10% for high-grade infiltrating tumors.

CHAPTER 21

The Lower Urinary Tract and Male Genital System

The Lower Urinary Tract
(p. 1024)

URETERS (p. 1024)

Congenital Anomalies (p. 1024)

Congenital anomalies are seen in 2% to 3% of autopsies and for the most part are of only incidental interest. However, *ureteropelvic junction narrowing or obstruction* can cause hydronephrosis; such narrowing may be congenital or acquired. In the latter case, obstruction occurs due to disorganized smooth muscle at the junction, excess stromal collagen deposition, or rarely extrinsic compression by aberrant polar renal vessels.

Tumors and Tumor-Like Lesions (p. 1025)

These lesions can be urothelial or connective tissue in origin and have morphologic features analogous to the same tumors in the renal pelvis and bladder.

Obstructive Lesions (p. 1025)

The major causes of ureteral obstruction are listed in Table 21–1.
Sclerosing retroperitoneal fibrosis (p. 1026) is a rare cause of obstruction and hydronephrosis. It is characterized by ill-defined fibrous masses that arise over the sacral promontory, encircle the lower abdominal aorta, and extend laterally

TABLE 21–1 **Major Causes of Ureteral Obstruction**

Intrinsic	

Calculi	Of renal origin, rarely more than 5 mm in diameter
	Larger renal stones cannot enter ureters
	Impact at loci of ureteral narrowing—
	  ureteropelvic junction, where ureters cross iliac
	  vessels, and where they enter bladder—and
	  cause excruciating "renal colic"

Strictures	Congenital or acquired (inflammations)
Tumors	Urothelial carcinomas arising in ureters Rarely, benign tumors or fibroepithelial polyps
Blood clots	Massive hematuria from renal calculi, tumors, or papillary necrosis
Neurogenic	Interruption of the neural pathways to the bladder
Extrinsic	
Pregnancy	Physiologic relaxation of smooth muscle or pressure on ureters at pelvic brim from enlarging fundus

Periureteral
  inflammation
	Salpingitis, diverticulitis, peritonitis, sclerosing
	  retroperitoneal fibrosis

Endometriosis	With pelvic lesions, followed by scarring
Tumors	Cancers of the rectum, bladder, prostate, ovaries, uterus, cervix, lymphomas, sarcomas

through the retroperitoneum to enclose and encroach on the ureters. Microscopically, the fibrosis is marked by a prominent inflammatory infiltrate of lymphocytes, often with germinal centers, plasma cells, and eosinophils. Sometimes, foci of fat necrosis and granulomatous inflammation are also present. In some cases, a specific cause can be identified; however, 70% of cases have no obvious cause and are considered idiopathic (*Ormond's disease*).

URINARY BLADDER (p. 1026)

Congenital Anomalies (p. 1026)

Diverticula (outpouchings of the bladder wall between the criss-crossing muscle bundles) can arise as congenital defects but more commonly are acquired in the setting of persistent urethral obstruction. They become sites of urinary stasis and predispose to infection as well as the formation of bladder calculi. They also predispose to vesicoureteric reflux; rarely, carcinomas can arise within them.

Exstrophy of the bladder is due to a defect in the anterior abdominal wall, where the bladder communicates directly through a large defect with the body surface or lies as an exposed sac. Chronic infections supervene, and there is an increased incidence of carcinoma, mostly adenocarcinoma.

Inflammations (p. 1027)

Acute and Chronic Cystitis (p. 1027)

Urinary tract infections (UTI) are discussed extensively in Chapter 20. The symptoms caused by cystitis include urinary frequency, lower abdominal pain, and pain or burning on urination (dysuria). In addition to the common agents of infectious cystitis (*E. coli, Proteus, Klebsiella,* and *Enterobacter*), several points are worth mentioning:

- *Tuberculous cystitis* can be a sequel to renal tuberculosis.
- *Candida* and *Cryptococcus* can cause cystitis in immunosuppressed patients or those receiving long-term antibiotics.
- *Schistosomiasis* (predisposing to bladder cancer) is common in Middle Eastern countries, notably Egypt.
- Adenovirus, *Chlamydia, Mycoplasma,* and radiation can also cause cystitis.
- *Chemotherapeutic agents* such as cyclophosphamide and busulfan produce hemorrhagic cystitis.
- The cystitis associated with long-term indwelling catheters results in mucosal bulges into the lumen, forming polyps *(polypoid cystitis),* a lesion that should not be mistaken for papillary carcinoma.

Special Forms of Cystitis (p. 1027)

- *Interstitial cystitis* (p. 1027) is a form of chronic cystitis, occurring usually in women, and causing pain and dysuria. In the early (nonclassic) form of interstitial cystitis, submucosal hemorrhages are noted. In the late (classic) phase, there is localized ulceration *(Hunner ulcer)* with inflammation and fibrosis of all bladder wall layers. Although mast cells are characteristic of this disease, there is no uniformity in the literature as to their specificity and diagnostic utility.
- *Malakoplakia* (p. 1027) is a type of chronic bacterial cystitis characterized by soft, yellow, slightly raised mucosal plaques, 3 to 4 cm in diameter. The plaques consist of lymphocytes and foamy histiocytes, the latter containing periodic acid–Schiff (PAS)-positive granules and *targetoid* intracellular structures called *Michaelis-Gutmann bodies.* The intracellular material represents incompletely digested bacteria. Identical lesions occur in the colon, lungs, bones, kidney, prostate, and epididymis and are sometimes associated with immunosuppression. *E. coli* is the most common causal organism.

Metaplastic Lesions (p. 1028)

Cystitis Glandularis and Cystitis Cystica (p. 1028)

In these common lesions nests of transitional epithelium *(Brunn nests)* grow downward into the lamina propria and undergo transformation into cuboidal or columnar epithelium lining *(cystitis glandularis)* or cystic spaces *(cystitis cystica).* Typical goblet cells are sometimes present, and the epithelium resembles intestinal mucosa *(intestinal metaplasia).* Both variants are common microscopic incidental findings in relatively normal bladders but are more prominent in inflamed and chronically irritated bladders. In contrast to earlier reports, lesions exhibiting extensive intestinal metaplasia have been shown not to be associated with an increased risk for the development of adenocarcinoma.

Nephrogenic Metaplasia (Nephrogenic Adenoma) (p. 1028)

Nephrogenic metaplasia represents a urothelial reaction to injury; the overlying urothelium may be focally replaced by papillary structures with cuboidal epithelium. An underlying tubular proliferation in the lamina propria and superficial detrusor muscle results and can histologically mimic a malignant process.

Neoplasms (p. 1028)

About 95% of bladder tumors are of epithelial origin, the remainder being mesenchymal.

Urothelial (Transitional Cell) Tumors (p. 1028)

Urothelial tumors represent about 95% of all bladder tumors and run the gamut from small benign lesions that may never recur, to tumors of low or indeterminate malignant potential, to lesions that invade the bladder wall and frequently metastasize. Many are multifocal at presentation. Although most commonly seen in the bladder, any of the urothelial lesions described here may be seen at any site where there is urothelium, from the renal pelvis to the distal urethra.

There are two distinct precursor lesions to invasive urothelial carcinoma. The more common precursor lesions are noninvasive papillary tumors. These lesions demonstrate a range of atypia, and several grading systems exist to reflect their biologic behavior. The other precursor lesion to invasive urothelial cancer is flat urothelial carcinoma, which is simply referred to as *carcinoma in situ* (CIS). This lesion is by definition high grade and hence not assigned a grade. *Squamous cell carcinomas* represent about 3% to 7% of bladder cancers in the United States, but in countries endemic for urinary schistosomiasis, they occur much more frequently. *Adenocarcinomas* of the bladder are rare and histologically are identical to adenocarcinomas seen in the gastrointestinal tract. Some arise from urachal remnants or in association with intestinal metaplasia (discussed earlier).

In about 50% of patients with invasive bladder cancer, the tumor is already invasive into the bladder wall at the time of presentation; nevertheless, precursor lesions may not be apparent. It is presumed that the precursor tumor was destroyed by the high-grade invasive component, which typically appears as a large ulcerated mass. Although invasion into the lamina propria worsens the prognosis, the major decrease in survival is associated with tumor invading the muscularis propria (detrusor muscle). Once muscularis propria invasion occurs, there is a 50% 5-year mortality rate. The most recent classification of papillary urothelial tumors adopted by the World Health Organization (WHO) recognizes a rare benign papilloma, a group of papillary urothelial neoplasms of low malignant potential, and two grades of carcinoma (low and high grade).

In most analyses, less than 10% of low-grade papillary cancers invade, but as many as 80% of high-grade papillary urothelial carcinomas are invasive. Aggressive tumors may extend not only into the bladder wall, but the more advanced stages invade the adjacent prostate, seminal vesicles, ureters, and retroperitoneum, and some produce fistulous communications to the vagina or rectum. About 40% of these deeply invasive tumors metastasize to regional lymph nodes. Hematogenous dissemination, principally to the liver, lungs, and bone marrow, generally occurs late, and only with highly anaplastic tumors.

Morphology

Papillary lesions appear as red elevated excrescences varying from less than 1 cm to large masses greater than 5 cm in diameter. Multicentric origins often produce separate tumors. As noted, the histologic changes encompass a spectrum from benign papillomas to highly aggressive anaplastic cancers. Overall, the majority of papillary tumors are low grade. Most arise from the lateral or posterior walls at the bladder base.

Carcinoma in Situ

Carcinoma in situ (CIS) is defined by the presence of any cytologically malignant cells present within a flat urothelium. A common feature analogous to high-grade papillary urothelial carcinoma is the lack of cohesiveness that leads to the shedding of malignant cells into the urine (which may be detectable on urine cytology). CIS usually appears as an area of mucosal reddening, granularity, or thickening without producing an evident intraluminal mass. It is commonly multifocal and may involve most of the bladder surface and extend into the ureters and urethra. Although CIS is most often found in bladders harboring well-defined urothelial carcinoma, about 1% to 5% of cases occur in the absence of such tumors. If untreated, 50% to 75% of CIS cases progress to invasive cancer.

Epidemiology and Pathogenesis

The incidence of carcinoma of the bladder resembles that of bronchogenic carcinoma, higher in men than in women, higher in industrialized versus developing nations, and affecting urban dwellers more often than rural dwellers. About 80% of patients are between 50 and 80 years old. Factors implicated in the causation of urothelial carcinoma include:

• Cigarette smoking
• Industrial exposure to arylamines, particularly 2-naphthylamine
• *Schistosoma haematobium* infections in areas where these are endemic (Egypt, Sudan)
• Heavy long-term exposure to cyclophosphamide, an immunosuppressive agent
• Prior exposure of the bladder to radiation

The cytogenetic and molecular alterations are heterogeneous, but most tumors, even when multicentric, are clonal. Particularly common (occurring in 30%–60% of tumors) are chromosome 9 monosomy or 9p/9q deletions. The 9p deletions involve the tumor-suppressor gene *p16* (*MTS1*), which encodes an inhibitor of a cyclin-dependent kinase INK4a. Additionally, many invasive urothelial carcinomas show 17p deletions, including *p53* mutations or deletions, suggesting that *p53* alterations contribute to urothelial carcinoma progression. Interestingly, *13q* deletions involving the *retinoblastoma gene* are also frequently present in invasive tumors.

Clinical Features

Bladder tumors produce painless hematuria, sometimes with frequency and urgency. About 60% of neoplasms, when first discovered, are single, and 70% are localized to the bladder. Patients with urothelial tumors, whatever their grade, have a tendency to develop new tumors after excision, and recurrences may exhibit a higher grade. Recurrent tumors reflect in some cases new tumors and in other instances they share the same clonal abnormalities as the initial tumor and thus represent a true recurrence of the initial lesion from shedding and implantation of the original tumor cells.

The extent of spread at the time of initial diagnosis of invasive urothelial cancer is the most important factor in determining prognosis. Thus, staging, in addition to grade, is critical in the assessment of bladder neoplasms. Prognosis depends on the histologic grade of the tumor and on the stage when it is first diagnosed. Papillomas, papillary urothelial neoplasms of low malignant potential, and low-grade papillary urothelial cancer yield a 98% 10-year survival rate regardless of the number of recurrences; only a few patients (<10%) have progression of their disease to higher grade lesions. In contrast, only about 40% of individuals with an initial high-grade cancer survive 10 years; the tumor progresses in 65%.

Bladder cancer therapy depends on the grade and stage, and whether the lesion is flat or papillary. For small localized papillary tumors that are not high grade, the initial diagnostic transurethral resection is all that is done. Patients are closely followed with periodic cystoscopic and urine cytologic examinations for the rest of their lives for recurrent tumor. After the biopsy site had healed, patients who are at high risk of recurrence or progression (CIS; papillary tumors which are either high grade, multifocal, have a history of rapid recurrence, or associated with lamina propria invasion) receive topical immunotherapy consisting of intravesicle installation of an attenuated strain of tuberculous bacillus called *bacillus Calmette-Guérin (BCG)*. Radical cystectomy is typically performed for: (i) tumor invading the muscularis propria; (ii) CIS or high-grade papillary cancer refractory to BCG; or (iii) CIS extending into the prostatic urethra and extending down the prostatic ducts, where BCG will not come into contact with the neoplastic cells. Advanced bladder cancer is treated by chemotherapy.

URETHRA (p. 1034)

Inflammations and Tumors and Tumor-Like Lesions (p. 1034)

Urethritis can be caused by gonococci and nongonococci. The nongonococcal forms include *E. coli,* other enteric organisms, *Chlamydia,* and *Mycoplasma.* A *caruncle* is a red, polypoid inflammatory tumor, 1 to 1.5 cm in diameter, of the external urethral meatus in women; excision is curative. Malignant tumors are rare, usually squamous cell carcinoma.

⊙ The Male Genital Tract (p. 1034)

PENIS (p. 1034)

Congenital Anomalies (p. 1035)

A variety of abnormalities occur in size and form, including aplasia or hypoplasia; hypertrophy; duplication; and more commonly, *hypospadias, epispadias,* and *phimosis.*

Hypospadias and Epispadias (p. 1035)

Malformations of the urethral groove and canal may produce abnormal urethral orifices involving the *ventral* or *dorsal* aspects of the penis, designated *hypospadias* or *epispadias*, respectively. These can be associated with other urogenital malformations, including *undescended testes,* and can produce lower urinary tract *obstruction* and *sterility.*

Phimosis (p. 1035)

Phimosis designates an abnormally small orifice in the prepuce; it may arise as a primary developmental defect but is more frequently secondary to inflammation. Phimosis predisposes to secondary *infections* and *carcinoma,* owing to chronic accumulation of secretions and other debris under the foreskin. *Paraphimosis* refers to abnormal, painful swelling of the glans penis after forceful retraction of a phimotic prepuce; it may cause urethral obstruction.

Inflammations (p. 1035)

Inflammations characteristically involve both the glans penis and the prepuce.

- *Nonspecific* inflammatory processes and specific *sexually transmitted diseases* (e.g., syphilis, gonorrhea, chancroid, lymphopathia venereum, genital herpes, granuloma inguinale) can occur.
- *Balanoposthitis* refers to nonspecific infection of the glans penis and prepuce, generally associated with *phimosis* or a *redundant prepuce;* there is resultant chronic accumulation of smegma. It can be caused by a wide variety of bacteria, fungi, mycoplasmas, and chlamydiae.

Tumors (p. 1035)

Tumors of the penis include benign tumors, carcinoma in situ, and malignant tumors.

Benign Tumors (p. 1035)

Condyloma Acuminatum (p. 1035)

- Condyloma acuminatum is a benign epithelial proliferation caused by *human papillomavirus* (HPV), especially types 6 and 11.
- Condyloma acuminatum may involve mucocutaneous genital surfaces of either sex; *sexual contact* is the most common mode of transmission. It occurs most frequently after puberty; presence in a prepubertal child should arouse suspicion of sexual abuse.
- Gross morphology is that of a sessile or pedunculated papillary excrescence, often involving the coronal sulcus or inner surface of the prepuce.
- Histologic characteristics include branching stromal papillae covered by hyperplastic stratified squamous epithelium, often associated with prominent hyperkeratosis. Vacuolation of superficial epithelial cells *(koilocytosis)* is common. Maturation of epithelial cells is orderly, in contrast to *carcinoma in situ.*

- Lesions are benign; they may recur owing to persistent HPV infection.

Malignant Tumors (p. 1036)

Carcinoma in Situ (p. 1036)

Variants of *carcinoma in situ* on the penis include Bowen disease and bowenoid papulosis.

Bowen Disease (p. 1036)

Bowen disease can occur in the genital region in both men and women, generally over age 35. In men, the disease presents most commonly as solitary or multiple thickened, gray-white or red shiny plaques over the penile shaft. Microscopically there is marked epithelial atypia with complete loss of normal surface maturation but *no invasion* of underlying stroma. Transition to invasive squamous cell carcinoma occurs in approximately 10% of cases.

Bowenoid Papulosis (p. 1036)

Bowenoid papulosis presents as multiple, pigmented papular lesions on external genitalia; it may grossly mimic condyloma acuminatum. Patients are generally younger than those with Bowen disease. Bowenoid papulosis is histologically indistinguishable from Bowen disease, but evolution into invasive carcinoma is rare.

Squamous Cell Carcinoma (p. 1036)

- Squamous cell carcinoma accounts for 1% of cancers in men in the United States; prevalence is higher in regions where circumcision is not routinely practiced. Most cases occur between ages 40 and 70.
- Potential causes include *carcinogens* within smegma accumulating under the foreskin and HPV types 16 and 18.
- Squamous cell carcinoma typically presents as epithelial thickening on the glans or inner surface of the prepuce, progressing to ulceroinfiltrative or exophytic growth eroding the penile tip, shaft, or both.
- Histologic appearance is identical to squamous cell carcinomas involving other cutaneous sites.
- Clinical course is characterized by slow growth. Metastases typically occur to regional (inguinal and iliac) lymph nodes, and distant metastases are uncommon. The 5-year survival rate is 66% for lesions confined to the penis and 27% with regional node involvement.
- Verrucous carcinoma is an uncommon well-differentiated form of invasive squamous cell carcinoma with low malignant potential.

TESTIS AND EPIDIDYMIS (p. 1037)

Congenital Anomalies (p. 1037)

Anomalies include cryptorchidism, aplasia, fusion (synorchism), and a variety of developmental cysts.

Cryptorchidism (p. 1037)

Cryptorchidism affects 1% of 1-year-old boys and represents *failure of descent;* testes may be found anywhere along the normal path of descent, from the abdominal cavity to the inguinal canal.

- Most cases are idiopathic; other causes include:

  Genetic abnormalities (e.g., trisomy 13)
  Hormonal abnormalities

- Most cases are unilateral; 25% are bilateral.
- Histologic changes may be apparent as early as 2 years of age, including *decreased germ cell development, thickening* and *hyalinization* of seminiferous tubular basement membrane, interstitial *fibrosis,* and relative sparing of Leydig cells. Regressive changes may also occur in the contralateral descended testis.
- Clinical significance is related to high prevalence of *inguinal hernias, sterility,* and an increased incidence of *testicular neoplasms;* surgical correction (orchiopexy) in most studies has been found to decrease the likelihood of sterility if performed early. To what extent the risk of cancer is reduced (which may occur in either testis) following orchiopexy is unclear.

Regressive Changes (p. 1038)

Atrophy (p. 1038) may be secondary to cryptorchidism, vascular disease, inflammatory disorders, hypopituitarism, malnutrition, obstruction of outflow of semen, elevated levels of female sex hormones (endogenous or exogenous), persistently elevated levels of follicle-stimulating hormone, exogenous androgenic steroids, radiation, and chemotherapy.

- Atrophy may also be encountered as a *primary developmental abnormality* in patients with Klinefelter syndrome.
- Morphologic alterations are identical to those seen in cryptorchidism.

Inflammations (p. 1039)

Inflammatory conditions are generally more common in the epididymis than in the testis. However, some infections (notably syphilis) can begin in the testis with secondary involvement of the epididymis. Inflammatory diseases include *nonspecific* epididymitis and orchitis, *granulomatous (autoimmune)* orchitis, and several *specific* infectious diseases (e.g., gonorrhea, mumps, tuberculosis, syphilis).

Nonspecific Epididymitis and Orchitis (p. 1039)

These conditions are often associated with infection of the *urinary tract,* with secondary infection of the epididymis via the vas deferens or lymphatics of the spermatic cord. Causes vary with the age of the patient and include:

- Gram-negative rods associated with genitourinary malformations in pediatric patients
- *Chlamydia trachomatis* and *Neisseria gonorrhoeae* in sexually active men younger than age 35
- *E. coli* and *Pseudomonas* species in older men

Nonspecific interstitial congestion, edema, and neutrophilic infiltrates occur in the early stages, with subsequent tubular involvement; severe cases may progress to generalized suppuration of the entire epididymis. Inflammation can extend to the testis via efferent ductules or local lymphatic channels. Scarring of the testis and epididymis may occur with resultant *infertility*. Leydig cells are less severely affected, and sexual potency generally is not disturbed.

Granulomatous (Autoimmune) Orchitis (p. 1039)

Granulomatous orchitis is an uncommon cause of *unilateral testicular enlargement* in middle-aged men. It has a possible *autoimmune* origin.

- Most cases present with sudden onset of a tender testicular mass, sometimes associated with fever; it may be painless in some patients and difficult to distinguish from testicular neoplasia.
- The lesions closely resemble tubercles but differ in that the granulomatous reaction is present diffusely throughout the testis confined to the seminiferous tubules.

Specific Inflammations (p. 1039)

Gonorrhea (p. 1039)

- Most cases of gonorrhea represent *retrograde extension* of infection from the posterior urethra to the prostate, seminal vesicles, and epididymis.
- The inflammatory pattern is identical to that seen in nonspecific epididymitis and orchitis (discussed previously); infection may extend to the testis and produce suppurative orchitis in untreated cases.

Mumps (p. 1039)

- Mumps orchitis is uncommon in children, but develops in 20% to 30% of postpubertal males infected with mumps.
- Orchitis typically develops about 1 week after onset of parotid inflammation; it can precede parotitis or occur in the absence of parotitis in a minority of patients.
- Orchitis is not usually associated with sterility, owing to unilateral testicular involvement and the patchy, predominantly interstitial pattern of inflammation.

Tuberculosis (p. 1039)

- Inflammation almost always begins in the *epididymis*, with secondary involvement of the testis.
- There is granulomatous inflammation associated with caseous necrosis, identical to active tuberculosis in other sites.

Syphilis (p. 1040)

- Inflammation virtually always begins as *orchitis*, with secondary involvement of the epididymis; it may present as isolated orchitis, without involvement of adnexal structures. Orchitis can occur in both congenital and acquired syphilis.
- Syphilis can produce nodular *gummas* or *diffuse interstitial inflammation*. Interstitial changes include edema, lymphoplasmacytic inflammatory cells, and typical obliterative endarteritis.

Vascular Disturbances (p. 1040)

Torsion (p. 1040)

Vascular disturbances, referred to as *torsion,* occur secondary to twisting of the spermatic cord, with resultant *venous obstruction;* arteries may also be occluded but often remain patent because of thicker walls.

There are two types of testicular torsion:

- *Neonatal torsion* occurs either *in utero* or shortly after birth. It lacks any associated anatomic defect to account for its occurrence.
- *Adult torsion* is typically seen in adolescence presenting as sudden onset of testicular pain. In contrast to neonatal torsion, adult torsion results from a bilateral anatomic defect where the testis has increased mobility, giving rise to what is termed the *bell-clapper abnormality.*

Torsion often occurs without any inciting injury; sudden pain heralding the torsion may even occur during sleep. Torsion is one of the few urologic emergencies. If the testis is explored surgically and manually untwisted within approximately 6 hours after the onset of torsion, there is a good chance that the testis will remain viable. In order to prevent the catastrophic occurrence of subsequent torsion in the contralateral testis, the testis unaffected by torsion is surgically fixed to the scrotum (orchiopexy).

Changes range from congestion and interstitial hemorrhage to extensive hemorrhagic necrosis, depending on the duration and severity of the process.

Testicular Tumors (p. 1040)

A wide range of histologic types of testicular tumors give rise to many different classification schemes. However, tumors are generally divided into two major groups:

- *Germ cell tumors* (accounting for approximately 95% of cases)
- *Nongerminal tumors* (stromal or sex cord tumors)

Most germ cell tumors are aggressive lesions, although the clinical outlook has improved considerably with current therapies.

Germ Cell Tumors (p. 1040)

The incidence of germ cell tumors is approximately 6:100,000 men annually, with a peak incidence between ages 15 and 34. Germ cell tumors account for 10% of cancer deaths in this age group.

Classification and Histogenesis

Diverse classification schemes are based on a wide spectrum of morphologic patterns and variable concepts of histogenesis. Testicular germ cell neoplasms may contain a *single* histologic pattern (40% of cases) or a *mixture* of patterns (60% of cases). Most tumors arise from a focus of intratubular germ cell neoplasia (ITGCN). The neoplastic germ cells may give rise to *seminoma* or transform into a *totipotential* neoplastic cell (embryonal carcinoma) capable of further differentiation. Germ cell neoplasms accordingly may be divided broadly into

TABLE 21–2 **Pathologic Classification of Common Testicular Tumors**

Germ Cell Tumors
Seminoma
Spermatocytic seminoma
Embryonal carcinoma
Yolk sac (endodermal sinus) tumor
Choriocarcinoma
Teratoma

Sex Cord–Stromal Tumors
Leydig cell tumor
Sertoli cell tumor

seminomas and *nonseminomatous tumors.* The *World Health Organization classification* of testicular neoplasms (Table 21–2) is the most widely used classification scheme.

Pathogenesis

Several risk factors are important:

- *Cryptorchidism* is associated with 10% of testicular tumors.
- *Genetic factors* may be significant. There is a higher risk of testicular neoplasia among siblings of patients with testicular tumors; some familial clustering has been reported. Significant racial differences also exist (e.g., rare in African blacks).
- *Testicular dysgenesis* includes testicular feminization and Klinefelter syndrome.
- Cytogenetic abnormalities involving *chromosome 12* are common; *i(12p)* is present in 90% of testicular germ cell tumors. In the remaining cases, extra genetic material derived from 12p is found in other chromosomes, thus strongly implicating genes located on the short arm of chromosome 12.

Seminoma (p. 1041)

Seminoma accounts for 50% of all testicular germ cell tumors; it is the most likely germ cell neoplasm to present with a single histologic pattern.

- Peak incidence is in the 30s.
- Variants include:

Classic seminoma (95% of seminomas)
Spermatocytic seminoma (5%; discussed later)

- Histologically identical tumors may occur in the ovary *(dysgerminomas)* and central nervous system *(germinomas).*

Seminoma presents as a homogeneous, lobulated, gray-white mass, generally devoid of hemorrhage or necrosis; the tunica albuginea usually remains intact. *Microscopically,* the mass is composed of large polyhedral *seminoma cells* containing abundant clear cytoplasm, large nuclei, and prominent nucleoli; cytoplasmic glycogen is typically present. A fibrous stroma of variable density divides the neoplastic cells into irregular *lobules;* an accompanying *lymphocytic infiltrate* (usually T cell) is present in most cases; granulomas may also be present. Neoplastic giant cells and syncytial cells resembling placental syncytiotrophoblasts may be seen in some cases; human chorionic gonadotropin (hCG) is present in such cells and presumably accounts for the minimally elevated serum hCG levels demonstrable in some patients with pure seminoma. The tumor cells contain placental alkaline phosphatase. Classic seminoma cells do not contain α-fetoprotein (AFP).

Spermatocytic Seminoma (p. 1042)

Spermatocytic seminomas are uncommon neoplasms, occurring in *patients older* than those with classic seminoma.

- These are *indolent* growths, with virtually no tendency to metastasize.
- Lesions tend to be larger than those of classic seminoma. Lesions are composed of a *mixed* population of cells, including smaller (6–8 mm) cells resembling secondary spermatocytes (hence the *spermatocytic* designation), medium-sized (15–18 mm) cells, and scattered giant cells.
- In contrast to classic seminomas, spermatocytic seminomas arise only in the testes and are not associated with other germ cell tumors.

Embryonal Carcinoma (p. 1043)

Embryonal carcinoma has a peak incidence between 20 and 30 years; these cancers are more *aggressive* than seminoma, although developments in chemotherapy have improved the prognosis considerably.

- Lesions may be small and confined to the testis; most examples are poorly demarcated, gray-white masses punctuated by foci of hemorrhage, necrosis, or both. They may extend through the tunica albuginea into the epididymis or spermatic cord.
- Microscopically, they are composed of primitive epithelial cells with indistinct cell borders, forming irregular sheets, tubules, alveoli, and papillary structures. Mitotic figures and neoplastic giant cells are common; syncytial cells positive for hCG and AFP may be detected.

Yolk Sac Tumor (p. 1043)

Yolk sac tumor is the most common testicular neoplasm in infants and young children; synonyms include *infantile embryonal carcinoma* and *endodermal sinus tumor.* Prognosis in children before 3 years is good. Most adult cases occur as a component of a *mixed* germ cell neoplasm.

- Pure forms present as infiltrative, homogeneous, yellow-white mucinous lesions.
- Microscopically, they are composed of cuboidal neoplastic cells arrayed in a lacelike (reticular) network; solid areas and papillae may also be seen. Structures resembling primitive glomeruli *(Schiller-Duval bodies)* are seen in 50% of cases. Eosinophilic, hyaline globules containing immunoreactive *AFP* and *α_1-antitrypsin* are present within and around the neoplastic cells.

Choriocarcinoma (p. 1043)

Choriocarcinoma is a highly malignant neoplasm composed of both cytotrophoblastic and syncytiotrophoblastic elements.

- Similar neoplasms may occur in the ovary, placenta, or ectopic pluripotential germ cell rests in other sites (e.g., mediastinum, abdomen). This neoplasm is rare in pure form within the testis; it is more often encountered as a component of a *mixed germ cell neoplasm*.

- The primary testicular neoplasm is often quite small, even in the presence of widespread systemic metastases. The gross appearance ranges from a bulky, hemorrhagic mass to an inconspicuous lesion replaced by a fibrous scar.
- Histologically, it is composed of polygonal, comparatively uniform cytotrophoblastic cells growing in sheets and cords, admixed with multinucleated syncytiotrophoblastic cells. hCG is readily demonstrable within the cytoplasm of the syncytiotrophoblastic elements.

Teratoma (p.1044)

Teratoma is a neoplasm exhibiting evidence of simultaneous differentiation along endodermal, mesodermal, and ectodermal lines. They can occur at any age.

- Teratomas are composed of a haphazard array of *differentiated* mesodermal (e.g., muscle, cartilage, adipose tissue), ectodermal (e.g., neural tissue, skin), and endodermal (e.g., gut, bronchial epithelium) elements.
- In the child, differentiated mature teratomas may be expected to behave as benign tumors, and almost all these patients have a good prognosis.
- In the postpubertal male, all teratomas are regarded as malignant and capable of metastatic behavior regardless of whether the elements are mature or immature. Consequently, it is not critical to note immaturity in a testicular teratoma in a postpubertal male.
- *Teratoma with malignant transformation* is characterized by non–germ cell malignancy (i.e., carcinoma, sarcoma, neuroblastoma, Wilms tumor) developing within a teratoma. When the non–germ cell component spreads outside the testis it does not respond to chemotherapy and the only hope for cure resides in the local resectability of the tumor.

Mixed Tumors (p. 1045)

Mixed tumors account in aggregate for approximately 50% of germ cell neoplasms.

- Histologic patterns are variable; the most common includes a mixture of teratoma, embryonal carcinoma, yolk sac tumor, and hCG-containing giant cells.
- *Teratocarcinoma* designates neoplasms containing both teratoma and embryonal carcinoma. Metastases from such lesions may contain virtually any germ cell element, including elements not present in the primary tumor.

Clinical Features of Germ Cell Neoplasms

- Most cases present with *painless enlargement of the testis;* neoplasia should be considered in the differential diagnosis of *all* testicular masses, even those that are painful. Clinical evaluation, however, does not reliably distinguish between the various types of germ cell tumors.
- Biopsy of a testicular neoplasm is associated with a risk of tumor spillage which would necessitate excision of the scrotal skin in addition to orchiectomy. Consequently, the standard management of a solid testicular mass is radical orchiectomy based on the presumption of malignancy.
- *Lymphatic* metastases most commonly go to *retroperitoneal para-aortic* nodes but may occur in more distant sites (e.g., mediastinal and supraclavicular nodes); the *lungs* are the most common site for *hematogenous* metastases, followed by

liver, brain, and bone. The histologic appearance of metastases may be identical to that of the primary tumor or may contain other germ cell elements (e.g., teratomatous metastases in a patient with a primary embryonal carcinoma).

- The biologic behavior of nonseminomatous germ cell tumors (NSGCTs) is, in general, more aggressive than that of seminomas. Roughly 70% of seminomas present with localized (clinical stage I) disease; in contrast, 60% of NSGCTs present with advanced (stage II or III) disease. Extensive metastases may be present even with small primary lesions, particularly in the case of choriocarcinoma.
- Clinical staging is as follows:

  Stage I: Tumor confined to the testis
  Stage II: Metastases limited to retroperitoneal nodes below the diaphragm
  Stage III: Metastases outside the retroperitoneal nodes or above the diaphragm

- Several peptides may be produced by germ cell neoplasms and can be detected in body fluids by sensitive assays; AFP (α-fetoprotein) and hCG (human chorionic gonadotropin) are the most commonly assayed. Lactate dehydrogenase, although not specific for testicular tumors, is produced by tumor cells, and the degree of elevation provides a rough measure of tumor burden. Serum markers are of value to (i) evaluate testicular masses; (ii) *stage* germ cell tumors; (iii) assess tumor burden; and (iv) monitor the response of a germ cell tumor to therapy.
- Seminoma, which is extremely radiosensitive and tends to remain localized for long periods, has the best prognosis. More than 95% of patients with stage I and II disease can be cured. Among nonseminomatous tumors, the histologic subtype does not influence the prognosis significantly, and hence these are treated as a group. Although they do not share the excellent prognosis of seminoma, approximately 90% of patients with nonseminomatous tumors can achieve complete remission with aggressive chemotherapy, and most can be cured. Pure choriocarcinoma has a dismal prognosis. However, when it is a minor component of a mixed germ cell tumor, the prognosis is not so adversely affected. With all testicular tumors, distant metastases, if present, usually occur within the first 2 years after treatment.

Tumors of Sex Cord–Gonadal Stroma (p. 1046)

Classification of sex cord tumors is based on differentiation into Leydig or Sertoli cells.

Leydig (Interstitial) Cell Tumors (p. 1046)

These tumors are relatively uncommon neoplasms, accounting for 2% of all testicular tumors; most occur between the ages 20 to 60 years, but they may be found at any age.

- Tumors may elaborate androgens or mixtures of androgens and other steroids (estrogens, corticosteroids).
- Clinical manifestations include a *testicular mass* and changes referable to *hormonal abnormalities* (e.g., gynecomastia, sexual precocity in prepubertal boys).
- Tumors are grossly circumscribed nodules with a homogeneous, golden brown cut surface. Microscopically, they are composed of polygonal cells with abundant granular,

eosinophilic cytoplasm and indistinct cell borders. Lipochrome pigment, lipid droplets, and eosinophilic Reinke crystalloids are commonly present. Ten percent of tumors invade or metastasize.

Sertoli Cell Tumors (Androblastoma) (p. 1046)

These tumors are uncommon neoplasms, composed of Sertoli cells.

- Tumors may elaborate androgens or estrogens but rarely in sufficient quantity to produce precocious masculinization or feminization.
- Tumors present as homogeneous gray-white to yellow masses of variable size. The microscopic picture is dominated by cells with tall, columnar cytoplasm, often forming cords reminiscent of immature seminiferous tubules. Most are benign; 10% demonstrate invasion or metastases.

Testicular Lymphomas (p. 1046)

Testicular lymphomas account for 5% of all testicular neoplasms; they are the most common testicular neoplasm in patients older than age 60. Most are diffuse, large cell, non-Hodgkin lymphomas and disseminate widely; the prognosis is accordingly poor.

Miscellaneous Lesions of the Tunica Vaginalis (p. 1047)

- *Hydrocele:* Accumulation of serous fluid within the tunica vaginalis, either secondary to generalized edema or due to incomplete closure of the processus vaginalis. A hydrocele may become secondarily infected.
- *Hematocele:* Accumulation of blood within the tunica vaginalis secondary to trauma, torsion, or hemorrhage; a generalized bleeding diathesis; or, rarely, invasion of the tunica by neoplasms.
- *Chylocele:* Accumulation of lymphatic fluid within the tunica vaginalis, secondary to lymphatic obstruction (e.g., in patients with elephantiasis).
- *Spermatocele:* Local accumulation of semen in the spermatic cord, generally within a dilated duct in the head of the epididymis.
- *Varicocele:* Local accumulation of blood within a dilated vein in the spermatic cord.

PROSTATE (p. 1047)

Major disorders of the prostate include inflammations (prostatitis), nodular hyperplasia, and carcinoma.

Inflammations (p. 1047)

Conditions include acute bacterial prostatitis, chronic bacterial prostatitis, chronic abacterial prostatitis, and granulomatous prostatitis.

Acute Bacterial Prostatitis (p. 1048)

- Most cases are caused by organisms associated with urinary tract infections (e.g., *E. coli* and other gram-negative rods), *Enterococcus,* or *Staphylococcus aureus.*

- Organisms reach the prostate via *direct extension* from the urethra or urinary bladder or by *lymphatic* or *hematogenous seeding* from more distant sites. This may follow *catheterization or surgical manipulation* of the urethra or prostate.
- Acute bacterial prostatitis presents with fever, chills, dysuria, and a boggy, markedly tender prostate. Diagnosis is based on clinical features and urine culture.

Chronic Bacterial Prostatitis (p. 1048)

- Chronic bacterial prostatitis may be asymptomatic or associated with low back pain, suprapubic and perineal discomfort, and dysuria; it is frequently associated with a history of *recurrent urinary tract infections* caused by the same organism.
- *Diagnosis* is established by demonstration of leukocytes in expressed prostatic secretions and positive bacterial cultures in prostatic secretions and urine; most cases are caused by organisms similar to those responsible for acute prostatitis.
- Most cases appear *insidiously,* without a history of acute prostatitis.

Chronic Abacterial Prostatitis (p. 1048)

- This is the most common form of prostatitis, typically affecting sexually active men.
- Manifestations are similar to those of chronic bacterial prostatitis but *without* a history of recurrent urinary tract infections.
- Expressed prostatic secretions contain more than 10 leukocytes per high-power field, but cultures are uniformly *negative.*

Granulomatous Prostatitis (p. 1048)

Granulomatous prostatitis can have a specific etiology when an infectious agent can be identified. In the United States, the most common cause is related to bladder installation of bacillus Calmette-Guérin (BCG) for treatment of superficial bladder cancer. BCG is an attenuated tuberculous strain that yields a histologic picture in the prostate indistinguishable from that seen with systemic tuberculosis. However, in this setting, the finding of prostatic granulomas is of no clinical significance and requires no treatment.

Nonspecific granulomatous prostatitis is relatively common and represents a reaction to secretions from ruptured prostatic ducts and acini.

Morphology

Acute prostatitis cases are associated with variable degrees of edema, congestion, and neutrophilic infiltration of parenchyma; neutrophils may also be present in glandular lumens. Severe cases are associated with a variable degree of parenchymal necrosis and abscess formation.

The histologic diagnosis of "chronic prostatitis," both bacterial and abacterial, should be restricted to those cases of inflammatory reaction in the prostate characterized by the aggregates of numerous lymphocytes, plasma cells, and macrophages (as well as neutrophils) only in the setting of clinical signs and symptoms of chronic prostatitis. Isolated lymphoid aggregates may be encountered in otherwise normal glands in elderly patients.

Benign Enlargement (p. 1048)

Nodular Hyperplasia (Benign Prostatic Hyperplasia) (p. 1048)

Nodular hyperplasia is present in approximately 20% of men at age 40 years, increasing to 70% by age 60 years and to 90% by age 70 years. Only 50% of those who have microscopic evidence of nodular hyperplasia have clinically detectable enlargement of the prostate; of these individuals, only 50% develop clinical symptoms. Nodular hyperplasia of prostate is a problem of enormous magnitude with approximately 30% of white American males over 50 years of age having moderate to severe symptoms. *No relationship* has been established between benign prostatic hyperplasia (BHP) of the prostate and prostatic carcinoma.

Pathogenesis

Dihydrotestosterone (DHT), a metabolite of testosterone, is the ultimate mediator of prostatic growth. It is synthesized in the prostate from circulating testosterone by the action of the enzyme 5α-reductase, type 2. While DHT appears to be the major trophic factor mediating prostatic hyperplasia, estrogens also participate, and stromal-epithelial interactions mediated by peptide growth factors also contribute. Clinical symptoms of lower urinary tract obstruction are due to smooth muscle-mediated contraction of the prostate. The tension of prostate smooth muscle is mediated by the α_1-adrenoreceptor localized to the prostatic stroma.

Morphology

- *Grossly,* the gland is enlarged by nodules of variable size arising in the transition zone (periurethral region). Nodules arising lateral to the urethra may compress the urethral lumen to a slitlike orifice; those arising more medially may project directly into the floor of the proximal urethra, contributing to obstruction. In other cases, nodules project into the lumen of the bladder and produce a ball-valve obstruction at the mouth of the urethra. Cut surface demonstrates well-demarcated nodules involving the inner portion of the prostate.
- *Microscopically,* nodules are composed of variable mixtures of proliferating *glands* and *fibromuscular stroma;* cystic dilation of glandular elements is common and contributes to the nodularity. Although the epithelium is characteristically heaped into numerous papillary buds and infoldings, this finding is not specific for BPH. Glands are lined by two layers of cells: a basal layer of low cuboidal epithelium covered by a layer of columnar secretory cells. Other changes include areas of *squamous metaplasia* and *infarcts.*

Clinical Features

Manifestations related to *urinary tract obstruction* include:

- Urinary frequency, nocturia, and difficulty starting and stopping the stream of urine

- Acute urinary retention
- Chronic urinary stasis with resultant bacterial overgrowth and urinary tract infection
- Chronic obstruction resulting in a variety of secondary structural alterations, including:

  Hypertrophy of the urinary bladder
  Urinary bladder diverticula
  Hydronephrosis

Tumors (p. 1050)

Adenocarcinoma (p. 1050)

Prostatic carcinoma is the *most common* form of cancer in men; currently, it is the second leading cause of cancer death among men. Approximately 180,000 new cases are detected annually. Postmortem and surgical biopsy material indicates an even larger number of *incidental* prostatic carcinomas.

- Prostatic carcinoma occurs predominantly in men over age 50.
- The disease is rare in Asians; it is more common in blacks than in whites.
- The *etiology* remains unknown; clinical and epidemiologic data suggest that advancing age, race, *hormonal influences,* genetic factors, and environmental factors (e.g., diet) all contribute.

  A role for *hormonal influences,* in particular, is suggested by the retardation of the growth of some prostatic carcinomas by antiandrogen therapy.

  In 10% of white American men, prostate cancer occurs in a familial form; in a third of these cases, a cancer susceptibility gene has been mapped to 1q24-25.

  Disease incidence increases when individuals migrate from a low-incidence area to a high-incidence locale; the observation suggests environmental influences. Several candidate factors have been suggested (e.g., dietary fat consumption) but no causality has been demonstrated. Other dietary products may prevent, inhibit, or delay progression of prostate cancer; these include lycopenes (found in tomatoes), vitamin A, vitamin E, selenium, and soy products.

  Morphology

Most cases (70%) arise in the peripheral zone of the prostate, particularly in the *posterior* region, facilitating palpation during rectal examination. Primary lesions characteristically are grossly poorly demarcated, firm, and yellow. Locally advanced cases may infiltrate the seminal vesicles and urinary bladder; invasion of the rectum is uncommon.

- *Lymphatic metastases* occur initially in obturator nodes, followed by spread to perivesical, hypogastric, iliac, presacral, and para-aortic nodes. *Hematogenous dissemination* occurs primarily to bone, most often in the form of *osteoblastic* metastases.
- Microscopically the vast majority of prostatic carcinomas are *adenocarcinomas,* ranging from well-differentiated lesions to poorly differentiated neoplastic cells forming sheets and cords. Well-differentiated lesions may be difficult to distinguish from benign mimickers of prostate cancer.

- In general the diagnosis is made based on a constellation of architectural, cytologic, and ancillary findings. In contrast to nodular hyperplasia, cancerous glands are smaller and more *closely spaced* and are lined by a *single layer* of epithelial cells.
- Invasion of perineural spaces aids in the diagnosis of malignancy.
- High-grade prostatic intraepithelial neoplasia (PIN) consists of preexisting benign glands with an intra-acinar proliferation of cells that demonstrate malignant nuclear features. High-grade PIN represents the precursor of most invasive carcinomas.

Grading and Staging

The *Gleason system* stratifies prostate cancers into five patterns on the basis of glandular patterns, without regard to cytologic features.

- Pattern 1 represents the most well differentiated tumors, in which the neoplastic glands are uniform and round in appearance and are packed into well-circumscribed nodules.
- By contrast, pattern 5 tumors show no glandular differentiation, and the tumor cells infiltrate the stroma in the form of cords, sheets, and nests. The other patterns fall in between.
- Most tumors contain more than one pattern; the pathologist assigns a dominant pattern and then the second most prevalent pattern. The primary and secondary patterns are added to obtain a combined Gleason score. Tumors with only one pattern are treated as if their primary and secondary patterns are the same, and, hence, the number is doubled. Thus, under this schema the most well-differentiated tumors have a Gleason score of 2 (1 + 1) and the least-differentiated tumors merit a score of 10 (5 + 5). Gleason scores are often combined into groups with similar biologic behavior: 2 to 4 representing well-differentiated cancer; 5 to 6 intermediate-grade cancer; 7 moderate to poorly differentiated cancer; and 8 to 10 high-grade cancer.
- Staging of prostatic cancer is also important in the selection of the appropriate form of therapy and in establishing a prognosis. The most common staging system is the TNM system.

  Stage T1 refers to cancer found incidentally either on transurethral resection (TURP) done for BPH symptoms (T1a and T1b depending on the extent and grade) or on needle biopsy typically performed for elevated serum PSA levels (stage T1c).

  Stage T2 is organ-confined cancer.

  Stage T3a and *T3b* tumors show extraprostatic extension, with and without seminal vesicle invasion, respectively.

  Stage T4 reflects direct invasion of contiguous organs. Any spread of tumor to the lymph nodes regardless of extent is eventually associated with a fatal outcome, such that the staging system merely records the presence or absence of this finding (N0/N1).

Clinical Features

In cases diagnosed in *asymptomatic* patients (stage T1), the prognosis is generally favorable for stage T1a and more ominous for T1b. Patients with clinically localized disease do not have urinary symptoms, and the lesion is discovered by the finding of a suspicious nodule on rectal examination or elevated serum prostate-specific antigen level (discussed later).

- Patients with clinically advanced prostatic cancer may present with urinary symptoms, such as difficulty in starting or stopping the stream, dysuria, frequency, or hematuria. Some patients come to attention because of back pain caused by vertebral metastases. *The finding of osteoblastic metastases in bone is virtually diagnostic of prostate cancer in men.* The outlook for these patients is universally fatal.

- Digital rectal examination may detect some early prostatic carcinomas because of their posterior location, although the test suffers from both low sensitivity and specificity. While there are characteristic findings of prostate cancer on prostatic imaging studies, the poor sensitivity and specificity of these tests also limit their diagnostic utility. A transrectal *biopsy is required to confirm the diagnosis.* Because microscopic metastases are usually missed by radiologic studies, most centers use pelvic lymphadenectomy as a staging procedure. Osseous metastases may be detected by skeletal surveys or the much more sensitive radionuclide bone scanning.

- The treatment and prognosis of prostatic carcinoma are influenced primarily by the stage of the disease. Localized (clinical stage T1 or T2) disease is treated primarily with *surgery or radiotherapy* with a 15-year survival rate of 90%.

- Many prostate cancers have a relatively indolent course; thus, it may take 10 years to see benefit from surgery or radiotherapy, and watchful waiting is an appropriate treatment for many older men (or those with significant comorbidity). External beam radiotherapy is also used to treat prostate cancer that is too locally advanced to be cured by surgery. *Hormonal* treatment includes orchiectomy or the administration of synthetic analogues of luteinizing hormone–releasing hormone; it is used primarily in patients with advanced disease or combined with radiotheraphy for local disease.

Prostate-Specific Antigen (p. 1054). Prostate-specific antigen (PSA) is used in the diagnosis and management of prostate cancer. PSA is a product of prostatic epithelium and is normally secreted in the semen. Serum levels of PSA are elevated to a lesser extent in benign nodular hyperplasia than prostate cancer, although there is considerable overlap. In most laboratories, a serum level of 4 ng/mL is reported on laboratory reports as a cutoff point between normal and abnormal. However, this simplified approach to serum PSA tests is dangerous and has lead to the delay in diagnosis of many prostate cancers. Several refinements in the estimation and interpretation of PSA values have been proposed (see below).

- *PSA is organ-specific, yet not cancer-specific.* Other factors such as BPH, prostatitis, infarct, and instrumentation of the prostate can increase serum PSA levels. Furthermore, 20% to 40% of patients with organ-confined prostate cancer have a PSA value of 4.0 ng/mL or less.

- *PSA density (PSAD)* factors out the contribution of benign prostatic tissue to serum PSA levels. Serum PSAD reflects the serum PSA level divided by the size of the prostate as estimated by radiological studies, resulting in PSA levels produced per gram of prostate tissue.

- *Age-specific PSA upper reference ranges* are based on measurements of serum PSA levels in a large group of men of varying ages without prostate cancer. As men age, their prostates tend to enlarge with BPH, with corresponding higher serum PSA levels. A serum PSA value of 3.5 (although within normal reference intervals) is a worrisome finding in a man in his 40s, and warrants additional evaluation.
- *PSA velocity (rate of change of PSA)* reflects the finding that men with prostate cancer demonstrate an increased rate of rise in PSA as compared to men who do not have prostate cancer. For this test to be valid, multiple measurements need to be made over a period of 1 to 2 years.
- *Percentage of free PSA* (free PSA/total PSA × 100) measures the fraction of serum PSA bound to α_1-antichymotrypsin and a minor free fraction. Percentage of free PSA is lower in men with prostate cancer than in men with benign prostatic diseases.
- Monitoring PSA levels is useful in assessing response to therapy or progression of disease.

CHAPTER 22

The Female Genital Tract

INFECTIONS OF THE FEMALE GENITAL TRACT
(p. 1062)

Infections Involving the Lower and Upper Genital Tract (p. 1064)

Pelvic Inflammatory Disease (p. 1064)

A variety of organisms can infect the lower and upper genital tract. *Pelvic inflammatory disease* (PID) refers to an ascending infection that begins in the vulva or vaginal glands but then spreads upward through the entire genital tract, potentially involving all structures. There are at least three known causes of PID:

- The *gonococcus* (most common), as part of a gonorrheal infection
- Postabortal and postpartum infection, usually caused by staphylococci, streptococci, coliform bacteria, or *Clostridium perfringens*
- Chlamydial infection

Gonococcal inflammation begins in Bartholin glands, in Skene ducts and periurethral glands, or occasionally in the endocervical glands. The organisms then spread upward over the mucosal surfaces, eventually involving fallopian tubes and tubo-ovarian regions. Gonococcal disease is characterized by an acute suppurative reaction, largely confined to the superficial mucosa and underlying submucosa.

Acute suppurative salpingitis is the most significant pathologic lesion. This can cause salpingo-oophoritis, pyosalpinx (pus in the distended tubes), and tubo-ovarian abscesses. Untreated or poorly treated infection results in chronic salpingitis, with tubo-ovarian adhesions and fibrosis of the fallopian tube, occlusion of its lumen, and resultant infertility.

In *postabortal* and *postpartum PID*, infection spreads through the uterine wall to involve the serosa and peritoneum.

Bacteremia is a frequent complication of this type of PID. Other PID complications include:

- Peritonitis
- Intestinal obstruction
- Infertility
- Ectopic tubal pregnancy

VULVA (p. 1065)

Bartholin Cysts (p. 1065)

Bartholin cysts result from inflammatory occlusion of the main ducts of the Bartholin vulvovaginal glands. Gonorrheal and other infections can cause inflammatory obstruction, which also occasionally produces abscesses that must be drained. Uninflamed cysts are lined by transitional or flattened epithelium.

Vulvodynia (p. 1065)

Vulvodynia (formerly *vestibular adenitis*) is characterized by vulvar pain, erythema. Some cases are associated with erythema and inflammation. The cause is unknown and therapy is often surgical.

Non-Neoplastic Epithelial Disorders (p. 1065)

These benign mucosal alterations of the vulva should be differentiated from more ominous dysplasias and cancer (p. 1042). There are two main varieties:

Lichen sclerosus (p. 1066) consists of yellowish blue papules or macules that eventually coalesce into thin, gray, parchment-like areas. Microscopically, there is epithelial thinning and subepithelial fibrosis (and occasionally marked hyperkeratosis) and mononuclear perivascular reaction. The cause is unknown.

Lichen simplex chronicus (p. 1066) is the physiologic outcome to rubbing the vulvar mucosa in response to pruritus and is characterized by thickened epithelium *(acanthosis)*, hyperkeratosis, and leukocytic dermal inflammation. These lesions appear as white plaques, traditionally termed *leukoplakia*. There are numerous underlying causes, including irritant exposure, dermatitis, and preinvasive or invasive neoplasia. Biopsy is indicated for all such lesions. Neither lichen sclerosus nor simplex chronicus is classified as premalignant per se but cytogenetic abnormalties, including *p53* mutations, may precede the onset of atypia in these lesions. Thus, they are considered "risk factors" for vulvar neoplasia.

Neoplasms (p. 1066)

Benign Tumors (p. 1067)

Papillary Hidradenoma (p. 1067)

This benign tumor arises from modified apocrine sweat glands. It presents as a sharply circumscribed nodule consisting of tubular ducts lined by nonciliated columnar cells atop a layer of flattened myoepithelial cells.

Condyloma Acuminatum (p. 1067)

Condyloma acuminatum is a wartlike, verrucous lesion caused by sexually transmitted human papillomavirus (HPV) types 6 or 11; it occurs on the vulva, perineum, vagina, and (rarely) cervix. Histologically, the lesions consist of a sessile or branching epithelial proliferation of stratified squamous epithelial cells, some of which may display perinuclear cytoplasmic clearing with nuclear atypia *(koilocytotic atypia)*. However, koilocytotic atypia is not a prerequisite for the diagnosis. Flat or macular condylomas associated with other HPV types are also benign.

Premalignant and Malignant Neoplasms (p. 1067)

Carcinoma and Vulvar Intraepithelial Neoplasia (p. 1067)

Vulvar intraepithelial neoplasia (VIN) is a premalignant, intramucosal squamous neoplasm that frequently precedes invasive carcinoma. Classic VINs are caused by sexually transmitted HPV 16, are multicentric, demonstrate marked nuclear atypia, and are synonymous with carcinoma in situ *(Bowen disease)*. Cancer risk increases with age, and spontaneous regression is more common in younger patients. These lesions typically occur in the fourth to fifth decades; a proportion progress to invasive carcinomas in the fifth to seventh decades.

Differentiated (simplex) VINs are usually HPV-negative and associate with lichen sclerosus or lichen simplex chronicus. These precancers usually arise after menopause, are well differentiated, exhibit primarily basal atypia and abnormal keratinization, and may progress to well-differentiated (keratinizing) carcinomas in the sixth to eighth decades.

Prognosis (and staging) of vulvar carcinomas depends on size, depth of invasion, and ultimately, lymph node status. Metastasis to regional lymph nodes indicates a poor prognosis. Rare variants (e.g., *verrucous carcinoma*) behave in a locally aggressive fashion but usually do not metastasize.

Extramammary Paget Disease (p. 1068)

Extramammary Paget disease appears as a red, crusted, sharply demarcated, maplike area, mostly on the labia majora. Histologically there are large, anaplastic, sometimes vacuolated tumor cells lying singly or in small clusters within the epidermis and its appendages. The tumor cells are mucin-positive. Most lesions are confined to the epidermis.

- In contrast to Paget disease of the nipple (Chapter 23), in which 100% of cases have an underlying ductal breast carcinoma, an underlying vulvar sweat gland adenocarcinoma is uncommon in vulvar Paget disease. Rarely, invasion of the epithelium by other carcinomas (such as urothelial cancers) may mimic Paget disease.
- Other vulvar carcinomas include basal cell carcinoma, adenocarcinoma arising in Bartholin glands or sweat glands, and malignant melanoma; the latter has a poor prognosis.

VAGINA (p. 1070)

Premalignant and Malignant Neoplasms
(p. 1071)

Vaginal Intraepithelial Neoplasia and Squamous Cell Carcinoma (p. 1071)

Primary vaginal carcinomas are rare. The most common type is *squamous cell carcinoma,* accounting for 95% of cases. The peak incidence is between 60 and 70 years of age; 1% to 2% of women with cervical carcinoma develop vaginal carcinoma. Grossly, the lesions are either plaquelike or occasionally fungating. They invade the cervix and perivaginal structures, such as the urethra, urinary bladder, and rectum.

Adenocarcinoma (p. 1071)

Vaginal adenocarcinomas are rare but epidemiologically important because of the increased frequency of clear cell adenocarcinoma in young women whose mothers were treated with diethylstilbestrol (DES) during pregnancy (for a threatened abortion). Only 0.14% of DES-exposed young women developed adenocarcinoma during the years following maximum use of the drug. These tumors are composed of glands lined by vacuolated, glycogen-containing clear cells. Currently, clear cell carcinoma is extremely uncommon.

Embryonal Rhabdomyosarcoma (p. 1071)

Embryonal rhabdomyosarcoma is an uncommon, highly malignant vaginal tumor in infants and children consisting of embryonal rhabdomyoblasts. The tumors are polypoid, bulky masses with grapelike clusters that may protrude from the vagina. The tumor cells are small, have oval nuclei, and have small protrusions of cytoplasm from one end (*tennis-racket* cells).

CERVIX (p. 1072)

Inflammations (p. 1072)

Acute and Chronic Cervicitis (p. 1072)

Cervicitis may be caused either by specific infections, such as gonococci, chlamydia, *Trichomonas vaginalis, Candida,* and *Mycoplasma,* or by endogenous vaginal aerobes and anaerobes, including streptococci, enterococci, *Escherichia coli,* and staphylococci (nonspecific cervicitis).

- *Acute cervicitis* is most commonly encountered postpartum and is characterized by acute infiltration of neutrophils beneath the lining mucosa.
- *Chronic cervicitis* is far more common and reflects the changes that occur in the cervix over reproductive life in response to a milieu produced by bacterial growth and alterations in pH. Features include squamous metaplasia, chronic inflammation, and columnar cell proliferation (microglandular change). Metaplasia leads to progressive obliteration of the endocervical papillae and obstruction of gland crypts to form nabothian cysts.

- Chronic cervicitis is benign and common. However, if the epithelial response to inflammation is exuberant *(reactive atypia)*, it may be confused with cervical intraepithelial neoplasia (CIN).

Tumors

Endocervical Polyps (p. 1073)

Endocervical polyps are benign tumors made up of connective tissue stroma harboring dilated glands and covered by endocervical epithelium. Although rare, the most important tumor that must be excluded is a well-differentiated mixed epithelial mesenchymal tumor (adenosarcoma).

Intraepithelial and Invasive Squamous Neoplasia (p. 1073)

Cervical intraepithelial neoplasia (CIN) is usually caused by cancer-related (high-risk) human papillomaviruses and peaks in incidence in the second to third decades. CIN is essentially a sexually transmitted disease, linked to HPV via the classic risk factors of early age of intercourse, greater number of sexual partners, and sexual partners who have had multiple prior partners.

Most HPVs have been isolated from cervical cancers, including types 16, 18, 31, 33, 35, 39, 45, 51, 52, 53, 56, 58, 59, and others. These "high-risk" HPVs are found in over 70% of CIN lesions (including milder forms such as CIN I; see below) and in over 95% of cervical cancers. Each year over 1 million women develop CIN, but less than 12,000 develop cancer, a testimony to the effective removal of the virus by the host immune system and Papanicolaou smear screening for the preinvasive lesions.

Cervical Intraepithelial Neoplasia (p. 1075)

Progression from CIN to cancer takes on average over 12 years and the risk of progression increases with higher grade CINs (CIN III or *carcinoma in situ*). The average age of women with CIN is 25 to 30 years and of women with cervical cancer, 40 to 45 years. *Risk of progression to malignancy is proportional to the grade of CIN and type of HPV, but the rates of progression are not uniform.* Carcinoma in situ is clearly a precursor of invasive carcinoma, the latter developing in up to 70% of women followed without treatment after a diagnosis of carcinoma in situ.

The oncoproteins (E6 and E7) of high-risk HPVs deregulate the cell cycle, produce genomic instability, and increase telomerase expression. All these molecular events promote neoplastic cell growth. Low risk HPVs (HPV 6 or 11) do not possess these properties and typically give rise to benign condylomas.

Morphology

CINs are classified according to the degree of epithelial maturation and the distribution of cytologic atypia:

- *CIN I* (including condyloma), in which the atypia is predominantly in the superficial cell layers (koilocytosis), with preservation of epithelial maturation

- *CIN II,* in which the atypia is conspicuous in both the superficial and the basal cell layers; there is decreasing maturation
- *CIN III,* in which the atypia is in all cell layers; there is minimal or no maturation (carcinoma in situ)

Squamous Cell Carcinoma (p. 1076)

Invasive cervical carcinoma manifests itself in three gross morphologic patterns: exophytic or fungating, ulcerating, and infiltrative. Histologically, 65% of tumors are large cell, nonkeratinizing, and moderately well differentiated. Some 25% are large and keratinizing, and the rest are composed of small, poorly differentiated squamous cells.

Staging for Cervical Cancer

0: Carcinoma in situ
I: Carcinoma confined to the cervix

    IA: Preclinical carcinoma diagnosed only by microscopy
      IA1: less than 3.0 mm in depth by 7.0 mm in length
      IA2: 3.0 to 5.0 mm in depth
    IB: Histologically invasive carcinoma greater than 5 mm in depth

II: Carcinoma extends beyond the cervix but not into the pelvic wall; into the vagina but not the lower third
III: Carcinoma extends to the pelvic wall or lower third of the vagina
IV: Carcinoma has extended beyond the pelvis

Five-year survival rates for squamous cell carcinoma depend on the stage:

0: 100% cure
I: 80% to 90%
II: 75%
III: 35%
IV: 10% to 15%

Of cervical carcinomas, 25% consist of adenocarcinomas, adenosquamous carcinomas, and undifferentiated carcinomas. The latter are termed *neuroendocrine carcinomas.* All nonsquamous carcinomas are strongly associated with HPV type 18.

BODY OF UTERUS AND ENDOMETRIUM (p. 1079)

Functional Endometrial Disorders (Dysfunctional Uterine Bleeding) (p. 1081)

The most common gynecologic problem in women during active reproductive life is excessive bleeding during or between menstrual periods. The causes of abnormal bleeding are many and vary among women of different age groups (Table 22–1). In many instances, bleeding is a result of a well-defined organic lesion, such as a submucosal leiomyoma, endometrial polyp, or chronic endometritis. The largest single group is so-called dysfunctional uterine bleeding, defined as abnormal bleeding in the absence of an organic lesion.

Important causes of dysfunctional uterine bleeding include:

- Hyperestrogenic states, associated with disturbances in ovarian function with anovulation, such as polycystic ovarian

TABLE 22-1 **Causes of Abnormal Uterine Bleeding by Age Group**

Age Group	Causes
Prepuberty	Precocious puberty (hypothalamic, pituitary, or ovarian origin)
Adolescence	Anovulatory cycle, coagulation disorders
Reproductive age	Complications of pregnancy (abortion, trophoblastic disease, ectopic pregnancy)
	Organic lesions (leiomyoma, adenomyosis, polyps, endometrial hyperplasia, carcinoma)
	Anovulatory cycle
	Ovulatory dysfunctional bleeding (e.g., inadequate luteal phase)
Perimenopausal	Anovulatory cycle
	Irregular shedding
	Organic lesions (carcinoma, hyperplasia, polyps)
Postmenopausal	Organic lesions (carcinoma, hyperplasia, polyps)
	Endometrial atrophy

disease, cortical stromal hyperplasia, and functioning ovarian tumors
- Other endocrine disorders, such as thyroid or adrenal disease or pituitary tumors
- Disturbances in coagulation or less well understood phenomena that lead to a loss of endometrial structural integrity

Morphologically, hyperestrogenic states produce cystic glandular changes associated with sporadic endometrial breakdown and bleeding. Other conditions may produce breakdown in the absence of any visible endometrial abnormality.

Inflammation (p. 1083)

Chronic endometritis (p. 1083) occurs (with decreasing frequency) in:
- Patients with *Chlamydia* and other intrauterine infections, including women suffering from chronic PID
- Postabortal or postpartal endometrial cavities, usually as a result of retained gestational tissue
- Patients with intrauterine contraceptive devices
- Rarely, patients with endometrial tuberculosis

In about 15% of patients, there is no predisposing condition, and the cause is unknown. Chronic endometritis is associated clinically with abnormal endometrial bleeding and histologically with infiltration of plasma cells and macrophages into the endometrium.

Endometriosis and Adenomyosis (p. 1083)

Endometriosis is defined as endometrial glands or stroma in abnormal locations *outside* the uterus. This condition can involve the ovaries, uterine ligaments, rectovaginal septum, pelvic peritoneum, laparotomy scars, and, rarely, the umbilicus, vagina, vulva, or appendix.
- Endometriosis presents clinically as severe dysmenorrhea and pelvic pain and *is a common cause of female infertility.*

- Endometrial foci are under the influence of ovarian hormones and therefore undergo cyclic menstrual changes with periodic bleeding.
- A definite histologic diagnosis requires two of the three following features:
  Endometrial glands in the ectopic lesions
  Stroma in the ectopic lesions
  Hemosiderin pigment in the ectopic lesions

Adenomyosis refers to nests of endometrium in the myometrium of the uterine wall. The condition causes uterine enlargement and irregular thickening of the uterine wall and is diagnosed histologically by the finding of endometrial stroma and glands in the myometrium.

Endometrial Polyps (p. 1085)

Endometrial polyps are sessile tumors composed of endometrial glands and stroma. They may be associated with hyperestrogenism or tamoxifen therapy. These polyps are usually benign but occasionally may harbor endometrial hyperplasia or cancer.

Endometrial Hyperplasia (Endometrial Intraepithelial Neoplasia) (p. 1085)

Endometrial hyperplasia is an important cause of abnormal uterine bleeding, and can result from a variety of disordered glandular and stromal growth patterns. A subset, defined as endometrial intraepithelial neoplasia (EIN), is considered a risk factor for endometrial carcinoma. The risk of carcinoma increases as a function of the degree of atypia. Both *endometrial hyperplasia and adenocarcinoma* (p. 1086) are associated with hyperestrogenism, microsatellite instability, and mutations in the *PTEN* gene.

Historically, there are three general categories of endometrial hyperplasia:

- *Simple hyperplasia without atypia* (also known as *cystic* or *mild hyperplasia*), containing benign cystically dilated glands. These are not neoplastic and are synonymous with anovulatory changes.
- *Complex hyperplasia,* in which glands of varying size are crowded together into clusters *of closely opposed glands.* Some of these are neoplastic (and contain *PTEN* mutations and are considered EIN).
- Complex hyperplasia with atypia, in which the gland crowding is accompanied by cytologic changes. Most hyperplasias in this category are neoplastic (EIN) and many contain *PTEN* mutations.

Malignant Tumors of the Endometrium (p. 1086)

Carcinoma of the Endometrium (p. 1086)

Carcinoma of the endometrium accounts for 7% of all invasive cancers in women. The peak age incidence is 55 to 65 years. There are two epidemiologic and pathophysiologic categories:

- Endometrioid adenocarcinomas, associated with obesity, diabetes, hypertension, infertility, and unopposed estrogen, containing mutations in *PTEN* and microsatellite instability, and often a preexisting EIN. These tumors are often associated with other forms of metaplasia.
- Papillary serous adenocarcinomas, associated with older age, often arising in endometrial polyps, or the endometrial surface epithelium, with multiple *p53* mutations.

Morphology

Grossly, endometrial carcinoma presents either as a localized polypoid tumor or as a diffuse spreading lesion involving the entire endometrial surface. *Histologically,* most endometrial carcinomas are adenocarcinomas. Biologically, the endometrioid tumors are well differentiated, closely resembling normal endometrial glands, with *squamous, secretory,* or *mucinous* differentiation (metaplasia). More aggressive neoplasms are poorly differentiated carcinomas, including *clear cell carcinomas* and *papillary serous carcinomas.*

Clinical Features

The patient usually presents with abnormal bleeding or an abnormal Papanicolaou smear. The prognosis depends on the state of the disease and is excellent in patients in whom the carcinoma is confined to the corpus uteri itself. However, serous tumors, like their counterparts in the ovary, can spread quickly, even when noninvasive.

Tumors of the Endometrium With Stromal Differentiation (p. 1088)

Malignant mixed mesodermal (mixed müllerian) tumors are relatively rare tumors derived from primitive stromal cells, originally derived from müllerian mesoderm. They consist of malignant glandular and stromal elements; the stromal sarcomatous elements may show muscle, cartilage, and osteoid differentiation. Grossly, the tumors protrude into the endometrial cavity and vagina and are bulky and polypoid.

Clinically, the tumors occur in postmenopausal women and are associated with postmenopausal bleeding. They are highly malignant and have a 5-year survival rate of 25%. *Endometrial stromal tumors* are varied and include the following types:

- *Benign stromal nodules:* Discrete nodules of stromal neoplasia within the myometrium.
- *Endometrial stromal sarcoma:* Well and poorly differentiated stromal neoplasms. These may penetrate into lymphatic channels (formerly classified as endolymphatic stromal myosis).
- *High-grade sarcomas, not otherwise specified:* High-grade unclassified tumors capable of widespread metastases.

Tumors of the Myometrium (p. 1089)

Leiomyomas (p. 1089)

Leiomyomas are the most common tumors in women, composed of benign masses of smooth muscle cells. They are most common in women in active reproductive life, are related to estrogenic stimulation, and are associated with a number of specific cytogenetic abnormalities.

Morphology

Lesions are sharply circumscribed, discrete, round, firm, gray-white nodules that occur within the myometrium (intramural), beneath the serosa (subserosal), or immediately beneath the endometrium (submucosal). They may undergo cystic degeneration and calcification. Leiomyomas may be asymptomatic or may be associated with abnormal uterine bleeding, pain, urinary bladder disorders, and impaired fertility. Malignant transformation is extremely rare.

Leiomyosarcomas (p. 1090)

Leiomyosarcomas are uncommon malignancies that form bulky, fleshy masses in the uterine wall. They are differentiated from benign leiomyomas by the presence of:

- Over 10 mitoses per 10 high-power fields, with or without cellular atypia
- Between 5 and 10 mitoses per 10 high-power fields with cellular atypia

These tumors disseminate throughout the abdominal cavity and aggressively metastasize. The 5-year survival rate is 40%. A subset of smooth muscle tumors display some but not all of the features of malignancy and are classified as of uncertain malignant potential.

FALLOPIAN TUBES (p. 1091)

Inflammations (p. 1091)

Suppurative salpingitis is due to infection with pyogenic organisms, including streptococci, staphylococci, and gonococci, and is part of PID. *Tuberculous salpingitis* is due to hematogenous spread of tuberculosis into the tubes and is sometimes associated with tuberculosis of the endometrium and peritoneum. Both forms of salpingitis are associated with infertility.

Tumors and Cysts (p. 1091)

Tumors of the fallopian tubes are rare. The most common is an *adenocarcinoma*, which resembles serous adenocarcinoma of the ovary. Recently, adenocarcinoma of the fallopian tube has been associated with *BRCA1* and *BRACA2* mutations; many arise in the fimbriated portion of the tube.

OVARIES (p. 1092)

Non-Neoplastic and Functional Cysts (p. 1092)

Follicular and Luteal Cysts (p. 1092)

These cysts are common, measure 1 to 8 cm in diameter, and are lined by follicular or luteinized cells. They may be asymptomatic or may rupture, causing a peritoneal reaction and pain.

Polycystic Ovaries and Stromal Hyperthecosis
(p. 1092)

Polycystic ovarian disease *(PCOD; Stein-Leventhal syndrome)* is a disorder of young women associated with oligomenorrhea, infertility, hirsutism, obesity, persistent anovulation, and fibrotic cystic ovaries. Patients exhibit insulin resistance, excessive production of androgens, increased conversion of androgen to estrogen, and inappropriate gonadotropin production by the pituitary. The ovaries are large; white; studded with subcortical cysts 0.5 to 1 cm in diameter; and covered by a thickened, fibrosed outer tunica. The pathogenesis is unknown, but PCOD is an important cause of infertility.

Ovarian Tumors (p. 1093)

Ovarian tumors are common forms of neoplasia in women and arise from the surface or subsurface epithelium, germ cells, or sex cord–stroma (Tables 22–2 and 22–3). The malignant tumors collectively account for about 6% of all cancers in women. Risk factors include nulliparity, family history, and specific inherited mutations (*BRCA1* and *BRCA2*).

Tumors of Müllerian Epithelium (p. 1094)

Serous Tumors (p. 1095)

Serous tumors are the most common cystic neoplasms. Cysts are lined by tall, columnar, ciliated epithelial cells and filled with serous fluid. *Serous tumors can be:*

- Benign (60%)
- Frankly malignant (25%)
- Of low malignant potential (also called *borderline*) (15%)

They present grossly as large (up to 40 cm in diameter) spherical or ovoid masses. The benign cystadenomas have a smooth and glistening inner lining. The *cystadenocarcinomas* often have small, mural, solid nodularities, papillary projections, and capillary invasion.

- Approximately 20% of benign tumors, 30% of borderline tumors, and 66% of malignant forms are bilateral.
- In benign tumors, the lining epithelium is composed of a single layer of tall, columnar, ciliated epithelial cells with small, microscopic papillae.
- Frankly malignant cystadenocarcinomas have multilayered epithelium with many papillary areas and large, solid epithelial masses with atypical cells focally invading the stroma.
- Tumors of low malignant potential show epithelial atypia and solid areas but no obvious invasion of the stroma.
- A proportion of borderline tumors demonstrate complex micropapillary epithelial architecture without invasion. These are variously termed *complex borderline tumors* or *low-grade micropapillary carcinomas.*

Prognosis in all of the foregoing groups is linked to stage. Borderline or micropapillary serous tumors may implant on the peritoneum. The presence of "invasive" implants heralds a poorer outcome in these patients.

Mucinous Tumors (p. 1097)

In contrast to serous neoplasms, 80% of mucinous tumors are benign, and only 5% to 10% are malignant.

TABLE 22–2 **Ovarian Neoplasms (1993 WHO Classification)**

Surface Epithelial-Stromal Tumors
Serous tumors
  Benign (cystadenoma)
  Cystadenoma of borderline malignancy
  Malignant (serous cystadenocarcinoma)
Mucinous tumors, endocervical-like and intestinal type
  Benign
  Of borderline malignancy
  Malignant
Endometrioid tumors
  Benign
  Of borderline malignancy
  Malignant
  Epithelial-stromal
    Adenosarcoma
    Mesodermal (müllerian) mixed tumor
  Clear cell tumors
    Benign
    Of borderline malignancy
    Malignant
  Transitional cell tumors
    Brenner tumor
    Brenner tumor of borderline malignancy
    Malignant Brenner tumor
    Transitional cell carcinoma (non-Brenner type)

Sex Cord–Stromal Tumors
Granulosa-stromal cell tumors
  Granulosa cell tumors
  Tumors of the thecoma-fibroma group
Sertoli-stromal cell tumors; androblastomas
Sex cord tumor with annular tubules
Gynandroblastoma
Steroid (lipid) cell tumors

Germ Cell Tumors
Teratoma
  Immature
  Mature (adult)
    Solid
    Cystic (dermoid cyst)
  Monodermal (e.g., struma ovarii, carcinoid)
Dysgerminoma
Yolk sac tumor (endodermal sinus tumor)
Mixed germ cell tumors

Malignant, Not Otherwise Specified

Metastatic Nonovarian Cancer (From Nonovarian Primary)

Data from the WHO Classification. (Courtesy Dr. Robert Scully, Massachusetts General Hospital, Boston, MA.)

- *Grossly* the tumors tend to produce large cystic masses (exceeding the size of serous tumors), often multiloculated and filled with sticky, gelatinous fluid. Less than 10% of primary (originating in the ovary) tumors are bilateral, usually falling into the "müllerian" mucinous group.
- *Histologically,* the tumors lined by tall, columnar intestinal-type epithelium are called *intestinal-type mucinous cystomas.* Those with papillary architecture and focal cilia are termed *müllerian mucinous tumors,* which may be associated with endometriosis. Cystadenocarcinomas are usually of the intestinal type, and display solid tumor growth and invasion of stroma.

TABLE 22–3 **Frequency of Major Ovarian Tumors**

Type	Percentage of Malignant Ovarian Tumors	Percentage That Are Bilateral
Serous	40	
Benign (60%)		25
Borderline (15%)		30
Malignant (25%)		65
Mucinous	10	
Benign (80%)		5
Borderline (10%)		10
Malignant (10%)		<5
Endometrioid carcinoma	20	40
Undifferentiated carcinoma	10	—
Clear cell carcinoma	6	40
Granulosa cell tumor	5	5
Teratoma		15
Benign (96%)		
Malignant (4%)	1	Rare
Metastatic	5	>50
Others	3	—

- Borderline mucinous tumors exhibit complex growth analogous to serous tumors, but lack solid growth or stromal infiltration.
- Primary ovarian mucinous tumors may seed the peritoneal cavity with multiple implants. However, this scenario is more characteristic of metastatic tumors originating in the appendix, large intestine, pancreas, or biliary tree.

Endometrioid Tumors (p. 1097)

Endometrioid tumors account for 20% of all ovarian cancers and are distinguished from serous and mucinous tumors by the close resemblance of tubular glands to benign or malignant endometrium. Up to 50% of these tumors are associated with endometriosis of the ovary. In 15% to 30% of endometrioid carcinomas, independent endometrial carcinomas appear.

Grossly, the ovarian lesions are a combination of solid and cystic masses. Of these carcinomas, 40% are bilateral, and histologically the glandular patterns bear a strong resemblance to endometrial adenocarcinoma.

Brenner Tumors (p. 1098)

These tumors are usually small, solid tumors characterized by dense fibrous stroma and nests of transitional cells resembling urinary transitional or rarely columnar epithelium. They are occasionally encountered in the wall of mucinous cystadenomas and are usually unilateral; the vast majority are benign.

Clinical Course, Detection, and Prevention of Surface Epithelial Tumors (p. 1098)

All large epithelial tumors cause similar symptoms, including lower abdominal pain, abdominal enlargement, and gastrointestinal and urinary complaints. Resected benign tumors represent a cure. Carcinomas in time extend through the capsule (or originate on the surface) and seed the peritoneal cavity, occasionally causing massive ascites.

Mucinous and endometrioid carcinomas are not infrequently confined to the ovaries. Serous carcinomas are usually detected after they have spread to the peritoneal surfaces. Close surveillance of patients with a familial history validates the origin of these tumors from the ovarian surface and, in some cases, the fallopian tube mucosa prior to more distant spread.

Germ Cell Tumors (p. 1099)

Germ cell tumors represent 15% to 20% of all ovarian tumors. They are similar to germ cell tumors in men and are presumed to arise from totipotential germ cells capable of differentiating into the three germ cell layers.

Teratomas (p. 1099)

Teratomas are divided into mature and monodermal (specialized) teratomas.

Mature (Benign) Teratomas (p. 1099). Most mature teratomas are cystic, relatively small, and known as *dermoid cysts*. They are lined by skin with adnexal structures and filled with hair-bearing sebaceous secretion. The tumors are bilateral in 10% to 15% of cases and histologically reveal epidermis, hair follicles, and other skin adnexae, as well as tooth structures. Cartilage, bone, thyroid tissue, and other organ formations can also be found.

Dermoid cysts are clinically benign and are cured by resection. About 1% undergo malignant transformation of any of the component elements but most commonly develop into squamous cell carcinoma.

Monodermal or Specialized Teratomas (p. 1100). Monodermal teratomas differentiate along the line of a single abnormal tissue. The most common is struma ovarii, composed entirely of mature thyroid tissue. Another example is the ovarian carcinoid, similar to carcinoids elsewhere.

Immature (Malignant) Teratomas (p. 1100). These rare tumors differ from benign teratomas in that embryonic (rather than adult) elements derived from more than one of the three germ layers are usually present. These tumors are most common in adolescents and young women.

- *Grossly,* the tumors are bulky and predominantly solid with areas of necrosis and hemorrhage.
- *Microscopically,* there are varied amounts of immature tissue differentiating toward cartilage, glands, bone, muscle, nerve, and other tissues. Extraovarian spread of immature teratomas depends primarily on the degree of immaturity of the tissues. Most are malignant, grow rapidly, and metastasize widely. They can be cured with chemotherapy if treated early.

Dysgerminoma (p. 1101)

Dysgerminoma is the ovarian counterpart of testicular seminoma. The tumors are uncommon and may occur in childhood or in the teens and 20s. Most are nonfunctional.

Of lesions, 80% to 90% are unilateral. The tumors are solid, yellowish white to gray-pink, and fleshy. Histologically, they consist of sheets and cords of large vesicular cells separated by scant fibrous stroma.

All dysgerminomas are malignant, but only about one third are highly aggressive. They are also radiosensitive and chemosensitive and thus have a relatively good prognosis if treated early.

Endodermal Sinus (Yolk Sac) Tumor (p. 1101)

This rare tumor is derived from multipotential embryonal carcinoma cells differentiating toward yolk sac structures. The tumor consists histologically of cystic spaces into which protrude papillary projections with central blood vessels enveloped by immature epithelium. Intracellular and extracellular hyalin droplets are characteristic, and can contain α-fetoprotein. The tumors occur in children and young women and grow rapidly and aggressively.

Choriocarcinoma (p. 1101)

Choriocarcinoma arises in the ovary from the teratogenous development of germ cells. Most such tumors exist in combination with other germ cell tumors. *Histologically,* they are identical to the more common placental lesions and, analogous to gestational choriocarcinoma, elaborate chorionic gonadotropins (p. 1076). Ovarian choriocarcinomas are highly malignant, metastasize widely, and are much more resistant to chemotherapy than their placental counterparts.

Sex Cord–Stromal Tumors (p. 1102)

These tumors originate either from the sex cords of the embryonic gonad or from the stroma of the ovary. The tumors are frequently functional and mostly have feminizing effects.

Granulosa-Theca Cell Tumors (p. 1102)

These tumors are composed of various combinations of granulosa and theca cells. Two thirds occur in postmenopausal women.

* The tumors are usually unilateral and solid and have a white-yellow coloration. The granulosa cell component consists of small cuboidal-to-polygonal cells growing in cords, sheets, or strands; the thecal cell components are composed of sheets of plump spindle cells closely resembling those of a fibroma. Thecal cells contain lipid droplets.
* Granulosa-theca cell tumors have the potential to elaborate large amounts of estrogen and thus to produce precocious sexual development and endometrial hyperplasia; they predispose to endometrial carcinoma.
* All granulosa cell tumors are potentially malignant, with clinical malignancy occurring in 5% to 25%. They are slow growing, however, and the 10-year survival rate is almost 85%. Pure thecomas are benign.

Fibroma-Thecomas (p. 1103)

Fibroma-thecomas are common forms of ovarian neoplasms. They are usually unilateral, solid, hard, gray-white masses made up histologically of well-differentiated fibroblasts. Of fibromas, 40% are associated with hydrothorax (usually right-sided) and ascites *(Meigs syndrome).*

Sertoli–Leydig Cell Tumors (Androblastomas) (p. 1103)

These tumors recapitulate the cells of the testes and commonly produce masculinization or defeminization. They are usually unilateral and consist histologically of tubules composed of Sertoli cells or Leydig cells interspersed with stroma.

Metastatic Tumors (p. 1104)

Metastases of abdominal and breast tumors to the ovary are common. *Krukenberg tumor* refers to metastatic ovarian cancer (usually bilateral) composed of mucin-producing signet cells that metastasize from the gastrointestinal tract, mostly the stomach. *Pseudomyxoma peritonei* also occurs with well-differentiated appendiceal tumors (see Chapter 17). Breast metastases may be conspicuous or detected on microscopic examination only.

GESTATIONAL AND PLACENTAL DISORDERS
(p. 1104)

Gestational and placental disorders can be divided into disorders of early and late pregnancy.

Disorders of Early Pregnancy (p. 1105)

Ectopic Pregnancy (p. 1105)

Ectopic pregnancy denotes implantation of the embryo in a site other than the uterus—most commonly the fallopian tubes (90%) but also rarely in the ovary or abdominal cavity. Predisposing factors include PID with chronic salpingitis and peritubular adhesions, but 50% occur in apparently normal tubes. Tubal pregnancy has one of four outcomes:

- Intratubal hemorrhage with the formation of hematosalpinx
- Tubal rupture with intraperitoneal hemorrhage
- Spontaneous regression with resorption of the products of conception
- Extrusion into the abdominal cavity (tubal abortion)

Tubal rupture is a medical emergency characterized by an acute abdomen and shock. Early diagnosis is critical and can be suggested by high human chorionic gonadotropin (hCG) levels, ultrasonographic findings, and an endometrial biopsy specimen showing decidual changes and absent chorionic villi.

Disorders of Late Pregnancy (p. 1105)

Placental Inflammations and Infections (p. 1106)

Placental infection occurs by two pathways:

- Ascending infections via the birth canal are most common, resulting in infection of the chorionic membranes (acute chorioamnionitis) and both a maternal (subchorionitis) and fetal (umbilical cord vasculitis) inflammatory response.
- Hematogenous (transplacental) infections derived from a maternal septicemia, including listeria, streptococcus, and TORCH (toxoplasma, rubella, syphilis, cytomegalovirus, herpes) are characterized by villous inflammation (villitis) and acute intervillositis.

Toxemia of Pregnancy (Preeclampsia and Eclampsia) (p. 1106)

Toxemia of pregnancy refers to a symptom complex characterized by hypertension, proteinuria, and edema (preeclampsia). Eclampsia is the severe form associated with convulsions and coma. Toxemia occurs in 6% of pregnancies, usually in the last trimester, and is most common in primiparas.

Pathogenesis

The pathogenesis is unclear. It is thought, however, that primary causes, such as immune or genetic factors, result in mechanical or functional obstruction of uterine spiral arterioles. One theory proposes that inadequate implantation results in decreased uteroplacental perfusion and placental ischemia. This situation results in increased production of vasoconstrictors (e.g., thromboxane, angiotensin) and decreased vasodilators (e.g., prostaglandin I_2, prostaglandin E_2), leading to arterial vasoconstriction and systemic hypertension. Recently, another mechanism has been proposed. Abnormal increases in an antiangiogenic factor sFlt-1 and reductions in proangiogenic factors vascular endothelial-derived growth factor (VEGF) and placental growth factor (PIGF) have been shown to predate and accompany the onset of toxemia. The implication is that placental vascular growth may be terminated prematurely by factor imbalance.

The resulting *placental ischemia* causes endothelial injury and activation of disseminated intravascular coagulation, accounting for the decreased glomerular filtration rate and proteinuria, central nervous system disturbances, abnormal liver function tests, and fibrin thrombi and ischemia in most other organs.

Clinical Features

Preeclampsia usually occurs after the 32nd week of pregnancy and is characterized by hypertension, edema, proteinuria, headaches, and visual disturbances. Mild toxemia can be controlled by bed rest, diet, and antihypertensive agents, but delivery is the only definitive treatment for established preeclampsia and eclampsia.

Gestational Trophoblastic Disease (p. 1110)

Gestational trophoblastic disease is a spectrum of tumors and tumor-like conditions of progressive malignant potential, characterized by proliferation of trophoblastic tissue. The lesions include hydatidiform mole (complete and partial), invasive mole, choriocarcinoma, and placental site trophoblastic tumor.

Hydatidiform Mole (Complete and Partial) (p. 1110)

Hydatidiform mole is characterized by cystic swelling of the chorionic villi, accompanied by variable trophoblastic proliferation; this is a common precursor of choriocarcinoma. Moles manifest in the fourth to fifth months of pregnancy with vaginal bleeding. There are two types of benign noninvasive moles, *complete* and *partial,* that can be differentiated by histologic, cytogenetic, and flow cytometric studies (Table 22–4). In a complete mole, one or two sperm fertilize an egg that has lost its chromosomes; all genetic material is therefore paternally derived. In a partial mole, an egg with normal chromosomal content is fertilized by one diploid or two haploid sperm to get a triploid complement of genetic material.

Morphology. *Grossly,* moles consist of masses of thin-walled, translucent, cystic, grapelike structures. Fetal parts are rarely seen in complete moles and are more common in partial

TABLE 22–4 **Features of Complete Versus Partial Hydatidiform Mole**

Feature	Complete Mole	Partial Mole
Karyotype	46,XX (46,XY)	Triploid
Villous edema	All villi	Some villi
Trophoblast proliferation	Diffuse, circumferential	Focal; slight
Atypia	Often present	Absent
Serum hCG	Elevated	Less elevated
hCG in tissue	++++	+
Behavior	2% choriocarcinoma	Rare choriocarcinoma

hCG, human chorionic gonadotropin.

moles. *Microscopically,* complete moles show hydropic swelling of villi, inadequate vascularization of villi, and significant trophoblastic proliferation. Partial moles show only focal edema and focal and slight trophoblastic proliferation. Most complete moles have diploid karyotypes, whereas partial moles are usually triploid. The two can also be distinguished by the expression of the normally maternally imprinted *p57* gene that is not expressed in the cytotrophoblast and stromal cells of the paternally derived mole.

Moles can be diagnosed by ultrasound examination and by quantitative analysis of serum hCG, revealing levels exceeding those produced by a normal pregnancy of similar age. Once complete moles are curetted, 80% to 90% do not recur, 10% develop into invasive moles, and 2.5% develop into choriocarcinoma. Follow-up with periodic determination of hCG is essential in these patients.

Invasive Mole (p. 1113)

An invasive mole penetrates and may even perforate the uterine wall, marked by active proliferation of both cytotrophoblasts and syncytiotrophoblasts. It does not metastasize. It is associated with a persistent elevated hCG level and varying degrees of luteinization of the ovaries. The tumor responds well to chemotherapy.

Choriocarcinoma (p. 1113)

Choriocarcinoma is a malignant tumor arising in 1:20,000 to 1:30,000 pregnancies in the United States, but it is much more common in some Asian and African countries. *About 50% arise in hydatidiform mole, 25% in previous abortions, 22% in normal pregnancies, and the rest in ectopic pregnancies.*

Morphology. *Grossly,* the tumor is large, soft, yellowish white, and fleshy with areas of necrosis and hemorrhage. *Histologically,* it consists of abnormal proliferations of both cytotrophoblasts and syncytiotrophoblasts. The tumor invades the underlying endometrium; penetrates blood vessels and lymphatics; and metastasizes to the lungs, bone marrow, liver, and other organs.

Clinical Features. Choriocarcinomas are manifested by vaginal bleeding and discharge that may appear in the course of an apparently normal pregnancy, after a miscarriage, or after curettage. hCG titers are elevated to levels above those seen in hydatidiform mole. When the condition is first discovered, widespread metastases may have already occurred. *Gestational* *choriocarcinomas are highly sensitive to chemotherapy,* and cures can be achieved even in patients with metastatic disease.

Placental Site Trophoblastic Tumor (p. 1114)

This rare tumor is composed of proliferating *intermediate trophoblasts* that are larger than cytotrophoblasts but mononuclear rather than syncytial. The lesion differs from that of choriocarcinoma in the absence of cytotrophoblastic elements and low levels of hCG production. Most are locally invasive only. Malignant variants are distinguished by a high mitotic index, extensive necrosis, and local spread. About 10% result in metastases and death.

CHAPTER 23

The Breast

Almost all breast lesions of clinical importance are carcinomas. Benign lesions present with similar clinical findings (palpable masses, nipple discharge, and mammographic abnormalities) and are typically encountered during investigation to exclude malignancy.

DISORDERS OF DEVELOPMENT (p. 1122)

Disorders of development include the following:

- *Milkline remnants* may give rise to supernumerary nipples or breast tissue from the axilla to the perineum. This tissue can undergo hyperplasia during pregnancy and can rarely be the site of breast cancer.
- *Congenital inversion* of the nipple may mimic inversion owing to retraction by an invasive carcinoma or inflammatory conditions.
- *Reduction or augmentation* are common surgical procedures to alter breast size or to reconstruct the breast after cancer surgery. Implants filled with saline or silicone are used to replace or augment breast tissue (see *http://www.fda.gov/cdrh/breastimplants/*).

CLINICAL PRESENTATIONS OF BREAST DISEASE (p. 1122)

- *Pain* is the most common breast symptom, but its causes are poorly understood. Fewer than 2% of women with pain will have cancer; the majority will also have a breast mass.
- *A palpable mass* is the second most common symptom. Most are simple cysts that can be completely aspirated with resolution of the mass. Masses become less common with age, while the likelihood of carcinoma increases (10% of masses in women under 40 are malignant compared to 60% of masses in women over 50). Over 90% of palpable carcinomas are invasive. These carcinomas average 2.4 cm in size and 58% have lymph node metastases.

- *Nipple discharge* is a less common complaint. It is most frequently due to an intraductal papilloma, but can be associated with carcinoma in a minority of women (e.g., 7% of women under 60 and 30% of women over 60). Carcinomas can be *in situ* or invasive.
- *Mammographic abnormalities* requiring biopsy occur in about 2% of screened asymptomatic women. A malignant lesion is found in 25% to 30% of cases. Densities due to malignancy will be invasive carcinoma in over 90% of cases (averaging 1.1 cm in size with a 14% incidence of lymph node metastases) and only rarely ductal carcinoma in situ (DCIS). Carcinomas associated with calcifications are due to DCIS in 71% of cases and small invasive carcinomas in the remainder (averaging 0.6 cm in size with a 6% incidence of lymph node metastasis).

INFLAMMATIONS (p. 1124)

Inflammatory conditions are rare except during lactation. Inflammatory carcinoma mimics inflammation by obstructing dermal lymphatics with tumor emboli and should always be suspected if a nonlactating woman develops a swollen erythematous breast.

Acute mastitis (p. 1125) is common complication during lactation, especially after the development of nipple fissures and infection by skin bacteria; the condition usually readily resolves with antibiotic treatment and continued breastfeeding.

Periductal mastitis (p. 1125) *(recurrent subareolar abscess, squamous metaplasia of lactiferous ducts, Zuska disease)* presents as a painful subareolar mass secondary to an inflammatory response to keratin debris from ruptured ducts lined by metaplastic keratin-producing cells. It is often complicated by formation of a periareolar fistulous tract. Treatment includes surgical excision of the involved ducts. Secondary infections by mixed anaerobes may occur. Almost all patients have a history of smoking.

Mammary duct ectasia (p. 1126) usually presents as a poorly defined periareolar mass with viscous nipple secretions. It is characterized by inspissation of secretions, duct dilation, and periductal inflammation.

Fat necrosis (p. 1126) after trauma, surgery, or radiation therapy is followed by inflammation and fibrosis and presents as a hard palpable mass or mammographic calcifications.

Granulomatous mastitis (p. 1126) can be associated with systemic diseases (sarcoidosis, Wegener granulomatosis) or be primary in the breast (granulomatous lobular mastitis).

BENIGN EPITHELIAL LESIONS (p. 1126)

Epidemiologic studies categorize these lesions according to the risk of subsequent development of invasive cancer in either breast (Table 23–1). However, it is worth highlighting that the majority of women with these changes *never develop breast cancer.*

CARCINOMA OF THE BREAST (p. 1129)

Breast carcinoma is the most common nonskin malignancy in women and about one third of affected women will succumb

TABLE 23-1 Breast Lesions and Relative Risk of Developing Invasive Carcinoma

Pathologic Lesion	Relative Risk of Developing Invasive Carcinoma	Breast at Risk	Modifiers of Risk
Nonproliferative Breast Changes	1.0	Neither	
Duct ectasia			
Cysts			
Apocrine change			
Mild hyperplasia			
Adenosis			
Fibroadenoma without complex features			
Proliferative Disease Without Atypia	1.5–2.0	Both breasts	Increased risk if there is a family history of breast carcinoma
Moderate or florid hyperplasia			Decreased risk 10 years after biopsy
Sclerosing adenosis			
Papilloma			
Complex sclerosing lesion (radial scar)			
Fibroadenoma with complex features			
Proliferative Disease With Atypia	4.0–5.0	Both breasts	Increased risk if there is a family history of breast carcinoma
Atypical ductal hyperplasia			Increased risk if premenopausal
Atypical lobular hyperplasia (ALH)			Decreased risk 10 years after biopsy for ALH
Carcinoma in Situ	8.0–10.0		
Lobular carcinoma in situ (LCIS)		Both breasts	Treatment (tamoxifen, bilateral mastectomy)
Ductal carcinoma in situ* (DCIS)		Ipsilateral breast	Treatment (tamoxifen, surgery to eradicate the lesion, radiation therapy)

*This risk applies to low-grade DCIS originally misdiagnosed as benign disease and followed without treatment. The risk for progression of high-grade DCIS is presumed to be greater than this.

to the disease. A woman who lives to age 90 has a one in eight chance of developing breast cancer.

Incidence and Epidemiology (p. 1130)

The incidence of breast cancer started to increase in the 1980s; this may be related to the introduction of regular mammographic screening at that time. As another effect of screening, the stage at which women are diagnosed has shifted downward to where the majority currently present with only DCIS or small invasive carcinomas without lymph node metastases. An effect on the death rate would not be expected for many years, as prolonged survival is possible, even with metastatic disease. Indeed, the death rate remained relatively constant until a steady decrease was documented in the 1990s. Hopefully, this trend will continue as a result of screening as well as better treatment.

Major risk factors for developing breast cancer (p. 1131) are as follows:

- *Age.* Breast cancer is rarely found before the age of 25 except in certain familial cases. The incidence increases throughout a woman's lifetime. The average age at diagnosis is 64 years.
- *Age at menarche.* Women who reach menarche before age 11 years have a 20% increased risk compared to women who achieve menarche after age 14 years. Late menopause also increases risk.
- *First live birth.* Women with a first full-term pregnancy before age 20 years have half the risk of nulliparous women or women with a first birth after the age of 35.
- *First-degree relatives with breast cancer.* Risk increases with the number of affected first-degree relatives, and 13% of women with cancer have such a history. About 25% of such women are carriers of specific germ-line mutations (Table 23–2). The remaining women presumably have combinations of genes conferring increased risk.
- *Breast biopsies.* A biopsy showing atypical hyperplasia increases the risk of developing carcinoma.
- *Race.* The risk of a 50-year-old woman for developing an invasive carcinoma in the next 20 years is 7% for white women, 5% for African-American women, and 4% for Hispanic women and Asian/Pacific Islanders. Although the risk for developing carcinoma is lower for African-Americans, these women frequently present at a more advanced stage and have an increased mortality rate. The reasons include social factors (e.g., access to health care) and biologic factors (e.g., the cancers tend to be poorly differentiated, lack hormone receptors, and have different *p53* mutations).

A modified interactive means to calculate the risk of developing cancer in the next 5 years (or by age 90), using the foregoing risk factors, is available at *http://bcra.nci.nih.gov/brc/*.

Additional factors increasing the risk of breast cancer include increased estrogen exposure (e.g., postmenopausal hormone therapy or obesity), radiation exposure at a young age (e.g., during the treatment of Hodgkin disease or after atom bomb exposure), carcinoma of the contralateral breast or endometrium, alcohol use, and residence in the United States or Europe. Factors decreasing risk include decreased estrogen exposure (e.g., due to prophylactic oophorectomy or

TABLE 23-2 Comparison of *BRCA1* and *BRCA2*

Feature	*BRCA1*	*BRCA2*
Chromosome	17q21	13q12.3
Gene size	81 kb	84 kb
Protein size	1863 amino acids	3418 amino acids
Function	Tumor suppressor	Tumor suppressor
	Transcriptional regulation	Transcriptional regulation
	Role in DNA repair	Role in DNA repair
Mutations	>500 identified	>300 identified
Mutations in population	About 0.1%	About 0.1%
Risk of breast cancer	60%–80%	60%–80%
Age at onset	Younger age (40s to 50s)	50 years
Families with breast cancer due to a single gene (%)	52%	32%
Families with breast and ovarian cancer (%)	81% (20%–40% risk)	14% (10%–20% risk)
Families with male and female breast cancer	<20%	76%
Risk of other tumors (varies with specific mutation)	Prostate, colon, pancreas	Prostate, pancreas, stomach, melanoma, colon
Mutations in sporadic breast cancer	Very rare (<5%)	Very rare (<5%)
Epidemiology	Specific mutations are found in certain ethnic groups	Specific mutations are found in certain ethnic groups
Pathology of breast cancers	Greater incidence of medullary carcinomas (13%), poorly differentiated carcinomas, ER-, PR-, and *Her2/neu*-negative carcinomas, carcinomas with *p53* mutations	Similar to sporadic breast cancers

Additional information about these genes can be found at *http://www.ncbi.nlm.nih.gov/*.

premenopausal obesity), and breastfeeding. Other possible risk factors including diet, exercise, and environmental toxins have been intensively investigated, but strong correlations have not been found.

Etiology and Pathogenesis (p. 1133)

The major risk factors for breast cancer are related to genetic factors and hormonal influences.

Hereditary Breast Cancer (p. 1133)

Approximately 3% to 10% of breast cancers are due to germ-line mutations in a single gene. About half are due to mutations in *BRCA1* and one-third to mutations in *BRCA2* (see Table 23–2). Mutations in *CHEK2*, *p53*, *PTEN*, and *LKB1/STK11* each account for fewer than 5% of cases. These genes act as autosomal dominant tumor suppressors (i.e., loss of function confers susceptibility); they code for multifunctional proteins involved in cell cycle control and regulation of genome integrity. Patients tend to present at younger ages, with multiple tumors, or tumors at multiple sites. The investigation of these genes has led to insights into the causes of sporadic breast cancer.

Obviously, this leaves roughly two thirds of familial breast cancer risk unexplained. A polygenic model in which many weakly penetrant genes confer an increased risk has been proposed.

Sporadic Breast Cancer (p. 1135)

The most important risk factors involve increased exposure to hormones, which could increase the risk of cancer by at least two mechanisms. Metabolites of estrogen can cause mutations or generate DNA-damaging free radicals. Via its hormonal actions, estrogen can also promote the proliferation of premalignant lesions, as well as cancers.

Mechanisms of Carcinogenesis (p. 1135)

Numerous cellular changes are found in breast carcinomas; these changes include decreased function of tumor suppressor genes and cell adhesion proteins, and increased expression of cell cycle proteins, angiogenic factors, and proteases. All these changes occur in some, but not all, carcinomas, suggesting that there are numerous possible pathways to malignancy.

It has been difficult to identify changes specific to invasive carcinoma that are not present in carcinoma in situ. It is conceivable that invasion occurs due to the loss of normal function in myoepithelial and stromal cells, rather than a gain in function by cancer cells.

The study of carcinogenesis has been greatly aided by the use of mRNA expression profiling, which allows the simultaneous evaluation of the relative abundance of thousands (and potentially all) gene transcripts. Such studies have been used to investigate types of breast cancer (e.g., hereditary versus sporadic tumors), prognosis, and response to therapy. However, not all changes in malignant cells are reflected by changes in mRNA (e.g., a point mutation can affect function without altering message levels); consequently, analogous techniques for analyzing DNA and proteins are under development.

Classification of Breast Carcinoma (p. 1138)

Breast carcinomas may be "in situ" (i.e., limited to ducts and lobules without the capacity to metastasize) or invasive (i.e., penetrate beyond the basement membrane with the possibility of metastasis). Different histologic types have characteristic clinical, biologic, and prognostic implications (Table 23–3).

Prognostic and Predictive Factors (p. 1146)

Major Prognostic Factors (p. 1146)

- *Invasive carcinoma or carcinoma in situ.* By definition, carcinoma in situ cannot cause death. Deaths associated with carcinoma in situ are due to the subsequent development of invasive carcinoma or the presence of an occult area of invasion. In contrast, about one third of women with invasive carcinoma will succumb to the disease.
- *Distant metastases.* Once distant metastases are present, cure is unlikely, although long-term remissions and palliation can be achieved. Common sites of metastasis are lungs, bone, liver, adrenal, brain, and meninges. Fortunately, fewer than 10% of women present with metastases to distant sites.
- *Lymph node metastases.* In the absence of distant metastases, lymph node status is the most important prognostic factor. If the nodes are free of carcinoma, 10-year disease-free survival rate is 70% to 80%, but it falls to 35% to 40% with one to three positive nodes, and to 10% to 15% with more than 10 positive nodes. Breast cancers drain to one or two "sentinel nodes" in the ipsilateral axilla that can be identified by colored dye or radioactive tracer. Women with negative sentinel nodes can be spared the morbidity of a full axillary dissection.
- *Tumor size.* The likelihood of metastasis increases with tumor size, but size is also an independent prognostic factor. Women with node-negative carcinomas smaller than 1 cm have a survival rate similar to women without breast cancer.

TABLE 23–3 **Distribution of Histologic Types of Breast Cancer**

Total Cancers	Percent
Carcinoma In Situ*	**15–30**
Ductal carcinoma in situ (DCIS)	80
Lobular carcinoma in situ (LCIS)	20
Invasive Carcinoma	**70–85**
No special type carcinoma ("ductal")	79
Lobular carcinoma	10
Tubular/cribriform carcinoma	6
Mucinous (colloid) carcinoma	2
Medullary carcinoma	2
Papillary carcinoma	1
Metaplastic carcinoma	<1

*The proportion of in situ carcinomas detected depends on the number of women undergoing mammographic screening and ranges from less than 5% in unscreened populations to almost 50% in patients with screen-detected cancers. Current observed numbers are between these two extremes.

The data on invasive carcinomas are modified from Dixon JM, et al: Long-term survivors after breast cancer. Br J Surg 72:445, 1985.

TABLE 23-4 **Staging of Breast Carcinoma**

Stage	Carcinoma	Lymph Node Metastasis	Distant Metastasis	5-Year Survival Rate
0	DCIS or LCIS	Absent	Absent	92%
I	Invasive ≤2 cm	Absent or <0.02 cm	Absent	87%
II	Invasive ≤5 cm or >5 cm	1 to 3 present Absent	Absent	75%
III	Invasive ≤5 cm or >5 cm or any size or locally advanced	≥4 present >1 present ≥10 present present or absent	Absent	46%
IV	Any size	Present or absent	Present	13%

DCIS, ductal carcinoma in situ; LCIS, lobular carcinoma in situ.
Adapted from Greene FL, et al: AJCC Cancer Staging Manual, 6th ed. New York, Springer-Verlag, 2003.

The majority of women with cancers larger than 2 cm will have lymph node metastases, and most of these women will die of the disease.

- *Locally advanced disease.* Carcinomas invading into the skin with ulceration, with satellite skin metastases, or with invasion into the chest wall have a worse prognosis. Fortunately, with greater awareness of breast cancer detection, such cases are now rare at initial presentation.
- *Inflammatory carcinoma.* Women presenting with an enlarged swollen erythematous breast due to carcinoma plugging vascular spaces in the skin have a very poor prognosis, with a 3-year survival rate of only 3% to 10%.

The preceding prognostic factors are used by the American Joint Committee on Cancer to divide breast carcinomas into the clinical stages shown in Table 23–4.

Minor Prognostic Factors (p. 1147)

These factors are used to determine which node-negative women might benefit from systemic therapy and to decide among treatment options.

- *Histologic subtypes.* In general, carcinomas classified as a special type of breast carcinoma have a better prognosis than those of no special type ("ductal"); the exception is metaplastic carcinomas, which have a worse prognosis.
- *Tumor grade.* The most widely used grading system ("Nottingham Prognostic Index") assesses tubule formation, nuclear pleomorphism, and mitotic rate to divide carcinomas into three grades.
- *Estrogen receptors (ERs) and progesterone receptors (PRs).* The presence of hormone receptors predicts the likelihood of response to hormone-based therapies (Table 23–5).
- *Her2/neu.* This protein is overexpressed in 20% to 30% of breast carcinomas and in general connotes a worse prognosis. In over 90% of these cancers, overexpression is due to amplification of the gene on 17q21. Overexpression can be detected either by immunohistochemistry (protein), or by FISH (*f*luorescence *i*n *s*itu *h*ybridization that allows an

TABLE 23-5 **Response to Hormone-Based Therapy**

Receptors	Percentage of Carcinomas	Response to Hormonal Treatment
ER+/PR+	83%	75%–80%
ER+/PR–	15%	25%–30%
ER–/PR+	5%	40%–45%
ER–/PR–	17%	<10%

ER, estrogen receptor; PR, progesterone receptor.

estimation of gene copy number) in order to predict response to trastuzumab *(Herceptin)*. Herceptin is a humanized monoclonal antibody for the treatment of patients whose tumors overexpress Her2/neu. As the first gene-targeted therapeutic agent for a solid tumor, the results have been very promising.

- *Lymphovascular invasion (LVI)*. Tumor cells can sometimes be seen in lymphatics in the breast and this finding is a poor prognostic factor in women without lymph node metastases.
- *Proliferative rate*. Proliferation can be measured by a variety of methods; a high proliferative rate is a poor prognostic factor. Mitotic counts are included as part of the standard grading system.
- *DNA content*. A DNA content equal to normal cells is a better prognostic factor than an abnormal DNA content. However, marked chromosomal abnormalities may be present, even if an overall change in DNA content cannot be detected.

Current therapeutic approaches include local and regional control, using combinations of surgery (mastectomy or breast conserving surgery) and postoperative radiation, and systemic control, using hormonal treatment, chemotherapy, or both. Newer therapeutic strategies include inhibition (by pharmacologic agents or specific antibodies) of membrane-bound growth factor receptors (e.g., Her2/neu), stromal proteases, and angiogenesis.

Stromal Tumors (p. 1149)

The breast-specific intralobular stroma gives rise to biphasic (stroma and epithelium) breast tumors, fibroadenomas, and phyllodes tumors. The interlobular stroma gives rise to benign and malignant tumors also occurring at other sites (e.g., lipomas and sarcomas).

Fibroadenomas (p. 1149)

Fibroadenomas are the most common benign tumor of the female breast, occurring most often during the reproductive period, and regressing and calcifying after menopause. Fibroadenomas present clinically as well-circumscribed palpable masses, ovoid mammographic densities, or mammographic calcifications. During pregnancy, fibroadenomas may grow in size and sometimes infarct. Although benign, they can exhibit proliferative changes and incur a slightly increased risk of cancer. Other benign, circumscribed mass-forming lesions of breast stroma include *pseudoangiomatous stromal hyperplasia (PASH)* and fibrous tumors.

Phyllodes Tumors (p. 1150)

Phyllodes tumors also arise from specialized breast stroma and are biphasic. They usually present as palpable masses in women aged 50 to 70. The stroma frequently overgrows the epithelial component, forming clefts and slits, and creating leaflike fronds of tumor (*phyllodes* means leaflike). Their cellularity, mitotic activity, stromal overgrowth, invasiveness, and possible heterologous elements differentiate them from fibroadenomas. Most phyllodes tumors behave in a benign fashion and can be cured by local excision. A few may recur locally after excision, and rare tumors metastasize hematogenously, usually to the lungs. Only the stromal component metastasizes.

Sarcomas (p. 1150)

Sarcomas occur rarely in the breast. The most common sarcoma is angiosarcoma, which arises as a primary tumor in young women, after radiation therapy for breast cancer, or in the skin of a chronically edematous arm after mastectomy (Stewart-Treves syndrome). Sarcomatous differentiation can also occur in phyllodes tumors and carcinomas (e.g., some metaplastic carcinomas).

Other Malignant Tumors of the Breast (p. 1151)

Lymphomas may arise primarily in the breast, or breasts may be secondarily involved by a systemic lymphoma; most are of large B-cell origin. Young women with Burkitt lymphoma may present with massive bilateral breast involvement and are often pregnant or lactating. Metastases to the breast are rare and most commonly arise from a contralateral breast carcinoma. The most frequent nonmammary metastases are from melanomas and lung cancers.

THE MALE BREAST (p. 1151)

Gynecomastia (p. 1151)

Gynecomastia is enlargement of the male breast. It is of chief importance as an indicator of an imbalance between estrogens and androgens. It may be found during puberty, in Klinefelter syndrome, due to hormone-producing tumors, in men with cirrhosis, or as a side effect of drugs. Histologically, there is proliferation of both epithelial and stromal components.

Carcinoma (p. 1152)

Carcinoma of the male breast is rare. Risk factors and prognostic factors are similar to those for women. Male breast cancer is strongly associated with *BRCA2*. The same histologic types of breast cancer are found in men and women. Because of the scant amount of surrounding breast tissue in men, carcinomas tend to invade skin and chest wall earlier and present at higher stages. Matched by stage, prognosis is similar in men and women.

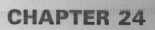

CHAPTER 24

The Endocrine System

The endocrine system is a highly integrated and widely distributed group of tissues that orchestrates a state of metabolic equilibrium *(homeostasis)* between the body's various organs. In endocrine signaling, secreted molecules (called *hormones*) act on target cells distant from the site of synthesis. Increased activity of the target tissue frequently then down-regulates the activity of the original gland that secreted the stimulating hormone—a process called *feedback inhibition.* Hormones are classified into broad categories depending on the type of receptor:

- Signaling molecules that interact with cell surface receptors

  Peptide hormones (e.g., growth hormone and insulin)
  Small molecules (e.g., epinephrine and histamine, derived from amino acids)

- Steroid hormones that diffuse across the plasma membrane and interact with intracellular receptors, which then activate specific gene expression

Endocrine diseases can be generally classified as:

- Diseases of hormone underproduction or overproduction.
- Diseases associated with the development of mass lesions. The mass lesions may be nonfunctional, or they may be associated with over- or underproduction of hormones.

PITUITARY GLAND (p. 1156)

The pituitary gland is at the base of the brain within the *sella turcica.* Along with the hypothalamus, the pituitary gland plays a critical role in the regulation of most other endocrine glands. It is composed of two morphologically and functionally distinct components:

1. Anterior lobe *(adenohypophysis)* comprises five cell types:

Somatotrophs, producing growth hormone (GH)

Lactotrophs, producing prolactin (Prl)

Corticotrophs, producing corticotropin and other hormones

Thyrotrophs, producing thyroid-stimulating hormone (TSH)

Gonadotrophs, producing follicle-stimulating hormone (FSH) and luteinizing hormone (LH)

The secretory activity of these hormones is normally regulated by stimulatory hypothalamic-releasing factors or an inhibitory factor (dopamine) controlling release of prolactin.

2. Posterior lobe *(neurohypophysis)* comprises modified glial cells (termed *pituicytes*) and axonal processes extending from the hypothalamus. The posterior pituitary stores two hormones, *oxytocin* and *vasopressin (antidiuretic hormone [ADH]).*

Clinical Manifestations of Pituitary Disease
(p. 1158)

Diseases of the pituitary are divided into those that primarily affect either the anterior or the posterior lobes.

• Diseases of the *anterior pituitary* can come to clinical attention as a result of either increased or decreased hormonal secretion (designated *hyperpituitarism* or *hypopituitarism,* respectively). In most cases, *hyperpituitarism* is intrinsic to the pituitary and is caused by a functional adenoma within the anterior lobe. *Hypopituitarism* can be caused by a variety of destructive processes, including ischemic injury, radiation, inflammatory reactions, and nonfunctioning neoplasms. In addition to endocrine abnormalities, diseases of the anterior pituitary may also be manifested by *local mass effects,* including radiographic enlargement of the sella turcica, visual field abnormalities resulting from encroachment of mass lesions on the visual pathways, and increased intracranial pressure.

• Diseases of the *posterior pituitary* can come to clinical attention because of increased or decreased secretion of one of its products (e.g., ADH).

Pituitary Adenomas and Hyperpituitarism
(p. 1158)

Excess production of anterior pituitary hormones is most often caused by an adenoma in the anterior lobe. Less commonly, excess production is due to primary hypothalamic disorders and *rarely* by carcinomas of the anterior pituitary. Functional pituitary adenomas are usually composed of a single cell type and produce a single predominant hormone (although some adenomas generate more than one hormone e.g., GH and Prl). Pituitary adenomas may be nonfunctional and cause hypopituitarism by destroying adjacent normal pituitary parenchyma. Pituitary adenomas are responsible for about 10% of intracranial neoplasms, and are discovered incidentally in some 25% of routine autopsies. They are usually found in adults with a peak incidence from ages 30 to 60.

Most pituitary adenomas are monoclonal in origin (even those that are plurihormonal) suggesting that most arise from a single somatic cell. Molecular studies demonstrate mutations in the gene encoding the α-subunit of G_s, a stimulatory G protein, in 40% of somatotroph adenomas. Mutations in the multiple endocrine neoplasia *(MEN)* 1 gene are seen in subsets of familial and sporadic pituitary tumors (see later discussion).

Morphology

Pituitary adenomas are divided into *microadenomas* (<10 mm in diameter) and *macroadenomas* (>10 mm in diameter). They are usually solitary and, in early stages, form discrete soft masses within the sella. Larger adenomas may compress or even infiltrate adjacent structures (e.g., cavernous sinus, base of brain, sphenoid bone), and such lesions are termed *invasive adenomas.*

Microscopically, adenomas are generally composed of uniform, *monomorphous* cell populations, in contrast to the normal pluricellular anterior pituitary. The neoplastic cells are arrayed in sheets, cords, nests, or papillae and have only a scanty reticulin network. Nuclear atypia, necrosis, and hemorrhage may all be present but do not imply malignancy. Ultrastructurally, variable numbers of membrane-bound *secretory granules* are present in the cytoplasm of most cells.

Prolactinomas (p. 1160)

Prolactinomas are the *most common* functional pituitary tumor, accounting for about 30% of all adenomas. Most are *macroadenomas,* composed of *sparsely granulated* acidophilic or chromophobic cells. Immunostaining for Prl is required to demonstrate the secretory product in histologic sections. Prl secretion by these adenomas is characterized by its *efficiency*—even microadenomas secrete sufficient Prl to cause hyperprolactinemia—and by its *proportionality*—serum Prl concentrations tend to correlate with the size of the adenoma.

Hyperprolactinemia can result from causes other than Prl-secreting pituitary adenomas. Physiologic hyperprolactinemia occurs in pregnancy, in which serum Prl levels increase throughout pregnancy, reaching a peak at delivery. Pathologic hyperprolactinemia can also result from *lactotroph hyperplasia* due to interference with normal dopamine inhibition of Prl secretion. This inhibition may occur as a result of damage to the dopaminergic neurons of the hypothalamus, pituitary stalk section (e.g., owing to head trauma), or drugs that block dopamine receptors on lactotroph cells. Any mass in the suprasellar compartment may disturb the normal inhibitory influence of the hypothalamus on Prl secretion, resulting in hyperprolactinemia—a phenomenon called the *stalk effect. Consequently, mild serum Prl elevations, even in a patient with a pituitary adenoma, does not necessarily indicate a Prl-secreting tumor.*

Clinical Features

Increased serum levels of Prl produce amenorrhea, galactorrhea, loss of libido, and infertility. The diagnosis of a pituitary adenoma is made more easily in women than in men because menses are more readily disrupted by hyperprolactinemia. Prl-secreting tumors underlie 25% of cases of amenorrhea. In contrast, in men and older women, the hormonal manifestations may be subtle, allowing the tumors to reach considerable size before being clinically detected.

Growth Hormone (Somatotroph Cell) Adenomas
(p. 1161)

GH-secreting tumors are the second most common type of functioning adenoma and are responsible for the vast majority of examples of *excess GH;* there is associated acromegaly or gigantism. Microscopically, GH-containing adenomas are composed of densely granulated cells, which appear acidophilic or chromophobic in routine sections; immunocytochemical stains demonstrate GH. Sparsely granulated variants contain a juxtanuclear "fibrous body" that is immunoreactive for cytokeratin.

Persistent hypersecretion of GH stimulates the hepatic secretion of insulin-like growth factor-1 (IGF-1), which causes many of the clinical manifestations. If somatotroph adenomas appear in children before the epiphyses have closed, the elevated levels of GH result in *gigantism.* This condition is characterized by a generalized increase in body size, with disproportionately long arms and legs. If increased GH first appears after epiphyseal closure, patients develop *acromegaly,* with enlargement of head, hands, feet, jaw, tongue, and soft tissues.

The goals of treatment are to (i) restore GH levels to normal; (ii) decrease symptoms referable to a pituitary mass lesion; and (iii) avoid hypopituitarism. Tumors can be surgically removed, or destroyed by radiation therapy, or GH secretion can be reduced by drug therapy.

Corticotroph Cell Adenomas (p. 1162)

Corticotroph cell adenomas are usually small microadenomas at the time of diagnosis. These tumors are basophilic or chromophobic. Immunostaining for corticotropin yields a strong reaction in basophilic adenomas. Chromophobic tumors are often larger and produce symptoms from local mass effects. *Crooke basophilic hyaline change* may be seen in the cytoplasm of corticotroph cells, including those in the non-neoplastic surrounding gland.

Excess production of corticotropin by the corticotroph adenoma leads to adrenal hypersecretion of cortisol with *hypercortisolism* (also known as *Cushing syndrome;* see later discussion). It can be caused by a wide variety of conditions in addition to corticotropin-producing pituitary tumors.

Other Anterior Pituitary Adenomas (p. 1162)

Pituitary adenomas may elaborate more than one hormone. As described earlier, somatotroph adenomas commonly contain immunoreactive Prl. In some tumors, designated *mixed adenomas,* more than one cell population is present. In other cases, a single cell type is apparently capable of synthesizing more than one hormone. A few additional comments should also be made:

• *Gonadotroph (LH- and FSH-producing) adenomas:* These adenomas make up 10% to 15% of pituitary adenomas. Gonadotroph adenomas are most frequently found in middle-aged men and women when the tumors become large enough to cause neurologic symptoms (e.g., impaired vision, headaches, diplopia, or pituitary apoplexy). Pituitary gonadotroph deficiencies also exist, most commonly impaired LH production. The result in men is low serum testosterone, causing decreased energy and libido. The result in premenopausal women is amenorrhea.

- *Thyrotroph (TSH-producing) adenomas:* These are rare, accounting for approximately 1% of all pituitary adenomas, and are rare causes of hyperthyroidism.
- *Nonfunctioning pituitary adenomas:* 25% of pituitary adenomas can be nonfunctioning; they include both nonsecretory *("silent")* variants of functioning adenomas, as well as true *hormone-negative* adenomas. The latter are unusual, and many pituitary tumors previously designated as "null cell" adenomas (because of inability to demonstrate any secretory product by routine techniques) are actually silent gonadotroph adenomas. Patients with nonfunctioning adenomas typically present with mass effects.
- *Pituitary carcinomas:* These tumors are quite rare, and most are not functional. The diagnosis of carcinoma requires the demonstration of metastases.

Hypopituitarism (p. 1162)

Hypopituitarism refers to decreased secretion of pituitary hormones; this can result from diseases of the hypothalamus or of the pituitary. To be symptomatic, 75% of the parenchyma must be destroyed or absent.

- *Tumors and other mass lesions:* Pituitary adenomas as well as metastatic malignancies and cysts can induce hypopituitarism. Any mass lesion in the sella can cause damage by exerting pressure on adjacent pituitary cells.
- *Pituitary surgery or radiation:* Surgical excision of a pituitary adenoma may inadvertently remove sufficient normal tissue to result in hypopituitarism. Radiation of the pituitary, used to prevent regrowth of residual tumor after surgery, can potentially damage the nonadenomatous pituitary tissue.
- *Rathke cleft cyst:* These cysts can accumulate proteinaceous fluid and expand, causing symptoms.
- *Pituitary apoplexy:* This is a sudden hemorrhage into the pituitary gland, often occurring into a pituitary adenoma. In its most dramatic presentation, apoplexy causes a rapid increase in the size of the tumor and the sudden onset of excruciating headache, diplopia resulting from pressure on the oculomotor nerves, and hypopituitarism.
- *Ischemic necrosis of the pituitary and Sheehan syndrome:* The anterior pituitary can tolerate ischemia reasonably well, although damage to more than 75% causes hypopituitarism. *Sheehan syndrome,* or postpartum necrosis of the anterior pituitary, is the most common form of clinically significant ischemic necrosis of the anterior pituitary. This syndrome results from sudden infarction of the anterior lobe precipitated by obstetric hemorrhage or shock. Pituitary necrosis can also be encountered in other conditions, such as disseminated intravascular coagulation or (more rarely) sickle cell anemia, elevated intracranial pressure, traumatic injury, and shock of any origin. The acutely infarcted adenohypophysis appears soft, pale, and ischemic or hemorrhagic. Over time, the ischemic area is resorbed and replaced by fibrous tissue.
- Rare genetic defects (mutations in the gene *Pit-1*) can cause hypopituitarism.

- *Empty sella syndrome:* Any condition that destroys part or all of the pituitary gland, such as ablation of the pituitary by surgery or radiation, can result in an *empty sella*. *Empty sella syndrome* refers to the presence of an enlarged, empty sella turcica that is not filled with pituitary tissue. There are two types:

  In *primary* empty sella, there is a defect in the *diaphragma sellae* that allows the arachnoid mater and cerebrospinal fluid to herniate into the sella, resulting in expansion of the sella and compression of the pituitary.

  In *secondary* empty sella, a mass, such as a pituitary adenoma, enlarges the sella but then is removed by surgery or radiation. Hypopituitarism results from the treatment of spontaneous infarction.

Posterior Pituitary Syndromes (p. 1163)

The posterior pituitary is composed of modified glial cells and axonal processes extending from nerve cell bodies in the supraoptic and paraventricular nuclei of the hypothalamus. These neurons produce two peptides: *ADH* and *oxytocin*. Oxytocin stimulates contraction of the uterine smooth muscle cells in the gravid uterus and those that surround the lactiferous ducts of the mammary glands. Inappropriate oxytocin secretion has not been associated with clinical abnormalities. ADH is a nonapeptide hormone synthesized predominantly in the supraoptic nucleus and is involved in the control of water conservation.

- *ADH deficiency (diabetes insipidus):* ADH deficiency causes diabetes insipidus, a condition characterized by excessive urination (polyuria) as a result of an inability of the kidney to resorb water properly from the urine, excessive thirst (polydipsia), and *hypernatremia*. It can result from multiple processes, including head trauma, tumors, and inflammatory disorders of the hypothalamus and pituitary, as well as surgical procedures involving these organs.
- *Syndrome of inappropriate ADH secretion (SIADH):* ADH excess causes resorption of excessive amounts of free water, resulting in *hyponatremia*. The most frequent causes of SIADH include the secretion of ectopic ADH by *malignant neoplasms* (particularly small cell carcinomas of the lung); non-neoplastic diseases of the lung (e.g., pulmonary tuberculosis, pneumonia); and local injury to the hypothalamus, posterior pituitary, or both. The clinical manifestations of SIADH are dominated by hyponatremia, cerebral edema, and resultant neurologic dysfunction.

Hypothalamic Suprasellar Tumors (p. 1164)

These tumors may induce hypofunction or hyperfunction of the anterior pituitary, diabetes insipidus, or combinations of these manifestations. The most commonly implicated lesions are *gliomas* (sometimes arising in the chiasm; Chapter 28) and *craniopharyngiomas*.

Craniopharyngiomas (p. 1164)

Craniopharyngiomas are derived from vestigial remnants of Rathke pouch. These slow-growing tumors account for about

5% of intracranial tumors. Most of these tumors are suprasellar, and they may encroach on the hypothalamus, third ventricle, or optic chiasm. Although they occur most commonly during childhood and adolescence, about 50% present after age 20. Children usually come to clinical attention because of endocrine deficiencies, such as growth retardation; adults present with visual disturbances.

Morphology

These tumors are characteristically cystic, and calcification is present in 75%. They are composed of a mixture of squamous epithelial elements and delicate reticular stroma, recapitulating the appearance of the enamel organ of a developing tooth. Intracystic components often include compact, lamellar keratin ("wet keratin") and a cholesterol-rich, thick brownish-yellow fluid that has been compared to "machinery oil." Malignancy is rare.

THYROID GLAND (p. 1164)

Thyroid follicular epithelial cells convert thyroglobulin into *thyroxine* (T_4) and lesser amounts of *triiodothyronine* (T_3) that are released into the systemic circulation. Most of the T_4 and T_3 are reversibly bound to circulating plasma proteins, such as thyroxine-binding globulin (TBG), for transport to peripheral tissues. In the periphery, the majority of free T_4 is deiodinated to T_3; the latter binds to thyroid hormone nuclear receptors in target cells with 10-fold greater affinity than T_4, and has proportionately greater activity. *The interaction of thyroid hormone with its nuclear thyroid hormone receptor (TR) results in the formation of a hormone-receptor complex that binds to thyroid hormone response elements (TREs) in target genes, regulating their transcription.* Thyroid hormone has diverse cellular effects, including increasing carbohydrate and lipid catabolism and stimulating protein synthesis in a wide range of cells. The net result of these processes is an increased basal metabolic rate.

Diseases of the thyroid are of great importance because they are relatively common in the general population, and most are amenable to medical or surgical management. They include conditions associated with excessive or deficient thyroid hormone production, and focal or diffuse mass lesions of the thyroid.

Hyperthyroidism (p. 1166)

Thyrotoxicosis is a hypermetabolic state caused by elevated circulating levels of free T_3 and T_4. Because it is caused most commonly by hyperfunction of the thyroid gland, it is often referred to as *hyperthyroidism*. Some of the more common causes of *primary* hyperthyroidism include:

- *Diffuse hyperplasia* of the thyroid associated with Graves disease (about 85% of cases)
- Hyperfunctional multinodular goiter
- Hyperfunctional *adenoma* of the thyroid

Secondary causes include thyrotroph pituitary adenomas. Inappropriate intake of exogenous thyroid hormone (as treatment for *hypo*thyroidism) and various inflammatory conditions of the thyroid are two common causes of thyrotoxicosis *not* associated with hyperactivity of the thyroid gland.

Clinical Features

The clinical manifestations of hyperthyroidism include changes referable to the *hypermetabolic state* induced by excess thyroid hormone as well as those related to overactivity of the *sympathetic nervous system.*

- *Cardiac manifestations are among the earliest and most consistent features of hyperthyroidism.* Patients with hyperthyroidism have increased cardiac output, due to both increased cardiac contractility and increased peripheral oxygen requirements. Tachycardia, palpitations, and cardiomegaly are common. Arrhythmias, particularly atrial fibrillation, occur frequently and are more common in older patients.
- *Ocular changes* often call attention to hyperthyroidism. A wide, staring gaze and lid lag are present owing to sympathetic overstimulation of the levator palpebrae superioris. Only patients with Graves disease have ophthalmopathy (see later).
- In the *neuromuscular system,* overactivity of the sympathetic nervous system produces tremor, hyperactivity, emotional lability, anxiety, inability to concentrate, and insomnia.
- The *skin* of thyrotoxic patients tends to be warm, moist, and flushed because of increased blood flow and peripheral vasodilation to increase heat loss. Infiltrative dermopathy is seen only in Graves hyperthyroidism (see below).
- In the *gastrointestinal system,* sympathetic hyperstimulation of the gut results in hypermotility, malabsorption, and diarrhea.
- *Apathetic hyperthyroidism* refers to thyrotoxicosis in the elderly when old age and various comorbidities blunt the typical features of thyroid hormone excess seen in younger patients.

The measurement of serum TSH concentration using sensitive TSH assays provides the most useful single screening test for hyperthyroidism, as its levels are decreased even at the earliest stages. A low TSH value is usually seen together with a correspondingly increased free serum T_4.

Hypothyroidism (p. 1167)

Hypothyroidism is caused by any structural or functional derangement that interferes with adequate production of thyroid hormone. As with hyperthyroidism, this disorder is divided into primary and secondary categories, depending on whether the hypothyroidism is intrinsic to the thyroid, or is a consequence of hypothalamic or pituitary disease.

- *Primary hypothyroidism* accounts for the vast majority of cases of hypothyroidism, and can be "goitrous" (accompanied by enlargement of thyroid gland) or "thyroprivic" (loss of thyroid parenchyma). The most common cause of goitrous hypothyroidism in iodine-sufficient areas of the world is *autoimmune thyroiditis,* most frequently due to *Hashimoto thyroiditis.* Other causes include dietary iodine deficiency–associated endemic goiter, inborn errors of metabolism, and drugs that block hormone synthesis (goitrogens). Thyroprivic hypothyroidism can follow thyroid surgery or radiation, can be due to an infiltrative disorder, or rarely can have a genetic basis.

- *Secondary hypothyroidism* is caused by TSH deficiency; *tertiary (central) hypothyroidism* is caused by thyrotropin-releasing hormone (TRH) deficiency.
- *Serum TSH level is the most sensitive screening test for hypothyroidsim.* The TSH level is increased in primary hypothyroidism owing to a loss of feedback inhibition of TRH and TSH production by the hypothalamus and pituitary, respectively.

Clinical Features

Clinical manifestations of hypothyroidism include *cretinism* if thyroid deficiency develops during the perinatal period or infancy, and *myxedema* in older children and adults.

Cretinism (p. 1168) may occur in both the *endemic* form, associated with dietary iodine deficiency and endemic goiter, and the *sporadic* form, often associated with a defect in hormone synthesis. Manifestations include impaired development of the skeletal and central nervous systems, with severe mental retardation, short stature, umbilical hernia, and coarse facial features including wide-set eyes and an enlarged, protruding tongue.

Myxedema (p. 1168) refers to hypothyroidism developing in the older child or adult. The older child shows signs and symptoms intermediate between those of the cretin and those of the adult with hypothyroidism; the latter is manifested by an insidious slowing of physical and mental activity, associated with fatigue, cold intolerance, and apathy. *Signs* include periorbital edema, coarsening of skin and facial features, cardiomegaly, pericardial effusion, hair loss, and accumulation of mucopolysaccharide-rich ground substance within the dermis *(myxedema)* and other tissues.

Thyroiditis (p. 1169)

Inflammation of the thyroid gland, or *thyroiditis,* encompasses a diverse group of disorders. These include conditions that result in acute illness with severe thyroid pain (e.g., infectious thyroiditis, subacute granulomatous thyroiditis) and disorders in which there is relatively little inflammation and the illness is manifested primarily by thyroid dysfunction (subacute lymphocytic [painless] thyroiditis and fibrous [Reidel] thyroiditis).

Acute infections may reach the thyroid gland via hematogenous spread or through direct seeding of the gland (e.g., via a fistula from the piriform sinus). Other infections of the thyroid are more chronic and include mycobacterial, fungal, and *Pneumocystis* infections that occur in immunocompromised patients. The inflammatory involvement may cause sudden onset of neck pain and tenderness in the area of the gland and is accompanied by fever, chills, and other signs of infection.

Hashimoto Thyroiditis (p. 1169)

Hashimoto thyroiditis is an insidiously developing condition; it is the most common cause of hypothyroidism in areas of the world where iodine levels are sufficient. It is characterized by gradual thyroid failure because of an autoimmune-mediated destruction of the thyroid gland. Hashimoto thyroiditis is most prevalent between ages 45 and 65 years, with a female predominance of 10:1 to 20:1. It is a major cause of nonendemic goiter in children.

Pathogenesis

Hashimoto thyroiditis is an autoimmune disease in which the immune system reacts against a variety of thyroid antigens. The overriding feature is progressive depletion of thyroid epithelial cells (thyrocytes) with replacement by mononuclear cell infiltrates and fibrosis. Multiple immunologic mechanisms contribute to the death of thyrocytes, although sensitization of autoreactive CD4+ T-helper cells to thyroid antigens appears to be the initiating event. The effector mechanisms for thyrocyte death includes CD8+ T cell–mediated cytotoxicity, cytokine-mediated cell death (e.g., interferon-γ), and antibody-dependent cell-mediated cytotoxicity (ADCC) caused by binding of antithyroid antibodies (*anti-TSH receptor antibodies, antithyroglobulin,* and *antithyroid peroxidase* antibodies) to thyrocyte surfaces. A genetic component is proposed based on family studies, high rates of concordance in monozygotic twins, and association with certain HLA subclasses (e.g., DR3 and DR5).

Morphology

The thyroid is diffusely—often asymmetrically—enlarged with an intact capsule. The parenchyma is generally paler than normal. Microscopic changes include an exuberant infiltrate of lymphocytes, plasma cells, and macrophages, even forming germinal centers; abundant eosinophilic granular cytoplasm in residual follicular cells (*Hürthle* cells or *oncocytes*); and delicate fibrosis. An *atrophic variant* is associated with more extensive fibrosis and less inflammation; the gland is often reduced in size.

Clinical Features

Hashimoto thyroiditis comes to clinical attention as painless enlargement of the thyroid, *usually associated with some degree of hypothyroidism* in a middle-aged woman. *Hyperthyroidism (hashitoxicosis)* may be seen early in the course of the disease, associated with the presence of anti-TSH receptor antibodies, but it is transient. Patients with Hashimoto thyroiditis are at increased risk for other *concomitant autoimmune diseases,* both endocrine (type 1 diabetes, autoimmune adrenalitis), and nonendocrine (systemic lupus erythematosus, myasthenia gravis, Sjögren syndrome). There is a small risk of subsequent lymphoma.

Subacute (Granulomatous) Thyroiditis (p. 1170)

Subacute (granulomatous) thyroiditis (also called *granulomatous thyroiditis* or *de Quervain thyroiditis*) occurs much less frequently than Hashimoto disease. It is most common between ages 30 and 50 and affects women considerably more often than men (3:1 to 5:1).

Pathogenesis

Subacute thyroiditis is caused by a *viral infection* or a postviral inflammatory process. The majority of patients have a history of an upper respiratory infection just before the onset of thyroiditis. Cases have been reported in association with coxsackievirus, mumps, measles, adenovirus, and other viral illnesses. There is an association with HLA-B35.

Morphology

Subacute thyroiditis is characterized by variable enlargement of the gland, which may be symmetric or irregular. Histologically, the changes are patchy and depend on the stage of the disease. Early lesions include *thyroid follicular disruption* with a *neutrophilic* infiltrate. Later, more characteristic features include aggregations of lymphocytes, histiocytes, and plasma cells around collapsed and damaged thyroid follicles. *Multinucleate giant cells* enclose naked pools or fragments of colloid.

Clinical Features

The presentation of subacute thyroiditis may be sudden or gradual. It is characterized by neck pain that can radiate to the jaw, throat, or ears, particularly when swallowing. Fever, fatigue, malaise, anorexia, and myalgia accompany the variable enlargement of the thyroid. The thyroid inflammation and the resultant hyperthyroidism are transient, usually diminishing in 2 to 6 weeks, even if the patient is not treated. It may be followed by a period of transient, usually asymptomatic hypothyroidism lasting from 2 to 8 weeks; recovery is virtually always complete.

Subacute Lymphocytic (Painless) Thyroiditis (p. 1171)

Subacute lymphocytic thyroiditis is an uncommon cause of hyperthyroidism or painless enlargement of the gland. It is most common in women in the postpartum period *(postpartum thyroiditis)*. Self-limited, it may be followed by *hypo*thyroidism. It is an inflammatory disorder of unknown etiology defined histologically by *nonspecific lymphoid infiltration* of the thyroid parenchyma; there is no germinal center formation or significant plasma cell infiltrate. No clear association with viral infection, subacute granulomatous thyroiditis, or Hashimoto disease has been described.

The principal clinical manifestation of painless thyroiditis is hyperthyroidism. Symptoms usually develop over 1 to 2 weeks and last from 2 to 8 weeks before subsiding. The patient may have any of the common findings in hyperthyroidism (e.g., palpitations, tachycardia, tremor, weakness, and fatigue).

Riedel Thyroiditis (p. 1171)

Riedel thyroiditis is an uncommon *fibrosing* process of unknown etiology associated with replacement of thyroid parenchyma by dense fibrous tissue penetrating the capsule and extending into *contiguous neck structures*. Manifestations include glandular atrophy and hypothyroidism. The disorder may be mistaken for an infiltrating neoplasm. It may be associated with idiopathic fibrosis in other sites.

Graves Disease (p. 1172)

The most common cause of endogenous hyperthyroidism, Graves disease is characterized by:

- *Hyperthyroidism* resulting from hyperfunctional, diffuse enlargement of the thyroid
- Infiltrative ophthalmopathy with resultant exophthalmos (in most, but not all, cases)
- Localized, infiltrative *dermopathy* sometimes called *pretibial myxedema* that is present in a minority of patients

Graves disease has a peak incidence between ages 20 and 40, with *women being affected up to seven times more often than men.* Graves disease is a common disorder present in 1.5% to 2.0% of U.S. women. Genetic factors are important in the onset of Graves disease; it is associated with HLA-B8 and DR3, polymorphisms in the cytotoxic T-lymphocyte–associated-4 *(CTLA-4)* locus and with *other autoimmune disorders,* including Hashimoto disease, pernicious anemia, and rheumatoid arthritis.

Pathogenesis

Graves disease is an autoimmune disorder resulting from autoantibodies to the TSH receptor, thyroglobulin, and to the thyroid hormones (T_3 and T_4).

- *Autoantibodies to the TSH receptor* (thyroid-stimulating immunoglobulin) are found in patients with Graves disease. The antibody is relatively specific for Graves disease, in contrast to thyroglobulin and thyroid peroxidase antibodies.
- *Thyroid growth-stimulating immunoglobulins* are directed against the TSH receptor and have been implicated in the proliferation of thyroid follicular epithelium.
- *TSH-binding inhibitor immunoglobulins* prevent TSH from binding normally to its receptor on thyroid epithelial cells. In so doing, these antibodies mimic the action of TSH, resulting in the stimulation of thyroid epithelial cell activity (other forms may actually *inhibit* thyroid cell function).

The trigger for the initiation of the autoimmune reaction in Graves disease remains uncertain, although the underlying mechanism is likely a breakdown in helper T-cell tolerance, causing production of anti-TSH autoantibodies. T cell–mediated autoimmunity against *orbital preadipocyte fibroblasts* expressing the TSH receptor may also play a role in the development of the *infiltrative ophthalmopathy* characteristic of Graves disease. In Graves ophthalmopathy, the volume of the retro-orbital connective tissues and extraocular muscles is increased owing to several causes, including (i) marked infiltration of the retro-orbital space by mononuclear cells, predominantly T cells; (ii) inflammatory edema and swelling of extraocular muscles; (iii) accumulation of extracellular matrix (ECM) components, specifically hydrophilic glycosaminoglycans (GAGs, e.g., hyaluronic acid and chondroitin sulfate); and (iv) increased numbers of adipocytes (fatty infiltration).

Morphology

The gland is mildly and *symmetrically enlarged,* with an intact capsule and soft parenchyma. Microscopic changes include diffuse *hypertrophy* and *hyperplasia* of follicular epithelium, manifested by crowding of the columnar cells into irregular papillary folds. Colloid is substantially decreased. Interfollicular parenchyma contains *hyperplastic lymphoid tissue* and increased numbers of blood vessels.

Preoperative therapy influences the histologic appearance:

- *Thiouracil* exaggerates hyperplasia.
- *Radioactive iodine* promotes devascularization, colloid accumulation, and follicular involution.

Changes in extrathyroidal tissue include generalized lymphoid hyperplasia, and both ophthalmopathy and dermopathy are characterized by lymphocyte infiltration and accumulation of hydrophilic GAGs.

Clinical Features

The clinical findings in Graves disease include changes referable to *thyrotoxicosis* as well as those associated uniquely with Graves disease—*diffuse hyperplasia of the thyroid, ophthalmopathy,* and *dermopathy.* Ophthalmopathy may be self-limited or may progress to severe proptosis despite control of the thyrotoxicosis. Laboratory values include *elevated free T_4 and T_3 levels* and depressed TSH levels. Because of ongoing thyroid follicle stimulation, *iodine uptake is elevated,* and *radioiodine scans show a diffuse iodine uptake.*

Diffuse and Multinodular Goiters (p. 1173)

Enlargement of the thyroid, or *goiter,* is the most common manifestation of thyroid disease. *The presence of goiter reflects impaired synthesis of thyroid hormone,* most often due to dietary iodine deficiency.

Diffuse Nontoxic (Simple) Goiter (p. 1174)

This form diffusely involves the entire gland without producing nodularity. Because the enlarged follicles are filled with colloid, the term *colloid goiter* has been applied to this condition. It occurs in both an endemic and a sporadic distribution.

- *Endemic goiter* occurs in geographic areas where the soil, water, and food supply contain only low levels of iodine. Such conditions are particularly common in mountainous areas of the world, including the Alps, Andes, and Himalayas. The lack of iodine leads to decreased synthesis of thyroid hormone and a *compensatory increase in TSH,* leading to follicular cell hypertrophy and hyperplasia and goitrous enlargement. With increasing dietary iodine supplementation, the frequency and severity of endemic goiter have declined significantly.
- *Sporadic goiter* occurs less frequently than does endemic goiter. There is a striking female preponderance and a peak incidence in young adult life. Sporadic goiter can be caused by a number of conditions, including the ingestion of substances that interfere with thyroid hormone synthesis (goitrogens, found in a variety of vegetables and plants). In other instances, goiter may result from hereditary enzymatic defects that interfere with thyroid hormone synthesis, transmitted as autosomal recessive conditions. These defects in thyroid hormone synthesis include defects in iodine transport, organification, dehalogenation, and iodotyrosine coupling.

Morphology

Two stages can be identified in the evolution of diffuse nontoxic goiter: the *hyperplastic stage* and *colloid involution.* In the hyperplastic stage, the thyroid gland is diffuse and symmetrically enlarged. Initial histologic changes include *hypertrophy* and *hyperplasia* of follicular epithelium with *scant colloid.* Later changes (as thyroid hormone demand is met) include colloid accumulation and variable atrophy of follicular epithelium. If thyroid hormone demand decreases, the stimulated follicular epithelium involutes to form an enlarged, colloid-rich gland *(colloid goiter).*

Clinical Features

The vast majority of patients with simple goiters are clinically euthyroid. Therefore, the clinical manifestations are primarily related to *mass effects* from the enlarged thyroid gland. Hypothyroidism is more common in children with underlying biosynthetic defects.

Multinodular Goiter (p. 1174)

Recurrent episodes of stimulation and involution of a diffuse goiter generate a more irregular enlargement of the thyroid, termed *multinodular goiter.* Most long-standing simple goiters convert into multinodular goiters. They may be nontoxic or may induce thyrotoxicosis (toxic multinodular goiter). Multinodular goiters produce the most extreme thyroid enlargements and are frequently mistaken for neoplastic involvement. *Mutations in proteins of the TSH signaling pathway (leading to constitutive activation) have been identified in a subset of toxic goiters.*

Morphology

Multinodular goiters are multilobulated, asymmetrically enlarged glands. Glands may become massively enlarged (>2000 gm). The pattern of enlargement is quite irregular and can produce lateral pressure on the trachea and esophagus. In other instances, the goiter grows behind the sternum, trachea, and clavicles to produce the so-called *intrathoracic* or *plunging goiter.* The irregular *nodularity* of the gland is associated with focal hemorrhage, fibrosis, calcification, and cystic change. Histologic changes include a variable degree of *colloid* accumulation, follicular *epithelial hyperplasia,* and follicular *involution* with focal intervening areas of scarring and hemorrhage.

Clinical Features

- Occasionally, abnormal thyroid function is a result of hyperactivity of a focal nodule with resultant *thyrotoxicosis* (rarely associated with hypothyroidism).
- Problems related to *mass effect* include cosmetic deformity, esophageal compression with dysphagia, tracheal compression, and, occasionally, obstruction of the superior vena cava. Hemorrhage into goiter may cause pain and contribute to mass effect.
- Most patients are euthyroid, but in a substantial minority of patients, a hyperfunctioning nodule may develop within a long-standing goiter, resulting in *hyperthyroidism* (toxic multinodular goiter). This condition, known as *Plummer syndrome,* is not accompanied by the infiltrative ophthalmopathy and dermopathy of Graves disease. As previously mentioned, goiter may be associated with clinical evidence of *hypothyroidism* in specific clinical settings. Radioiodine

uptake is uneven, reflecting varied levels of activity in different regions. Hyperfunctioning nodules concentrate radioiodine and appear "hot." Distinction between multinodular goiter and neoplasm may be difficult, especially in patients with a dominant mass.

Neoplasms of the Thyroid (p. 1175)

Solitary thyroid nodules are present in 1% to 10% of the U.S. population, although the estimated incidence is significantly higher in endemic goitrous regions. Single nodules are about four times more common in women than in men; the incidence increases throughout life. Most solitary thyroid nodules prove to be benign, either follicular adenomas or localized, non-neoplastic conditions (e.g., nodular hyperplasia, simple cysts, or focal thyroiditis).

Fortunately, benign solitary nodules outnumber thyroid carcinomas by a ratio of nearly 10:1. Several clinical criteria may provide a clue as to the nature of the thyroid nodule:

- *Solitary nodules* are more likely to be neoplastic than are multiple nodules.
- *Nodules in younger patients* (<40 years old) are more likely to be neoplastic than those in older patients.
- *Nodules in men* are more likely to be neoplastic than are those in women.
- A history of *radiation treatment* to the head and neck region is associated with an increased incidence of thyroid malignancy.
- Nodules that take up radioactive iodine in imaging studies (*hot* or functioning nodules) are more likely to be benign.
- *Fine-needle aspiration* biopsy is often useful in the evaluation of thyroid nodules.

Adenomas (p. 1175)

Adenomas of the thyroid are discrete, solitary masses. There are multiple histologic variants, all representing *follicular neoplasms*. Although the vast majority of adenomas are nonfunctional, a small proportion produces thyroid hormones and cause clinically apparent thyrotoxicosis ("toxic adenomas"). Adenomas are rarely the precursors of cancer.

Pathogenesis

The *TSH receptor signaling pathway* plays an important role in the pathogenesis of toxic adenomas. *Activating somatic mutations in one of two components of this signaling system* (the TSH receptor itself or the α-subunit of G_s) cause chronic cAMP pathway stimulation, generating cells that acquire a growth advantage. This results in clonal expansion of specific epithelial cells within the follicular adenoma; these can autonomously produce thyroid hormone and cause symptoms of thyroid excess. Overall, mutations leading to constitutive cAMP activation appear to be the cause of 50% to 75% of autonomously functioning thyroid adenomas. Less is known about the pathogenesis of nonfunctioning adenomas.

Morphology

The typical thyroid adenoma is a well-demarcated, solitary lesion, occasionally accompanied by fibrosis, hemorrhage, or calcification. It is sharply demarcated from the adjacent parenchyma by a well-defined fibrous capsule. The tumor compresses the surrounding gland, which is notable for the absence of multinodularity (unlike goiters). Microscopically, the constituent cells often form uniform-appearing follicles that contain colloid. The follicular growth pattern within the adenoma is usually quite distinct from the adjacent non-neoplastic thyroid, and this is another distinguishing feature from multinodular goiters. *Hürthle cell* adenomas feature granular, eosinophilic cells containing abundant mitochondria. Careful evaluation of the integrity of the capsule is critical in the distinction of follicular adenomas from follicular carcinomas; the latter demonstrate capsular and vascular invasion.

Clinical Features

A thyroid adenoma typically presents as a painless mass that must be differentiated from a carcinoma. Most adenomas take up less radioactive iodine than does normal thyroid parenchyma. On radionuclide scanning, therefore, adenomas appear as *cold* nodules relative to the adjacent thyroid. Up to 10% of cold nodules eventually prove to be malignant. By contrast, malignancy is rare in *hot* nodules. *Owing to the need for evaluating capsular integrity, the definitive diagnosis of adenomas can be made only after careful histologic examination of the resected specimen.*

Carcinomas (p. 1177)

Carcinomas of the thyroid are relatively uncommon in the United States, accounting for about 1.5% of all cancers. Most cases occur in adults, with a female predominance. Most (90%–95%) are *well-differentiated lesions* and are therefore relatively not aggressive. The major subtypes of thyroid carcinoma and their relative frequencies include

* Papillary carcinoma: 75% to 85%
* Follicular carcinoma: 10% to 20%
* Medullary carcinoma: 5%
* Anaplastic carcinomas: <5%

Pathogenesis

Several factors—both genetic and environmental—are implicated in thyroid cancer pathogenesis. The major *environmental risk factor* predisposing to thyroid cancer is exposure to *ionizing radiation,* particularly during the first 2 decades of life. The major *genetic abnormalities* associated with carcinoma subtypes include the following:

* *Follicular carcinomas* arise via two distinct, nonoverlapping molecular pathways:

  Mutations in the *RAS* family of oncogenes (roughly 50% of cancers)

  t(2;3)(q13;p25) translocations, resulting in fusion of *PAX-8,* a paired homeobox gene with the peroxisome proliferator-activated receptor γ1 *(PPARγ1),* a nuclear hormone receptor implicated in terminal differentiation of cells (approximately 33% of cases)

* *Papillary carcinomas* also arise via two distinct, nonoverlapping molecular pathways:

  Rearrangements of the *RET* tyrosine kinase receptors (chromosome 10q) or *NTRK1* (neurotrophic tyrosine kinase receptor 1) (chromosome 1q), placing the tyrosine kinase domain of these genes under the transcriptional control of constitutively active genes. In the case of RET, novel fusion genes so formed are as known as *ret/PTC* [*ret/papillary* thyroid carcinoma]). *RET* and *NTRK1* abnormalities together account for roughly 50% of papillary cancers

Approximately 33% to 50% of papillary thyroid carcinomas harbor an activating mutation in the *BRAF* gene, specifically, a valine to glutamic acid missense mutation at codon 599 of the *BRAF* gene (V599E).

- *Medullary carcinomas* arise from the parafollicular C cells in the thyroid. Familial medullary thyroid carcinomas occur in multiple endocrine neoplasia type 2 (see later), and are associated with germline *RET* protooncogene mutations; *RET* mutations are also seen in nonfamilial (sporadic) medullary thyroid cancers.
- *Anaplastic carcinomas* are characterized by inactivating *p53* mutations, rarely seen in the other thyroid cancer types.

Papillary Carcinoma (p. 1178)

The most common form of thyroid cancer, papillary carcinoma occurs at any age but most commonly affects women aged 20 to 50; these account for the vast majority of thyroid carcinomas associated with previous exposure to ionizing radiation.

Morphology. The tumors are solitary or multifocal lesions that may infiltrate the adjacent parenchyma and are sometimes associated with calcification or cystic change. The microscopic appearance ranges from lesions that are predominantly *papillary* in architecture to those with mostly *follicular* elements (follicular variant of papillary carcinoma). *The diagnosis of papillary carcinoma is based on nuclear features* (see later discussion) *even in the absence of papillary architecture.*

Histologic features include:

- Hypochromatic empty nuclei devoid of nucleoli *(Orphan Annie eyes)* and nuclear grooves (the diagnostic features of papillary carcinomas)
- Eosinophilic intranuclear inclusions (cytoplasmic invaginations)
- Psammoma bodies (concentric calcifications)

Histologic variants of papillary carcinoma include:

- *Encapsulated variant* (well-encapsulated, thyroid-confined, with excellent prognosis)
- *Follicular variant* (distinguished by nuclei resembling true follicular carcinoma, and carrying a worse prognosis)
- *Tall cell variant* (tall columnar cells with intensely eosinophilic cytoplasm; tend to occur in older individuals, and are usually associated with prominent vascular invasion, extrathyroidal extension, and cervical and distant metastases)
- *Diffuse sclerosing variant* (does not present as a mass, but rather bilateral goiter; extensive, diffuse fibrosis, often associated with a prominent lymphocytic infiltrate, simulating Hashimoto thyroiditis; prominent Psammoma bodies)
- *Hyalinizing trabecular tumors* (organoid growth pattern; intra- and extracellular hyalinization; may be encapsulated [adenomas], or infiltrative [carcinomas]).

Clinical Features. Most papillary carcinomas present as asymptomatic thyroid nodules, but because of their great propensity for lymphatic invasion, the first manifestation may be a mass in a cervical lymph node. The tumor involves *regional nodes* in 50% of cases at time of diagnosis, although distant metastases are uncommon at presentation (5%). The carcinoma, typically a single nodule, moves freely during swallowing and is not distinguishable from a benign nodule. Hoarseness, dysphagia, cough, or dyspnea suggests advanced disease. Prognosis is generally excellent (>95% survival rate at 10 years); unfavorable factors include age above 40 years, the presence of extrathyroidal extension, and distant metastases.

Follicular Carcinomas (p. 1180)

Follicular carcinomas account for 10% to 20% of thyroid cancers. These tumors have a peak incidence in the 40s to 50s and a female predominance (3:1). There is an increased prevalence in areas of dietary *iodine deficiency,* suggesting that multinodular goiter may predispose to follicular carcinoma.

Morphology. Follicular carcinomas are single nodules that may be well-circumscribed or infiltrative. *Minimally invasive follicular carcinomas* may be exceedingly difficult to distinguish from follicular adenomas, and require extensive sampling of the thyroid–tumor interface. In contrast, extensive invasion of adjacent thyroid parenchyma or extrathyroidal tissues makes the diagnosis of carcinoma obvious in *widely invasive follicular carcinomas.* Microscopically, architecture of the tumors may vary considerably; the nuclear features noted in papillary carcinomas are absent. Most have a microfollicular pattern, with relatively uniform, colloid-filled follicles reminiscent of normal thyroid. Other patterns include a trabecular and sheetlike architecture. Some variants contain large numbers of eosinophilic cells resembling Hürthle cells.

Clinical Features. The majority of metastases are *hematogenous* (bone, lungs, liver). The prognosis is largely dependent on the extent of invasion at presentation, with approximately 75% to 80% of patients with widely invasive follicular carcinomas developing metastases, and up to half succumbing to their disease within 10 years. This is in stark contrast to minimally invasive follicular carcinoma, which has a 10-year survival rate of over 90%. Better-differentiated lesions may take up *radioactive iodine,* which may be used to identify and palliate metastatic lesions.

Medullary Carcinomas (p. 1182)

These *neuroendocrine* neoplasms originate from the parafollicular or C cells, of the thyroid. The cells of medullary carcinomas, similar to normal C cells, secrete *calcitonin* and possibly other secretory products. The tumors arise sporadically in about 80% of cases. The remainder occurs in the setting of MEN syndrome 2A or 2B, or as familial tumors without an associated MEN syndrome (familial medullary thyroid carcinoma, or FMTC). Mutations in the *RET* protooncogene play an important role in the development of both familial and sporadic medullary carcinomas. Peak incidence is age 40 to 60 for sporadic and FMTC cases and 20 to 40 for MEN-associated cases.

Morphology. Medullary carcinomas can arise as a solitary nodule or may present as multiple lesions involving both lobes of the thyroid. Sporadic cases tend to originate in one lobe, whereas familial cases are usually bilateral and multicentric. Microscopic features include polygonal to spindle-shaped cells arrayed in nests, trabeculae, and, occasionally, follicles. *Amyloid deposits,* derived from altered calcitonin molecules, are present in the adjacent stroma in many cases. Foci of *C-cell hyperplasia* are often present in familial cases but are typically absent in sporadic cases.

Clinical Features. Clinical features vary, depending on whether the case is sporadic or familial.

- *Sporadic cases* usually present as a thyroid mass, sometimes associated with dysphagia, hoarseness, or cough; occasional cases may present with manifestations related to the secretion of a peptide product (e.g., diarrhea resulting from calcitonin or vasoactive intestinal polypeptide).
- *Familial cases* are usually detected through screening of asymptomatic relatives of affected patients for abnormal serum calcitonin levels.
- In the spectrum of biologic virulence, familial medullary thyroid carcinomas are fairly indolent lesions, sporadic medullary carcinomas and those associated with MEN-2A are of intermediate aggressiveness, while MEN-2B tumors have a particularly poor outcome, with a propensity for early metastases via the bloodstream.

Anaplastic Carcinomas (p. 1183)

These aggressive undifferentiated tumors of the thyroid follicular epithelium account for less than 5% of thyroid carcinomas and are most common in elderly patients, particularly in areas of endemic goiter.

Morphology. Microscopically, these neoplasms are composed of highly anaplastic cells, which have one of three histologic patterns:

- Large, pleomorphic giant cells
- Spindle cells with a sarcomatous appearance
- Small anaplastic cells resembling those seen in small cell carcinomas arising in other sites

Clinical Features. The tumors have a dismal prognosis. Dissemination is common, but death is usually attributable to aggressive local growth.

Congenital Anomalies (p. 1183)

Thyroglossal duct (cyst) is the most common clinically significant congenital anomaly. It may present at any age, and arises as a remnant of the tubular development of the thyroid gland (e.g., a midline cyst or mass anterior to the trachea). Histologic features include squamous epithelium in segments occurring high in the neck and thyroidal acinar epithelium in lesions arising more inferiorly. Lymphocytic infiltrates are often conspicuous. They may become infected and form abscess cavities; rarely, they can give rise to carcinoma.

PARATHYROID GLANDS (p. 1183)

Parathyroid activity is controlled by the level of free (ionized) calcium in the bloodstream. Decreased levels of free calcium stimulate the synthesis and secretion of *parathyroid hormone* (PTH). The net result of these activities is an increase in the serum level of free calcium that inhibits further PTH secretion in a classic feedback loop. The metabolic functions of PTH in supporting serum calcium level include:

- Activating osteoclasts, thereby mobilizing calcium from bone
- Increasing renal tubular reabsorption of calcium, thereby conserving free calcium
- Increasing vitamin D conversion to its active $1,25\text{-}(OH)_2D_3$ form in the kidneys
- Increasing urinary phosphate excretion, thereby lowering serum phosphate level
- Augmenting gastrointestinal calcium absorption

Hypercalcemia is one of a number of changes induced by elevated PTH and is a relatively common complication of malignancy. In fact, *malignancy is the most common cause of clinically apparent hypercalcemia;* primary hyperparathyroidism (see later discussion) is a more common cause of *asymptomatic* hypercalcemia. Hypercalcemia of malignancy is due to increased bone resorption and subsequent release of calcium, occurring through two mechanisms:

- *Osteolytic metastases and local release of cytokines:* RANKL (*receptor activator of nuclear factor κB ligand*) is secreted by tumor cells and peritumoral stromal cells in metastatic foci, and activates an osteoclastic pathway by binding to the RANK receptor on osteoblast cell surfaces.
- *Release of PTH-related protein (PTHrP):* The most frequent cause of hypercalcemia in nonmetastatic solid tumors (e.g., squamous cell cancers) is PTHrP release.

Hyperparathyroidism (p. 1184)

Hyperparathyroidism occurs in two major forms, *primary* and *secondary*. The first condition represents an autonomous overproduction of PTH, whereas the latter condition typically occurs secondary to chronic renal insufficiency.

Primary Hyperparathyroidism (p. 1185)

Primary hyperparathyroidism is one of the most common endocrine disorders; it is an important cause of *hypercalcemia*. The frequency of the various lesions underlying parathyroid hyperfunction is as follows:

- Adenoma: 75% to 80%
- Primary hyperplasia (diffuse or nodular): 10% to 15%
- Parathyroid carcinoma: less than 5%

The annual incidence of primary hyperparathyroidism is roughly 25 cases per 100,000 in United States and Europe; most cases occur in patients over 50 years old, with a 3 : 1 female predominance. In over 95% of cases, the disorder is caused by sporadic parathyroid adenomas or sporadic hyperplasia.

Familial hyperparathyroidism can arise in the backdrop of:

- *Multiple endocrine neoplasia-1* (MEN-1): Primary hyperparathyroidism (including parathyroid adenomas and hyperplasia) occurs as a component of MEN-1 syndrome, associated with germ line *MEN-1* gene mutations.
- *Multiple endocrine neoplasia-2* (MEN-2): Primary hyperparathyroidism occurs as a component of MEN-2A syndrome, associated with germ line *RET* mutations.

- Familial hypocalciuric hypercalcemia (FHH) is an autosomal dominant disorder characterized by enhanced parathyroid function due to decreased sensitivity to extracellular calcium. Mutations in the parathyroid calcium-sensing receptor gene *(CASR)* on chromosome 3q are a primary cause for this disorder. *CASR* mutations have not been described in sporadic parathyroid tumors.

Among the *sporadic adenomas,* there are two notable tumor-specific (i.e., not germ line) chromosome defects in genes that appear related to the clonal origin of some of these tumors:

- *Parathyroid adenoma 1 (PRAD 1): PRAD 1* encodes cyclin D1, a major regulator of the cell cycle. Cyclin D1 is overexpressed in approximately 40% of parathyroid adenomas.
- *MEN-1:* Approximately 20% to 30% of sporadic adenomas demonstrate homozygous inactivation of the *MEN-1* gene.

Morphology

The morphologic changes seen in primary hyperparathyroidism involve not only the parathyroid glands but also all other organs affected by hypercalcemia.

- *Parathyroid adenomas* are almost always *solitary,* averaging 0.5 to 5.0 gm, and are surrounded by a delicate capsule. In contrast to primary hyperplasia, the remaining glands are usually normal or somewhat shrunken in size as a result of feedback inhibition by the elevations in serum calcium. Microscopically, parathyroid adenomas are composed of predominantly *chief cells* arrayed in uniform sheets, trabeculae, or follicles; foci of oxyphil cells may be present.
- *Primary hyperplasia* may occur sporadically, or in association with the MEN syndromes. It usually involves *all glands* histologically, although *asymmetric* involvement may be seen, particularly in cases of nodular hyperplasia. The combined weight of the affected glands rarely exceeds 1.0 gm. Microscopically, the most common pattern seen is that of chief cell hyperplasia, involving the glands in a diffuse or multinodular pattern. As for adenomas, stromal fat is inconspicuous within hyperplastic foci.
- *Parathyroid carcinoma* may be a fairly circumscribed lesion that is difficult to distinguish from an adenoma, either grossly or microscopically. These tumors enlarge one parathyroid gland and consist of gray-white, irregular masses sometimes exceeding 10 gm. The cells of parathyroid carcinomas are usually uniform and not too dissimilar from normal parathyroid cells. Diagnosis of malignancy is based on the presence of *local invasion, metastases,* or both.
- Other organs:

  Skeletal changes include osteoclast activation causing bone resorption. In severe cases, the marrow of affected bones contains increased amounts of fibrous tissue accompanied by foci of hemorrhage and cyst formation *(osteitis fibrosa cystica).*

  Hypercalcemia favors formation of urinary tract stones *(nephrolithiasis),* calcification of the renal interstitium and tubules *(nephrocalcinosis),* and metastatic calcifications in other tissues.

Clinical Features

Primary hyperparathyroidism usually presents in two general ways:

- *Asymptomatic hyperparathyroidism:* Routine serum calcium determinations in medical evaluations have resulted in the diagnosis of most cases of primary hyperparathyroidism at an early stage. In patients with primary hyperparathyroidism, serum PTH levels are inappropriately elevated for the level of serum calcium, whereas PTH levels are low to undetectable in the hypercalcemia resulting from nonparathyroid diseases.
- *Symptomatic primary hyperparathyroidism:* The signs and symptoms of hyperparathyroidism reflect the combined effects of increased PTH secretion and hypercalcemia. Primary hyperparathyroidism has been traditionally associated with a constellation of symptoms including *painful bones, renal stones, abdominal groans, and psychic moans.* The clinical manifestations affect multiple systems and include:

  Bone disease: bone pain, secondary to fractures of bones weakened by osteoporosis

  Renal disease: nephrolithiasis (renal stones) with attendant pain and obstructive uropathy

  Gastrointestinal disturbances: constipation, nausea, peptic ulcers, pancreatitis, and gallstones

  Central nervous system alterations: depression, lethargy, and eventually seizures

  Neuromuscular abnormalities: complaints of weakness, fatigue

  Cardiac manifestations: aortic and mitral valve calcifications

Secondary Hyperparathyroidism (p. 1187)

Secondary hyperparathyroidism is caused by any condition associated with a chronic depression in the serum calcium level because low serum calcium leads to compensatory parathyroid overactivity. *Renal failure is, by far, the most common cause of secondary hyperparathyroidism.* The pathogenesis in renal failure is related to phosphate retention and hypocalcemia, with compensatory hypersecretion of PTH. Impaired gastrointestinal calcium absorption because of reduced $1,25\text{-}(OH)_2D_3$ synthesis and skeletal resistance to the effects of PTH and vitamin D may also contribute. *Morphology* of parathyroid glands is identical to that of primary hyperplasia. Skeletal changes, including osteitis fibrosa cystica (usually not as severe as that in primary disease) and osteomalacia, are present, and *metastatic calcifications* may be seen in many tissues (vascular calcification may occasionally result in significant ischemic damage to skin, a process referred to as *calciphylaxis*). The condition may remit with correction of underlying renal failure. Occasionally, an *autonomous adenoma* may develop (*tertiary* hyperparathyroidism).

Hypoparathyroidism (p. 1188)

Hypoparathyroidism has multiple causes:

- It may be surgically induced.
- It is caused by congenital absence of all glands (e.g., DiGeorge syndrome).
- Familial hypoparathyroidism is often associated with chronic mucocutaneous candidiasis and primary adrenal insufficiency; this syndrome is known as autoimmune polyen-

docrinopathy syndrome type 1 (APS1) and is caused by mutations in the autoimmune regulator *(AIRE)* gene.
*   *Idiopathic hypoparathyroidism* most likely is an autoimmune disorder with isolated parathyroid destruction.

Clinical Features

*   *Neuromuscular manifestations,* such as tetany, muscle cramps, carpopedal spasms, laryngeal stridor, and convulsions
*   *Mental status changes,* such as irritability or psychosis
*   *Intracranial manifestations,* such as parkinsonian-like movement disorders and elevated intracranial pressure with papilledema
*   *Ocular* changes with calcification of the lens leading to cataract formation
*   *Cardiac* conduction defects, which produce a characteristic electrocardiographic QT interval prolongation

Pseudohypoparathyroidism (p. 1188)

The pathogenesis of pseudohypoparathyroidism is related to mutations in *GNAS1,* the gene encoding $G_s\alpha$, a G-protein that mediates PTH action on cells. As a result, there is loss of responsiveness to PTH in target tissues. This situation results in hypocalcemia, compensatory parathyroid hyperfunction, and a variety of skeletal and developmental abnormalities. Patients with this disorder may have short stature, round face, short neck, and short metacarpals and metatarsals.

THE ENDOCRINE PANCREAS (p. 1189)

Diabetes Mellitus (p. 1189)

Diabetes mellitus is not a single disease entity, but rather a *group of metabolic disorders sharing the common underlying feature of hyperglycemia.* The net effect is a chronic disorder of carbohydrate, fat, and protein metabolism with long-term complications affecting the *blood vessels, kidneys, eyes,* and *nerves.* Worldwide, over 140 million people suffer from diabetes, making this one of the most common noncommunicable diseases.

Diagnosis (p. 1190)

Normal glucose homeostasis is tightly regulated by three interrelated processes: glucose production in the liver, glucose uptake and utilization by peripheral tissues (chiefly skeletal muscle), and actions of insulin and counterregulatory hormones, including glucagons. Blood glucose values are normally maintained in a very narrow range, usually 70 to 120 mg/dL. The diagnosis of diabetes mellitus is established by demonstrating elevations of blood glucose by any one of three criteria:

*   Random glucose level at or over 200 mg/dL, with classical signs and symptoms (discussed subsequently)
*   Fasting glucose level at or over 126 mg/dL
*   Abnormal oral glucose tolerance test (OGTT), in which the glucose level is at or over 200 mg/dL 2 hours after a standard carbohydrate load

Classification (p. 1190)

The vast majority of cases of diabetes fall into one of two broad classes. Table 24–1 lists the broad etiologic classification of diabetes mellitus, while Table 24–2 summarizes the differences between type 1 and type 2 diabetes.

TABLE 24–1 **Classification of Diabetes Mellitus**

1. **Type 1 diabetes** (β-cell destruction, leads to absolute insulin deficiency)
   Immune-mediated
   Idiopathic

2. **Type 2 diabetes** (insulin resistance with relative insulin deficiency)

3. **Genetic defects of β-cell function**
   Maturity-onset diabetes of the young (MODY), caused by mutations in:
      Hepatocyte nuclear factor 4α [HNF-4α] (MODY1)
      Glucokinase (MODY2)
      Hepatocyte nuclear factor 1α [HNF-1α] (MODY3)
      Insulin promoter factor [IPF-1] (MODY4)
      Hepatocyte nuclear factor 1β [HNF-1β] (MODY5)
      Neurogenic differentiation factor 1 [Neuro D1] (MODY6)
   Mitochondrial DNA mutations

4. **Genetic defects in insulin processing or insulin action**
   Defects in proinsulin conversion
   Insulin gene mutations
   Insulin receptor mutations

5. **Exocrine pancreatic defects**
   Chronic pancreatitis
   Pancreatectomy
   Neoplasia
   Cystic fibrosis
   Hemochromatosis
   Fibrocalculous pancreatopathy

6. **Endocrinopathies**
   Acromegaly
   Cushing syndrome
   Hyperthyroidism
   Pheochromocytoma
   Glucagonoma

7. **Infections**
   Cytomegalovirus
   Coxsackie virus B

8. **Drugs**
   Glucocorticoids
   Thyroid hormone
   α-interferon
   Protease inhibitors
   β-adrenergic agonists
   Thiazides
   Nicotinic acid
   Phenytoin

9. **Genetic syndromes associated with diabetes**
   Down syndrome
   Kleinfelter syndrome
   Turner syndrome

10. **Gestational diabetes mellitus**

Data from the Report of the Expert Committee on the Diagnosis and Classification of Diabetes Mellitus. Diabetic Care 25(Suppl 1):S5–S20, 2002.

TABLE 24–2 Type 1 Versus Type 2 Diabetes Mellitus (DM)

Feature	Type 1 DM	Type 2 DM
Clinical	Onset: <20 years	Onset: >30 years
	Normal weight	Obese
	Markedly decreased blood insulin	Increased blood insulin (early); normal to moderate decreased insulin (late)
	Anti-islet cell antibodies	No anti-islet cell antibodies
	Ketoacidosis common	Ketoacidosis rare; nonketotic hyperosmolar coma
Genetics	30%–70% concordance in twins	50%–90% concordance in twins
	Linkage to MHC class II HLA genes	No HLA linkage
		Linkage to candidate diabetogenic genes (PPAR-γ, calpain 10)
Pathogenesis	Autoimmune destruction of β cells mediated by T cells and humoral mediators (TNF, IL1, NO)	Insulin resistance in skeletal muscle, adipose tissue and liver
	Absolute insulin deficiency	β-cell dysfunction and relative insulin deficiency
Islet cells	Insulitis early	No insulitis
	Marked atrophy and fibrosis	Focal atrophy and amyloid deposition
	β-cell depletion	Mild β-cell depletion

- *Type 1 diabetes* is characterized by an absolute deficiency of insulin secretion caused by pancreatic β-cell destruction. It is also termed *insulin-dependent diabetes mellitus* (IDDM). Type 1 diabetes accounts for approximately 10% of all cases.
- *Type 2 diabetes* is caused by a combination of peripheral resistance to insulin action and an inadequate compensatory response of insulin secretion by the pancreatic β cells ("relative insulin deficiency"). It is also called *non-insulin-dependent diabetes mellitus* (NIDDM). Approximately 80% to 90% of patients have type 2 diabetes.

Normal Insulin Physiology (p. 1190)

Insulin is an *anabolic* hormone, necessary for uptake of glucose and amino acids by peripheral tissues (especially skeletal and heart muscle, and adipose tissue), glycogen formation in the liver and skeletal muscles, glucose conversion to triglycerides, and protein synthesis. In addition to these metabolic effects, insulin has several mitogenic functions, including initiation of DNA synthesis in certain cells and stimulation of their growth and differentiation. Glucose itself is the most important stimulus for insulin synthesis and release. A rise in blood glucose levels results in glucose uptake into pancreatic β cells, facilitated by an insulin-independent, glucose-transporting protein, GLUT-2. Intracellular glucose metabolism and ATP (adenosine triphosphate) generation then inhibits an ATP-sensitive K+ channel on the β-cell membrane, with resultant membrane depolarization, influx of Ca^{2+} ions, and an *immediate phase* of preformed insulin hormone release. If the secretory stimulus persists, a delayed and protracted response follows that involves *active synthesis of insulin.* Other agents, including intestinal hormones and certain amino acids (leucine and arginine), stimulate insulin release, but not synthesis. The metabolic and mitogenic actions of insulin are mediated by the hormone binding to the tetrameric insulin receptor, with consequent activation of mitogen-activated protein kinase (MAPK) and phosphatidylinositol-3-kinase (PI-3K) signaling pathways.

Pathogenesis of Type 1 Diabetes Mellitus (p. 1192)

This form of diabetes results from a severe lack of insulin caused by an autoimmune destruction of islet β cells. Type 1 diabetes most commonly develops in childhood, becomes manifest at puberty, and is progressive with age.

Mechanisms of β-Cell Destruction (p. 1193)

* *T lymphocytes* react against β-cell antigens and cause cell damage. These T cells include:

  CD4+ T cells of the T_H1 subset causing tissue injury by activating macrophages, with the macrophages causing damage in a characteristic delayed-type hypersensitivity response

  CD8+ cytotoxic T lymphocytes that directly kill β cells and also secrete cytokines that activate macrophages

* Locally produced *cytokines* damage β cells. Among the cytokines implicated in the cell injury are IFN-γ, produced by T cells, and TNF and IL1, produced by macrophages that are activated during the immune reaction.

* *Autoantibodies* against islet cells and insulin are also detected in the blood of 70% to 80% of patients. The autoantibodies are reactive with a variety of β-cell antigens, including the enzyme glutamic acid decarboxylase (GAD). In susceptible children who have not developed diabetes (e.g., relatives of patients), the presence of antibodies against islet cells is predictive of the development of IDDM.

Genetic Susceptibilty (p. 1194)

Type 1 diabetes has a complex pattern of genetic associations, with at least 20 genetic loci potentially contributing to the altered host immune tolerance that eventually results in autoimmunity. By far the most important genetic association is with the class II major histocompatibility complex (MHC) HLA locus. Between 90% and 95% of whites with type 1 diabetes have HLA-DR3 or DR4 haplotypes. Certain alleles within these haplotypes, such as DQβ1*0302 allele, demonstrate an even greater degree of association with type 1 diabetes. Non-MHC genes associated with disease susceptibility include the insulin gene itself, and the gene encoding the T-cell inhibitory receptor CTLA-4.

Environmental Factors (p. 1194)

Several viral agents have been implicated as potential triggers for an autoimmune attack, including coxsackieviruses, mumps, measles, cytomegalovirus, rubella, and infectious mononucleosis. One postulate is that the viruses produce proteins that mimic self-antigens, and the immune response to the viral protein cross-reacts with the self-tissue *(molecular mimicry).*

Pathogenesis of Type 2 Diabetes Mellitus (p. 1194)

Type 2 diabetes mellitus is by far the more common type, with an even greater role for genetic susceptibility. The disease appears to result from a collection of multiple genetic defects, each contributing its own predisposing risk and modified by environmental factors. Unlike type 1, there is no evidence to suggest an autoimmune basis to type 2 diabetes. The two main metabolic defects that characterize type 2 diabetes are *insulin resistance* and *β-cell dysfunction.*

Insulin Resistance (p. 1195)

Insulin resistance is a decreased ability of peripheral tissues to respond to insulin. Functional studies in individuals with insulin resistance demonstrate numerous quantitative and qualitative abnormalities of the insulin signaling pathway, including down-regulation of the insulin receptor, decreased insulin receptor phosphorylation and tyrosine kinase activity, and reduced levels of active intermediaries in the insulin signaling pathway. It is recognized that insulin resistance is a complex phenomenon, influenced by a variety of genetic and environmental factors. Genetic factors associated with insulin resistance remain largely a mystery, as mutations in the insulin receptor itself account for a very small minority of patients with type 2 diabetes (discussed later).

Among environmental factors, *obesity has the strongest association.* The association of obesity with type 2 diabetes has been recognized for decades, and insulin resistance is the underlying basis. The risk for diabetes increases as the body mass index (a measure of body fat content) increases, suggesting a dose-response relationship between body fat and insulin resistance. Possible factors influencing insulin resistance in obesity include high circulating and intracellular levels of free fatty acids that can interfere with insulin function ("lipotoxicity") and a variety of cytokines released by adipose tissue ("adipokines") including *leptin, adiponectin,* and *resistin.* The peroxisome proliferator-activated receptor gamma (PPAR-γ), an adipocyte nuclear receptor activated by a new class of antidiabetic agents called *thiazolidinediones,* can modulate gene expression in adipocytes, eventually leading to reduction of insulin resistance.

β-Cell Dysfunction (p. 1196)

β-Cell dysfunction is manifested as inadequate insulin secretion in the face of insulin resistance and hyperglycemia. β-Cell dysfunction is both *qualitative* (loss in the normal pulsatile, oscillating pattern of insulin secretion and attenuation of the rapid first phase of insulin secretion triggered by elevation in plasma glucose) as well as *quantitative* (decreased β-cell mass, islet degeneration, and deposition of islet amyloid).

Monogenic Forms of Diabetes (p. 1197)

Monogenic forms of diabetes result from either a primary defect in β-cell function, or a defect in insulin/insulin receptor signaling.

- *Maturity-onset diabetes of the young* (MODY): MODY is a primary defect in β-cell function that occurs without β-cell loss, affecting either β-cell mass or insulin transcription; six distinct genetic defects have been identified thus far (see

Table 24–1). Approximately 2% to 5% of diabetics fall under one of the six known categories of MODY. MODY is characterized by:

Autosomal dominant inheritance as a monogenic defect, with high penetrance

Early onset, usually before age 25, as opposed to after age 40 for most patients with type 2 diabetes

Absence of obesity

Lack of islet cell autoantibodies and insulin resistance syndrome

- *Mitochondrial diabetes:* Diabetes is rarely (<1% cases) associated with point mutations in a mitochondrial tRNA gene, tRNA[Leu(UUR)]
- *Insulin gene or insulin receptor mutations:* Mutations that affect *insulin processing* from its precursor (proinsulin), or those that affect *insulin structure* and binding to its receptor are a rare cause of diabetes. *Insulin receptor* mutations that affect receptor synthesis, insulin binding, or receptor tyrosine kinase activity can result in mild to severe insulin resistance and type 2 diabetes.

Pathogenesis of the Complications of Diabetes
(p. 1197)

Metabolic Complications

Insulin is a major anabolic hormone; deranged insulin function affects glucose, fat, and protein metabolism. Counterregulatory hormones (e.g., GH, epinephrine) are secreted unopposed; peripheral tissues cannot accumulate glucose. Excess glycosuria induces osmotic diuresis and *polyuria,* with profound loss of water and electrolytes. Intense thirst *(polydipsia)* develops, with increased appetite *(polyphagia),* completing the classic diabetic triad.

- *Diabetic ketoacidosis* occurs almost always in type 1 diabetes as a result of severe insulin deficiency and absolute or relative increases in glucagon: excessive release of free fatty acids from adipose tissue and hepatic oxidation generates ketone bodies (butyric acid and acetoacetic acid). Ketonemia and ketonuria, with dehydration, can cause life-threatening *systemic metabolic ketoacidosis.*
- *Nonketotic hyperosmolar coma* usually develops in type 2 diabetics in the setting of severe dehydration (from sustained hyperglycemic diuresis) and an inability to drink water.

Long-Term Complications

The morbidity associated with long-standing diabetes of either type results from a number of serious complications, involving both large and medium-sized muscular arteries *(macrovascular disease),* as well as capillary dysfunction in target organs *(microvascular disease).* Macrovascular disease causes *accelerated atherosclerosis* among diabetics, resulting in increased risk of myocardial infarction, stroke, and lower extremity gangrene. The effects of microvascular disease are most profound in the retina, kidneys, and peripheral nerves, resulting in *diabetic retinopathy, nephropathy,* and *neuropathy,* respectively. At least three distinct metabolic pathways appear to be involved in the pathogenesis of long-term diabetic complications:

- *Nonenzymatic glycosylation:* Glucose chemically attaches to amino groups of proteins, reflected in *glycated hemoglobin* (HbA$_{1c}$) blood levels. With glycation of collagens and other long-lived proteins, *irreversible advanced glycation end products (AGE)* accumulate over the lifetime of blood vessel walls. AGE formation of proteins, lipids, and nucleic acids leads to:

  Protein cross-linking, trapping (among others) plasma lipoproteins in vessel walls

  Reduction in normal proteolysis

  AGE binding to cell receptors, inducing a variety of (undesired) biologic activities

- *Intracellular hyperglycemia with disturbances in polyol pathways:* Some tissues (nerve, lens, kidney, blood vessels) do not require insulin for glucose uptake and thus accumulate increased intracellular glucose by mass action. This glucose is then metabolized to *sorbitol* and then *fructose,* so that an equilibrium with extracellular solute is not achieved. The accompanying osmotic load leads to influx of water and osmotic cell injury. Sorbitol also decreases phosphoinositide metabolism and signal transduction.

- *Activation of protein kinase C:* Activation of intracellular protein kinase C (PKC) by calcium ions and the second messenger diacylglycerol (DAG) is an important signal transduction pathway in many cellular systems. Intracellular hyperglycemia stimulates the *de novo* synthesis of DAG from glycolytic intermediates, and hence activates PKC. The downstream effects of PKC activation are numerous:

  Production of the pro-angiogenic molecule vascular endothelial growth factor (VEGF), implicated in the neovascularization characterizing diabetic retinopathy

  Increased deposition of ECM and basement membrane material

  Production of the pro-coagulant molecule plasminogen activator inhibitor-1 (PAI-1), leading to reduced fibrinolysis and possible vascular occlusive episodes

Morphology of Diabetes and Its Late Complications (p. 1199)

Pancreas (Variable)

There is a reduction in number and size of islets (especially type 1 diabetes mellitus), *insulitis* (a heavy lymphocytic infiltrate within and about islets) in newly symptomatic type 1 diabetics, β-cell degranulation and fibrosis of islets, and deposition of extracellular amyloid (*amylin* protein), especially in longstanding type 2 diabetes.

Diabetic Macrovascular Disease

Accelerated *atherosclerosis* in the aorta and large and medium-sized arteries increases the risk for myocardial infarction, cerebral stroke, aortic aneurysms, and gangrene of the lower extremities. *Hyaline arteriolosclerosis,* the vascular lesion associated with hypertension, is more prevalent and more severe in diabetics.

Diabetic Microangiopathy

One of the most consistent morphologic features of diabetes is *diffuse thickening of basement membranes.* The thickening is most evident in the capillaries of the skin, skeletal muscle, retina, renal glomeruli, and renal medulla. It may affect nonvascular structures, such as renal tubules, Bowman capsule, peripheral nerves, and placenta. It should be noted that despite the increase in the thickness of basement membranes, diabetic capillaries are more leaky than normal to plasma proteins. The microangiopathy underlies the development of diabetic nephropathy, retinopathy, and some forms of neuropathy.

Diabetic Nephropathy

The kidneys are the most severely damaged organ in diabetics, and renal failure is a major cause of death.

- *Glomerular involvement:* diffuse mesangial sclerosis, nodular glomerulosclerosis (Kimmelstiel-Wilson lesion), or exudative lesions, resulting in progressive proteinuria and chronic renal failure
- *Vascular effects:* arteriosclerosis, including benign nephrosclerosis with hypertension
- *Infection:* urinary tract infections, with *pyelonephritis* and sometimes *necrotizing papillitis*

Diabetic Ocular Complications

Diabetic retinopathy affects the majority of diabetics. *Nonproliferative retinopathy* consists of intraretinal and preretinal hemorrhages, exudates, edema, thickening of retinal capillaries, and microaneurysms. *Proliferative retinopathy* is the process of neovascularization and fibrosis of the retina, which has a high propensity to cause blindness.

Diabetic Neuropathy

A *symmetric peripheral neuropathy* affecting motor and sensory nerves of the lower extremities is attributable to Schwann cell injury, myelin degeneration, and axonal damage. *Autonomic neuropathy* may lead to sexual impotence and bowel and bladder dysfunction. Focal neurologic impairment *(diabetic mononeuropathy)* is most likely due to microangiopathy.

Clinical Features of Diabetes (p. 1202)

Type 1 Diabetes Mellitus

Type 1 diabetes was traditionally thought to occur primarily in those under age 18, but is now known to occur at any age. In the initial 1 to 2 years following manifestation of overt type 1 diabetes, the exogenous insulin requirements may be minimal to none secondary to ongoing endogenous insulin secretion (referred to as the *"honeymoon period"*); shortly thereafter, however, any residual β-cell reserve is exhausted and insulin requirements increase dramatically. Type 1 diabetes is dominated by *signs of altered metabolism:* polyuria, polydipsia, and polyphagia. Despite an increased appetite, catabolic effects prevail, resulting in weight loss and muscle weakness. *Chemical indices* include ketoacidosis, low or absent plasma insulin, and elevated plasma glucose. Metabolic derangement and insulin need are directly related to physiologic stress, including deviations from normal dietary intake, increased physical activity, infections, and surgery.

Type 2 Diabetes Mellitus

Type 2 diabetes mellitus patients are usually older than age 40, with polydipsia and polyuria and, frequently, obesity. Metabolic derangements are usually mild, and most frequently, the diagnosis is made after routine blood or urine testing in asymptomatic persons. *Nonketotic hyperosmolar coma* can occur in elderly individuals who become dehydrated secondary to osmotic diuresis and lack adequate water intake.

Complications of Both Types of Diabetes

- In both forms of long-standing diabetes, *cardiovascular disease* events such as myocardial infarction, renal vascular insufficiency, and cerebrovascular accidents are the most common causes of death. In most instances, these complications appear approximately 15 to 20 years after hyperglycemic onset. The impact of cardiovascular disease can be gauged from the fact that it accounts for up to 80% of deaths in type 2 diabetes; in fact, diabetics have a 3 to 7.5 times greater incidence of death from cardiovascular causes compared to the nondiabetic population.
- *Diabetic nephropathy* is a leading cause of end-stage renal disease in the United States. The earliest manifestation of diabetic nephropathy is the appearance of low amounts of albumin in the urine ($\geq$30 mg/day, but less than 300 mg/day), or *microalbuminuria*. Without specific interventions, approximately 80% of type 1 diabetics and 20% to 40% of type 2 diabetics will develop *overt nephropathy with macroalbuminuria* ($\geq$300 mg/day) over the next 10 to 15 years, usually accompanied by the appearance of hypertension.
- Approximately 60% to 80% of patients develop some form of *diabetic retinopathy* approximately 15 to 20 years after diagnosis. This disease is currently the fourth leading cause of acquired blindness in the United States. In addition, diabetics have a predisposition to *cataracts* and *glaucoma*.
- Diabetics are plagued by enhanced susceptibility to *infections* of the skin and to tuberculosis, pneumonia, and pyelonephritis.

Pancreatic Endocrine Neoplasms (p. 1205)

Pancreatic endocrine neoplasms (PENs), also known as islet cell tumors, are rare compared with tumors of the exocrine pancreas. PENs may be hormonally functional or nonfunctional, single or multiple, benign or malignant. *Unequivocal criteria for malignancy* include:

- Metastases to regional lymph nodes or distant organs (including the liver)
- Angioinvasion
- Gross invasion of adjacent viscera

Other *features suggestive of malignancy* include invasion beyond the tumor capsule into the pancreatic parenchyma, a high mitotic index, tumor necrosis, and significant cellular atypia. In general, tumors smaller than 2 cm tend to behave in an indolent manner, but there are significant exceptions to this rule. Finally, the functional status of the tumor may have some import on prognosis as approximately 90% of insulinomas are benign, while 60% to 90% of other functioning and nonfunctioning pancreatic endocrine neoplasms tend to be malignant.

Hyperinsulinism (Insulinoma) (p. 1205)

β-Cell tumors are the most common PEN subtype. Tumors may elaborate sufficient insulin to cause hypoglycemia; symptomatic attacks occur with serum glucose below 50 mg/dL.

Morphology

Most are solitary lesions, although multiple tumors or tumors ectopic to the pancreas may be encountered. Bona fide carcinomas (about 10% of cases) are diagnosed on the basis of criteria for malignancy listed above. β-cell tumors are usually less than 2 cm in diameter, usually encapsulated, firm, yellow-brown nodules composed of cords and nests of well-differentiated β cells, with typical β-cell granules by electron microscopy.

Clinical Features

Symptoms of insulinomas include hypoglycemia-induced confusion, stupor, and loss of consciousness. Attacks are promptly relieved by glucose feeding or infusion. Hyperinsulinism may also be caused by *diffuse hyperplasia of the islets,* most commonly seen in neonates and infants secondary to maternal diabetes, Beckwith-Wiedemann syndrome, and rare metabolic disorders.

Zollinger-Ellison Syndrome (Gastrinomas) (p. 1206)

Zollinger-Ellison syndrome comprises a triad of recalcitrant peptic ulcer disease, gastric hypersecretion, and an endocrine cell tumor elaborating gastrin.

Morphology

Gastrinomas are just as likely to arise in the duodenum and peripancreatic soft tissues as in the pancreas (so-called "gastrinoma triangle"). In approximately 25% of patients, gastrinomas arise in conjunction with other endocrine tumors, thus conforming to the MEN-1 syndrome; MEN-1-associated gastrinomas are frequently multifocal, while sporadic gastrinomas are usually single. The histologic and ultrastructural features are similar to normal intestinal and gastric G cells.

Clinical Features

The duodenal and gastric ulcers are often *multiple;* although they are identical to those found in the general population, they are often *intractable* to usual modalities of therapy. In addition, ulcers may also occur in *unusual locations* such as the jejunum; when intractable jejunal ulcers are found, Zollinger-Ellison syndrome should be considered. More than 50% of the patients have diarrhea; in 30% it is the presenting symptom. Sixty percent of gastrinomas are malignant, with spread to lymph nodes and metastasis; 40% are benign. Surgical removal of gastrinomas is extraordinarily difficult; recurrence of symptoms postsurgically is quite common.

Other Rare Pancreatic Endocrine Neoplasms (p. 1207)

Elaboration of multiple hormones is occasionally seen in *multihormonal tumors:* insulin, glucagon, gastrin, corticotropin, melanocyte-stimulating hormone, vasopressin, norepinephrine, and serotonin.

- *α-cell tumors (glucagonomas):* associated with extremely high plasma glucagon levels, mild features of diabetes mellitus, migratory necrotizing skin erythema, and anemia. These tumors are seen in perimenopausal and postmenopausal women.
- *δ-cell tumors (somatostatinomas):* associated with high plasma somatostatin levels. These tumors have features of diabetes mellitus, cholelithiasis, steatorrhea, and hypochlorhydria.
- *VIPoma (diarrheogenic islet cell tumor):* watery diarrhea, hypokalemia, achlorhydria; associated with neural crest tumors.
- *Pancreatic carcinoid tumors:* serotonin-producing; rare.
- *Pancreatic polypeptide-secreting islet cell tumors:* rare, asymptomatic.

ADRENAL CORTEX (p. 1207)

Adrenocortical Hyperfunction (Hyperadrenalism) (p. 1207)

There are three basic types of corticosteroids elaborated by the adrenal cortex (glucocorticoids, mineralocorticoids, and sex steroids) and three distinctive hyperadrenal clinical syndromes:

- Cushing syndrome (excess cortisol)
- Hyperaldosteronism
- Adrenogenital syndromes (excess androgens)

Hypercortisolism (Cushing Syndrome) (p. 1207)

Hypercortisolism is caused by an elevation in glucocorticoid levels. There are *multiple etiologies:*

- Administration of exogenous glucocorticoids, the most common cause
- Primary hypothalamic-pituitary diseases associated with corticotropin hypersecretion
- Hypersecretion of cortisol by an adrenal adenoma, carcinoma, or nodular hyperplasia
- The secretion of ectopic corticotropin by a nonendocrine neoplasm

Pituitary hypersecretion of corticotropin (also called *Cushing disease*) is encountered most commonly in young adult life with a female predominance (5:1). It accounts for 70% to 80% of cases of *endogenous* hypercortisolism. Most cases are associated with a corticotropin-producing *pituitary adenoma; corticotroph hyperplasia* accounts for 15% of cases. The adrenals are bilaterally hyperplastic, and elevated serum corticotropin is usually readily detectable.

Primary *adrenal neoplasms,* such as adrenal adenoma, carcinoma, and primary cortical hyperplasia, account, in aggregate, for 10% to 20% of cases of endogenous Cushing syndrome. These lesions are independent of corticotropin because the adrenals function autonomously. Adenomas and carcinomas are equally common in adults; carcinomas predominate in children. Hypercortisolism is usually more marked with carcinomas than with adenomas or hyperplasia. In patients with a unilateral neoplasm, the contralateral adrenal cortex is usually atrophic because of *corticotropin suppression* and low levels of corticotropin.

Ectopic corticotropin secretion by nonpituitary tumors accounts for 10% of cases of endogenous Cushing syndrome and is seen most commonly in men 40 to 60 years old. It is most commonly associated with *small cell carcinoma of lung,* carcinoid tumors of the bronchus or pancreas, medullary carcinoma of the thyroid, and islet cell tumors of the pancreas (e.g., gastrinomas). It may rarely be associated with *ectopic secretion of corticotropin-releasing factor,* with resultant overproduction of corticotropin and hypercortisolism. The adrenals are bilaterally hyperplastic.

Determining the cause of Cushing syndrome depends on measuring the level of serum corticotropin and determining urinary steroid excretion after administration of dexamethasone to suppress corticotropin levels. These results coupled with imaging of pituitary and adrenals are necessary to characterize Cushing syndrome fully.

Morphology

The pituitary shows *Crooke hyaline change* within basophils caused by elevated glucocorticoid levels. The morphology of the adrenal glands depends on the cause of the hypercortisolism. *Diffuse adrenal cortical hyperplasia* is present in 60% to 70% of cases of Cushing syndrome; the glands are enlarged and affected bilaterally. *Nodular adrenal cortical hyperplasia* is present in 15% to 20% of cases; the appearance of the cortex between nodules is identical to that in diffuse hyperplasia, suggesting that nodular hyperplasia probably evolves from the latter. *Corticotropin levels are elevated* in most cases of hyperplasia. *Adrenal cortical adenomas and carcinomas* resemble nonfunctional cortical neoplasms (described later). Lesions occur most commonly from 30 to 60 years of age, with a female predominance. Adenomas are generally small and well circumscribed; carcinomas tend to be larger and unencapsulated. The zona reticularis and fasciculata of the adjacent residual cortex and the contralateral gland are *atrophic;* the zona glomerulosa is intact.

Clinical Features of Cushing Syndrome (see Table 24–9, p. 1209 of *Robbins and Cotran Pathologic Basis of Disease,* 7th ed.)

- Central obesity (85%–90%)
- Moon facies (85%)
- Weakness and fatigability (85%)
- Hirsutism (75%)
- Hypertension (75%)
- Plethora (75%)
- Glucose intolerance/diabetes (75%/20%)
- Osteoporosis (75%)
- Neuropsychiatric abnormalities (75%–80%)
- Menstrual abnormalities (70%)
- Cutaneous striae (50%)
- Delayed wound healing/bruisability

Primary Hyperaldosteronism (p. 1210)

Primary hyperaldosteronism is characterized by chronic excess aldosterone secretion. Excessive levels of aldosterone cause sodium retention and potassium excretion, with resultant hypertension and hypokalemia. Primary hyperaldosteronism indicates an autonomous overproduction of aldosterone, with resultant suppression of the renin-angiotensin system and decreased levels of plasma renin activity. It can be caused by

- An aldosterone-producing adrenocortical neoplasm; a solitary aldosterone-secreting adenoma accounts for about 80% of cases *(Conn syndrome).*
- Primary adrenocortical hyperplasia *(idiopathic hyperaldosteronism);* the genetic basis of idiopathic hyperaldosteronism is not clear, although it is possibly caused by an overactivity of the aldosterone synthase gene, *CYP11B2.*
- *Glucocorticoid-remediable hyperaldosteronism* is an uncommon cause of familial primary hyperaldosteronism, and a *chimeric gene* formed by fusion between *CYP11B1* (the 11β-hydroxylase gene) and *CYP11B2* (the aldosterone synthase gene) is often responsible. The activation of aldosterone secretion comes under the influence of corticotropin and hence is suppressible by exogenous administration of glucocorticoids.

In *secondary hyperaldosteronism,* aldosterone release occurs in response to activation of the renin-angiotensin system and is encountered in conditions such as congestive heart failure, decreased renal perfusion, and pregnancy.

Morphology

Aldosterone-producing adenomas are usually *solitary, small, encapsulated lesions;* they occur more commonly on the left side. *Peak incidence* is between ages 30 and 50, usually in women. They may be buried within the adrenal and not apparent externally; the cut surface is usually bright yellow, reflecting high lipid content. Constituent lipid-laden cells more often resemble cells of zona fasciculata than zona glomerulosa (the normal source of aldosterone). A characteristic feature of aldosterone-producing adenomas is the presence of PAS-reactive, eosinophilic, laminated cytoplasmic inclusions, known as *spironolactone bodies* (originally described after treatment with the antihypertensive medicine, spironolactone). *Bilateral idiopathic hyperplasia* is characterized by hyperplasia of cells resembling normal zona glomerulosa, interspersed with nodules resembling zona fasciculata.

Clinical Features

The clinical manifestations of primary hyperaldosteronism are those of hypertension and hypokalemia. Hypokalemia results from renal potassium wasting and can cause a variety of neuromuscular manifestations, including weakness, paresthesias, visual disturbances, and occasionally tetany. Sodium retention increases the total body sodium and expands the extracellular fluid volume, resulting in hypertension.

Adrenogenital Syndromes (p. 1211)

Disorders of sexual differentiation, such as virilization in the female and precocious puberty in the male, may be caused by primary gonadal or adrenal disorders:

- Androgen-secreting adrenal cortical *neoplasms* are more likely to be an *androgen-secreting adrenal carcinoma* than an adenoma.
- *Congenital adrenal hyperplasia* (CAH) represents a group of autosomal recessive, inherited metabolic errors, each characterized by a deficiency or total lack of a particular enzyme involved in the biosynthesis of cortical steroids, particularly cortisol. Steroidogenesis is then channeled into other pathways leading to increased production of androgens and accounting for the virilization. Certain enzymatic defects may also be associated with *salt wasting* resulting from impaired aldosterone production.

21-Hydroxylase Deficiency (p. 1212)

Defective conversion of progesterone to 11-deoxycorticosterone by 21-hydroxylase (CYP21B) accounts for 85% to 90% of cases of congenital adrenal hyperplasia. All adrenogenital syndromes are autosomal recessive disorders. Three distinctive syndromes are described:

- Salt-wasting adrenogenitalism is associated with a complete absence of hydroxylase activity and resultant mineralocorticoid and cortisol deficiency syndrome usually recognized after birth, with virilization in females, salt wasting, hyponatremia, hyperkalemia, and cardiovascular collapse.
- Simple virilizing adrenogenitalism without salt wasting is associated with incomplete loss of hydroxylase activity. Thus, the level of aldosterone is mildly reduced, testosterone is increased, and corticotropin is elevated, with resultant adrenal hyperplasia.
- Nonclassic adrenogenitalism implies mild disease that may be entirely asymptomatic or associated only with symptoms of androgen excess during childhood or puberty.

Morphology

Changes include substantial, *bilateral* adrenal enlargement; the cortex is widened and nodular and appears brown because of lipid depletion. In addition to cortical abnormalities, *"adrenomedullary dysplasia"* (characterized by incomplete migration of the chromaffin cells to the center of the gland) has also been recently reported in patients with classic salt-wasting 21-hydroxylase deficiency.

Clinical Features

Clinical features are determined by the specific enzyme deficiency and include abnormalities related to *androgen excess* versus *aldosterone* and *glucocorticoid deficiency*. CAH should be suspected in any neonate with ambiguous genitalia; severe enzyme deficiency in infancy can be a life-threatening condition with vomiting, dehydration, and salt wasting. In the milder variants, women may present with delayed menarche, oligomenorrhea, or hirsutism. Patients with CAH are treated with exogenous glucocorticoids. Mineralocorticoid supplementation is required in the salt-wasting variants of CAH.

Adrenal Insufficiency (p. 1214)

Primary Acute Adrenocortical Insufficiency (p. 1214)

Primary acute adrenocortical insufficiency can be caused by any lesion of the adrenal cortex that impairs corticosteroid production or may be secondary to corticotropin deficiency. Patterns include:

- Primary acute adrenocortical insufficiency (adrenal crisis)
- Primary chronic adrenocortical insufficiency (Addison disease)
- Secondary adrenocortical insufficiency

Acute adrenal cortical insufficiency can occur in a variety of settings, including:

- A *sudden increase in glucocorticoid requirements* in patients with chronic adrenocortical insufficiency
- *Rapid withdrawal of steroids* from patients with adrenal suppression secondary to long-term glucocorticoid therapy or *failure to increase steroid doses* in adrenalectomized patients during episodes of stress
- *Massive destruction* of the adrenals (e.g., neonatal adrenal hemorrhage, postsurgical disseminated intravascular coagulation, Waterhouse-Friderichsen syndrome)

Waterhouse-Friderichsen Syndrome (p. 1214)

This uncommon but catastrophic syndrome is characterized by:

- Overwhelming septicemic infection usually caused by *meningococci,* less often by other virulent bacteria (pneumococci, gonococci, staphylococci)
- Rapidly progressive hypotension and shock
- Disseminated intravascular coagulation with purpura
- Massive adrenal hemorrhage with adrenal insufficiency
- Common occurrence in *children* but may occur at any age

Morphologic changes are those of *massive, bilateral adrenal hemorrhage,* which begins in the medulla. The cause of the hemorrhage is unclear but may involve direct bacterial seeding of adrenal vessels, disseminated intravascular coagulation, endotoxin-induced vasculitis, or a hypersensitivity vasculitis. The clinical course can be devastatingly abrupt unless recognition is prompt and appropriate therapy provided.

Primary Chronic Adrenocortical Insufficiency (Addison Disease) (p. 1215)

This uncommon condition occurs most often in adults who suffer destruction of at least 90% of the adrenal cortex. *Causes are multiple,* including the following:

- *Autoimmune adrenalitis* accounts for 60% to 70% of cases of Addison disease. Autoimmune adrenalitis can occur in one of three clinical settings:

  Autoimmune polyendocrinopathy syndrome type 1 (APS1) is caused by mutations in the autoimmune regulator-1 *(AIRE1)* gene on chromosome 21q22, and is characterized by chronic mucocutaneous candidiasis and abnormalities of skin, dental enamel, and nails (ectodermal dystrophy), occurring in association with a combination of organ-specific autoimmune disorders (autoimmune adrenalitis, autoimmune hypoparathyroidism, idiopathic hypogonadism, pernicious anemia).

  APS2 presents as a combination of adrenal insufficiency with autoimmune thyroiditis or type 1 diabetes and is not known to be a monogenic disorder.

  Isolated autoimmune Addison disease.

- Infectious processes, particularly tuberculosis and those caused by fungi such as *Histoplasma capsulatum* and *Coccidioides immitis,* may destroy the adrenals.
- Patients with the acquired immunodeficiency syndrome (AIDS) are at risk for developing adrenal insufficiency from complicatioins of their disease (cytomegalovirus, *Mycobacterium avium-intracellulare,* Kaposi sarcoma).
- *Metastatic neoplasms* are an uncommon cause of adrenal insufficiency. Common primary tumors include carcinomas of the lung and breast.
- *Rare genetic disorders of adrenal insufficiency* include adrenal hypoplasia congenita (AHC) and adrenoleukodystrophy.

Morphology

Morphologic features vary, depending on the underlying disease (e.g., metastatic neoplasm, tuberculous granulomas). *Autoimmune adrenalitis* usually produces small glands, lipid depletion of adrenal cortex, and a variable lymphocytic infiltrate in cortex; the medulla is spared.

Clinical Features

Features of Addison disease include weakness, fatigue, anorexia, hypotension, nausea, vomiting, and cutaneous hyperpigmentation. Laboratory values include elevated levels of corticotropin, hyperkalemia, and low sodium (hyponatremia), associated with volume depletion and hypotension.

Secondary Adrenocortical Insufficiency (p. 1216)

Secondary adrenocortical insufficiency can be caused by any disorder of the hypothalamus or pituitary causing *decreased corticotropin production.* It is distinguished from primary hypoadrenalism by the following:

- Absence of hyperpigmentation (corticotropin and precursor peptides with melanocyte-stimulating activity are not elevated in secondary cases).
- Normal or near-normal aldosterone levels (aldosterone production is independent of corticotropin; severe hyponatremia and hyperkalemia are *not* features of secondary adrenocortical insufficiency).

Corticotropin deficiency may be isolated or associated with decreased levels of other pituitary hormones (panhypopituitarism). Morphologically, this condition is characterized by variable degrees of atrophy of the adrenal cortex, with *sparing of the zona glomerulosa and medulla.*

Adrenocortical Neoplasms (p. 1217)

In addition to hyperplasias and neoplasms associated with steroid production, nonfunctional adrenal cortical neoplasms also may occur.

- *Adrenal adenomas* are typically poorly encapsulated, yellow-orange lesions; they may lie within the cortex or protrude into the medulla or the subcapsular region. Larger lesions may contain areas of hemorrhage, cystic change, and calcification. Adjacent adrenal cortex is of normal thickness (in contrast to atrophic changes seen adjacent to functional adenomas).

- *Adrenal cortical carcinomas* are highly malignant neoplasms, usually of large size at the time of diagnosis. Lesions are predominantly yellow on cut surface but usually contain areas of hemorrhage, cystic change, and necrosis. Histologically, cells range from well differentiated to markedly anaplastic; they may be difficult to differentiate from metastatic cells. The tumors commonly invade vascular channels, with metastases to regional and periaortic lymph nodes and to viscera, especially lung. They are more likely to be functional than adenomas and are therefore often associated with virilism or other clinical manifestations of hyperadrenalism.

Other Lesions of the Adrenal (p. 1218)

Advancements in medical imaging and greater utilization of abdominal computed tomographic (CT) scans have led to the incidental discovery of adrenal masses in asymptomatic individuals. The prevalence of "adrenal incidentalomas" discovered by CT scans is in the order of 0.5% to 2% in the general population, but the probability of finding an incidental mass rises to over 6% in individuals over the age of 70 years. Fortunately, *the vast majority of adrenal incidentalomas are nonsecreting cortical adenomas.*

ADRENAL MEDULLA (p. 1218)

The adrenal medulla is structurally and functionally distinct from the cortex. Most adrenal medullary disorders are *neoplasms,* the most significant of which are pheochromocytomas, neuroblastomas, and ganglioneuromas. Neuroblastomas and ganglioneuromas are discussed elsewhere (Chapter 10).

Pheochromocytomas (p. 1219)

Pheochromocytomas are relatively uncommon neoplasms associated with *catecholamine production* and *hypertension* (account for 0.1%–0.3% of all cases of hypertension). Pheochromocytomas usually subscribe to a convenient *"rule of 10s"*:

- *10% of pheochromocytomas arise in association with one of several familial syndromes,* including MEN-2A and MEN-2B syndromes (described later), type I neurofibromatosis (neurofibromatosis, café au lait spots, schwannomas, meningiomas, gliomas, pheochromocytomas), von Hippel–Lindau syndrome (visceral cysts, renal cell carcinomas, pheochromocytomas, angiomatosis, cerebellar hemangioblastoma), and Sturge-Weber syndrome (cavernous hemangiomas in trigeminal nerve distribution, pheochromocytomas).
- *10% of pheochromocytomas are extra-adrenal,* occurring in sites such as the organ of Zuckerkandl and the carotid body, where they are usually called *paragangliomas.*
- *10% of nonfamilial adrenal pheochromocytomas are bilateral;* this figure may rise to 70% in cases that are associated with familial syndromes.
- 10% of *adrenal pheochromocytomas are biologically malignant,* although the associated hypertension represents a serious and potentially lethal complication of even "benign"

tumors. Frank malignancy is somewhat more common (20%–40%) in tumors arising in extra-adrenal sites.

* *10% of adrenal pheochromocytomas arise in childhood,* usually the familial subtypes, and with a strong male preponderance. The nonfamilial pheochromocytomas most often occur in adults between ages 40 and 60, with a slight female preponderance.

Morphology

Tumors vary widely in size (1 gm to 4 kg). The cut surface is usually pale gray or brown and is often associated with hemorrhage, necrosis, or cystic change. Usually, the tumors are highly vascular. Fixation of tumor in a dichromate fixative (e.g., Zenker) causes it to turn brown-black because of oxidation of catecholamines (hence the term *chromaffin*). *Microscopically,* the tumors are composed of polygonal to spindle-shaped chromaffin cells or chief cells, clustered with the sustentacular cells into small nests or alveoli (zellballen), by a rich vascular network. Cellular and nuclear pleomorphism is common, and *there is no single histologic feature that can reliably predict clinical behavior in pheochromocytomas.* Large tumor size; *extensive* vascular, capsular, or periadrenal adipose tissue invasion; increased mitotic index (>3 per 10 high-power fields) or atypical mitotic figures; confluent ("sheetlike") tumor necrosis; high cellularity and large tumor nests; cellular monotony; and spindle-cell morphology have been associated with an aggressive behavior. The only reliable criterion of malignancy is metastasis, most commonly to lymph nodes, liver, lungs, and bones.

Clinical Features

The dominant clinical feature in patients with pheochromocytoma is *hypertension*. Classically, this feature is described as an abrupt, precipitous elevation in blood pressure, associated with tachycardia, palpitations, headache, sweating, tremor, and a sense of apprehension. Paroxysmal release of catecholamines may also be associated with episodic headache, anxiety, sweating, tremor, visual disturbances, abdominal pain, and nausea. Sometimes the hypertension is stably elevated. The hypertension may be associated with other organ dysfunction, including congestive heart failure, myocardial infarcts, cardiac arrhythmia, and cerebral hemorrhage. Cardiac complications are attributed to ischemic myocardial damage secondary to catecholamine-induced vasoconstriction *(catecholamine cardiomyopathy)*. Preoperative diagnosis is based on laboratory evaluation, including measurement of urinary catecholamines and their metabolites, plasma catecholamine assays, and radiographic imaging studies.

Tumors of Extra-Adrenal Paraganglia
(p. 1221)

Pheochromocytomas that develop in paraganglia other than the adrenal medulla are often designated *paragangliomas.* Paragangliomas may arise in any organ that contains paraganglionic tissue. Tumors arising in the carotid body are designated *carotid body* tumors, whereas those originating in the jugulotympanic body are sometimes referred to as *chemodectomas.*

The tumors occur most commonly in patients in their teens to 20s and are *multicentric* in 15% to 25% of cases. They are *malignant* in 20% to 40% of cases; 10% of the tumors metastasize widely.

Morphology

Tumors are usually firm, 1- to 6-cm lesions, often densely adherent to adjacent tissues. They are composed of well-differentiated neuroendocrine cells arrayed in nests or cords, separated by prominent fibrovascular stroma. Tumors may contain mitotic figures and may exhibit substantial pleomorphism.

Multiple Endocrine Neoplasia Syndromes
(p. 1221)

Multiple endocrine neoplasias (MEN) are a group of genetically inherited diseases resulting in proliferative lesions (hyperplasia, adenomas, and carcinomas) of multiple endocrine organs (summarized in Table 24–3). Tumors arising in MEN settings have certain distinctive features, including:

* These tumors occur at a *younger age* than sporadic cancers.
* They arise in *multiple endocrine organs,* either *synchronously* (at the same time) or *metachronously* (at different times).
* Even in one organ, the tumors are often *multifocal.*
* The tumors are usually preceded by an *asymptomatic stage of endocrine hyperplasia* involving the cell of origin of the tumor. For example, patients with MEN-1 syndrome develop varying degrees of islet cell hyperplasia, some of which progress to pancreatic tumors.
* These tumors are usually *more aggressive* and *recur* in a higher proportion of cases than similar endocrine tumors that occur sporadically.

Multiple Endocrine Neoplasia, Type 1 (p. 1221)

MEN-1, or *Wermer syndrome,* is characterized by the 3 "Ps":
* *Parathyroid hyperplasia* or *multiple adenomas* are seen in 90% to 95% of cases, appearing by age 40 to 50.
* *Pancreatic lesions* include endocrine tumors, which may secrete a variety of peptide hormones (pancreatic polypeptide being most common overall, while gastrin and insulin are the most frequent hormones associated with clinical symptoms).
* *Pituitary adenomas* are present in 10% to 15% of cases, frequently as prolactinoma.
* Additional tumors include duodenal gastrinomas, carcinoid tumors, and thyroid and adrenocortical adenomas.

The etiology involves germ line mutations in the *MEN-1* gene on chromosome 11q11-13, encoding a 610–amino acid product known as *menin.* The dominant clinical manifestations of MEN-1 syndrome are usually defined by the peptide hormones and include such abnormalities as recurrent hypoglycemia in insulinomas and recurrent peptic ulcers in patients with gastrin-secreting neoplasms (Zollinger-Ellison syndrome).

TABLE 24-3 **Multiple Endocrine Neoplasia (MEN) Syndromes**

	MEN-1	MEN-2A	MEN-2B
Pituitary	Adenomas		
Parathyroid	Hyperplasia +++ Adenomas +	Hyperplasia +	
Pancreatic islets	Hyperplasia ++ Adenomas ++ Carcinomas +++		
Adrenal	Cortical hyperplasia	Pheochromocytoma ++ C-cell hyperplasia +++	Pheochromocytoma +++ C-cell hyperplasia +++
Thyroid		Medullary carcinoma +++	Medullary carcinoma +++
Extraendocrine changes			Mucocutaneous ganglioneuromas Marfanoid habitus
Mutant gene locus	MEN1	RET	RET

Relative frequency: +, uncommon; +++, common.

Multiple Endocrine Neoplasia, Type 2 (p. 1222)

MEN-2 is subclassified into three distinct syndromes: MEN-2A, MEN-2B, and familial medullary thyroid cancer.

MEN-2A or *Sipple syndrome* is clinically and genetically distinct from MEN-1 and has been linked to germ line activating mutations of the *RET protooncogene* on chromosome 10. MEN-2A is characterized as follows:

- *Medullary thyroid carcinomas* arise in 100% of patients and are usually multifocal. C-cell hyperplasia is almost always present. In addition to *calcitonin,* medullary carcinomas may elaborate other biologically active peptides. Most tumors pursue a malignant course, and prophylactic thyroidectomy is recommended for germ line *RET* mutation carriers.

- *Pheochromocytomas* are present in 50% of patients, are often bilateral, and may be extra-adrenal. Most lesions are clinically benign.

- *Parathyroid hyperplasias* are found in 10% to 20% of cases with evidence of hypercalcemia or renal stones.

MEN-2B is clinically similar to MEN-2A, with additional features of *neuromas* or *ganglioneuromas* involving lips, oral cavity, eyes, respiratory tract, gastrointestinal tract, urinary bladder, and other sites, and a *marfanoid habitus,* with long axial skeletal features and hyperextensible joints. A single amino acid change in *RET* ($RET^{Met918Thr}$), distinct from the mutational spectra seen in MEN-2A, appears to be responsible for virtually all cases of MEN-2B.

Familial medullary thyroid cancer is a variant of MEN-2A, with a strong predisposition to thyroid malignancy but without the other clinical manifestations.

PINEAL GLAND (p. 1223)

Pineal region neoplasms account for less than 1% of brain tumors; they include both *germ cell* tumors (resembling those arising in the gonads) and neoplasms of *pineal parenchymal origin.*

Pinealomas (p. 1223) are classified as *pineoblastomas* or *pineocytomas,* depending on the level of differentiation.

- *Pineoblastomas* occur predominantly in the pediatric population and are composed of *primitive embryonal cells* reminiscent of cerebellar medulloblastomas (i.e., a "small blue cell" tumor). They may *invade* local structures and *metastasize* via cerebrospinal fluid pathways. Most patients die within 1 to 2 years.

- *Pineocytomas* are more common in adults and are composed of a variable mixture of *glial* and *neuronal* elements, recapitulating the structure of the mature pineal gland. There is prolonged survival (average 7 years).

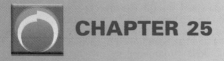

CHAPTER 25

The Skin

THE SKIN: MORE THAN A MECHANICAL BARRIER (p. 1228)

More than just a passive barrier to fluid loss and mechanical injury, skin is composed of interdependent cell types all contributing to its *protective* function:

- *Squamous epithelial cells (keratinocytes)* make up the majority of epidermal cells and the major mechanical barrier; they are also a source of cytokines that regulate the cutaneous environment.
- *Melanocytes* produce *melanin* pigment to screen ultraviolet light.
- *Langerhans cells:* Dendritic cells process and present antigen to activate the immune system.
- *Neural end organs* detect pain and temperature.
- *Sweat glands* permit cooling.
- *Hair follicles* elaborate hair shafts and are repositories for epithelial stem cells.

Definitions

Macroscopic Terms (p. 1229):

Blister Common term for vesicle or bulla

Bulla Elevated fluid-filled lesion larger than 5 mm

Excoriation Linear, traumatic lesion resulting in epidermal breakage (i.e., a deep scratch)

Lichenification Thick, rough skin with prominent skin markings, often due to repeated rubbing

Macule Flat, circumscribed area distinguished from surrounding skin by coloration

Nodule Elevated solid area larger than 5 mm

Onycholysis Loss of nail substance

Papule Elevated solid area 5 mm or smaller

Plaque Elevated flat-topped lesion larger than 5 mm

Pustule Discrete, pus-filled raised area

Scale Dry, platelike excrescence resulting from aberrant cornification

Vesicle Elevated fluid-filled lesion 5 mm or smaller

Wheal Pruritic, erythematous elevated area resulting from dermal edema

Microscopic Terms (p. 1230):

Acantholysis Loss of intercellular connections between keratinocytes

Acanthosis Epidermal hyperplasia

Dyskeratosis Abnormal keratinization below the stratum corneum

Erosion Focal, incomplete loss of epidermis

Exocytosis Inflammatory cells infiltrating the epidermis

Hyperkeratosis Stratum corneum thickening, often with aberrant keratinization

Lentiginous Linear pattern of melanocyte proliferation in the epidermal basal cell layer; may be reactive or neoplastic

Papillomatosis Elongation or widening of the dermal papillae

Parakeratosis Abnormal retention of nuclei in stratum corneum

Spongiosis Epidermal intercellular edema

Ulceration Focal, complete loss of epidermis; may include dermis and subcutaneous fat

Vacuolization Vacuoles within or adjacent to cells

DISORDERS OF PIGMENTATION AND MELANOCYTES (p. 1230)

Vitiligo (p. 1230)

Vitiligo is a common disorder presenting as irregular, well-demarcated macules (few to many centimeters) devoid of pigmentation. It occurs in all races but is most apparent in darkly pigmented individuals. It often involves the wrists, axillae, and perioral, periorbital, and anogenital regions.

Pathogenesis

- Autoimmune etiology (best supported by the data, including melanocyte autoantibodies and T-cell, macrophage, or Langerhans cell abnormalities)
- Neurohumoral factors
- Toxic intermediates in melanin synthesis

Morphology

Histologically, loss of melanocytes is seen. This finding contrasts with some forms of *albinism,* in which melanocytes are present but nonfunctional.

Freckles (Ephelis) (p. 1231)

Freckles are common pigmented lesions of childhood: tan-red to brown macules, measuring 1 to 10 mm, occurring after sun exposure, and fading and recurring with subsequent cycles of winter and summer.

Morphology

Histologically, there is a normal melanocyte number (possibly slight hypertrophy) but increased melanin within basal keratinocytes.

Melasma (p. 1231)

Melasma refers to mask-like facial hyperpigmentation, typically seen in hyperestrogenic states such as pregnancy. It presents as blotchy, irregular, ill-defined macules. Sunlight accentuates the pigmentation, which usually fades postpartum. Melasma is caused by enhanced melanin transfer (and accumulation) from melanocytes to other cell types.

Morphology

Histologically, melasma is characterized by:

- Increased melanin deposition in basal layers *(epidermal type)*
- Papillary dermal macrophage phagocytosis of melanin released from the epidermis (i.e., pigment incontinence *[dermal type]*)

Lentigo (p. 1232)

Lentigo (plural, *lentigines*) is a common, benign, hyperpigmented macule (5–10 mm) in skin and mucous membranes, most often occurring in infancy and childhood. In contrast to freckles, lentigines do not darken with sun exposure. The cause and pathogenesis are unknown.

Morphology

Histologically, there is linear basal hyperpigmentation resulting from melanocyte hyperplasia, often with elongation and thinning of rete ridges.

Melanocytic Nevus (Pigmented Nevus, Mole) (p. 1232)

Melanocytic nevus specifically refers to a group of congenital or acquired *melanocyte neoplasms*. Clinically, common acquired nevocellular nevi are well-demarcated, uniformly tanbrown papules measuring 6 mm or less; features of common variants are described in Table 25–1.

Pathogenesis

- Melanocytes of nevocellular nevi derive from basal cells that have transformed into round-oval cells with uniform nuclei and inconspicuous nucleoli.
- Nevi initially form nests along the dermoepidermal junction: *junctional nevi.*
- Eventually, most junctional nevi also extend nests and cords into the underlying dermis: *compound nevi.*
- In mature lesions, the epidermal component may be lost: *dermal nevi.*
- With extension into the dermis, the *nevus cells undergo* maturation, becoming nonpigmented and resembling neural

TABLE 25–1 Variant Forms of Nevocellular Nevi

Nevus Variant	Diagnostic Architectural Features	Diagnostic Cytologic Features	Clinical Significance
Congenital nevus	Deep dermal and sometimes subcutaneous growth around adnexa, neurovascular bundles, and blood vessel walls	Identical to ordinary acquired nevi	Present at birth; large variants have increased melanoma risk
Blue nevus	Non-nested dermal infiltration, often with associated fibrosis	Highly dendritic, heavily pigmented nevus cells	Black-blue nodule; often confused with melanoma clinically
Spindle and epithelioid cell nevus (Spitz nevus)	Fascicular growth	Large, plump cells with pink-blue cytoplasm; fusiform cells	Common in children; red-pink nodule; often confused with hemangioma clinically
Halo nevus	Lymphocytic infiltration surrounding nevus cells	Indentical to ordinary acquired nevi	Host immune response against nevus cells and surrounding normal melanocytes
Dysplastic nevus	Large, coalescent intraepidermal nests	Cytologic atypia	Potential precursor of malignant melanoma

tissue. This is diagnostically important because *melanomas usually show no maturation.*

Clinical Features

Nevocellular nevi are significant largely as a model of tumor progression and possibly for cosmetic reasons.

Dysplastic Nevi (p. 1233)

Dysplastic nevi arise as a manifestation of an autosomal dominant (gene on chromosome 1) predisposition to develop atypical acquired nevi; these may evolve into malignant melanoma (50% of affected individuals by age 59 years). Dysplastic nevi may also occur as isolated sporadic lesions with a low risk of malignant transformation. Usually, these lesions are larger than typical acquired nevi (>5 mm) and may occur as hundreds of irregular macules or plaques with pigment variegation on both sun-exposed and nonexposed skin (in contrast to typical moles).

Morphology

Histologically, there is cytologic and architectural atypia, with enlarged and fused epidermal nevus cell nests, lentiginous melanocytic hyperplasia, linear papillary dermal fibrosis, and pigment incontinence.

Clinical Features

The risk of developing melanoma *(heritable melanoma syndrome)* is increased for unaffected skin as well as for areas with preexisting nevi. However, most dysplastic nevi are clinically stable.

Malignant Melanoma (p. 1234)

Malignant melanoma is a relatively common neoplasm, currently increasing in incidence; sun exposure is an important pathogenic factor, and lightly pigmented individuals are at greater risk than darkly pigmented persons. Hereditary substrates (e.g., dysplastic nevus syndrome) also increase the risk. These pruritic, variegated, irregular maculopapular lesions are most commonly found on skin but occasionally involve the mucosae, conjunctiva, orbit, nail beds, esophagus, and leptomeninges. In contrast to benign nevi, melanomas may be black, brown, red-blue, or gray.

Diagnostically important is a change in coloration. Typically a melanoma initially extends horizontally within the epidermis and superficial dermis *(radial growth phase)* during which time it does not metastasize. Specific types of radial growth phase melanomas (e.g., *lentigo maligna* and *superficial spreading*) are defined by architectural and cytologic features and exhibit different biologic behaviors. Eventually a *vertical growth phase* evolves, with extension into the deep dermis, loss of cellular maturation, and development of a metastatic capacity. The clinical behavior (e.g., *probability of metastasis*) is determined by the characteristics and measured depth of invasion of the vertical growth; prediction of the clinical outcome can be further refined by the mitotic rate and extent of lymphocytic infiltrates.

Morphology

Histologically, melanoma cells are larger than nevus cells, with irregular nuclei and prominent eosinophilic nucleoli; they grow as loose nests lacking the typical features of melanocyte maturation. Mitoses, often atypical, are uncommon in both radial and ventrical growth phases.

BENIGN EPITHELIAL TUMORS (p. 1237)

These benign tumors are common, generally biologically inconsequential lesions derived from keratinocytes or skin appendages.

Seborrheic Keratoses (p. 1237)

Seborrheic keratoses are spontaneous lesions, most often occurring in middle-aged and older individuals and most numerous on the trunk (also called *senile keratoses*). Similar smaller facial lesions in nonwhites are called *dermatosis papulosa nigra.* They may occur spontaneously in large numbers as part of a paraneoplastic syndrome *(sign of Leser-Trélat),* possibly as a result of tumor elaboration of growth factors (e.g., transforming growth factor-α).

Morphology

Grossly, seborrheic keratoses are uniform, tan-brown, velvety or granular round plaques millimeters to several centimeters in diameter; keratin-filled plugs may be evident.

Histologically, seborrheic keratoses are sharply demarcated, exophytic lesions with hyperplasia of variably pigmented basaloid cells and *hyperkeratosis;* there are occasional keratin-filled *horn cysts.* When irritated and inflamed, the basaloid cells undergo squamous differentiation. When associated with hair follicle epithelium, lesions are endophytic, growing downward *(inverted follicular keratoses).*

Acanthosis Nigricans (p. 1237)

Acanthosis nigricans refers to thickened, hyperpigmented zones, typically in flexural areas (axilla, groin, neck, anogenital region), associated with benign and malignant conditions elsewhere in the body.

- The *benign* type makes up 80% of all cases; it develops gradually, usually arising in childhood through puberty.

  It is an autosomal dominant trait with variable penetrance
  It occurs in association with obesity or endocrine disorders (especially diabetes and pituitary or pineal tumors).
  It can be a component of certain rare congenital disorders.

- The *malignant* type arises in middle-aged and older individuals, often in association with an occult adenocarcinoma (possibly due to tumor elaboration of epidermal growth factors).

Morphology

Histologically, both types are characterized by hyperkeratosis, with prominent rete ridges and basal hyperpigmentation (without melanocyte hyperplasia).

Fibroepithelial Polyp (p. 1238)

Also called *acrochordon, squamous papilloma,* or *skin tag,* fibroepithelial polyps are found on the neck, trunk, face, or intertriginous zones and are exceptionally common benign lesions in middle-aged and older individuals. These are soft, flesh-colored tumors attached by a slender fibrovascular stalk covered by benign epidermis. They may be associated with pregnancy, diabetes, or intestinal polyposis.

Epithelial Cysts (Wens) (p. 1238)

Epithelial cysts are common lesions presenting as well-circumscribed, firm, subcutaneous nodules, formed by downgrowth and cystic expansion of the epidermal or follicular epithelium.

Morphology

Histologically, they are subdivided on the basis of the cyst wall characteristics. All are filled with keratin and variable amounts of lipid and debris from sebaceous secretions.

- *Epidermal inclusion cysts:* The wall is almost identical to normal epidermis.
- *Pilar (trichilemmal) cysts:* The wall resembles follicular epithelium (i.e., without a granular cell layer).
- *Dermoid cysts:* The wall is similar to epidermis but with multiple skin appendages, especially hair follicles.
- *Steatocystoma multiplex:* The wall resembles sebaceous gland ductal epithelium with numerous compressed sebaceous lobules (frequently occurs as a dominantly inherited lesion).

Adnexal (Appendage) Tumors (p. 1238)

Adnexal tumors are typically benign neoplasms arising from skin appendages. Although most are localized and not aggressive, others can be confused with cutaneous malignancies; a subset can be malignant (e.g., *sebaceous carcinoma* arising in eyelid meibomian glands). Certain of these tumors have a mendelian pattern of inheritance and occur as multiple disfiguring lesions; in other instances, they can serve as markers for visceral malignancies (e.g., multiple trichilemmomas and breast cancer occurring in *Cowden syndrome*).

Morphology

Nondescript flesh-colored solitary to multiple papules and nodules are seen. Occasionally they show a predilection for specific anatomic sites (e.g., *eccrine poromas* on palms and soles).

- *Cylindromas* occur typically as multiple coalescing nodules of basaloid cells with apocrine differentiation on the scalp and forehead *(turban tumor).*
- *Syringomas* usually occur as multiple, small, tan papules near the lower eyelids composed of tadpole-shaped islands of basaloid epithelium with focal eccrine differentiation.
- *Trichoepitheliomas* usually present as multiple flesh-colored papules on the face, scalp, neck, and upper trunk; proliferations of basaloid cells form hair follicle-like structures.

- *Trichilemmomas* are proliferations of cells resembling the uppermost portion of the hair follicle.
- *Hidradenoma papilliferum* occurs on the face and scalp; it is composed of ducts and papillae lined by apocrine-type cells.

Keratoacanthoma (p. 1239)

Keratoacanthoma is a self-limited, often *spontaneously resolving,* rapid-growing lesion, typically occurring in sun-exposed skin of whites 50 years of age and older, in men more often than women. Most have detectable p53 oncoprotein (occasionally with mutations), suggesting that these may represent a form of *squamous cell carcinoma* (see later discussion) that regresses because of host-tumor interactions.

Morphology

Grossly, keratoacanthomas appear as flesh-colored, dome-shaped nodules with central keratin-filled craters, often on the face or hands, measuring 1 cm to several centimeters.

Histologically, cup-shaped epithelial proliferations are seen, often with atypical cells, enclosing a central keratin-filled plug. The pattern of keratinization recapitulates the normal hair follicle (no granular cell layer). Minimal inflammation occurs during the rapid proliferative phase, but as the lesion matures, dermal inflammation and fibrosis supervene, with eventual regression and disappearance.

PREMALIGNANT AND MALIGNANT EPIDERMAL TUMORS (p. 1240)

Actinic Keratosis (p. 1240)

Actinic keratosis refers to a premalignant dysplastic lesion (not to be confused with seborrheic keratosis) associated with chronic sun exposure, especially in light-skinned individuals. Ionizing radiation, hydrocarbons, and arsenicals may induce similar lesions. Because many undergo malignant transformation, local eradication is indicated.

Morphology

Grossly, these lesions are usually smaller than 1 cm, tan-brown, red, or flesh-colored, with a rough consistency. Hyperkeratosis may produce cutaneous horns.

Histologically, there is cytologic atypia in the lower epidermis, frequently with basal cell hyperplasia and dyskeratosis. Intercellular bridges are present. *Hyperkeratosis* and *parakeratosis* may be present, or there may be epidermal atrophy. The dermis contains thickened, blue-gray elastic fibers *(elastosis),* resulting from aberrant synthesis by sun-damaged fibroblasts.

Squamous Cell Carcinoma (p. 1241)

The most common tumor of sun-exposed skin of older individuals, squamous cell carcinoma occurs more frequently in men than in women, with the exception of lower leg lesions. *Sunlight (specifically ultraviolet irradiation)* is the greatest predisposing factor, primarily by directly damaging DNA and causing mutations. Ultraviolet light also causes immunosuppression by injuring antigen-presenting Langerhans cells and augmenting the development of suppressor T lymphocytes. Other predisposing factors include industrial carcinogens (tars), chronic skin ulcers, old burn scars, draining osteomyelitis, ionizing radiation, and (for oral mucosa) tobacco or betel nut chewing. Immunosuppression (as a consequence of chemotherapy or tissue transplantation) and xeroderma pigmentosum (an inherited defect in DNA repair, Chapter 7) increase tumor risk; human papillomavirus (e.g., HPV 36) may also occasionally contribute.

Morphology

Grossly, in situ squamous cell carcinoma appears as well-demarcated, red, scaling plaques. *Invasive lesions* are nodular, variably hyperkeratotic, and prone to ulceration. Mucosal involvement is manifested as white thickening called *leukoplakia.* Most tumors remain localized, with less than 5% metastasis to regional nodes at the time of resection.

Microscopically, in situ carcinoma has full-thickness epidermal atypia (versus actinic keratosis, which has only basal atypia). *Invasive tumors* vary from well differentiated (with prominent keratinization) to highly anaplastic with necrosis and abortive keratinization.

Basal Cell Carcinoma (p. 1242)

Basal cell carcinomas are common, slow-growing tumors, typically found in sun-exposed skin; *they rarely metastasize.* Immunosuppression and xeroderma pigmentosum increase the incidence.

Morphology

Grossly, basal cell carcinomas appear as pearly papules or expanding plaques; some are melanin pigmented. Advanced lesions ulcerate, and there can be extensive local invasion, termed *rodent ulcer.*

Microscopically, there is uniform, rather monotonous basal cell proliferation, either as *multifocal superficial growths* over a large area (several centimeters) of skin or as *nodules* extending deeply into the dermis. Anaplasia, mitoses, and tumor giant cells are absent.

Merkel Cell Carcinoma (p. 1244)

Merkel cells are functionally obscure epidermal, neural crest–derived cells (possibly involved in lower animal tactile sensation). Merkel cell carcinoma is a rare, potentially lethal tumor composed of small, round malignant cells containing neurosecretory-type cytoplasmic granules that closely resemble small cell carcinoma in the lung.

Molecular Genetics of Skin Cancer (p. 1244)

Much has been learned about the molecular underpinnings of skin cancers from otherwise rare hereditary cancer syndromes that also happen to have frequent skin manifestations (Table 25–2).

TABLE 25-2 A Survey of Familial Cancer Syndromes with Cutaneous Manifestations

Disease	Inheritance	Chromosomal Location	Gene/Protein	Function/Manifestation
Ataxia-telangiectasia	AR	11q22.3	AT/AT[†]	DNA repair after radiation injury; p53 signaling/neurologic and vascular lesions
Nevoid basal cell carcinoma syndrome	AD	9q22.3	PTCH//PTCH	Developmental gene/multiple basal cell carcinomas; jaw cysts, etc.
Cowden syndrome	AD	10q23	PTEN, MMAC1/PTEN, TEP1, MMAC1	Lipid/protein phosphatase/benign follicular appendage tumors (trichilemmomas); internal adenocarcinoma
Familial melanoma syndrome	AD	9p21	CDKN2/p16INK4	Inhibits CDKs from phosphorylating Rb, thus arresting cell cycle/melanoma
			CDKN2/p14ARF	Binds MDM2 and thus, preserves p53/melanoma
Muir-Torre syndrome	AD	2p22	hMSH2/hMSH2	Involved in DNA mismatch repair/benign and malignant sebaceous tumors; internal adenocarcinoma
Neurofibromatosis I	AD	17q11.2	NF1/neurofibromin	Negatively regulates Ras family of signal molecules/neurofibromas
Neurofibromatosis II	AD	22q12.2	NF2/merlin	Integrates cytoskeletal signaling/neurofibromas and acoustic neuromas
Tuberous sclerosis	AD	9q34	TSC1/hamartin	Interacts with tuberin; function unknown
		16p13.3	TSC2/tuberin	Interacts with hamartin; may regulate Ras proteins/angiofibromas, mental retardation
Xeroderma pigmentosum	AR	9q22 and others	XPA/XPA and others	Nucleotide excision repair/melanoma and nonmelanoma skin cancers

AD, Autosomal dominant; AR, autosomal recessive.
[†]By convention, genes are italicized and proteins are not italicized.

Nevoid Basal Cell Carcinoma Syndrome

Nevoid basal cell carcinoma syndrome (NBCCS; also known as basal cell nevus syndrome or Gorlin syndrome) is a rare (1:56,000) autosomal dominant disorder characterized by multiple basal cell carcinomas, usually manifesting before age 20. Patients also develop medulloblastomas, ovarian fibromas, odontogenic keratocysts, pits of the palms and soles, and multiple developmental abnormalities.

The responsible *PTCH* gene on chromosome 9q22.3 is the human homologue for the *Drosophila* developmental gene *patched;* it encodes for a receptor for the protein product of the *sonic hedgehog gene (SHH)*. Normally, the PTCH protein binds to another transmembrane protein (SMO) preventing it from activating multiple downstream regulatory pathways. When *SHH* and PTCH interact, SMO is released to trigger downstream target activation, including transcription factors important for cell cycle regulation. Germ line mutations of *PTCH* (as in NBCSS) or sporadic mutations in *PTCH* or *SMO* (as in sporadic basal cell carcinoma) lead to the increased incidence of basal cell carcinomas. In *xeroderma pigmentosum,* a disorder of DNA repair, UV-induced DNA damage frequently leads to basal cell carcinomas secondary to *PTCH* or *p53* mutations.

Melanomas

Approximately 10% to 15% of melanomas arise in a familial setting, frequently when there are large numbers of dysplastic nevi. *Familial melanoma syndrome (FMS)* does not have a straightforward mendelian mode of inheritance, but the main locus of the genetic predisposition has been mapped to chromosome 9p21 involving the cyclin-dependent kinase inhibitor 2. *CDNK2* is frequently deleted in melanomas, leading to relatively unrestricted RB phosphorylation, E2F release, and uncontrolled cell proliferation.

TUMORS OF THE DERMIS (p. 1247)

Benign Fibrous Histiocytoma (Dermatofibroma) (p. 1247)

Benign fibrous histiocytoma describes a heterogeneous group of benign, indolent neoplasms of dermal fibroblasts and histiocytes. Lesions are usually seen in adults and frequently appear on the legs of young to middle-aged women. Histogenesis is unknown, although antecedent trauma and aberrant healing are often implicated. Benign fibrous histiocytoma should not be confused with clinically aggressive malignant fibrous histiocytoma, arising in skin and extracutaneous sites.

Morphology

Grossly, there are tan-brown, sometimes tender, usually firm papules, which may achieve several centimeters in diameter. Lateral compression causes them to dimple inward.

Histologically, the most common form is the *dermatofibroma,* composed of spindle-shaped fibroblasts in a well-defined, mid-dermal nonencapsulated mass, frequently extending into the subcutaneous fat. Other variants have conspicuous foamy histiocytes with fewer fibroblasts or have numerous blood vessels and hemosiderin deposits *(sclerosing hemangioma)*.

Dermatofibrosarcoma Protuberans (p. 1248)

This well-differentiated, slow-growing fibrosarcoma of the skin is locally aggressive but rarely metastasizes.

Morphology

Grossly, these are firm, solid nodules arising as protuberant, occasionally ulcerated aggregates within an indurated plaque, typically on the trunk.

Microscopically, these cellular neoplasms are composed of radially oriented (storiform) fibroblasts; mitoses are not as numerous as in fibrosarcoma. The overlying epidermis is thinned, and there often is microscopic extension into subcutaneous fat.

Xanthomas (p. 1248)

Xanthomas are not true neoplasms but rather focal accumulations of foamy histiocytes. They may be idiopathic or associated with familial or acquired hyperlipidemias or lymphoproliferative disorders. *Microscopically,* all lesions are characterized by variably cellular dermal aggregates of macrophages with vacuolated cytoplasm containing cholesterol, phospholipids, and triglycerides. They may be subdivided on the basis of the gross appearance and associated hyperlipidemias:

- *Eruptive xanthoma:* Sudden showers of yellow papules wax and wane with plasma triglyceride and lipid levels; they occur on the buttocks, posterior thighs, knees, and elbows *(hyperlipidemia types I, IIB, III, IV, and V).*
- *Tuberous xanthoma:* Yellow, flat-round nodules occur over the joints, especially knees and elbows *(types IIA and III).*
- *Tendinous xanthoma:* Yellow nodules occur over the Achilles tendon and finger extensor tendons *(types IIA and III).*
- *Plane xanthoma:* Linear yellow lesions are found in skin folds, especially palmar creases *(type III).* Occasionally plane xanthoma is associated with primary biliary cirrhosis *(type IIA).*
- *Xanthelasma:* Soft, yellow plaques occur on the eyelids (types IIA and III, or without lipid abnormality).

Dermal Vascular Tumors (p. 1248)

Hemangiomas and malignant vascular tumors, Kaposi sarcoma, and bacillary angiomatosis are discussed in Chapter 11. *Capillary hemangiomas* are the most common form of cutaneous vascular tumors. Occurring throughout life as dark pink papules, *histologically* there are well-demarcated clusters of endothelium-lined and blood-filled vascular spaces in the dermis.

TUMORS OF CELLULAR IMMIGRANTS TO THE SKIN (p. 1249)

These tumors are proliferative disorders of cells that have arisen elsewhere but that have homed to the skin (e.g., Langerhans cells, T lymphocytes, and mast cells).

Langerhans Cell Histiocytosis (p. 1249)

The systemic pattern of histiocytosis is discussed in Chapter 14. The *cutaneous form* may present as solitary or multiple papules or nodules or as scaling erythematous plaques resembling seborrheic dermatitis.

Morphology

Histologic lesions include variable numbers of eosinophils and diffuse to granulomatous dermal infiltrates of round-ovoid mononuclear cells with indented, bland nuclei; occasionally the mononuclear cells have foamy, xanthoma-like cytoplasm. Ultrastructural demonstrations of Birbeck granules and immunohistochemical documentation of CD1 antigens on the infiltrating cells confirm their Langerhans cell derivation.

Mycosis Fungoides (Cutaneous T-Cell Lymphoma) (p. 1249)

Various patterns may be seen:
- A chronic proliferative process—*mycosis fungoides*
- A nodular eruptive variant—*mycosis fungoides d'emblée*
- A form with an aggressive course called *adult T-cell leukemia* or *lymphoma* (attributed to human T-cell lymphotropic virus type 1)

Mycosis fungoides arises primarily in the skin and generally remains localized there for many years. *Sézary syndrome* occurs with seeding of the blood by malignant T cells, accompanied by diffuse erythema and scaling *(erythroderma)*; it represents evolution into a more generalized T-cell leukemia or lymphoma.

Morphology

Grossly, mycosis fungoides initially presents as eczema-like lesions, evolving into scaly, red-brown patches or plaques, and eventually into fungating nodules (up to 10 cm) on the trunk, extremities, face, and scalp. Nodular cutaneous growth correlates with deep dermal invasion and the onset of lymph node and visceral involvement.

The *histologic hallmark* of mycosis fungoides is the *Sézary-Lutzner cell,* a malignant CD4+ (T-helper) cell with a hyperconvoluted or *cerebriform* nucleus. These typically form bandlike dermal infiltrates with invasion by single cells or small clusters into the epidermis *(Pautrier microabscesses).*

Mastocytosis (p. 1250)

This family of rare disorders is characterized by cutaneous (and occasionally visceral) mast cell proliferation. Symptoms reflect the consequences of mast cell degranulation, with release of histamine (e.g., pruritus, flushing, rhinorrhea, or dermal edema and erythema). The dermal change results in a *wheal* when lesional skin is rubbed *(Darier sign)* and *dermatographism* when evoked in normal skin. Rarely, epistaxis or gastrointestinal bleeding occurs secondary to heparin release from the mast cells.

Urticaria pigmentosa (50% of all cases) is an exclusively cutaneous form of mastocytosis, with a generally favorable prognosis, occurring mainly in children. Systemic mastocytosis occurs in 10% of patients, usually adults, and carries a much poorer prognosis. The *pathogenesis* (at least in some cases) is due to point mutations of the c-*KIT* proto-oncogene, resulting in activation of the KIT tyrosine kinase that directs mast cell growth and differentiation.

Morphology

Grossly, skin lesions of urticaria pigmentosa and systemic mastocytosis are multiple, round-oval, nonscaling, red-brown papules and plaques.

Microscopically, variable dermal fibrosis, edema, eosinophils, and numerous mast cells may be seen.

DISORDER OF EPIDERMAL MATURATION (p. 1251)

Ichthyosis (p. 1251)

One of many disorders that impair epidermal maturation, ichthyosis is actually a collection of generally hereditary (autosomal dominant, recessive, or X-linked) clinical entities, presenting at or near birth with marked hyperkeratosis grossly resembling fish scales (hence the name). Acquired variants exist and may be associated with various malignancies. The disorder is clinically grouped according to the mode of inheritance and clinical and histologic features. The primary defect in most forms is increased cell-cell adhesion resulting in abnormal desquamation and consequently scale formation.

Morphology

Microscopically, ichthyosis is characterized by accrual of compacted stratum corneum, with minimal inflammation and subtle changes in epidermal and stratum granulosum thickness.

Acute Inflammatory Dermatoses (p. 1252)

Acute inflammatory dermatoses constitute an enormous family of conditions, mediated by local or systemic immunologic factors and characterized by short-lived lesions (days to weeks) marked by mononuclear cell infiltrates with associated edema and occasionally local tissue damage.

Urticaria (p. 1252)

Urticaria (also known as "hives") is a common disorder, typically occurring in young adults and marked by focal mast cell degranulation, with histamine-mediated dermal pruritus, edema, and wheal formation. Individual lesions develop and regress within hours, but sequential lesions may occur for months. *Angioedema* is related but is distinguished by *dermal* and *subcutaneous fat* edema.

Pathogenesis

Most lesions are mediated by antigen-specific IgE, but *IgE-independent urticaria* can occur by direct chemical-induced mast cell degranulation in sensitive patients or by suppression of prostaglandin synthesis (i.e., with aspirin). Persistent urticaria may reflect an inability to clear the inciting antigen or can reflect cryptic collagen vascular disorders or Hodgkin lymphoma.

Hereditary angioneurotic edema consists of recurrent attacks of angioedema with gastrointestinal tract and laryngeal involvement. It is due to deficient C1 esterase inhibitor and unregulated activation of the early complement components.

Morphology

Grossly, lesions vary from small, pruritic papules to large edematous plaques. Sites of predilection include any area exposed to pressure, such as the trunk, distal extremities, and ears.

Microscopically, there is a sparse mononuclear perivascular infiltrate associated with edema and occasionally with dermal eosinophils but no evidence of increased mast cell numbers.

Acute Eczematous Dermatitis (p. 1253)

Acute eczematous dermatitis refers to a variety of pathogenically unique conditions, all with similar histologic features. Five types, distinguished primarily by their clinical features, are described in Table 25–3. Many forms of *eczema* constitute a cutaneous delayed-type hypersensitivity response, with pathogenesis attributed to cytokine release and nonspecific recruitment of the bulk of the inflammatory cells.

Morphology

Grossly, all types of acute eczema are pruritic, red, papulovesicular to blistered, oozing, and subsequently crusted lesions (e.g., contact hypersensitivity to poison ivy). With chronic exposure, lesions may evolve into psoriasis-like scaling plaques. Bacterial superinfection produces a yellow crust *(impetiginization)*.

Histologically, there is initially *spongiosis;* with progressive fluid accumulation, keratinocytes splay apart, and intraepidermal vesicles form. There is also a dermal perivascular lymphocytic infiltrate with mast cell degranulation and papillary dermal edema. Lesions resulting from drug hypersensitivity may have eosinophils. In chronic lesions, the vesicular phase is replaced with progressive *acanthosis* and *hyperkeratosis.*

Erythema Multiforme (p. 1255)

Erythema multiforme is an uncommon, self-limited hypersensitivity response to certain drugs or infections or to systemic disorders (malignancy or collagen vascular diseases), characterized by extensive epidermal degeneration and necrosis. It is due to CD8+ T cell–mediated cytotoxicity and has similarities to other immunologic cutaneous disorders, such as graft-versus-host disease and skin allograft rejection.

TABLE 25–3   Classification of Eczematous Dermatitis

Type	Cause or Pathogenesis	Histology*	Clinical Features
Contact dermatitis	Topically applied antigens	Spongiotic dermatitis	Marked itching, burning, or both; requires antecedent exposure
Atopic dermatitis	Unknown; may be heritable	Spongiotic dermatitis	Erythematous plaques in flexural areas; family history of eczema, hay fever, or asthma
Drug-related eczematous dermatitis	Systemically administered antigens or haptens (e.g., penicillin)	Spongiotic dermatitis; infiltrate often deeper with abundant eosinophils	Temporal relationship to drug administration; remits with cessation of drug
Eczematous insect bite reaction	Locally injected antigen or toxin	Spongiotic dermatitis; wedge-shaped infiltrate; many eosinophils	Papules, nodules, and plaques with vesicles; may be linear when multiple
Photoeczematous eruption	Ultraviolet light	Spongiotic dermatitis; infiltrate that diminishes gradually with depth	Occurs at sites of sun exposure; may require associated exposure to systemic or topical antigen; photopatch testing may help in diagnosis
Primary irritant dermatitis	Repeated trauma or chemical irritants (as in detergent)	Spongiotic dermatitis in early stages; acanthosis predominates in later stages	Localized mechanical or chemical irritants (nonimmunologic)

*All types, with time, may develop chronic changes, with prominent acanthosis of the epidermal layer.

Morphology

Grossly, lesions are *multiform* and include macules, papules, vesicles, and bullae as well as characteristic *targets* consisting of red maculopapular lesions with central pallor. Symmetric involvement of the extremities is common.

Microscopically, early lesions of erythema multiforme show dermal-epidermal junction and superficial perivascular lymphocytic infiltrates with dermal edema and focal basal keratinocyte degeneration and necrosis. *Exocytosis* is associated with epidermal necrosis, blistering, and shallow erosions. *Target lesions* show central epidermal necrosis with associated perivenular inflammation.

Clinical Features

A severe, febrile form typically occurring in children is called *Stevens-Johnson syndrome;* it is marked by erosions and hemorrhagic crusting of the lips, oral mucosa, conjunctiva, urethra, and anogenital regions. Bacterial superinfection may be life threatening.

Toxic epidermal necrolysis is another variant, characterized by diffuse mucocutaneous epithelial necrosis and sloughing; it is clinically analogous to extensive third-degree burns.

Chronic Inflammatory Dermatoses (p. 1256)

These persistent inflammatory disorders (months to years) are characterized by excessive or abnormal scaling and shedding *(desquamation)*. These dermatoses are to be distinguished from noninflammatory scaling lesions, such as *ichthyosis* (see previous discussion).

Psoriasis (p. 1256)

Psoriasis is a common disorder (1%–2% of the U.S. population). An association with certain human leukocyte antigen (HLA) types suggests a genetic component; the genesis of new lesions at sites of trauma *(Koebner phenomenon)* suggests a role for exogenous stimuli. Nonspecific damage to the stratum corneum may unmask new antigens with subsequent antibody deposition and secondary complement-mediated injury. Alternatively, lesions may evolve at sites of abnormally reactive endothelium. Lymphocytes from psoriatic patients also induce dermal angiogenesis and keratinocyte growth, suggesting that the disease may actually be a manifestation of systemic immune dysfunction.

Psoriasis may be associated with other diseases, including myopathies, enteropathies, acquired immunodeficiency syndrome (AIDS), and mild to deforming arthritis (resembling rheumatoid arthritis).

Morphology

Grossly, findings include the following:

- Well-demarcated, salmon-pink plaques with silvery scaling usually occur on the elbows, knees, scalp, lumbosacral area, intergluteal cleft, and glans penis. *Annular, linear, gyrate,* or *serpiginous* variations occur.
- Psoriasis may also present as total body scaling and erythema—*erythroderma.*

- Nail changes (discoloration, pitting, onycholysis) occur in 30% of patients.
- *Pustular psoriasis* is a rare variant in which multiple small pustules form on erythematous plaques; when generalized, it can be life threatening.

Microscopically, there is marked acanthosis with rete elongation and mitoses well above the basal layer. The stratum granulosum is thinned or absent, with extensive overlying parakeratosis. Epidermis over the dermal papillae is thinned; dilated vessels in these papillae yield pinpoint bleeds when the overlying scale is removed *(Auspitz sign).*

Aggregates of epidermal neutrophils occur within small spongiotic foci in the stratum spinosum *(spongiform pustules)* or within the parakeratotic stratum corneum *(Munro microabscesses).* Larger, abscess-like accumulations may also occur in pustular psoriasis.

Seborrheic Dermatitis (p. 1257)

Seborrheic dermatitis is even more common than psoriasis; although it typically involves cutaneous areas that have high densities of sebaceous glands (e.g., scalp, forehead, nasolabial folds, and presternal), it is not a disease primarily of sebaceous glands. The etiology is unknown, although the efficacy of antifungal agents suggests that lipophilic yeasts (e.g., *Malassezia furfur)* may be involved.

Morphology

Lesions are macules and papules on a greasy yellow erythematous base, often with scaling and crusting. Dandruff is the common clinical expression of scalp seborrheic dermatitis.

Histologically, early lesions resemble spongiotic dermatitis, while later lesions are more suggestive of acanthotic psoriasis. Mounds of perakeratosis admixed with acute inflammatory cells accumulate around hair follicles, with an overall superficial perivascular infiltrate of neutrophils and lymphocytes.

Lichen Planus (p. 1258)

Lichen planus is a self-limited disease that after 1 to 2 years generally leaves only postinflammatory hyperpigmentation. Oral lesions may persist longer and occasionally become malignant. The *pathogenesis* is unknown, but T-cell infiltrates with Langerhans cell hyperplasia are seen, and cell-mediated immune injury to basal cells is suspected. Koebner phenomenon occurs in lichen planus.

Morphology

Grossly, lesions are *pruritic, purple, polygonal papules* that may coalesce into *plaques;* lesions are often highlighted by white dots or lines called *Wickham striae.* Lesions are typically multiple and symmetrically distributed, often on the wrists and elbows and on the glans penis; oral mucosal lesions are generally white and netlike. A form with preferential involvement of hair follicle epithelium is called *lichen planopilaris.*

Histologically, there is a dense, bandlike dermal-epidermal junction lymphocytic infiltrate with basal cell degeneration and necrosis and jagged rete sawtoothing. Necrotic basal cells may be sloughed into inflamed papillary dermis, forming *colloid* or *Civatte bodies.* Lesions are also typified by chronic changes, including acanthosis, hyperkeratosis, and thickening of the granular cell layer.

Lupus Erythematosus (p. 1258)

Systemic lupus erythematosus (SLE) is detailed elsewhere (Chapter 6). *Discoid lupus erythematosus (DLE) is a localized cutaneous form without systemic manifestations.* Although patients with DLE rarely progress to develop systemic disease, one third of patients with SLE develop DLE-like skin pathology. Thus, evaluation of the cutaneous lesions *alone* does not distinguish the two entities. The *pathogenesis* of DLE involves immune complex–mediated and, to a lesser extent, cell-mediated injury to pigment-containing basal cells (Chapter 6).

Morphology

Grossly, skin lesions of both SLE and DLE include an ill-defined malar erythema (more characteristic of SLE) or sharply demarcated *discoid* erythematous scaling plaques with zones of irregular pigmentation and small keratotic plugs in hair follicles. Sun exposure exacerbates the lesions.

Microscopically, DLE is marked by dermal-epidermal junction, perivascular, and periappendiceal lymphocytic infiltrates. Preferential infiltration of subcutaneous fat is called *lupus profundus.* There are also basal cell vacuolization, epidermal atrophy, and variable hyperkeratosis.

By immunofluorescence, lesions show a *granular* band of immunoglobulin and complement along the dermal-epidermal and dermal-follicular junctions *(lupus band test).*

Blistering (Bullous) Diseases (p. 1259)

These diseases are *primary* blistering disorders, as opposed to vesicles and bullae that occur as a *secondary* phenomenon in a variety of unrelated conditions. The level within the skin where the blister occurs is critical in diagnosis (Fig. 25–1).

Pemphigus (p. 1260)

This rare autoimmune disorder typically occurs in patients from ages 30 to 60, with no gender predilection. Patients have circulating antibodies to keratinocyte intercellular cement component (desmoglein 3, a component of desmosomes); binding of these antibodies triggers release of plasminogen activator by keratinocytes, leading to the acantholytic breakdown of the desmosomes. There are four clinical and pathologic variants, depending on the level of the blister (and presumably the fine specificity of the autoantibody):

- *Pemphigus vulgaris* accounts for 80% of pemphigus. This disorder involves the oral mucosa, scalp, face, intertriginous zones, trunk, and pressure points. Lesions are superficial, easily ruptured blisters that leave shallow, crusted erosions. If untreated, it is almost uniformly fatal.
- *Pemphigus vegetans* is a rare form presenting with large, moist verrucous plaques studded with pustules, typically in flexural and intertriginous zones.
- *Pemphigus foliaceus* is a more benign form occurring epidemically in South America and sporadically elsewhere. Lesions occur mainly on the face, scalp, and upper trunk.

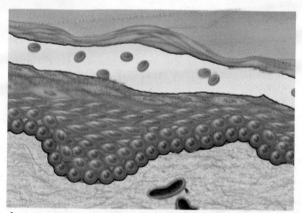

A. Subcorneal

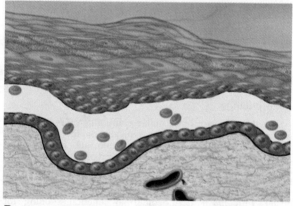

B. Suprabasal

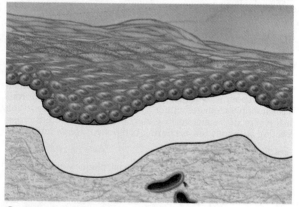

C. Subepidermal

FIGURE 25–1 Schematic representation of sites of blister formation. *A,* In a subcorneal blister, the stratum corneum forms the roof of the bulla (as in impetigo or pemphigus foliaceus). *B,* In a suprabasal blister, a portion of epidermis, including the stratum corneum, forms the roof (as in pemphigus vulgaris). *C,* In a subepidermal blister, the entire epidermis separates from the dermis (as in bullous pemphigoid and dermatitis herpetiformis).

Bullae are extremely superficial, leaving only slight erythema and crusting after rupture.

- *Pemphigus erythematosus* is a localized, milder variant of pemphigus foliaceus, typically involving only a malar distribution.

Morphology

Microscopically, all variants are characterized by *acantholysis* with intercellular clefting and eventually broad-based, *intraepithelial* blisters. For pemphigus vulgaris and vegetans, the separation occurs immediately above the basal layer *(suprabasal blister),* leaving an intact layer of basal cells, described as a row of *tombstones;* in the foliaceus variant, only the stratum granulosum is involved. With anti-immunoglobulin or anticomplement immunofluorescence, netlike *(reticular)* staining may be seen in the epidermis, outlining each keratinocyte.

Bullous Pemphigoid (p. 1261)

Bullous pemphigoid is a relatively common autoimmune blistering disease of skin and mucosa typically affecting elderly individuals. It is caused by antibodies to hemidesmosome proteins responsible for attaching basal cells to the basal membrane; the antibodies cause injury by secondary complement activation and granulocyte recruitment.

Morphology

Grossly, there are tense bullae containing clear fluid measuring 4 to 8 cm in diameter, typically on the inner thigh, forearm flexor surfaces, lower abdomen, and intertriginous zones; oral mucosa is involved in one third of patients. The blisters do not rupture as easily as those in pemphigus and, if uninfected, heal without scarring.

Microscopically, there is a subepidermal nonacantholytic blister with *linear* dermoepidermal junction staining for immunoglobulin and complement. There is a variable, mostly superficial, perivascular infiltrate of lymphocytes, eosinophils, and neutrophils.

Dermatitis Herpetiformis (p. 1262)

Dermatitis herpetiformis is a rare disorder, typically occurring in patients aged 20 to 40, seen more often in men than in women. It is associated with specific HLA types and with celiac disease (Chapter 17). Both cutaneous and gastrointestinal lesions respond to a gluten-free diet. Dermatitis herpetiformis is presumably mediated either by immune complex deposition in the skin or by gliadin (a gluten protein) antibodies cross-reacting with junction-anchoring components (e.g., reticulin).

Morphology

Grossly, intensely pruritic, urticarial plaques and grouped vesicles, characteristically symmetric, involve the extensor surfaces, upper back, and buttocks.

Microscopically, neutrophils and fibrin accumulate in the tips of dermal papillae *(microabscesses)* with overlying basal vacuolization and microscopic blisters coalescing to large subepidermal blisters. Immunofluorescence shows granular immunoglobulin A (IgA) deposits at the dermal papillae tips.

Noninflammatory Blistering Diseases:
Epidermolysis Bullosa, Porphyria (p. 1263)

Noninflammatory blistering diseases are primary disorders with vesicles and bullae not mediated by inflammatory mechanisms.

Epidermolysis bullosa (p. 1263) refers to a pathogenetically unrelated group of disorders that have in common neonatal blistering at pressure sites or trauma. The *junctional type* shows blistering at the lamina lucida in otherwise histologically normal skin. The scarring *dystrophic type* shows blistering beneath the lamina densa that presumably is due to defective anchoring fibrils. The *simplex type* results from epidermal basal cell degeneration.

Porphyria (p. 1263) refers to a group of inborn or acquired disturbances of porphyrin metabolism (there are five major types). Porphyrins are the ring structures that bind the metal ions in hemoglobin, myoglobin, and cytochromes. The pathogenesis is unknown. The cutaneous lesions consist of urticaria and vesicles that are exacerbated by sun exposure and heal without scarring.

Morphology

Microscopically, there are subepidermal vesicles with associated marked superficial dermal vascular thickening.

DISORDERS OF EPIDERMAL APPENDAGES
(p. 1264)

Acne Vulgaris (p. 1264)

Acne vulgaris is a common, chronic, inflammatory dermatosis affecting hair follicles, typically occurring in the middle to late teens, seen in males more than females, presumably secondary to hormonal changes and alterations in hair follicle maturation. It may be induced or exacerbated by sex hormones, corticosteroids, occupational exposure (coal tars), or occlusive conditions (heavy clothes). There may be a heritable component.

Pathogenesis

Speculatively, acne involves bacterial (*Propionibacterium acnes*) lipase degradation of sebaceous oils to form highly irritating fatty acids. Antibiotics (e.g., tetracyclines) may be effective by inhibiting the lipase activity. The vitamin A derivative 13-*cis*-retinoic acid has also shown efficacy.

Morphology

Grossly, noninflammatory acne is characterized by *open comedones* (follicular papules with central black keratin plugs) and *closed comedones* (follicular papules with central plugs trapped beneath the epidermis and therefore not visible). The latter may rupture with inflammation. *Inflammatory acne* shows erythematous papules, nodules, and pustules.

Histologically, comedones are composed of expanding masses of lipid and keratin at the midportion of hair follicles, with follicular dilation and epithelial and sebaceous gland atrophy. There is a variable lymphohistiocytic infiltrate, but with rupture there is extensive acute and chronic inflammation, occasionally with ensuing scar formation.

Panniculitis (p. 1265)

Panniculitis is inflammation of subcutaneous fat; it may be acute or chronic, and commonly involves the lower extremities. A rare form of panniculitis, *Weber-Christian disease (relapsing febrile nodular panniculitis)* occurs as crops of erythematous plaques or nodules, mainly on the legs, associated with deep lymphohistiocytic infiltrates and occasional giant cells. *Factitial panniculitis* (from self-administered foreign substances), deep mycotic infections in immunocompromised hosts, and occasionally disorders such as SLE may mimic the clinical and histologic appearance of primary panniculitis.

Erythema Nodosum and Erythema Induratum (p. 1265)

Common forms of panniculitis can affect:
- Connective tissue septa *(erythema nodosum)*
- Fat lobules *(erythema induratum)*

Erythema nodosum is more common than erythema induratum. It typically has an acute onset and may be idiopathic or occur in association with specific drugs, infections, sarcoidosis, inflammatory bowel disease, or visceral malignancy. It presents with ill-defined, exquisitely tender erythematous nodules, occasionally with fever and malaise. With time, old lesions flatten and become ecchymotic without scarring, while new lesions develop. Deep wedge biopsy shows distinctive early septal widening (edema, fibrin deposition, and neutrophil infiltration) and lymphohistiocytic infiltration (occasionally with giant cells and eosinophils) without vasculitis.

Erythema induratum is an uncommon form of panniculitis, typically affecting adolescents and menopausal women. It may represent a primary vasculitis of subcutaneous fat with subsequent inflammation and necrosis of adipose tissue. It presents as an erythematous, slightly tender nodule that eventually ulcerates and scars. Early lesions show necrotizing vasculitis in small to medium-sized vessels in deep dermis and subcutis. Eventually the fat lobules develop granulomatous inflammation and necrosis.

Infection and Infestation (p. 1265)

The following is a representative sampling of infectious cutaneous lesions:

Verrucae (Warts) (p. 1265)

Verrucae are common, spontaneously regressing (6 months to 2 years) lesions, typically seen in children and adolescents. They are caused by papillomaviruses, transmitted by direct contact.

Verrucae are subdivided on the basis of clinical morphology and anatomic location. Certain lesions are typically caused by particular papillomavirus types. For example, types 6, 11, 16, and 18 are associated with anogenital warts. Type 16 is associated with anogenital wart dysplasia and *in situ* squamous cell carcinoma of the genitalia.

- *Verruca vulgaris* is the most common type of wart, most frequently seen on the dorsum of the hand. Grossly, these lesions are gray-white to tan, flat to convex, 0.1- to 1-cm papules with a rough pebbly surface.
- *Verruca plana (flat wart)* usually occurs on the face or dorsum of the hand. Grossly, they are flat, smooth, tan papules that are smaller than those of verruca vulgaris.
- *Verruca plantaris (soles) or palmaris (palms)* appears as rough, scaly lesions 1 to 2 cm in diameter that may coalesce and be confused with calluses.
- *Condyloma acuminatum (anogenital and venereal warts)* appears as soft, tan, cauliflower-like masses measuring up to many centimeters in diameter.

Morphology

Microscopically, all variants have undulant *(verrucous)* epidermal hyperplasia and superficial keratinocyte perinuclear vacuolization *(koilocytosis).* Electron microscopy reveals numerous viral particles within nuclei.

Molluscum Contagiosum (p. 1266)

This common, self-limited disease is caused by a poxvirus, transmitted by direct contact.

Morphology

Grossly, firm, pruritic, pink to skin-colored, umbilicated papules 0.2 to 2 cm are seen on the trunk or anogenital regions. Cheesy material containing diagnostic molluscum bodies can be expressed from the central umbilications.

Microscopically, there is cuplike verrucous epidermal hyperplasia with pathognomonic *molluscum bodies*—large (up to 35 mm) eosinophilic cytoplasmic inclusions in the stratum granulosum or stratum corneum containing numerous virions.

Impetigo (p. 1267)

Impetigo refers to streptococcal or staphylococcal skin infection seen in normal children or sick adults, especially on the face and hands. It begins as an erythematous macule that progresses to small pustules and eventually to a shallow erosion with a honey-colored crust.

Morphology

Microscopically, there are subcorneal pustules filled with neutrophils and gram-positive cocci, with accompanying dermal inflammation. Pustule rupture releases serum and necrotic debris to form the characteristic crust.

Superficial Fungal Infections (p. 1267)

Superficial fungal infections are typically caused by dermatophytes (fungi growing in soil and on animals) and are *confined to the nonviable stratum corneum.*

- *Tinea capitis* is typically noted in children. It causes asymptomatic hairless patches on the scalp, associated with mild erythema, crusting, and scale.
- *Tinea barbae* is an uncommon dermatophytosis of the beard area in adult men.
- *Tinea corporis* is a common superficial dermatophytosis of the body, especially in children. Predisposing factors are

excessive heat or humidity, exposure to infected animals, and chronic dermatophytosis of the feet or nails. This typically presents with an expanding erythematous plaque with an elevated scaling border *(ringworm)*.

- *Tinea cruris* is typically found in the inguinal areas of obese men during warm weather. It occurs as moist red patches with raised scaling borders.
- *Tinea pedis (athlete's foot)* is characterized by erythema and scaling, beginning in the webbed spaces between the digits, usually toes. It affects up to 40% of individuals at some time in their lives. Most of the inflammation is due to secondary bacterial superinfection.
- *Tinea versicolor* is due to *Malassezia furfur* and typically is found on the upper trunk. This displays characteristic groups of various-sized hyperpigmented or hypopigmented macules with a peripheral scale.
- *Onychomycosis* is a nail dermatophytosis characterized by discoloration, thickening, and deformity of the nail plate.

There is histologic variability, but basically, these reactive epidermal changes are similar to a mild eczematous dermatitis. Fungal organisms—*present in the stratum corneum*—are revealed by special stains. Identification and cultures may be obtained by superficial scraping of affected areas.

Arthropod Bites, Stings, and Infestations (p. 1268)

Arthropod-associated lesions are bites, stings, and infestations associated with arachnids (spiders, scorpions, ticks, mites), insects (lice, bees, fleas, flies, and mosquitos), and chilopods (centipedes). Reactions range from minimal to fatal. Gross bites range from urticarial lesions and inflamed papules or nodules to expanding, erythematous plaques (e.g., *erythema migrans* in the case of the bite from the tick vector for Lyme disease). Arthropod-associated pathologies include the following:

- A direct irritant effect of insect parts or secretions
- Immediate (IgE-mediated, including anaphylaxis) or delayed (cell-mediated) hypersensitivity responses to body parts or secretions
- Specific effects of venom:

  Black widow spider venom causes pain and cramping.
  Brown recluse spider venom produces significant tissue necrosis, often requiring radical surgical excision of involved areas.

- Lesions associated with secondary invaders (bacteria, rickettsiae, parasites)

Pediculosis (p. 1268) is a pruritic dermatosis caused by the head, body, or crab louse. The insect or its eggs can usually be seen attached to hair shafts. Scalp pediculosis is complicated by impetigo and cervical lymphadenopathy, especially in children. Body lice may be accompanied by excoriations and hyperpigmentation.

Scabies (p. 1268) refers to a pruritic dermatosis caused by the mite *Sarcoptes scabiei*. The female burrows beneath the stratum corneum, producing linear, poorly defined furrows on the interdigital skin, palms, and wrists and on the periareolar skin in women and in the scrotal folds in men.

Although arthropod bites have a variable histologic pattern, there is classically a *wedge-shaped dermal perivascular lymphohistiocytic and eosinophilic infiltrate*. There may be a highly focal central zone of epidermal necrosis with birefringent insect mouth parts delineating the bite site. In some lesions, there is an urticaria-like response. In others there is a florid inflammatory infiltrate or spongiosis resulting in intraepidermal blisters.

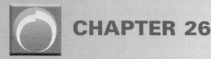

CHAPTER 26

Bones, Joints, and Soft Tissue Tumors

BONES (p. 1274)

Developmental (Genetic) and Acquired Abnormalities in Bone Cells, Matrix, and Structure (p. 1278)

- Developmental anomalies are frequently genetically based and manifest during early stages of bone formation; acquired diseases are usually detected in adulthood.
- Molecular-pathogenic classification of genetic disorders is based on the functional properties of the involved gene or protein (Table 26–1).

Malformations and Diseases Caused by Defects in Nuclear Proteins and Transcription Factors (p. 1279)

Synpolydactyly (for example) is caused by a mutation in the homeobox HOXD-13 transcription factor. The mutation manifests as an extra digit between the third and fourth digits with some fusion of the fingers.

Diseases Caused by Defects in Hormones and Signal Transduction Mechanisms (p. 1279)

Achondroplasia (for example) is the most common form of dwarfism. It results from a defect in paracrine cell signaling in growth plate cartilage, namely a genetic derangement in the gene that codes for FGF receptor 3 located on chromosome 4. Some cases are familial, but most are acquired mutations.

- Anatomically, the growth plates are shortened and disordered, resulting in abnormally short extremity bones. Because appositional growth is not affected, bones are of normal width and the skull appears comparatively enlarged.

TABLE 26-1 Molecular Genetics of Diseases of the Skeleton

Human Disorder	Gene Mutation	Affected Molecule	Phenotype
Defects in Transcription Factors Producing Abnormalities in Mesenchymal Condensation and Related Cell Differentiation			
Synpolydactyly	HOXD-13	Transcription factor	Extra digit with fusion
Waardenburg syndrome	PAX-3	Transcription factor	Hearing loss, abnormal pigmentation, craniofacial abnormalities
Greig syndrome	GL13	Transcription factor	Synpolydactyly, craniofacial abnormalities
Campomelic dysplasia	SOX9	Transcription factor	Sex reversal, abnormal skeletal development
Oligodontia	PAX9	Transcription factor	Congenital absence of teeth
Nail-patella syndrome	LMX1B	Transcription factor	Hypoplastic nails, hypoplastic or aplastic patellae, dislocated radial head, progressive nephropathy
Holt-Oram syndrome	TBX5	Transcription factor	Congenital abnormalities, forelimb anomalies
Ulnar-mammary syndrome	TBX3	Transcription factor	Hypoplasia or absent ulna, 3rd–5th digits, breast, and teeth, delayed puberty
Cleidocranial dysplasia	CBFA1	Transcription factor	Abnormal clavicles, wormian bones, supernumerary teeth
Defects in Extracellular Structural Proteins			
Osteogenesis imperfecta types 1–4	COL1A1	Type 1 collagen	Bone fragility, hearing loss, blue sclerae
	COL1A2		Dentinogenesis imperfecta
Achondrogenesis II	COL2A1	Type 2 collagen	Short trunk, severely shortened extremities, relatively enlarged cranium, flattened face
Hypochondrogenesis	COL2A1	Type 2 collagen	Short trunk, shortened extremities, relatively enlarged cranium, flattened face
Stickler dysplasia	COL2A1	Type 2 collagen	Myopia, retinal detachment, hearing loss, flattened face, premature osteoarthritis
Multiple epiphyseal dysplasia	COL9A2	Type 9 collagen	Short or normal stature, small epiphyses, early onset osteoarthritis
Schmid metaphyseal chondrodysplasia	COL10A1	Type 10 collagen	Mild short stature, bowing of lower extremities, coxa vara, metaphyseal flaring

Continued

TABLE 26-1 Molecular Genetics of Diseases of the Skeleton—cont'd

Human Disorder	Gene Mutation	Affected Molecule	Phenotype
Defects in Hormones and Signal Transduction Mechanisms Producing Abnormal Proliferation or Maturation of Chondrocytes and Osteoblasts			
Brachydactyly type C	CDMP1	Signaling molecule	Shortened metacarpals and phalanges
Jansen metaphyseal chondroplasia	PTHrp receptor	Receptor	Short bowed limbs, clinodactyly, facial abnormalities, hypercalcemia, hypophosphatemia
Achondroplasia	FGFR3	Receptor	Short stature, rhizomelic shortening of limbs, frontal bossing, midface deficiency
Hypochondroplasia	FGFR3	Receptor	Disproportionate short stature, micromelia, relative macrocephaly
Thanatophoric dwarfism	FGFR3	Receptor	Severe limb shortening and bowing, frontal bossing, depressed nasal bridge
Crouzon syndrome	FGFR2	Receptor	Craniosynostosis

Adapted from Mundlos S, Olsen BR: Heritable diseases of the skeleton. Part I: Molecular insights into skeletal development—transcription factors and signaling pathways. FASEB J 11:125–132, 1997; Mundlos S, Olsen BR: Heritable diseases of the skeleton. Part II: Molecular insights into skeletal development—matrix components and their homeostasis. FASEB J 11:227–233, 1997; Superti-Furga A et al: Molecular-pathogenetic classification of genetic disorders of the skeleton. Am J Med Genet 106:282–293, 2001.

- Heterozygotes have normal longevity with easily recognizable disease because head and body are too large for the markedly shortened extremities. Mental, sexual, and reproductive development are normal.
- Thanatophoric dwarfism, the most common form of lethal dwarfism, is caused by a different mutation in FGF receptor 3, and the dysfunctional growth plates produce micromelic shortening of the limbs, relative macrocephaly, and a constricted thoracic cage that causes death soon after birth.

Diseases Associated With Defects in Extracellular Structural Proteins (p. 1279)

Osteogenesis imperfecta, or *brittle bone disease,* refers to a group of closely related genetic disorders caused by qualitatively or quantitatively abnormal type I collagen synthesis (constitutes about 90% of the organic matrix of bone). The underlying genetic defect is a mutation in the genes that code for the alpha 1 and alpha 2 chains of the collagen molecule. Consequently, the bones are prone to fracture.

- Based on the specific biosynthetic abnormality, four major subsets of osteogenesis imperfecta are classified; some have well-defined modes of inheritance and phenotypic changes, and others are less well characterized.
- Syndromes range from one variant (type II) that is uniformly fatal in the perinatal period (from multiple bone fractures) to other variants marked by increased predisposition to fracture but compatible with survival.
- Morphologically, the basic change is osteopenia (too little bone), with marked thinning of the cortices and rarefaction of the trabeculae.

Diseases Associated With Defects in Folding and Degradation of Macromolecules (p. 1281)

Mucopolysaccharidoses are a group of lysosomal storage diseases caused by deficiencies in enzymes (mainly acid hydolases) that degrade the various mucopolysaccharides (e.g., dermatan sulfate, heparan sulfate, others). Chondrocytes play a role in mucopolysaccharide metabolism; consequently, in these disorders there are abnormalities in hyaline cartilage, including growth plates, costal cartilages, and articular surfaces. Patients are frequently of short stature and have malformed bones as well as other cartilage abnormalities.

Diseases Associated With Defects in Metabolic Pathways (Enzymes, Ion Channels, and Transporters) (p. 1281)

Osteopetrosis refers to a group of rare genetic diseases characterized by reduced osteoclastic activity resulting in diffuse skeletal sclerosis with loss of the medullary cavity (with impaired hematopoiesis). Despite *too much bone,* it is brittle and fractures like chalk.

- Severe forms are clinically evident at birth and are associated with anemia, neutropenia, infections, and eventually death.
- Patients with benign forms of the disease are predisposed to fractures.

- The underlying genetic defect is aberrant osteoclast function resulting in reduced bone resorption and an increase in bone mass.
- The nature of the genetic defect has been identified for some forms; these include mutations in the genes that code for carbonic anhydrase II and CIC-7 chloride channel.

Diseases Associated With Decreased Bone Mass
(p. 1282)

Osteoporosis refers to a reduction in bone mass owing to small but incremental losses occurring with the constant turnover of bone. This common condition is seen most often in the elderly of both sexes but is more pronounced in post-menopausal women. Osteoporosis may occur as a primary disorder of obscure origin or as a secondary complication of a large variety of diseases (Table 26–2). Osteoporosis becomes clinically significant when it induces vertebral instability with back pain and increases the risk for fractures of hips, wrists, and vertebral bodies.

Pathogenesis

The cause of senile and postmenopausal osteoporosis is multifactorial and different aspects contribute to the loss of bone

TABLE 26–2 **Categories of Generalized Osteoporosis**

Primary
Postmenopausal
Senile
Idiopathic

Secondary
Endocrine Disorders

Hyperparathyroidism
Hypo-hyperthyroidism
Hypogonadism
Pituitary tumors
Diabetes, type 1
Addison disease

Rheumatologic Disease Drugs

Anticoagulants
Chemotherapy
Corticosteroids
Anticonvulsants
Alcohol

Neoplasia

Multiple myeloma
Carcinomatosis

Gastrointestinal

Malnutrition
Malabsorption
Hepatic insufficiency
Vitamin C, D deficiencies

Miscellaneous

Osteogenesis imperfecta
Immobilization
Pulmonary disease
Homocystinuria
Anemia

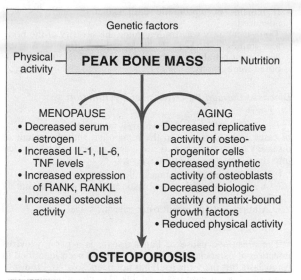

FIGURE 26–1 Pathophysiology of postmenopausal and senile osteoporosis.

mass (Fig. 26–1). In essence, genetic factors determine the peak bone mass achieved in young adulthood. Thereafter, aging-related slowing of osteoblast formation and function, decreased biologic activity of matrix bound growth factors and diminished physical activity results in senile osteoporosis. In postmenopausal osteoporosis there is also an increase in osteoclastic activity induced by decreased serum estrogen levels. The diminished estrogen levels result in increased secretion of interleukins 1 and 6 (IL1, IL6) and tumor necrosis factor (TNF) by blood monocytes. These cytokines are potent stimulators of osteoclast recruitment and activity by increasing the levels of RANK and RANKL and reducing osteoprotegrin (OPG). Compensatory osteoblastic activity occurs, but it does not keep pace with the bone loss. Accumulating evidence indicates that estrogen replacement therapy coupled with calcium supplementation, when begun during or soon after the onset of the menopause, can slow or prevent the abnormal loss of bone.

Morphology

In postmenopausal and senile osteoporosis, the entire skeleton is involved, but patients may have localized disease due to immobilization or extremity paralysis.

- Cortex and trabeculae are thinned, and haversian systems are widened.
- Residual bone is of normal composition.

Clinical Features

Osteoporosis causes pain due to microfractures. It results in loss in height and stability of the vertebral column, and particularly predisposes to fractures of femoral necks, wrists, and vertebrae. The condition is difficult to diagnose for the following reasons:

- It remains asymptomatic until skeletal fragility is well advanced.
- There is no easy way to determine the severity of the bone loss (radiographs are unreliable with less than 40% bone loss); most reliable are absorptiometry and quantitive computed tomography.

Diseases Caused by Osteoclast Dysfunction
(p. 1284)

Paget disease (osteitis deformans) is monostotic in about 15% of cases and polyostotic in the remainder, with the extent of disease varying from site to site. Paget disease can be divided into the following sequential stages:

1. An initial osteolytic stage, followed by
2. A mixed osteolytic-osteoblastic stage, evolving ultimately into
3. A burnt-out, quiescent osteosclerotic stage

Pathogenesis

The presumed cause of Paget disease is a paramyxovirus infection of osteoclasts. Viral particles have been identified in osteoclasts but the virus itself has not been isolated. Predisposition of Paget disease has been linked to chromosome 18q.

Morphology

- The *osteolytic phase* is marked by resorption by numerous, overly large osteoclasts (some containing >100 nuclei).
- The *mixed phase* has new disordered, predominantly woven bone formation (but some lamellar). The new bone is poorly mineralized, and is therefore soft and porous, lacking structural stability, and thus, the bone is vulnerable to fracture or deformation under stress. In this stage, units of lamellar bone are deposited in a *tile-like or mosaic pattern, which is pathognomonic of Paget disease.* Adjacent marrow is fibrotic.
- Eventually, after many years, a *burnt-out phase* supervenes, marked predominantly by bone sclerosis composed of a mosaic pattern of lamellar bone with coarsely thickened trabeculae and cortices.

Clinical Features

- Patients may demonstrate fractures, nerve compression, osteoarthritis, and skeletal deformities (e.g., tibial bowing, skull enlargement).
- Any bone can be involved, and coarsening of the facial bones *may produce* leontiasis ossea (lion-like facies). Less commonly, the vascularity of polyostotic lesions can cause high-output heart failure. Occasionally, in about 1% of patients, secondary sarcoma develops.

Diseases Associated With Abnormal Mineral Homeostasis (p. 1287)

Rickets and Osteomalacia (p. 1287)

Rickets in growing children and osteomalacia in adults are caused by defects in matrix mineralization and frequently result from either vitamin D deficiency or phosphate depletion. Causes of vitamin D deficiency include:

- Dietary deficiency
- Inadequate sunlight exposure
- Malabsorption of vitamin D, calcium, or phosphate
- Derangements in conversion of vitamin D to active metabolites (e.g., in renal disease)
- End-organ resistance
- Rare hereditary or acquired disorders of vitamin D metabolism

Morphology. The fundamental defect in osteomalacia or rickets is failure to mineralize bone; this causes excess unmineralized matrix and abnormally wide osteoid seams.

Clinical Features. In the growing child, the skeleton is weak with bowing of legs and deformities of ribs, skull, and other bones. In adults—after bone growth has ceased—it results in no skeletal deformities, but does cause *osteopenic osteomalacia*.

Hyperparathyroidism (p. 1287)

Hyperparathyroidism, either primary or secondary (as occurs with renal failure), leads to the following:

- Increased levels of parathyroid hormone (PTH) occur.
- Increased osteoclastic activity occurs, with resorption of bone and peritrabecular fibrosis (osteitis fibrosa).
- Unabated bone resorption predisposes to microfractures, fibrosis, and secondary hemorrhage with formation of cysts within the marrow cavity (*osteitis fibrosa cystica* or *von Recklinghausen disease of bone*).
- Bone loss is particularly evident by x-ray as *subperiosteal bone resorption* along the radial aspect of the middle phalanges of the index and middle fingers and distal clavicles, and loss of the lamina dura about the tooth sockets.
- So-called "brown tumors" (resembling reparative giant cell granulomas) also occur within the bones; paradoxically, soft tissue metastatic calcifications sometimes appear. The bone changes completely regress with control of hyperparathyroidism.

Renal Osteodystrophy (p. 1287)

Renal osteodystrophy refers to a complex set of bone changes appearing in most patients with chronic renal failure: increased osteoclastic activity, delayed matrix mineralization (osteomalacia), osteosclerosis, growth retardation, and osteoporosis.

- With protracted skeletal disease, metastatic calcifications can also develop in the skin, eyes, arterial walls, and joints.
- Other factors that contribute to the bone changes include metabolic acidosis and iron and aluminum deposition in bone (derived from dialysate, and interfering with matrix mineralization).

Fractures (p. 1288)

Speed of healing and perfection of fracture repair depend on the type of fracture and whether the break has occurred in normal bone or in previously diseased bone (i.e., *pathologic fracture*).

- Well-aligned, *incomplete* (greenstick), and *closed* (intact skin) fractures heal most rapidly, with potentially complete reconstitution of the preexisting architecture.

- *Comminuted* (splintered bone) and *compound* (open skin wound) fractures heal much more slowly, with poorer end results.

Morphology

Fracture healing is regulated by cytokines and growth factors, and is a continuous process proceeding through three distinct stages:

- *Organization of the hematoma* at the fracture site, leading to a soft, organizing, *procallus*
- Conversion of the procallus to a *fibrocartilaginous callus* composed of reactive mesenchymal cells
- Replacement of the latter by an *osseous callus,* which is eventually remodeled along lines of weight bearing to complete the repair

If the fracture has been well aligned and the original weight-bearing strains are restored, virtually perfect repair is accomplished. Imperfect results are seen when there is malalignment, comminution, inadequate immobilization of fracture site, infection, and superimposed systemic abnormality (e.g., atherosclerosis, avitaminosis, dietary deficiency, osteoporosis).

Osteonecrosis (Avascular Necrosis) (p. 1289)

Infarction of bone and marrow is relatively common and can occur in the medullary cavity of the metaphysis or diaphysis and the subchondral region of the epiphysis. The mechanisms leading to the local ischemia include:

- Vascular interruption (fracture)
- Thrombosis and embolism *(caisson disease)*
- Vessel injury (vasculitis, radiation therapy)
- Vascular compression (possibly steroid-induced necrosis)
- Venous hypertension

Among the aforementioned mechanisms, steroid-induced necrosis is most common. Many cases are idiopathic and have no known etiology.

Morphology

A local geographic area of pale yellow infarction is seen in marrow (the cortex is usually not affected because of its collateral blood flow). The necrotic region is marked by death of osteocytes, empty lacunae, and necrotic fat cells. Creeping substitution with living tissue occurs from the margin of the infarct. In subchondral infarcts, the articular cartilage may collapse into the necrotic bone.

Clinical Features

Patients may be asymptomatic, but subchondral lesions often cause joint pain and predispose to subsequent osteoarthritis.

Infections—Osteomyelitis (p. 1290)

Pyogenic Osteomyelitis (p. 1290)

Pyogenic osteomyelitis results from bacterial seeding of bone by:

- Hematogenous spread
- Extension from a contiguous infection
- Open fracture or surgical procedure

Blood-borne infections are common causes of osteomyelitis, and *Staphylococcus aureus* (often penicillin resistant) is most often implicated (although other pathogens can clearly be involved). For obscure reasons, patients with sickle cell anemia are prone to *Salmonella* infections.

Extension of infection or traumatic inoculation is frequently associated with mixed infections, including anaerobes.

Basically, the suppurative reaction is associated with ischemic necrosis, fibrosis, and bony repair.

- Necrosis of a bone segment may produce a *sequestrum*.
- Subperiosteal new bone produces an *involucrum* that encloses and envelops the inflammatory focus.
- Chronic cases may lead to bone deformities and sinus tracts. Small walled-off intracortical abscesses are known as a *Brodie abscess* (sometimes sterile).

Clinical Features

Pyogenic osteomyelitis is an acute febrile illness with local pain, tenderness, and heat. Subtle lesions, however, may present as unexplained fever in infants or localized pain without fever in adults. During the first 10 days, x-ray changes may be minimal, but radionuclide studies often show localized uptake of tracers. Complications include fracture, amyloidosis, bacteremia with endocarditis, and development of squamous cell carcinoma in sinus tract.

Tuberculous Osteomyelitis (p. 1291)

Tuberculous osteomyelitis has experienced a resurgence in developed countries attributed to the influx of immigrants from developing countries and the greater numbers of immunosuppressed patients. It remains common in developing nations where pulmonary and gastrointestinal tuberculosis are still prevalent.

- It arises as a blood-borne infection, which is much more destructive and resistant to control than suppurative diseases.
- In the spine, it is called *Pott disease*.
- It produces typical granulomatous reaction with caseous necrosis.

Skeletal Syphilis (p. 1292)

Although rare in the United States, syphilitic bone disease can occur in either congenital or acquired forms.

- *Congenital* syphilis appears at birth and is marked by periostitis. On x-ray, a *crew haircut–like* appearance of new bone formation on cortex is produced. *Saber shin* results when the tibia is involved.

- *Acquired* syphilis appears in the tertiary stage of disease. It may be manifested as periostitis but more often by bone gummas.

Bone Tumors and Tumor-Like Lesions
(p. 1292)

There is a great diversity of benign and malignant tumors of bone (Table 26–3). Since certain tumors tend to occur within certain age groups and at particular locations, the patient's age, the location of the neoplasm, as well as its radiologic appearance are all very important.

Bone-Forming Tumors (p. 1293)

Osteoma (p. 1293)

This bosselated, sessile tumor is attached to a bone surface. It is usually composed of well-formed cortical-type bone; its trabecular counterpart is the bone island.

- Osteomas protrude from cortical surfaces, most often the skull and facial bones.
- These tumors are of little clinical significance unless their location (e.g., nasal sinus, inner table of the skull) compromises local organ function, or produces cosmetic deformities.
- Multiple osteomas are seen in the setting of *Gardner syndrome* (Chapter 17).

Osteoid Osteoma and Osteoblastoma (p. 1293)

An *osteoid osteoma* is a small, benign neoplasm without malignant potential; 90% occur in persons between their teens

TABLE 26–3 **Classification of Primary Tumors Involving Bones**

Histologic Type	Benign	Malignant
Hematopoietic (40%)		Myeloma
		Malignant lymphoma
Chondrogenic (22%)	Osteochondroma	Chondrosarcoma
	Chondroma	Dedifferentiated chondrosarcoma
	Chondroblastoma	Mesenchymal chondrosarcoma
	Chondromyxoid fibroma	
Osteogenic (19%)	Osteoid osteoma	Osteosarcoma
	Osteoblastoma	
Unknown origin (10%)	Giant cell tumor	Ewing tumor
		Giant cell tumor
		Adamantinoma
Histiocytic origin	Fibrous histiocytoma	Malignant fibrous histiocytoma
Fibrogenic	Metaphyseal fibrous defect (fibroma)	Desmoplastic fibroma
		Fibrosarcoma
Notochordal		Chordoma
Vascular	Hemangioma	Hemangioendothelioma
		Hemangiopericytoma
Lipogenic	Lipoma	Liposarcoma
Neurogenic	Neurilemmoma	

Data on percentage of each type from Unni KK: Dahlin's Bone Tumors, 5th ed. Philadelphia, Lippincott-Raven, 1996, p 4; by permission of Mayo Foundation.

and 20s. The tumors are usually about 1 cm in diameter, and are most often located near the ends of the tibia and femur (although all bones have been involved).

• They are painful (classically there is night pain relieved by aspirin) and appear on x-ray as a small radiolucent nidus within cortex surrounded by densely reactive sclerotic bone.
• Histologically, the tumor consists of haphazardly oriented trabeculae of woven bone rimmed by numerous osteoblasts and surrounded by highly vascular loose connective tissue enclosed by abundant reactive bone.

The morphologically related *osteoblastoma* is usually a mixed lytic and blastic tumor having the same histologic appearance as osteoid osteoma but usually with a smaller amount of surrounding reactive bone. Osteoblastoma is associated with persistent dull achy pain.

Larger than osteoid osteomas (>2 cm), osteoblastomas tend to be located in the posterior elements of the vertebrae and long bones. They are considered benign, but can locally recur; rarely, some transform to osteosarcoma.

Osteosarcoma (p. 1294)

Osteosarcoma is a primary mesenchymal bone malignancy in which the neoplastic cells synthesize and secrete the organic components of bone matrix (that may or may not mineralize). There is no minimal amount of bone matrix required to classify the tumor as osteosarcoma, and therefore, the presence of any neoplastic bone, even if only microscopic, allows categorization as an osteosarcoma. These tumors also frequently exhibit areas that have chondroid and fibroblast differentiation.

• Excluding multiple myeloma, osteosarcoma is the most common form of primary bone cancer.
• Primary cases arise in otherwise normal underlying bone, mostly in persons younger than 20 years old.
• The metaphyseal region of long bones, especially around the knee, is a common site.
• Secondary osteosarcoma occurs mostly in older people (in both flat and long bones) and develops mainly in bones affected by a preexisting disease process (e.g., Paget disease, irradiation, infarction, infection, fracture, and benign tumors such as enchondroma, osteochondroma, or fibrous dysplasia).

Pathogenesis. Genetic, constitutional, and environmental influences are important.

Sporadic osteosarcomas result from a complex accrual of multiple genetic alterations, usually involving the inactivation of tumor suppressor genes and the overexpression of oncogenes. Osteosarcoma is also associated with genetic syndromes including the *Rothmund-Thomson syndrome* (mutation of chromosome 8q24.3 encoding a DNA helicase), *Bloom syndrome* (mutation of chromosome 15q26.1 encoding a DNA helicase), *Werner syndrome* (mutation of chromosome 8p11 encoding a DNA helicase), *Li-Fraumeni syndrome* (mutation of chromosome 17p13 encoding *p53,* a tumor suppressor gene), and retinoblastoma gene mutations. Patients with bilateral retinoblastoma have a several hundred-fold increased risk of developing osteosarcoma.

Constitutional influences include the fact that most osteosarcomas develop in the areas of greatest active bone growth.

Consequently, favored locations are adjacent to the growth plates of the distal femur and proximal tibia.

Irradiation is the most important *environmental factor* known to predispose to secondary osteosarcoma. Other diseases that result in chronic cell turnover in bone also increase the chances of developing osteosarcoma.

Morphology. From 80% to 90% of osteosarcomas arise in the medullary cavity of the metaphyseal ends of long bones and about 5% to 10% are surface based. The tumors are large, destructive, tan-white, gritty, and sometimes bloody and cystic masses.

- Most osteosarcomas are composed of large, hyperchromatic, and pleomorphic mitotically active tumor cells.
- Tumors may be largely osteoblastic, chondroblastic, or fibroblastic. Some may consist predominately of large blood-filled cysts (telangiectatic variant). *All form neoplastic bone that frequently has a coarse lace-like pattern.*
- Cortical penetration of tumor with periosteal elevation causes *Codman triangle,* an x-ray finding in some patients. Tumors rarely penetrate the epiphyseal plate.
- Extraskeletal osteosarcoma also can occur, but usually arises in deep soft tissues of elderly patients.

Clinical Features. Osteosarcomas present with local pain, tenderness, and swelling. They are biologically aggressive neoplasms, and are treated with surgery and chemotherapy.

- Osteosarcomas metastasize widely, usually first to lung but eventually to other organs and bones (lymph node metastases are rare).
- Surgery alone results in 20% 5-year survival rates, but surgery combined with chemotherapy yields 60% to 80% 5-year survival rates.
- Osteosarcomas of the jaw and the low-grade variants, *parosteal* (juxtacortical) and *intraosseous low-grade* osteosarcoma, have a better prognosis than does classic osteosarcoma.

Cartilage-Forming Tumors (p. 1296)

Osteochondroma (p. 1296)

Osteochondroma is also known as an *exostosis* and may occur as solitary sporadic lesions or in profusion as part of the syndrome of autosomal dominant *multiple hereditary exostosis.* Osteochondromas were previously believed to result from displacement of the lateral portion of the growth plate, which proliferated diagonal to the long axis of the bone and away from the nearby joint. More recent studies have identified specific cytogenetic abnormalities in the cartilage cap of osteochondromas supporting the theory that these lesions are neoplastic. The male-female ratio is 3:1.

- Osteochondromas typically develop in the metaphyseal region of long bones. Occasionally, the pelvis, scapula, and ribs are involved (rarely the small bones of the hands and feet).
- *Morphologically,* osteochondromas are mushroom-shaped surface protrusions, covered by perichondrium which overlies a cap of hyaline cartilage. The cartilage cap has the appearance of disorganized growth plate and undergoes enchondral ossification. The outer, well-formed cortices of

the stalk and medullary cavities of the cap are in continuity with cortex and marrow cavity of the underlying bone.

- Exostoses are usually discovered in late childhood or adolescence, often as chance x-ray findings.
- These are benign lesions; however—rarely in the hereditary or sporadic states—chondrosarcomas can arise.

Chondromas (p. 1296)

These benign tumors are composed of hyaline cartilage.

- Those within the bone are called *enchondromas*, and are thought to arise from remnants of epiphyseal cartilage. Approximately one third arise in the short tubular bones of the fingers and usually develop in young adults. Radiographically, they appear as well-circumscribed radiolucencies with scattered punctuate calcifications.
- Chondromas may be single or multiple. A nonfamilial multiple form is known as *enchondromatosis* or *Ollier disease,* and a familial form with multiple chondromas associated with hemangiomas is known as *Maffucci syndrome.*
- Sarcomatous transformation of solitary sporadic chondromas is uncommon, but with the multiple tumors in the systemic syndromes, sarcomatous transformation (usually chondrosarcoma) can occur.
- Chondromas are usually asymptomatic but may cause bone deformity, pain, and fracture. Lesions of the hands and feet are almost always innocuous but may recur when incompletely removed. Those in long bones raise the differential diagnosis of well-differentiated chondrosarcoma.

Chondroblastoma (p. 1297)

Chondroblastoma is an uncommon benign painful tumor almost invariably found in epiphyses of skeletally immature individuals (not to be confused with giant cell tumor or clear cell chondrosarcoma, both occurring in the same location but usually in older patients).

- The tumor cells are polygonal, arranged in sheets, and sometimes surrounded by a lacelike pattern of focally hyaline cartilage. Their nuclei are often deeply indented or longitudinally grooved.
- Multinucleated, osteoclast-like giant cells may be present and abundant enough to suggest a giant cell tumor of bone.
- The tumors are benign, but approximately 1% may develop metastases, usually after pathologic fracture or multiple recurrences. The metastases are cured by resection.

Chondromyxoid Fibroma (p. 1298)

This uncommon benign tumor is composed of chondroid, fibrous, and myxoid tissues.

- Chondromyxoid fibroma classically occurs in the metaphyses of the long bones about the knee, but any bone can be involved.
- There is a male preponderance, with most occurring during the teens and 20s.
- X-ray images show an eccentric circumscribed lucency and occasional calcifications.
- Because focal atypia can be marked, these tumors can be misdiagnosed as sarcomas.
- They are adequately treated by curettage and, despite possible recurrence, pose no threat.

Chondrosarcoma (p. 1298)

Chondrosarcoma occurs about half as often as osteosarcoma.

- Almost 90% arise *de novo* (primary); secondary chondrosarcomas arise in association with a preexisting enchondroma or osteochondroma.
- Most occur in middle to later life, the primary lesions being in the central skeleton (ribs, shoulder, and pelvic girdle) and around the knee. Lesions distal to the ankles and wrists are rare.
- Tumors are lobulated gray glistening and semitranslucent; necrosis and spotty calcification are frequently present.
- Distinction from enchondroma may be difficult in well-differentiated (grade I) tumors. An infiltrative growth pattern, hypercellularity, and anaplasia point toward chondrosarcoma.
- Equally difficult may be the differentiation of chondrosarcoma with ossification from osteosarcoma with chondroid differentiation. In chondrosarcomas, enchondral bone formation occurs at the edges of the cartilage; osteosarcomas have bone arising out of a background of cytologically malignant, osteoblastic-fibroblastic cells.
- X-ray images can be diagnostic. Classically, there is a localized area of lytic bone destruction punctuated by mottled densities from calcification or ossification. The tumor can extend for long distances in the medullary cavity, transgress the cortices, and form a soft tissue mass.
- All tumors require total removal; 5-year survival rates for grades I, II, and III (increasing cytologic anaplasia) are 90%, 81%, and 43%, respectively. None of the grade I lesions and 40% to 70% of the grade III lesions disseminate.

Fibrous and Fibro-Osseous Tumors (p. 1299)

Fibrous Cortical Defect and Nonossifying Fibroma (p. 1299)

These benign tumors are closely related. Nonossifying fiboma develops from a fibrous cortical defect that enlarges and extends into the medullary cavity. These lesions are some of the most common tumors of the skeleton. Radiographically, they are sharply defined, radiolucent, and typically arise in the metaphysis of the distal femur, proximal tibia, and fibula.

- Single (50%) or multiple and bilateral (50%)
- Does not transform to malignancy
- Generally asymptomatic but may (when large) lead to fracture
- Extremely common (reported in one third of normal children)
- Often spontaneously resolves

Fibrous Dysplasia (p. 1300)

Fibrous dysplasia refers to a localized, benign, progressive replacement of bone by a fibrous proliferation intermixed with poorly formed, haphazardly arranged trabeculae of woven bone. The latter are present in variable amounts, are not lined by osteoblasts, and form configurations likened to *Chinese characters*. There are three, somewhat overlapping, presentations:

- Involvement of a single bone *(monostotic):* 70%.
- Involvement of several or many bones *(polyostotic):* 25%.
- *Polyostotic disease associated with various endocrinopathies:* 3% to 5%. When accompanied by irregular skin pigmentation and precocious sexual development, it is termed *McCune-Albright syndrome.*
- The monostotic form is often asymptomatic, whereas the polyostotic form is frequently associated with deformities and fractures, especially of the craniofacial bones and the proximal femur (shepherd-crook deformity).
- The clinical course of the polyostotic forms is unpredictable.
- Rarely, secondary sarcoma develops, sometimes after irradiation.
- All forms result from a somatic (not hereditary) mutation occurring during embryogenesis involving a gene coding for a guanine nucleotide-binding G protein.

Fibrosarcoma and Malignant Fibrous Histiocytoma (p. 1301)

These tumors have overlapping clinical, radiographic, and pathologic features. Currently, malignant fibrous histiocytoma should be considered a sarcoma with a fibroblastic and myofibroblastic phenotype.

- Malignant fibrous histiocytoma and fibrosarcoma manifest as destructive, poorly defined, lytic masses that frequently extend into the soft tissues.
- Lesions usually arise *de novo*, but some arise on a background of Paget disease, bone infarcts, or prior radiation.
- They are large, solid gray-white masses. Fibrosarcoma is composed of cytologically malignant fibroblasts arranged in a herringbone pattern. More often, fibroblasts are moderately well differentiated but may be anaplastic.
- Malignant fibrous histiocytoma is composed of spindled fibroblasts in a storiform pattern admixed with bizarre multinucleated giant cells and neoplastic-appearing histiocytes (actually fibroblasts).
- Malignant fibrous histiocytoma is generally a high-grade pleomorphic tumor.
- These conditions may arise in soft tissues as well as in the metaphyses of long bones and pelvis.
- Prognosis depends on cytologic grade; high-grade tumors have a 20% 5-year survival rate.

Miscellaneous Tumors (p. 1301)

Ewing Sarcoma and Primitive Neuroectodermal Tumor (p. 1301)

Ewing sarcoma/primitive neuroectodermal tumor (PNET) is the prototypical malignant small round cell tumor that demonstrates varying degrees of neuroectodermal differentiation. Previously, Ewing sarcoma was considered undifferentiated, whereas PNET demonstrated neural differentiation. The tumor is characterized by a specific 11;22 chromosomal translocation.

- This tumor arises most often in children 10 to 15 years old; 80% are younger than 20 years.
- Boys are affected more often than girls; blacks are rarely affected.
- It is the second most common bone sarcoma in childhood.

- It arises in the medullary cavity in the diaphysis of long tubular bones, especially the femur, and flat bones of the pelvis.
- The tumor usually invades cortex and penetrates the periosteum to produce a soft tissue mass.
- It is composed of sheets of uniform small round cells that occasionally produce Homer-Wright pseudorosettes (tumor cells arrayed in a circle about a central fibrillary space).
- Cells have scant cytoplasm, which often contains glycogen.
- Generally, there is prominent necrosis in regions remote from vessels and little fibrous stroma.
- Frequently, the tumor metastasizes to other bones, lungs, or elsewhere.

Clinical Features. Ewing sarcoma/PNET presents as a painful, enlarging, warm, and swollen mass often suggesting an infection. The periosteal reaction produces layers of reactive bone deposited in an onion-skin fashion. With combined radiation, chemotherapy, and surgery, there is now a 75% 5-year survival rate.

Giant Cell Tumor (p. 1302)

Giant cell tumor of bone is a locally aggressive neoplasm found most often in the epiphyseal ends of long bones in adults 20 to 55 years old. More than half occur about the knees, but virtually any bone can be involved. Giant cell tumor of bone is *rare in skeletally immature people and infrequent in the elderly.*

Morphology
- The histologic pattern is one of uniformly distributed, osteoclast-like, multinucleated giant cells in a plump spindle-cell background.
- The neoplastic cell is the spindled stromal cell; the multinucleated cells are non-neoplastic.
- There may be foci of necrosis, hemorrhage, hemosiderin, or osteoid.

Clinical Features. X-ray images are distinctive (not pathognomonic), revealing large, lytic, eccentric lesions extending from the epiphysis into the diaphysis. Absent are stippling and calcifications.

- Histologic features do not allow prediction of which tumors will recur or metastasize. A rare lesion is overtly malignant from the outset.
- This biologic unpredictability complicates clinical management.

   The majority of tumors are localized and can be eradicated by curettage or conservative resections.

   From 40% to 60% recur locally.

   From 1% to 2% develop deceptively benign-looking metastases to the lungs.

Metastatic Disease (p. 1303)

In adults, more than half of skeletal metastases originate from cancers of the prostate, breast, kidney, and lung. In children, there is secondary involvement of skeleton, most commonly from neuroblastoma, Wilms tumor, osteosarcoma, Ewing sarcoma/PNET, and rhabdomyosarcoma. Most metastases to bone are lytic. The tumor cells elaborate prostaglandins, interleukins, and PTH-related protein that stimulate osteoclastic bone resorption. Osteosclerotic responses are most often induced by prostate and breast cancer by stimulating osteoblastic activity.

JOINTS (p. 1303)

Osteoarthritis (p. 1304)

Osteoarthritis or degenerative joint disease (DJD) is characterized by progressive deterioration and breakdown of articular cartilage, mainly in weight-bearing joints; this leads to subchondral bony thickening and bony overgrowths—osteophytes (spurs)—about the joint margins. DJD also causes the bony, knobby protrusions at the margins of the distal interphalangeal joints, creating nontender, subcutaneous Heberden nodes. The cause is unknown but is most likely related to metabolic and biochemical alterations.

DJD occurs in two clinical patterns:

- *Primary DJD* occurs *de novo*, mostly in men in midlife, somewhat later in women. Frequency increases with age to about 80% of those older than 70 years. Association between osteoarthritis and aging is nonlinear, the prevalence increasing exponentially beyond the age of 50.
- *Secondary DJD* appears at any age in a previously damaged or congenitally abnormal joint.

The relationship between age and previous injury suggests that *wear and tear* contributes to the genesis of this disease. Shoulders and elbows are often involved in baseball players, and knees in basketball players. Usually, knees and hands are more commonly involved in women and hips in men.

Pathogenesis

Pathogenesis is unknown but is clearly related to aging and injury; it is likely multifactorial.

- With aging, chondrocyte capacity to maintain cartilaginous matrix slows.
- Age-related changes include alterations in the content of proteoglycans and collagen within articular cartilage; ultimately, there is decreased resilience and increased vulnerability to injury.
- Under stresses of injury, chondrocytes elaborate IL1, which initiates matrix breakdown.
- Secondary mediators, such as TNF-α and transforming growth factor β, enhance chondrocyte lytic enzyme release, while inhibiting matrix synthesis.

Morphology

- Involvement usually is oligoarticular.
- Earliest changes are proteoglycan loss and decreased metachromasia of the articular cartilage, associated with areas of chondrocyte proliferation (*cloning*) and increased matrix basophilia.
- Thinning, fissuring, pitting, and flaking of the cartilage develop, followed by vertical clefts down to the subchondral bone.

- Flaking of the cartilage exposes underlying bone (eburnation); this appears ivory-like especially as continued joint motion polishes the surface.
- Subchondral fractures and microcysts typically develop.
- Synovium shows a mild chronic inflammatory infiltrate (nonspecific synovitis) and can develop osteocartilaginous metaplasia, fragments of which create osteocartilaginous loose bodies *(joint mice)* within the joint space.

Clinical Features

Although DJD may be asymptomatic, most patients experience morning stiffness in affected joints. There is usually no local heat or tenderness, but affected joints often show restricted range of motion, small effusions, and crepitus. Progressive reduction in mobility and increased painfulness with joint motion occur, but progression to bony ankylosis does not occur. Bone spurs and joint narrowing are apparent on x-rays. *There is no known way of preventing or arresting DJD.*

Rheumatoid Arthritis (p. 1305)

Rheumatoid arthritis (RA) is basically a severe form of chronic synovitis leading to destruction and ankylosis of affected joints. Blood vessels, skin, heart, lungs, nerves, and eyes may also be affected.

- About 1% of the world population suffers from rheumatoid arthritis.
- Women are affected three times more often than men.
- Peak prevalence is in the 20s to 30s.
- There is a familial association, and a link with HLA-DR4 or HLA-DR1.

Pathogenesis

The current best hypothesis regarding the pathogenesis of RA involves initiation by an arthritogenic antigen, possibly a microbial agent, in an immunogenetically susceptible host. After initial injury, a continuing autoimmune reaction ensues, in which T cells (CD4+) release cytokines and inflammatory mediators that ultimately destroy the joint.

- Linkage to HLA-DRB1 points to genetic susceptibility.
- Definitive microbial triggers are unknown, but Epstein-Barr virus is a prime suspect. Other agents, such as retroviruses, mycobacteria, *Borrelia,* and *Mycoplasma,* are also suspected.
- Once an inflammatory synovitis is initiated, an autoimmune reaction ensues: CD4+ cells are activated with release of many cytokines, particularly IL1 and TNF-α. These cells within joints mediate lysis of articular cartilage, initiate the inflammatory synovitis, and stimulate juxta-articular bone resorption.
- Autoantibodies are produced, some against autologous immunoglobulin G (IgG).
- Autoantibody against the Fc portion of autologous IgG is called *rheumatoid factor* (it is usually IgM, but sometimes IgG, IgA, or IgE).
- Rheumatoid factor contributes to the pathogenesis and indicates that humoral immune responses also play an important role in the disease.

Morphology

RA generally first affects small, proximal joints of the hands and feet but then may involve (usually symmetrically) the wrists, elbows, ankles, and knees.

- Well-developed lesions show villous hypertrophy of the synovium, synoviocytic hyperplasia, an intense lympho-plasmacytic and histiocytic synovial infiltrate, and numerous aggregates of organizing fibrin. Exuberant synovium is known as a *pannus*, which eventually fills the joint space, encroaching on the articular surfaces.
- Release of destructive enzymes (proteases and collagenases) and cytokines (particularly IL1 and TNF-α), and pannus formation destroy cartilage, leading to changes reminiscent of DJD but with fibrous and bony ankylosis. Neutrophils can be present in synovial fluid.
- Other features include *rheumatoid nodules* in subcutaneous tissues (these are areas of necrosis surrounded by a palisade of histiocytes at pressure points); acute vasculitis; and non-specific, fibrosing inflammatory lesions of lungs, pleura, pericardium, myocardium, peripheral nerves, and eyes.

Clinical Features

Clinical features are variable. Most patients experience a prodrome of malaise, fever, fatigue, and musculoskeletal pain before joint mobility is reduced.

- The lucky patient experiences mild transient disease without sequelae, but most have fluctuating disease with the greatest progression during the initial 4 to 5 years. In a minority, the onset is acute, with rapidly progressive limitation of motion and development of joint deformities.
- Characteristic deformities are radial deviation of the wrist with ulnar deviation of the fingers.
- Extra-articular manifestations are rarely the presenting features of the disease and tend to develop in patients with high rheumatoid factor titers (possibly related to deposition of circulating immune complexes).
- Some of the total morbidity of rheumatoid arthritis is caused by gastrointestinal bleeding from aspirin therapy, infections from steroid use, or amyloidosis in long-term severe disease.
- Variants of RA include *Felty syndrome* (features rheumatoid arthritis, splenomegaly, and neutropenia). RA also shares some features with the seronegative spondyloarthropathies.

Seronegative Spondyloarthropathies
(p. 1309)

Seronegative spondyloarthropathies are a group of diseases that develop in genetically predisposed individuals; they are initiated by environmental factors, especially prior infections or exposures. The manifestations are immune mediated. The seronegative arthropathies include ankylosing spondylitis, reactive arthritis (Reiter syndrome, enteropathic arthritis), psoriatic arthritis, and arthritis associated with inflammatory bowel disease. All have similar clinical features, and many are associated with HLA-B27, but all lack rheumatoid factor (hence the "seronegative" modifier).

- *Ankylosing spondylarthritis (Marie-Strümpell disease)* (p. 1309) is a chronic inflammatory joint disease of vertebrae and sacroiliac joints that usually occurs in males. It begins in adolescence after an infection and is suspected to be of immunogenetic origin, with autoantibodies directed at joint elements. It follows a chronic progressive course, with extension to hips, knees, and shoulders in one third of patients and sometimes uveitis, aortitis, and amyloidosis.

- Reiter syndrome comprises the triad of arthritis, nongonococcal urethritis or cervicitis, and conjunctivitis. Men are most often affected in their 20s to 30s, and most are positive for HLA-B27. The disease is caused by an autoimmune reaction initiated by prior infection, usually gastrointestinal or genitourinary. Ankles, knees, and feet may be affected, but in chronic disease, the spine is affected as well, reminiscent of ankylosing spondylitis. Extra-articular involvements include skin, eyes, heart, tendons, and muscles.

- *Psoriatic arthritis* (p. 1310) appears in about 5% of patients with psoriasis. The arthritis usually affects small joints of the hands and feet but may also extend to ankles, knees, hips, and wrists. Spinal disease occurs in about one quarter of the patients. Psoriatic arthritis is not as severe as RA, and there is less joint destruction.

- *Arthritis associated with inflammatory bowel disease* appears in 10% to 20% of patients with inflammatory bowel disease as a migratory oligoarthritis of the large joints and spine. It may resemble ankylosing spondylitis, but is generally less severe and remits spontaneously in a year or so.

Infectious Arthritis (p. 1310)

Infectious arthritis is uncommon but can rapidly destroy a joint to produce permanent loss of motion. Any of a great variety of microorganisms can seed the joint hematogenously or, more rarely, by direct inoculation or spread from a nearby focus of infection.

- *Suppurative arthritis* (p. 1310) is most commonly caused by gonococcus, staphylococcus, streptococcus, *Haemophilus influenzae,* and gram-negative coliforms. Individuals with sickle cell disease are prone to infection with salmonella. *H. influenzae* predominates in children younger than 2 years of age; *S. aureus* in older children and adults; and gonococcus in late adolescence and young adult life. In most instances, a single joint is affected, usually the knee, followed in frequency by hip, shoulder, elbow, wrist, and sternoclavicular joint. Gonococcal arthritis is mostly oligoarticular and often associated with a skin rash and a genetic deficiency of C5, C6, or C7.

- *Tuberculous arthritis* (p. 1310) is an insidious chronic arthritis from hematogenous spread or nearby tuberculous osteomyelitis. The most common site is the spine (Pott disease) followed by hip, knee, elbow, wrist, ankle, and sacroiliac joints. It tends to be a more destructive process than suppurative arthritis.

- *Lyme arthritis* (p. 1310) follows several days or weeks after the initial skin infection. The arthritis tends to be remitting and migratory and primarily involves large joints, especially the knees, shoulders, elbows, and ankles. The articular involvement morphologically resembles RA; in most cases, it clears spontaneously or with therapy, but in about 10% of patients, it results in permanent deformities.

Gout and Gouty Arthritis (p. 1311)

This group of conditions shares several characteristics:

* Hyperuricemia
* Attacks of acute arthritis triggered by crystallization of urates in joints
* Asymptomatic intervals
* Eventual development of chronic tophaceous gout and arthritis

Hyperuricemia is necessary for gout, but only a small fraction of hyperuricemic individuals develop gout. Most cases occur in men (after the 20s); women are almost never affected before menopause.

Pathogenesis

Primary and secondary forms exist:

* *Primary (90% of all cases):* The overwhelming majority are idiopathic (>95%), are of multifactorial inheritance, and are associated with overproduction of uric acid with normal or increased excretion or normal production of uric acid with underexcretion; alcohol use and obesity are predisposing factors. A small percentage of primary cases are associated with specific enzyme defects (e.g., X-linked, partial deficiency of hypoxanthine-guanine phosphoribosyltransferase [HGPRT]).
* *Secondary (10% of all cases):* Most are associated with increased nucleic acid turnover, which occurs with chronic hemolysis, polycythemia, leukemia, and lymphoma. Less commonly, drugs (especially diuretics, aspirin, nicotinic acid, and ethanol) or chronic renal disease leads to symptomatic hyperuricemia. Lead intoxication may induce *saturnine gout.* Rarely, the specific enzyme defects causing von Gierke disease (glycogen storage disease type I) and the Lesch-Nyhan syndrome (with a total lack of HGPRT seen only in men and associated with neurologic deficits) lead to gouty symptoms.

Morphology

Gouty arthritis represents an acute oligoarticular or monoarticular inflammatory synovitis initiated by urate crystal formation within joints.

* Needle-shaped crystals are birefringent with polarized light.
* The crystals activate factor XII (Hageman factor), with the production of chemoattractants (e.g., C3a and 5a) and inflammatory mediators. Neutrophils and macrophages accumulate in joints and phagocytose crystals, leading to release of lysosomal enzymes, toxic free radicals, IL1, IL6, IL8, TNF-α, prostaglandins, and leukotrienes, which collectively produce acute synovitis.
* Chronic arthritis evolves from the progressive precipitation of urates into the synovial linings of joints after recurrent attacks of acute arthritis.
* *The tophus is the pathognomonic lesion of gout*—a mass of urates, crystalline or amorphous, surrounded by an intense inflammatory reaction, composed of macrophages, lymphocytes, fibroblasts, and foreign body giant cells. Tophi tend to occur on the ear, in the olecranon and patellar bursae, and in periarticular ligaments and connective tissue.

- Three types of renal disease result from hyperuricemia:

  Acute uric acid nephropathy (intratubular urate deposition)
  Nephrolithiasis
  Chronic urate nephropathy (interstitial urate deposition)

Clinical Features

About 50% of the initial attacks of acute gouty arthritis involve the great toe or, less frequently, the instep, ankle, or heel.

- Sometimes physical or emotional fatigue, an alcoholic spree, or dietary overindulgence precedes an attack.
- The initial attack subsides spontaneously or with therapy, usually recurring within several months to a few years.
- Other joints become involved, and multiple recurrences lead to chronic gouty arthritis.
- About 90% of patients with chronic arthritis develop some renal impairment.
- Uricosuric therapy is effective in controlling gout.

Calcium Pyrophosphate Crystal Deposition Disease (Pseudogout) (p. 1314)

This form of acute or chronic arthritis is secondary to deposition of calcium pyrophosphate (chondrocalcinosis or pseudogout). *Many of the clinicopathologic features of this disease are similar to those of gout.* The crystals initially form in cartilage, and as the deposits enlarge they can rupture and shower the joint and synovium with billions of crystals that can induce further inflammatory reactions.

Pseudogout can be hereditary, sporadic, or associated with trauma or surgery. Calcium pyrophosphate crystals are frequently present in joint specimens from patients with DJD and in intervertebral disc material removed from patients with disc herniation.

- The deposits appear as oval aggregates (pools) of basophilic-staining rhomboid crystals. Whether these deposits cause the joint disease or are a secondary phenomenon is unclear.
- In pseudogout, almost any combination of joints as well as the intervertebral discs can be involved, but the knee is most frequently affected.
- Joint involvement may be transient, but about half the patients suffer significant joint damage.

Tumors and Tumor-Like Lesions (p. 1314)

Ganglion and Synovial Cyst (p. 1315)

A ganglion cyst is a small (1–1.5 cm), multiloculated, cavitated *(cystic)* lesion found in connective tissues of joint capsules or tendon sheaths.

- It arises from a focus of myxoid degeneration and softening of connective tissues. The cavities are cystic, not lined by epithelium, and they do not communicate with joint spaces.
- Favored location is the small joints of the wrist, where ganglions are palpated as a firm but yielding, pea-sized superficial nodule.
- The lesions are easily treatable by surgical removal; occasionally, they may erode underlying bone.

- Herniations of a synovium may occur, particularly into the popliteal space from the knee joint when there is a marked increase of intra-articular fluid or exudate, as in rheumatoid or suppurative arthritis. The herniations of the knee joints are known as synovial or Baker cysts.
- The anatomic changes are those of the underlying articular disease.

Pigmented Villonodular Synovitis and Giant Cell Tumor of Tendon Sheath (p. 1315)

Villonodular synovitis is the term for a group of closely related lesions involving synovial membranes and tendons, usually of peripheral joints.

- *Morphologically,* the lesions are made up of proliferating, mononuclear, polyhedral, synovial-like cells, fibroblasts, hemosiderin-laden histiocytes, and multinucleated, osteoclast-like cells.
- When the process is sharply localized and arising in a joint, it is referred to as *localized nodular synovitis;* if it arises in a tendon, it is a *localized nodular tenosynovitis or giant cell tumor of tendon sheath.* Tumors that more diffusely involve the synovial membrane (often with hemosiderin pigment) are called *pigmented villonodular synovitis.*
- Cytogenetic studies reveal a consistent abnormality strongly suggesting that these lesions are neoplasms and not manifestations of reactive processes.
- They can recur, especially the poorly localized forms, and cause destruction of underlying bone.

SOFT TISSUE TUMORS AND TUMOR-LIKE LESIONS (p. 1316)

Soft tissue tumors are "mesenchymal proliferations that arise in the extraskeletal nonepithelial tissue of the body, exclusive of the viscera, coverings of the brain, and lymphoreticular system." Soft tissue tumors are classified according to the normal tissue counterpart they recapitulate (Table 26–4). Some soft tissue tumors have specific chromosomal abnormalities (Table 26–5). Soft tissue tumors may be benign or malignant; most are benign with only a small minority being malignant (i.e., sarcomas, with the capacity to metastasize). Sarcomas are important because of their aggressive biologic potential. They may arise in any location, although about 40% occur in the lower extremity, especially the thighs, and 20% occur in the upper extremity, 10% in the head and neck, and 30% in the trunk and retroperitoneum. Critical to the clinical management of sarcomas are the following parameters:

- Size: the larger the mass, the poorer the outlook.
- Accurate histologic classification and grade: I through III are based largely on the degree of cytologic atypia, mitotic activity, and necrosis.
- Staging.
- Location of tumor: the more superficial, the better the prognosis.

TABLE 26–4 **Soft Tissue Tumors**

Tumors of Adipose Tissue
Lipomas
Liposarcoma

Tumors and Tumor-Like Lesions of Fibrous Tissue
Nodular fasciitis
Fibromatoses
   Superficial fibromatoses
   Deep fibromatoses
Fibrosarcoma

Fibrohistiocytic Tumors
Benign fibrous histiocytoma
Dermatofibrosarcoma protuberans
Malignant fibrous histiocytoma

Tumors of Skeletal Muscle
Rhabdomyoma
Rhabdomyosarcoma

Tumors of Smooth Muscle
Leiomyoma
Smooth muscle tumors of uncertain malignant potential
Leiomyosarcoma

Vascular Tumors
Hemangioma
Lymphangioma
Hemangioendothelioma
Hemangiopericytoma
Angiosarcoma

Peripheral Nerve Tumors
Neurofibroma
Schwannoma
Granular cell tumor
Malignant peripheral nerve sheath tumor

Tumors of Uncertain Histogenesis
Synovial sarcoma
Alveolar soft part sarcoma
Epithelioid sarcoma

Fatty Tumors (p. 1317)

Lipomas (p. 1317)

Lipomas are the most common benign soft tissue tumor of adults, arising in subcutaneous regions at any site but most commonly on the back, shoulder, and neck. They can also arise in skeletal muscle, mediastinum, retroperitoneum, or bowel wall.

Lipomas are delicately encapsulated, usually small tumors recapitulating normal, mature white adipose tissue. Uncommonly, atypical examples occur in subcutaneous locations, where they should not be mistaken for liposarcoma.

Liposarcomas (p. 1318)

Liposarcomas are much less common and tend to be big bulky masses. Liposarcomas appear virtually anywhere in the body without regard to adipose tissue. Most arise in deep soft tissues and pursue a course closely dependent on their morphologic features.

TABLE 26-5 **Chromosomal and Genetic Abnormalities in Soft Tissue Sarcomas**

Tumor	Cytogenetic Abnormality	Genetic Abnormality
Extraosseous Ewing sarcoma and primitive neuroectodermal tumor	t(11:22)(q24;q12)	FLI1-J-EWS fusion gene
	t(21:22)(q22;q12)	ERG-EWS fusion gene
	t(7;22)(q22;q12)	ETV1-EWS fusion gene
Liposarcoma—myxoid and round cell type	t(12:16)(q13;p11)	CHOP/TLS fusion gene
Synovial sarcoma	t(x;18)(p11;q11)	SYT-SSX fusion gene
Rhabdomyosarcoma—alveolar type	t(2;13)(q35;q14)	PAX3-FKHR fusion gene
	t(1;13)(p36;q14)	PAX7-FKHR fusion gene
Extraskeletal myxoid chondrosarcoma	t(9;22)(q22;q12)	CHN-EWS fusion gene
Desmoplastic small round cell tumor	t(11;22)(p13;q12)	EWS-WT1 fusion gene
Clear cell sarcoma	t(12;22)(q13;q12)	EWS-ATF1 fusion gene
Dermatofibrosarcoma protuberans	t(17:22)(q22;q15)	COLA1-PDGFB fusion gene
Alveolar soft part sarcoma	t(X;17)(p11.2;q15)	TFE3-ASPL fusion gene
Congenital fibrosarcoma	t(12;15)(p13;q23)	ETV6-NTRK3 fusion gene

- Well-differentiated (lipoma-like) liposarcoma is a low-grade tumor that is stubbornly recurrent, follows a protracted course, does not metastasize, and infrequently undergoes dedifferentiation.
- In contrast, myxoid/round cell liposarcoma, and pleomorphic liposarcoma are high-grade, aggressive sarcomas (40%–90% metastasize). The myxoid/round cell variant has a characteristic balanced 12:16 translocation.

Fibrous Tumors and Tumor-Like Lesions
(p. 1318)

Reactive Pseudosarcomatous Proliferations
(p. 1318)

Nodular Fasciitis (p. 1318)

Nodular fasciitis is a reactive, benign, fibroproliferative lesion, also known as pseudosarcomatous fasciitis, that is more commonly mistaken for a neoplasm than any other non-neoplastic condition.

- The lesions appear as palpable nodules or small masses, most often in the extremities in young and middle-aged adults of either sex.
- After a period of rapid growth (several weeks to a month), the tumors tend to plateau in size, indicating cessation of growth.
- *Morphologically,* they are composed of spindled fibroblasts and myofibroblasts in a loose myxoid background resem-

bling cultured fibroblasts. Some of the more active cells are enlarged and have prominent nuclei and nucleoli; mitoses are often present and may be numerous.

- Recurrence, even after incomplete excision, is exceedingly rare and should lead to a reappraisal of the original diagnosis.

Myositis Ossificans (p. 1319)

Myositis ossificans is often preceded by trauma, occurring most often in skeletal muscle but sometimes in subcutaneous fat.

- Favored locations are the extremities, particularly the quadriceps or brachialis muscle.
- The lesions are circumscribed but unencapsulated masses. Morphologically, they have a zonal pattern and are composed of a central region of proliferating fibroblasts and myofibroblasts in a myxoid stroma. This area merges with tissue that contains poorly formed trabeculae of woven bone, often mineralized, and rimmed by large metabolically active osteoblasts. The bone is most mature in appearance at the periphery and over time may closely resemble normal bone, including the presence of hematopoietic elements. Myositis ossificans should not be confused with osteogenic sarcoma.
- Mature lesions are completely ossified.

Fibromatoses (p. 1319)

Palmar, Plantar, and Penile Fibromatosis (p. 1319)

The *fibromatoses* encompass a group of fibroproliferative lesions with similar histopathologic features but variable clinical presentations.

- When on the palm, the process is known as *palmar fibromatosis (Dupuytren contracture)*.
- When on the foot, the process is known as *plantar fibromatosis*.
- When involving the penis, the process is known as *penile fibromatosis (Peyronie disease)*.

These lesions may recur after excision or spontaneously resolve in about 25% of patients.

Deep-Seated Fibromatosis (Desmoid Tumors) (p. 1319)

This locally aggressive tumor, unlike low-grade fibrosarcoma, does not have the capacity to metastasize. Mutations in the *APC* or beta-catenin genes are present in most tumors.

- It presents as an infiltrative mass in abdominal (affecting mothers in the perinatal period), extra-abdominal (affecting men and women equally), and intra-abdominal (Gardner syndrome) locations.
- It is composed of banal, *tame-looking* fibroblasts (actually myofibroblasts by electron microscopy) that are arranged in broad sweeping fascicles that infiltrate the neighboring tissues.
- Although curable by adequate excision, they stubbornly recur in the local site when incompletely removed.

Fibrosarcomas (p. 1320)

Fibrosarcomas occur in deep soft tissue and are gray, soft (fish-flesh consistency) masses with increased cellularity, anaplasia, high nuclear-cytoplasmic ratios, abundant mitotic figures, and *spindled growth in a herringbone pattern.*

- Fibrosarcomas often are large masses that appear deceptively encapsulated but are nonetheless infiltrative.
- Overall, 60% to 80% of patients survive 5 years with present methods of treatment.

Fibrohistiocytic Tumors (p. 1320)

Benign Fibrous Histiocytomas (Dermatofibroma) (p. 1320)

These distinctive unencapsulated but demarcated neoplasms are composed of a mixture of cells resembling fibroblasts, myofibroblasts, and histiocytes.

- Hemosiderin pigment, benign giant cells, and lipid-laden foamy cells are often present.
- Benign lesions predominantly occur in the skin and are most frequently referred to as *dermatofibromas.*

Malignant Fibrous Histiocytoma (p. 1321)

Malignant fibrous histiocytoma is one of the most common sarcomas of adulthood. Despite the name, the phenotype of the tumor is fibroblastic and not histiocytic. Recently, these lesions have been the center of controversy as some investigators believe that most represent poorly differentiated variants of other types of sarcomas.

- They typically develop during adulthood, arising in the deep soft tissues of the extremities, especially the thigh. Also, they may be limited to the subcutis or dermis (atypical fibroxanthoma).
- Most common subtypes are storiform-pleomorphic and myxoid (myxofibrosarcoma) variants. Many are high-grade.
- They can behave aggressively; they are appropriately treated with surgery, and in some circumstances chemotherapy and radiation.

Tumors of Skeletal Muscle (p. 1321)

Rhabdomyosarcoma (p. 1321) *is the most common soft tissue sarcoma of children.* These are subdivided into three major types based on morphologic features:

- Embryonal (including botryoid and spindle variants)
- Alveolar
- Pleomorphic

The botryoid pattern is basically a morphologic variant of the embryonal pattern, which in submucosal locations projects into a cavity (e.g., vagina, bladder, as grapelike masses [hence botryoid]).

- About 90% of embryonal and alveolar rhabdomyosarcomas occur before age 20 years. Embryonal rhabdomyosarcoma frequently arises in children in areas that do not contain an abundance of skeletal muscle such as the head and neck and urogenital regions. In contrast, alveolar rhabdomyosarcomas develop in older children, and are commonly centered in the deep skeletal muscle of the extremities.
- Embryonal and alveolar variants are poorly differentiated tumors composed of malignant small round blue cells. The tumors frequently demonstrate focal skeletal muscle

differentiation in the form of rhabdomyoblasts. These cells have abundant, eccentric, eosinophilic cytoplasm and can exhibit cross-striations.

- Rhabdomyoblastic differentiation may be apparent only with electron microscopic or immunohistochemical techniques (thick and thin filaments with cross striations or immunoperoxidase positivity with desmin, myogenin, and Myo D1). The alveolar variant is characterized by a 2:13 chromosomal translocation.
- The pleomorphic type is rare and occurs in patients older than 45 years. It is composed of large, atypical tumor cells, some showing abundant cytoplasm with cross-striations. This variant has a poor prognosis.
- The tumors are usually treated with surgery combined with chemotherapy and radiation. The alveolar and pleomorphic variants are the most aggressive types and have the worst prognosis.

Tumors of Smooth Muscle (p. 1322)

Leiomyoma (p. 1322)

Benign smooth muscle tumors occur predominantly in the female genital tract, particularly the uterus (Chapter 22), but they may also occur at other body sites where smooth muscle is well represented (e.g., scrotum, nipple, bowel wall).

Leiomyosarcoma (p. 1322)

- Leiomyosarcomas are uncommon; they occur more frequently in women than in men.
- Most develop in skin and deep soft tissue.
- They are usually large, soft, gray masses of spindle cells with cigar-shaped nuclei.
- Variants may be myxoid or epithelioid.
- Superficial lesions often can be excised; deep tumors are invasive and rarely resectable.

Synovial Sarcoma (p. 1323)

These tumors occur around joints (but not in joint spaces), in the parapharyngeal region, in the abdominal wall, and less commonly at other body sites.

- The highly distinctive feature of these infiltrative sarcomas (shared by mesotheliomas and carcinosarcomas) is their biphasic pattern of cell growth: there are distinct epithelial components forming glands and papillary patterns, admixed with well-defined spindle cell components.
- They range in behavior from aggressive lesions causing death within a few months to indolent tumors permitting cure or long-term survival (5-year survival rate is about 50%).
- Most have a reciprocal translocation between chromosomes X and 18 (p11.2;q11.2).

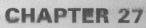

CHAPTER 27

Peripheral Nerve and Skeletal Muscle

NORMAL NEUROMUSCULAR FUNCTION
(p. 1326)

A *motor unit* consists of

- A single *lower motor neuron* (spinal anterior horn cell)
- The *axon* of that neuron
- The *muscle fibers* it innervates

There are more muscle fibers per motor unit in muscles with coarse movements (such as calf muscles with 1800 muscle fibers in each unit) than in those with refined movements (such as extraocular eye muscles with 10 muscle fibers in each unit). *Peripheral nerves* are composed of *myelinated* (2–15 μm) and *unmyelinated* (0.2–3 μm) *axons* and their investing Schwann cells grouped into fascicles by connective tissue sheaths:

- Epineurium—encloses the entire nerve
- Perineurium—encircles each fascicle
- Endoneurium—surrounds individual nerve fibers

Single Schwann cells myelinate axonal segments (internodes) separated by nodes of Ranvier. Protein synthesis does not occur in the axon; rather, axoplasmic flow delivers proteins and other substances synthesized in the perikaryon, and a retrograde transport system serves as a feedback to the cell body. The *perineurial barrier* is formed by the tight junctions between the perineurial cells. Endoneurial capillaries complete the *blood-nerve barrier.*

Skeletal muscles (muscle fibers) are syncytial cells with multiple nuclei located beneath the plasma membrane *(sarcolemma);* they contain identical repeating units *(sarcomeres)* of actin and myosin contractile proteins delimited by perpendicularly disposed Z bands (primarily α-actinin). In normal human muscle, there are two types of fibers with different functional characteristics and staining patterns (Table 27–1). All fibers of a given motor unit are of the same

659

TABLE 27–1 **Muscle Fiber Types**

Feature	Type 1	Type 2
Action	Sustained force	Sudden movements
Strength	Weight bearing	Purposeful motion
Enzyme content	NADH dark staining	NADH light staining
	ATPase at pH 4.2, dark staining	ATPase at pH 4.2, light staining
	ATPase at pH 9.4, light staining	ATPase at pH 9.4, dark staining
Lipids	Abundant	Scant
Glycogen	Scant	Abundant
Ultrastructure	Many mitochondria	Few mitochondria
	Wide Z-band	Narrow Z-band
Physiology	Slow-twitch	Fast-twitch
Color	Red	White
Prototype	Soleus (pigeon)	Pectoral (pigeon)

type; however, they are distributed across the cross-section of a muscle, giving a checkerboard pattern (when visualized using special stains).

General Reactions of the Motor Unit
(p. 1328)

Segmental Demyelination (p. 1328)

Loss of myelin occurs along discrete regions of axons from dysfunction of the Schwann cell or damage to the myelin sheath; no primary abnormality of the axon is present. With sequential episodes of demyelination and remyelination, layers of Schwann cell processes accumulate around the axon (onion bulbs).

Axonal Degeneration and Muscle Fiber Atrophy
(p. 1329)

Primary destruction of the axon occurs, with secondary disintegration of its myelin sheath. In the slowly evolving neuronopathies or axonopathies, evidence of myelin breakdown is scant because only a few fibers degenerate at a time. Wallerian degeneration is the acute reaction distal to a cut axon and consists of axonal and myelin breakdown with phagocytosis by macrophages.

Nerve Regeneration and Reinnervation of Muscle
(p. 1330)

Proximal stumps of degenerated axons can regrow, guided by Schwann cells vacated by degenerated axons. Regeneration occurs at a rate on the order of 2 mm per day and shows multiple, closely aggregated, thinly myelinated small-caliber axons (regenerating cluster). This regrowth of axons is a slow process, apparently limited by the rate of the slow component of axonal transport and the movement of tubulin, actin, and intermediate filaments.

Reactions of the Muscle Fiber (p. 1330)

- Denervation atrophy: Breakdown of myosin and actin, and shrinkage of muscle fibers to small, angulated shapes occur as a result of loss of innervation.

- *Reinnervation:* This occurs after nerve regeneration or, more commonly, when surviving axons sprout around denervated muscle cells and incorporate the fibers into their motor unit, imparting the same histochemical type to a group of contiguous fibers—*type grouping.*
- *Group atrophy:* This occurs when a type group becomes denervated.
- *Myopathic changes:* Varied patterns occur, including segmental necrosis, myophagocytosis, myocyte regeneration via satellite cells, increased central nuclei, and variation in fiber size.
- *Segmental necrosis:* Destruction of a portion of a myofiber may be followed by *myophagocytosis* as macrophages infiltrate the region.
- *Regeneration:* Peripherally located satellite cells proliferate and reconstitute a destroyed portion of the fiber. The regenerating fiber shows large internalized nuclei, prominent nucleoli, and basophilic cytoplasm laden with RNA.
- *Hypertrophy:* In response to increased load, large fibers may divide along a segment *(muscle fiber splitting)* so that, in cross-section, a single large fiber contains a cell membrane traversing its diameter, often with adjacent nuclei.

DISEASES OF PERIPHERAL NERVE (p. 1330)

Inflammatory Neuropathies (p. 1330)

Immune-Mediated Neuropathies (p. 1331)

- *Guillain-Barré syndrome* (acute inflammatory demyelinating polyradiculoneuropathy) (p. 1331) is a life-threatening ascending paralysis, with weakness beginning in the distal limbs but rapidly advancing to affect proximal muscles.

  Annual incidence in the United States is 1/100,000 to 3/100,000.

  Nerve conduction velocity is slowed and cerebrospinal fluid protein is elevated in the absence of increased cells.

  Pathologic features are segmental demyelination and chronic inflammatory cells involving the nerve roots and peripheral nerves.

  Guillain-Barré syndrome appears to be an immune-mediated disorder, often following a viral infection (cytomegalovirus, Epstein-Barr virus) or *Campylobacter jejuni.*

- *Chronic inflammatory demyelinating polyradiculoneuropathy* (p. 1331) is a mixed sensorimotor polyneuropathy similar to Guillain-Barré syndrome, but it follows a subacute or chronic course, usually with relapses and remissions. Peripheral nerves show recurrent demyelination and remyelination and "onion bulb" histologic changes.

Infectious Polyneuropathies (p. 1331)

- Direct infections of Schwann cells occur in leprosy (p. 387); the host response can be either limited *(lepromatous leprosy)* or vigorous *(tuberculoid leprosy).*
- After chickenpox, varicella-zoster virus produces latent infection of neurons in the sensory ganglia of the spinal cord and brain stem; subsequent reactivation leads to a painful

vesicular skin eruption in the distribution of sensory dermatomes *(shingles)*, most frequently thoracic or trigeminal.
- In contrast to these direct infectious processes, diphtheritic neuropathy results from the effects of the diphtheria exotoxin. It begins clinically with paresthesias and weakness and is characterized pathologically by segmental demyelination.

Hereditary Neuropathies (p. 1332)

Both strength and sensation are affected in the *hereditary motor and sensory neuropathies*.

Hereditary Motor and Sensory Neuropathy Type I (HMSN I)

Hereditary motor and sensory neuropathy type I (HMSN I) is the most common form (also known as *Charcot-Marie-Tooth disease,* hypertrophic form) and typically presents in young adults with weakness and calf atrophy. The disease is autosomal dominant, with multiple genetic forms. The most common genetic variant involves duplication of a portion of chromosome 17, including a myelin-specific protein gene, *PMP-22* (HMSN, type IA). Less commonly, there is a mutation of a gene on chromosome 1, coding for myelin protein zero (HMSN, type IB). An X-linked form involves gap junction protein connexin-32. Pathologically, the disease shows segmental demyelination and "onion bulb" histologic changes; the underlying common pathogenic feature involves repetitive demyelination.

Other Hereditary Motor and Sensory Neuropathies

- HMSN II is clinically similar, but exhibits axonal loss without demyelination. This neuronal type is also autosomal dominant (locus on chromosome 1). Nerves show axonal loss without nerve enlargement and no onion bulb histologic changes.
- Déjérine-Sottas disease (HMSN III) is an infantile, autosomal recessive neuropathy that may involve either *PMP-22* (on chromosome 17) or myelin protein zero (on chromosome 1). Onset is in infancy, with progressive upper and lower extremity weakness and muscle atrophy and greatly enlarged palpable nerves. Segmental demyelination is severe, with prominent onion bulbs.

In the *hereditary sensory and autonomic neuropathies,* symptoms are usually limited to numbness, pain, and autonomic dysfunction, such as orthostatic hypotension (Table 27–2). Some hereditary neuropathies are notable for the deposition of amyloid within the nerve; these *familial amyloid polyneuropathies* have a clinical presentation similar to that of the hereditary sensory and autonomic neuropathies. In other cases, inborn errors of metabolism cause prominent peripheral nerve manifestations (Table 27–3).

TABLE 27–2   Hereditary Sensory and Autonomic
Neuropathies

Disease and Inheritance	Gene and Locus	Clinical and Pathologic Findings
HSAN I; autosomal dominant	Serine palmitoyl-transferase, long-chain base, subunit 1 (*SPTLC1*) gene; 9q22.1–q22.3	Predominantly sensory neuropathy, presenting in young adults; axonal degeneration (mostly myelinated fibers)
HSAN II; autosomal recessive (some cases are sporadic)	Unknown	Predominantly sensory neuropathy, presenting in infancy; axonal degeneration (mostly myelinated fibers)
HSAN III (Riley-Day syndrome; familial dysautonomia; most often in Jewish children); autosomal recessive	Inhibitor of kappa light polypeptide gene enhancer in B cells, kinase complex-associated protein (*IKBKAP or IKAP*) gene; 9q31–q33	Predominantly autonomic neuropathy, presenting in infancy; axonal degeneration (mostly unmyelinated fibers); atrophy and loss of sensory and autonomic ganglion cells

Acquired Metabolic and Toxic Neuropathies
(p. 1334)

Peripheral Neuropathy in Adult-Onset Diabetes Mellitus (p. 1334)

Three principal patterns of neuropathy occur in diabetes mellitus:

- *Distal symmetric sensory or sensorimotor neuropathy* (most commonly a chronic axonal neuropathy with dramatic reduction of small myelinated and unmyelinated fibers)
- *Autonomic neuropathy* (affects about 20%–40% of diabetics)
- *Focal or multifocal asymmetric neuropathy* (mononeuropathy or multiple mononeuropathy), such as unilateral ocular nerve palsies with sparing of reflexes

Metabolic and Nutritional Peripheral Neuropathies (p. 1334)

Neuropathies are encountered in patients with renal failure (before dialysis), chronic liver disease, chronic respiratory insufficiency, and hypothyroidism. Axonal neuropathies also occur with deficiencies of thiamine, vitamin B_{12} (cobalamin) vitamin B_6 (pyridoxine), and vitamin E (α-tocopherol). The neuropathy caused by excessive alcohol consumption is often associated with thiamine deficiency.

Neuropathies Associated With Malignancy (p. 1334)

- *Direct effects:* Infiltration or compression of peripheral nerves by tumor may cause a mononeuropathy, brachial

TABLE 27-3 Hereditary Neuropathies Accompanying Inherited Metabolic Disease

Disease	Metabolic Defect	Inheritance	Clinical Findings	Pathologic Findings
Adrenoleukodystrophy	ATP-binding cassette, or ABC, transporter protein, subfamily D, member 1 (ALD protein, or *ABCD1*) gene; Xq28	X-linked; 4% of female carriers are symptomatic	Mixed motor and sensory neuropathy, adrenal insufficiency, spastic paraplegia; onset between 10 and 20 years for males with leukodystrophy, between 20 and 40 years for females with myeloneuropathy	Segmental demyelination, with onion bulbs; axonal degeneration (myelinated and unmyelinated); electron microscopy; linear inclusions in Schwann cells
Familial amyloid polyneuropathies	Transthyretin (*TTR*) gene (rarely other genes); 18q11.2–q12.1	Autosomal-dominant	Sensory and autonomic dysfunction; age at onset varies with site of mutation	Amyloid deposits in vessel walls and connective tissue with axonal degeneration
Porphyria, acute intermittent (AIP) or variegate coproporphyria	Enzymes involved in heme synthesis (acute intermittent porphyria—porphobilinogen deaminase deficiency; 11q24.1–q24.2)	Autosomal-dominant	Acute episodes of neurologic dysfunction, psychiatric disturbances, abdominal pain, seizures, proximal weakness, autonomic dysfunction; attacks may be precipitated by drugs	Acute and chronic axonal degeneration; regenerating clusters
Refsum disease	Peroxisomal enzyme phytanoyl CoA α-hydroxylase (*PAHX*) gene; 10pter–p11.2	Autosomal-recessive	Mixed motor and sensory neuropathy with palpable nerves; ataxia, night blindness, retinitis pigmentosa, ichthyosis; age at onset before 20 years (a genetically distinct infantile form also exists)	Severe onion bulb formation

plexopathy, cranial nerve palsy, or polyradiculopathies involving the lower extremities when the cauda equina is involved by meningeal carcinomatosis.
* Paraneoplastic syndromes:

Progressive sensorimotor neuropathy is most pronounced in the lower extremities, particularly with small cell lung carcinoma. Less commonly, a pure sensory neuropathy occurs as a result of loss of dorsal root ganglion cells and axonal loss in the posterior columns of the spinal cord. Patients often have a circulating polyclonal antibody directed against a neuronal protein (anti-Hu).

Peripheral neuropathy with deposition of light-chain amyloid in peripheral nerves (AL type) occurs in patients with plasma cell dyscrasias. Neuropathy may also be related to the binding of monoclonal immunoglobulin M (IgM) to myelin-associated glycoprotein (MAG) independent of amyloid deposition.

Toxic Neuropathies (p. 1335)

Peripheral neuropathies may occur after exposure to industrial or environmental chemicals, biologic toxins, heavy metals, or therapeutic drugs.

Traumatic Neuropathies (p. 1335)

* *Lacerations:* Neuropathies can follow cutting injuries or bone fractures in which sharp fragments of bone lacerate a nerve.
* *Avulsions:* Following application of tension to a nerve, neuropathies can occur as the result of a force applied to one of the limbs.
* *Traumatic neuromas:* Painful nodules of tangled axons and connective tissue from regenerating axonal sprouts of the proximal stump may occur after nerve transection.
* *Compression neuropathy (entrapment neuropathy):* Most commonly seen with the median nerve at the level of the wrist within the compartment delimited by the transverse carpal ligament *(carpal tunnel syndrome)*. This neuropathy is observed with any condition that can cause decreased space within the carpal tunnel, such as tissue edema; additional factors include pregnancy, degenerative joint disease, hypothyroidism, amyloidosis (especially that related to β_2-microglobulin deposition in renal dialysis patients), and excessive wrist usage.

Tumors of Peripheral Nerve (p. 1335)

These tumors are discussed in association with tumors of the central nervous system (Chapter 28).

DISEASES OF SKELETAL MUSCLE (p. 1335)

Denervation Atrophy (p. 1335)

Denervation atrophy is caused by any process that affects the anterior horn cell or its processes in the peripheral nervous system.

Spinal Muscular Atrophy (Infantile Motor Neuron Disease) (p. 1336)

Spinal muscular atrophy (SMA) refers to a group of autosomal recessive motor neuron diseases beginning in childhood or adolescence, with a locus on chromosome 5 (5q12.2-13.3). Histologic findings include large numbers of extremely atrophic fibers, often involving an entire fascicle of a muscle. The most common form *(Werdnig-Hoffmann disease, SMA type 1)* has onset at birth or within the first 4 months, with death within the first 3 years. SMA 2 and SMA 3 present at later ages, with shorter survival times in the earlier-onset form (SMA 2).

Muscular Dystrophies (p. 1336)

The muscular dystrophies are a heterogeneous group of inherited disorders, often beginning in childhood and characterized clinically by progressive muscular weakness and wasting.

X-Linked Muscular Dystrophy (Duchenne Muscular Dystrophy and Becker Muscular Dystrophy) (p. 1336)

Duchenne Muscular Dystrophy

Duchenne muscular dystrophy is the most common dystrophy (incidence about 1 : 3500 males). Affected boys are normal at birth but become weak by age 5 leading to wheelchair dependence by age 10 to 12. The disease progresses relentlessly until death by the early 20s. Weakness begins in the pelvic girdle muscles, extending to the shoulder girdle. Pathologic changes are also found in the heart, and cognitive impairment appears to be a component of the disease. Histopathologic abnormalities common to Duchenne muscular dystrophy and Becker muscular dystrophy include:

- *Variation in myofiber size* (diameter), owing to the presence of both small and giant fibers, sometimes with fiber splitting
- Increased numbers of internalized nuclei (beyond the normal range of 3%–5%)
- Degeneration, necrosis, and phagocytosis of muscle fibers
- Regeneration of muscle fibers
- Proliferation of endomysial connective tissue

The responsible gene is at Xp21 region; it encodes a 427-kD protein *(dystrophin)*, putatively responsible for transducing contractile forces from the intracellular sarcomeres to the extracellular matrix. Deletions represent a large proportion of patients, with frameshift and point mutations accounting for the rest. Muscle from patients with Duchenne muscular dystrophy has almost no detectable dystrophin by either staining or biochemical measurement.

Becker Muscular Dystrophy

Becker muscular dystrophy involves the same genetic locus as Duchenne muscular dystrophy but is less common and much less severe, with onset occurring later in childhood or in adolescence and having a slower, more variable rate of progression. Muscle from Becker muscular dystrophy patients has diminished amounts of dystrophin, usually of an abnormal molecular weight, reflecting mutations that allow synthesis of some protein.

Other X-linked Muscular Dystrophies

These disorders, such as Emery-Dreifuss muscular dystrophy, are caused by mutations affecting separate genes.

Autosomal Muscular Dystrophies (p. 1338)

Some autosomal muscular dystrophies affect specific muscle groups, and the specific diagnosis is based largely on the pattern of clinical muscle weakness (Table 27–4). A group of the autosomal muscular dystrophies are similar to the X-linked muscular dystrophies and are termed *limb girdle muscular dystrophies* (LGMDs).

Limb girdle muscular dystrophies (p. 1338) affect the proximal musculature of the trunk and limbs with either an autosomal dominant *(LGMD 1)* or a recessive *(LGMD 2)* inheritance. Mutations of proteins that interact with dystrophin have been identified in some of the LGMDs.

Myotonic Dystrophy (p. 1338)

Myotonic dystrophy is an autosomal dominant disease that tends to increase in severity and appear at a younger age in succeeding generations. Myotonic dystrophy presents with abnormalities in gait secondary to weakness of foot dorsiflexors; weakness progresses with atrophy of muscles of the face, and ptosis ensues. Other associated findings include cataracts, frontal balding, gonadal atrophy, cardiomyopathy, smooth muscle involvement, decreased plasma IgG, and an abnormal glucose tolerance test.

Myotonia, the sustained involuntary contraction of a group of muscles, is the cardinal neuromuscular symptom in this disease. Muscles show features of a dystrophy (similar to Duchenne muscular dystrophy) as well as a striking increase in the number of internal nuclei and *ring fibers,* with a subsarcolemmal band of cytoplasm that appears distinct from the center of the fiber. Myotonic dystrophy is the only dystrophy that shows pathologic changes in muscle spindles, with fiber splitting, necrosis, and regeneration.

The gene (19q13.2-13.3, coding for *myotonin-protein kinase*) contains a trinucleotide repeat. The disease state is caused by expansion of the repeat sequence (in normal subjects, <30 repeats are present, whereas in severely affected individuals, several thousand repeats may be present).

Ion Channel Myopathies (Channelopathies) (p. 1339)

- *Hypokalemic, hyperkalemic, and normokalemic periodic paralysis:* Relapsing episodes of hypotonic paralysis are associated with various levels of serum potassium. Hyperkalemic periodic paralysis is caused by mutations in a muscle sodium channel (gene on chromosome 17); periodic acid–Schiff (PAS)-positive vacuoles, especially evident during episodes of acute weakness, correspond to dilation of the sarcoplasmic reticulum.
- *Malignant hyperpyrexia (malignant hyperthermia):* This is an autosomal dominant syndrome with a dramatic

TABLE 27-4 Other Muscular Dystrophies

Disease and Inheritance	Gene and Locus	Clinical Findings	Pathologic Findings
Facioscapulohumeral muscular dystrophy, autosomal-dominant	Type 1A—deletion of variable number of 3.3-kb subunits of a tandemly arranged repeat (D4Z4) on 4q35 Type 1B (FSHMD1B)—locus unknown	Variable age at onset (most commonly 10–30 years); Weakness of muscles of face, neck, and shoulder girdle	Dystrophic myopathy, but also often including inflammatory infiltrates of muscle
Oculopharyngeal muscular dystrophy, autosomal-dominant	Poly(A)-binding protein-2 (PABP2) gene; 14q11.2–q13	Onset in midadult life; ptosis and weakness of extraocular muscles; difficulty in swallowing	Dystrophic myopathy, but often including rimmed vacuoles in type 1 fibers
Emery-Dreifuss muscular dystrophy; X-linked (mostly)	Emerin (EMD1) gene; Xq28	Variable onset (most commonly 10–20 years); prominent contractures, especially of elbows and ankles	Mild myopathic changes; absent emerin by immunohistochemistry
Congenital muscular dystrophies; autosomal-recessive (also called *muscular dystrophy, congenital*, subtypes MDC1A, MDC1B, MDC1C)	Type 1A (merosin-deficient type)— laminin α2 (merosin) gene; 6q22–q23 Type 1B—locus at 1q42; gene unknown Type 1C; fukutin-related protein gene; 19q13.3	Neonatal hypotonia, respiratory insufficiency, delayed motor milestones	Variable fiber size and extensive endomysial fibrosis

hypermetabolic crisis (tachycardia, tachypnea, muscle spasms, and later hyperpyrexia) triggered by anesthesia (ordinarily halogenated inhaled agents and succinylcholine).

Congenital Myopathies (p. 1340)

This group of muscle diseases is characterized by onset in early life of nonprogressive or slowly progressive, proximal or generalized muscle weakness, and hypotonia *(floppy babies)*, or severe joint contractures *(arthrogryposis)* (Table 27–5).

Myopathies Associated With Inborn Errors of Metabolism (p. 1341)

Myopathies are often associated with disorders of glycogen synthesis and degradation (Chapter 5) and can also result from disorders of mitochondrial function.

Lipid Myopathies (p. 1341)

The principal morphologic characteristic of lipid myopathies is vacuolar accumulation of lipid within myocytes, predominantly in type 1 fibers. Fatty acids are normally catabolized in mitochondria; the myopathies are caused by an abnormal carnitine transport system or deficiencies of the mitochondrial dehydrogenase enzyme systems leading to defective ATP (adenosine triphosphate) generation.

- *Fatty acid catabolism (β-oxidation)* begins with trans-esterification of acyl-CoA to carnitine (via carnitine palmitoyltransferase, CPT I), transport across the inner mitochondrial membrane, trans-esterification to acyl-CoA (CPT II), and catabolism to acetyl-CoA via acyl-CoA dehydrogenases. Lipid myopathies may occur due to deficiencies of CPTs, carnitine, or acyl-CoA dehydrogenases.
- *Carnitine palmitoyl transferase (CPT I) deficiency* may result in episodic acute myonecrosis *(rhabdomyolysis)* after prolonged exercise, with appearance of myoglobin in the urine. Renal failure can occur after massive episodes of rhabdomyolysis.

Mitochondrial Myopathies (Oxidative Phosphorylation Diseases) (p. 1341)

Mitochondrial genome (mtDNA) encodes one fifth of the proteins involved in mitochondrial oxidative phosphorylation as well as mitochondrial tRNA and rRNA. Diseases that involve mtDNA show maternal inheritance because the oocyte contributes the mitochondria to the embryo. Mitochondrial myopathies typically present in young adulthood, manifesting with proximal muscle weakness, sometimes with severe involvement of the eye musculature *(external ophthalmoplegia)*. Weakness may be accompanied by other neurologic symptoms, lactic acidosis, and cardiomyopathy. Pathologic findings include aggregates of abnormal mitochondria, causing irregular muscle fiber contour *(ragged red fibers* on trichrome stains). There are increased numbers of, and abnormalities in the shape and size of, mitochondria, some of which contain paracrystalline arrays (so-called *"parking lot inclusions"*) or alterations in the structure of cristae.

TABLE 27-5   Congenital Myopathies

Disease and Inheritance	Gene and Locus	Clinical Findings	Pathologic Findings
Central core disease: autosomal-dominant	Ryanodine receptor-1 (*RYR1*) gene; 19q13.1	Early-onset hypotonia and nonprogressive weakness; associated skeletal deformities; may develop malignant hyperthermia	Cytoplasmic cores are lightly eosinophilic and distinct from surrounding sarcoplasm; found only in type 1 fibers, which usually predominate, best seen on NADH stain
Nemaline myopathy; autosomal-dominant or autosomal-recessive	Autosomal-dominant (*NEM1*)—Tropomyosin 3 (*TPM3*) gene; 1q22.1 Autosomal-recessive (*NEM2*)—nebulin (*NEB*) gene; 2q22 Autosomal-dominant or recessive—skeletal muscle actin, α chain (*ACTA1*) gene; 1q42.1	Weakness, hypotonia, and delayed motor development in childhood; may also be seen in adults; usually nonprogressive; involves proximal limb muscles most severely; skeletal abnormalities may be present	Aggregates of subsarcolemmal spindle-shaped particles (*nemaline rods*); occur predominantly in type 1 fibers; derived from Z-band material (α-actinin) and best seen on modified Gomori stain
Myotubular (centronuclear) myopathy; X-linked (*MTM1*), autosomal-recessive, or autosomal-dominant	X-linked—myotubularin (*MTM1*) gene; Xq28 Autosomal-dominant—myogenic factor 6 (*MYF6*) gene; 12q21 Autosomal-recessive—locus and gene unknown	X-linked form presents in infancy with prominent hypotonia and poor prognosis; autosomal forms have limb weakness and are slowly progressive; autosomal-recessive form is intermediate in severity and prognosis	Abundance of centrally located nuclei involving the majority of muscle fibers; central nuclei are usually confined to type 1 fibers, which are small in diameter, but can occur in both fiber types

- One type of mutation involves the genes for mitochondrial proteins encoded by nuclear DNA and shows autosomal dominant or recessive inheritance.
- A second type of mutation involves *point mutation* in mtDNA and includes many mitochondrial encephalomyopathies; they tend to show maternal inheritance.
- A third subset of patients have *deletions* of mtDNA; many of these disorders show prominent involvement of extraocular muscles *(chronic progressive external ophthalmoplegia, Kearns-Sayre syndrome).*

Inflammatory Myopathies (p. 1342)

There are three subgroups of inflammatory muscle diseases:

- Infectious myositis (see Chapter 8)
- Systemic inflammatory diseases that involve muscle along with other organs (see Chapter 6)
- Noninfectious inflammatory muscle disease, including polymyositis, dermatomyositis, and inclusion body myositis (p. 1342)

Dermatomyositis (p. 1342)

Dermatomyositis is an inflammatory disorder of skin and muscle. Rash (lilac or heliotrope discoloration of upper eyelids with periorbital edema) can accompany or precede the muscle weakness, which usually involves proximal muscles first. There is an association with malignancy in adults; nearly 40% of adult patients with dermatomyositis have cancer; juvenile patients more frequently have vasculitis and calcinosis, and less frequently have cancer. Capillaries appear to be the primary target of immunologic attack. Histologic features include perivascular inflammatory infiltrates, atrophy of muscle fibers especially at the periphery of fascicles ("perifascicular atrophy"), and scattered necrotic muscle fibers. Immunosuppressive therapy is the optimal treatment.

Polymyositis (p. 1343)

In this inflammatory disorder of muscle, proximal muscles are affected first. Immune cell–mediated injury of myocytes appears to be the primary basis of polymyositis. Histologic features include endomysial inflammatory infiltrates, scattered necrotic muscle fibers, but not the perifascicular atrophy or perivascular inflammation of dermatomyositis. Immunosuppressive therapy is the optimal treatment.

Inclusion Body Myositis (p. 1343)

Unlike dermatomyositis or polymyositis, inclusion body myositis begins with involvement of distal muscles, especially extensors of the knee and flexors of the wrists. The disorder typically affects individuals over the age of 50. Histologic features include endomysial inflammatory infiltrates, and "rimmed vacuoles"—clear cytoplasmic vacuoles in myocytes surrounded by a thin rim of basophilic material. The vacuoles stain positively for amyloid with Congo red, and contain both β-amyloid protein and hyperphosphorylated tau. Immunosuppressive therapy is generally not beneficial (unlike other forms of noninfectious myositis).

Toxic Myopathies (p. 1343)

- *Thyrotoxic myopathy* (p. 1343): Acute or chronic, proximal muscle weakness sometimes presents before clinical thyroid dysfunction. In thyrotoxic periodic paralysis, weakness and hypokalemia occur.
- *Ethanol myopathy* (p. 1344): *Binge* drinking can produce an acute toxic syndrome of rhabdomyolysis with accompanying myoglobinuria; it can lead to renal failure.
- *Drug-induced myopathies* (p. 1344): Proximal muscle weakness and atrophy may occur in Cushing syndrome or during therapeutic administration of steroids. The severity of clinical disability is variable and is not directly related to the steroid level or the therapeutic regimen. It is characterized by atrophy that selectively involves type 2 fibers.

DISEASES OF THE NEUROMUSCULAR JUNCTION (p. 1344)

Myasthenia Gravis (p. 1344)

This autoimmune disease is characterized clinically by easy fatigability, ptosis, and diplopia resulting from an immune-mediated injury causing decreased numbers of muscle acetylcholine receptors (AChRs).

Pathogenesis

Antibodies to AChR are present in the serum of 85% to 90% of patients. These antibodies accelerate internalization and down-regulation of the AChR. Plasmapheresis can be effective treatment.

About 15% of patients have other autoimmune diseases, including autoimmune thyroid disease, rheumatoid arthritis, pernicious anemia, systemic lupus erythematosus, and other collagen vascular disorders.

Thymic hyperplasia is seen in about 65% to 75% of patients, and a thymoma is found in 15%. Resection of an intercurrent thymoma can improve symptoms.

Morphology

Morphologically, light microscopic examination of muscle is ordinarily unremarkable or may show disuse type 2 atrophy in severe cases; ultrastructurally, junctional folds are greatly reduced or abolished at the neuromuscular junction.

Lambert-Eaton Myasthenic Syndrome (p. 1344)

This paraneoplastic disorder of the neuromuscular junction occurs most commonly with small cell carcinoma of the lung (60% of cases); it differs from myasthenia gravis in having increased contractions with repeated stimuli. The causal autoantibody is directed against a presynaptic voltage-gated calcium channel so that each neuronal stimulus results in the release of fewer synaptic vesicles.

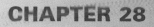

CHAPTER 28

The Central Nervous System

It is important to understand certain aspects of the central nervous system (CNS) to fully appreciate potential pathologies:

- Specific neurologic functions are often localized to distinct (often spatially clustered) groups of neurons; loss of these neurons produces clinical changes that may not be corrected by other neurons.
- Neurons are relatively unable to regenerate (focal destructive lesions cause permanent clinical deficits); stem cell populations are present but have limited capacity to replace neurons in most regions of the brain.
- Certain neurons have selective vulnerability to injury based on differences in structure and function.
- Physical restrictions of the skull and spine render the brain and spinal cord vulnerable to expansile pressure.
- The CNS has a distinct cerebrospinal fluid (CSF) circulation, lacks lymphatics, and has a functionally selective blood-brain barrier.
- The CNS has unique responses to injury and patterns of wound healing.

CELLS OF THE CENTRAL NERVOUS SYSTEM

Neurons (p. 1349)

Neurons vary in structure, functional interconnections, and biochemical properties.

- There are distinct topographic organizations of neurons in different areas: aggregates (nuclei, ganglia), elongated columns (the intermediolateral gray column of the spinal cord), and layers (the six-layered cerebral cortex).
- Some cortical and subcortical neurons and their projections are arranged somatotopically (e.g., the motor homunculus).

- Characteristic ultrastructural features common to many neurons include microtubules, neurofilaments, prominent Golgi apparatus and rough endoplasmic reticulum, and synaptic specializations.
- Immunohistochemical markers for neurons and their processes commonly used in diagnostic work include neurofilament protein, NeuN, and synaptophysin.

Glia (p. 1349)

Glial cells provide a support function for neurons and their cellular processes; they also have a primary role in repair, fluid balance, and energy metabolism.

Astrocytes (p. 1349)

Astrocytes have round-oval nuclei, finely stippled chromatin, and branching cytoplasmic processes; they contain the intermediate filament glial fibrillary acidic protein (GFAP). The processes (end feet) are directed toward capillaries, neurons, and the subpial and subependymal surfaces. Important normal functions include structural support, contributions to the blood-brain barrier, and action as metabolic buffers or detoxifiers.

Oligodendrocytes (p. 1350)

Oligodendrocytes have a lymphocyte-sized nucleus with densely packed chromatin and little cytoplasm visible on routine staining. They produce and maintain CNS myelin.

Ependymal Cells (p. 1350)

These cells form a single layer of cuboidal/columnar cells that line the ventricular system (and rest on subependymal glia). After injury, they do not regenerate, and the underlying subependymal glia proliferates, forming *ependymal granulations*.

Microglia (p. 1350)

Microglia are bone marrow–derived, CD68+ and CR3+ mononuclear cells (markers typical of peripheral macrophages); they contain a bean-shaped nucleus with minimal cytoplasm. They respond to injury by developing elongated nuclei (rod cells), forming aggregates about small foci of tissue necrosis (microglial nodules), or aggregating around dying neurons *(neuronophagia).*

Cellular Pathology of the Central Nervous System (p. 1350)

The CNS has distinct patterns of reaction to injury—mostly realated to changes in neurons and astrocytes.

Reactions of Neurons to Injury (p. 1350)

- *Axonal reaction:* After an axon is cut or damaged, cytoplasm around the nucleus becomes pale (chromatolysis) and swollen.

- *Acute cell injury (red neuron):* Intense eosinophilia of cytoplasm and pyknosis of the nucleus follows acute anoxia or ischemia.
- *Atrophy and degeneration:* Loss of neurons occurs without other recognized morphologic change (characteristic of slowly progressive neurologic diseases and system degenerations).
- Intraneuronal deposits occur in:
  aging (lipofuscin)
  disorders of metabolism (storage material)
  viral diseases (inclusion bodies)
  neurodegenerative diseases associated with aggregated proteins (Table 28–1)

Reactions of Astrocytes to Injury (p. 1351)

Astrocytes are the principal cells responsible for repair and scar formation in the brain. In damaged brain, they develop conspicuous eosinophilic cytoplasm *(gemistocytic astrocyte);* later, they form a network of cellular processes, a process referred to as *gliosis.*

Additional pathologic reactions include formation of the following structures:

- *Rosenthal fibers:* Elongated, eosinophilic structures, containing αB-crystallin, within astrocytic processes and found in long-standing gliosis, or pilocytic astrocytomas
- *Corpora amylacea:* Lamellated polyglucosan bodies increasing in number with advancing age
- *Alzheimer type II astrocytes:* Glia with an enlarged nucleus and pale chromatin, found in patients with hyperammonemia

COMMON PATHOPHYSIOLOGIC PHENOMENA
(p. 1352)

Three interrelated pathophysiologic phenomena of great significance are:
- Cerebral edema
- Herniations
- Hydrocephalus

Cerebral Edema (p. 1352)

The accumulation of extravascular fluid within the brain can cause life-threatening increased intracranial pressure because the intracranial compartment is a closed space. The blood-brain barrier closely regulates the movement of fluids and other substances in and out of the brain; tight junctions between brain capillary endothelial cells constitute an important component of the cellular barrier.

Three types of edema often occur in combination:

- *Vasogenic:* Accumulation of fluid outside the vascular compartment secondary to increased vascular permeability is commonly seen with cerebrovascular accidents, trauma, tumors, and infections. The brain is heavy, swollen, and softened; there is tissue vacuolation with preferential involvement of white matter.

TABLE 28–1 Neurodegenerative Diseases Associated With Aggregated Proteins

Disease	Protein	Normal Structure	Aggregate/Inclusion	Location
Transmissible spongiform encephalopathies (Prion disease)	Prion protein (PrP)	α-Helix and random coil	β-pleated sheet, proteinase K-resistant	Extracellular
Alzheimer disease	Amyloid precursor protein (APP)	α-Helix and random coil	β-pleated sheet, amyloid (fragment of APP)	Extracellular
Tauopathies and Alzheimer disease	Tau (microtubule binding protein)	3 and 4 repeat isoforms	Hyperphosphorylated aggregated protein	Intracellular
Parkinson disease	α-Synuclein	Random coil, repeats	Aggregated, Lewy bodies	Cytoplasmic
Multiple system atrophy	α-Synuclein	Random coil, repeats	Aggregated, glial cytoplasmic inclusions	Cytoplasmic
Huntington disease	Huntingtin	Trinucleotide repeats	Insoluble aggregates	Nuclear
Spinocerebellar ataxias	Ataxins	Trinucleotide repeats	Insoluble aggregates	Nuclear

Modified from Welch WJ, Gambetti P: Chaperoning brain diseases. Nature 392:23–24, 1998.

- *Cytotoxic:* Secondary to altered cell regulation of fluid, this form of edema is seen in anoxia or toxic/metabolic disturbances. The fluid is intracellular and tends to involve the gray matter.
- *Interstitial:* Transudation of fluid from the ventricular system occurs across the ependymal lining (characteristic of increased intraventricular pressure).

Raised Intracranial Pressure and Herniation (p. 1352)

The volume of the intracranial contents is fixed by the skull. As a result, the introduction of additional tissue or fluid (e.g., with space-occupying lesions, cerebral edema, or hydrocephalus) raises intracranial pressure. This can cause life-threatening herniation of the brain through openings of the dural partitions of the cranial cavity or across openings of the skull. The major herniations are as follows:

- *Subfalcine:* Cingulate gyrus herniates under the falx (can compromise the anterior cerebral artery).
- *Transtentorial:* Medial temporal lobe (uncus) passes over the free edge of the tentorium (can lead to distortion of the adjacent midbrain and pons and tearing of feeding vessels *[Duret hemorrhages]* or can compress the posterior cerebral artery).
- *Tonsillar:* Cerebellar tonsils herniate through the foramen magnum (can compress the medulla and compromise cardiorespiratory centers).

Hydrocephalus (p. 1353)

Obstruction of CSF flow leads to enlargement of the ventricles with an associated increase in the volume of CSF. Hydrocephalus is most often caused by congenital malformations and leptomeningeal or intraventricular tumors, hemorrhage, or infections.

There are two principal forms of hydrocephalus:

- *Noncommunicating hydrocephalus:* Blockage occurs anywhere along the ventricular system, usually the aqueduct or the foramina of Monro.
- *Communicating hydrocephalus:* Obstruction occurs along the subarachnoid path of CSF flow, including the sites of its resorption.

In infants and children in whom fusion of the cranial bones has not yet occurred, hydrocephalus produces enlargement of the head. In adults, hydrocephalus can lead to increased intracranial pressure.

Normal pressure hydrocephalus is a clinical syndrome typically found in elderly people and characterized by mental slowness, incontinence, and gait disturbances associated with a slowly evolving hydrocephalus. In diseases associated with extensive tissue loss, compensatory expansion of the entire CSF compartment results in *hydrocephalus ex vacuo.*

MALFORMATIONS AND DEVELOPMENTAL DISEASES (p. 1353)

Patterns of developmental malformation are largely determined by the gestational age of the fetus at the time of the injury. Etiologic factors include maternal and fetal infections, drugs, anoxia, ischemia, and genetic disorders. Major categories of CNS malformations are covered here.

Neural Tube Defects (p. 1353)

Failure of closure or reopening of the caudal portions of the neural tube results in malformation of the vertebral arches *(spina bifida)*. This can be associated with a disorganized segment of spinal cord and an overlying meningeal outpouching (myelomeningocele). Antenatal diagnosis can be made by imaging and maternal screening for α-fetoprotein. Folate deficiency during the initial weeks of gestation is a risk factor. *Anencephaly* is a malformation of the anterior end of the neural tube, resulting in failure of development of the cerebrum. *Encephalocele* is a malformed diverticulum of CNS tissue extending through a defect in the cranium.

Forebrain Abnormalities (p. 1354)

These abnormalities include megalencephaly and microencephaly (abnormally large or small brain volume), agyria and polymicrogyria (abnormally formed gyri), neuronal heterotopias (abnormal migration of neurons), holoprosencephaly (incomplete separation of the cerebral hemispheres), and agenesis of the corpus callosum.

Posterior Fossa Anomalies (p. 1355)

Chiari II malformation (Arnold-Chiari malformation) consists of a small posterior fossa, a malformed midline cerebellum with extension of the vermis through the foramen magnum, hydrocephalus, and a lumbar myelomeningocele. *Dandy-Walker malformation* is characterized by an enlarged posterior fossa, absent cerebellar vermis, and large midline cyst.

Syringomyelia and Hydromyelia (p. 1356)

These terms refer to expansion of the central canal of the spinal cord or formation of a cleftlike cavity in the cord. Most occur in the cervical region. Symptoms are loss of pain and temperature sensation in the upper extremities, absence of motor deficits, and retention of position sense.

PERINATAL BRAIN INJURY (p. 1356)

Cerebral palsy is a nonprogressive neurologic motor deficit, with onset during the perinatal period, associated with several pathologic findings:

- *Intraparenchymal hemorrhage* occurs within the germinal matrix, near the junction between the thalamus and caudate nucleus, and sometimes extends into the ventricular system.
- *Ischemic* infarcts can occur focally in the periventricular white matter *(periventricular leukomalacia)* or develop

throughout the hemispheres *(multicystic encephalopathy)*. Ischemia and hemorrhage are seen in premature newborn infants.

- *Ulegyria* (thin, gliotic gyri) and *status marmoratus* (neuronal loss and gliosis in the basal ganglia and thalamus associated with aberrant and irregular myelin formation) are also related to ischemic injury. Choreoathetosis and related movement disorders are important clinical sequelae.

TRAUMA (p. 1356)

There are four categories of brain trauma:
- Skull fractures
- Parenchymal injuries
- Traumatic vascular injury
- Spinal cord injury

Skull Fractures (p. 1357)

Skull fractures may cross sutures. Bone displacement into the cranial cavity (i.e., displaced fracture) sometimes occurs. The relative incidence varies depending on the location of the injury and the thickness of the bone.

Parenchymal Injuries (p. 1357)

Concussion (p. 1357)

A transient neurologic syndrome occurring after trauma, concussion is associated with loss of consciousness, respiratory arrest, and loss of reflexes. Amnesia for the event persists. Concussion is unassociated with permanent structural damage.

Direct Parenchymal Injury (p. 1357)

Bruises of gyral crests can occur either at the site of impact *(coup contusion)* or at a point opposite *(contrecoup contusion)*. Microscopically, these represent focal brain hemorrhage. After resolution, a depressed, yellowish glial scar extends to the pial surface *(plaque jaune)*. A *laceration* is a penetrating injury leading to tearing of tissue.

Diffuse Axonal Injury (p. 1358)

In roughly 50% of patients who become comatose after traumatic injury there is diffuse axonal injury (axonal swellings) and hemorrhages in the corpus callosum and brain stem *(white matter injury)*. Mechanical forces, including angular acceleration even in the absence of impact, damage the axons.

Traumatic Vascular Injury (p. 1359)

Depending on the anatomic position of the ruptured vessel, trauma-related hemorrhages are *epidural, subdural, subarachnoid,* and *intraparenchymal* (Fig. 28–1). Contusion of superficial cerebral tissue or, less frequently, cerebellar cortex is associated with disruption of small vessels within both the brain parenchyma and the overlying leptomeninges.

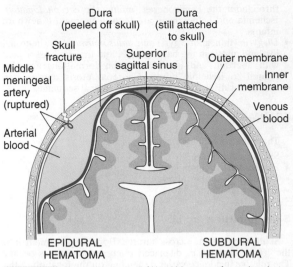

FIGURE 28–1 Epidural hematoma *(left)* in which rupture of a meningeal artery (usually associated with a skull fracture) leads to accumulation of arterial blood between the dura and skull. In a subdural hematoma *(right)*, damage to bridging veins between the brain and superior sagittal sinus leads to blood accumulation between the dura and the arachnoid.

Epidural Hematoma (p. 1359)

Arterial blood, usually from a fracture-related rupture of the middle meningeal artery, collects between the dura and the internal surface of the skull and compresses the brain. Patients are often lucid for several hours after the trauma. The lesion can expand rapidly, can cause increased intracranial pressure or herniation, and requires drainage to prevent coma and death.

Subdural Hematoma (p. 1359)

Venous blood from torn superficial bridging veins between the convexities and the dural venous sinuses collects in the space between the dura and the outer layer of the arachnoid. Chronic subdural hematomas may occur in older individuals and alcoholics, sometimes after relatively minor trauma. The treatment is surgical drainage acutely and removal of the associated granulation tissue *(membranes)* in longstanding lesions.

Spinal Cord Trauma (p. 1360)

Most injuries that damage the spinal cord are associated with displacement of the spinal column. In the acute phase, there is hemorrhage, necrosis, and white matter axonal swellings. Later the central necrotic lesion becomes cystic and gliotic, and the damaged ascending and descending white matter tracts undergo secondary degeneration.

CEREBROVASCULAR DISEASES (p. 1361)

Cerebrovascular diseases are the most prevalent neurologic disorders in terms of both morbidity and mortality. The major categories are:

- Hypoxia, ischemia, and infarction
- Intracranial hemorrhage
- Hypertensive cerebrovascular disease

Hypoxia, Ischemia, and Infarction (p. 1361)

Brain oxygen deprivation causes either generalized *(ischemic or hypoxic encephalopathy)* or focal ischemic necrosis *(cerebral infarction)*.

Hypotension, Hypoperfusion, and Low-Flow States (Global Cerebral Ischemia) (p. 1361)

Generalized hypoxia occurs with reduced blood oxygen content or with reduction of cerebral perfusion pressure, as with hypotension. *Watershed* or *border zone infarcts* occur with reduced perfusion in those regions of the brain and spinal cord that lie at the most distal edges of arterial supply (i.e., at the border zone between major vascular territories); the territory between the anterior and middle cerebral artery is most at risk.

Morphology

In the first 12 to 24 hours after injury, neurons show ischemic cell injury *(red neurons)*. The most susceptible regions are the pyramidal neurons of Sommer sector of the hippocampus (CA1), the Purkinje cell layer of the cerebellar cortex, and the pyramidal neurons in the neocortex *(pseudolaminar necrosis)*. Healing is characterized by gliosis.

Infarction From Obstruction of Local Blood Supply (Focal Cerebral Ischemia) (p. 1363)

Cerebral infarction from focal vascular obstruction can occur either from thrombotic or, more frequently, embolic arterial occlusion. These events manifest as a *stroke*—the sudden onset of a neurologic deficit with clinical manifestations referable to the anatomic location of the lesion. The deficit evolves over time, and the outcome is either permanent or can slowly improve over a period of months. Venous infarcts are often hemorrhagic; they occur after thrombotic occlusion of the superior sagittal sinus, or occlusion of the deep cerebral veins.

- *Thrombosis* (usually due to underlying atherosclerosis) most frequently affects the extracerebral carotid system and the basilar artery.
- *Embolism* most commonly involves the intracerebral arteries (most frequently the middle cerebral artery distribution). Emboli can originate from cardiac mural thrombi, valvular disease, and atrial fibrillation. Fragments of thrombotic material can also break off from arterial mural thrombi (most often in the carotid artery), or can arise as paradoxical emboli from the systemic venous circulation that access the cerebral vasculature via atrial or ventricular septal defects.

Morphology

Nonhemorrhagic infarcts (bland or anemic infarcts) are evident at 48 hours as pale, soft regions of edematous brain. The tissue then liquefies, and a fluid-filled cavity containing macrophages is lined by reactive glia. *Hemorrhagic infarcts,* characteristic of embolic occlusion with reperfusion injury, exhibit blood extravasation.

Intracranial Hemorrhage (p. 1365)

Nontraumatic intracranial hemorrhage can be:

- Intraparenchymal
- Subarachnoid
- Mixed (e.g., in vascular malformations)

Intracerebral (Intraparenchymal) Hemorrhage (p. 1366)

Intraparenchymal hemorrhage is the leading cause of death in stroke patients; *hypertension* is a predisposing factor in 80% of cases. *Hypertensive intracerebral hemorrhage* is most commonly observed in the putamen, thalamus, pontine tegmentum, and cerebellar hemispheres. Vascular rupture is believed to be due to arteriolar injury with formation of microaneurysms *(Charcot-Bouchard aneurysms). Lobar hemorrhages* involve areas supplied by hemispheric arteries and are due to amyloid angiopathy or hemorrhagic diatheses. In patients who survive, the hematoma is slowly resorbed over a period of months with some restitution of function.

Morphology

Macroscopically, acute hemorrhages exhibit extravasated blood with compression of the adjacent parenchyma. *Microscopically,* resolution shows an area of cavitary destruction of brain with a rim of gliotic tissue containing pigment-laden macrophages.

Subarachnoid Hemorrhage and Ruptured Saccular Aneurysms (p. 1366)

Subarachnoid hemorrhage occurs most often with rupture of a *berry aneurysm (saccular aneurysm, congenital aneurysm),* the most frequent type of intracerebral aneurysm (fusiform atherosclerotic aneurysms and mycotic aneurysms occur more rarely).

- Most berry aneurysms occur in the anterior circulation and are found near arterial branch points; 20% to 30% of patients have more than one.
- Most occur sporadically, but they also are associated with autosomal dominant polycystic kidney disease (Chapter 20).
- Hypertension and collagen disorders (Ehlers-Danlos syndrome, pseudoxanthoma elasticum, Marfan syndrome) predispose to their development.

The probability of rupture increases with the size of the lesion; aneurysms greater than 10 mm have a roughly 50% risk per year of bleeding. Rupture often occurs with acute increases in intracranial pressure, such as with straining at stool or sexual orgasm. Between 25% and 50% of patients die with the first rupture. Rebleeding is common in the survivors, and with each episode of bleeding, the prognosis is more grave. Blood in the subarachnoid space can lead to arterial vasospasm. Eventually, blood resorption may lead to meningeal fibrosis and hydrocephalus.

Morphology

At the neck of the aneurysm, the muscular wall and intimal elastic lamina are usually absent or fragmentary, and the wall of the sac is made up of thickened hyalinized intima. With acutely ruptured aneurysms, blood diffusely fills the subarachnoid spaces.

Vascular Malformations (p. 1367)

There are several types of vascular malformations.

- *Arteriovenous malformations:* Arteriovenous malformations are tangles of numerous, abnormally tortuous and misshapen vessels, containing arteries and veins without an intervening capillary bed, most often in middle cerebral artery territory. Men are affected twice as frequently as women; the lesion is most often recognized clinically between ages 10 and 30, presenting as a seizure disorder, intracerebral hemorrhage, or subarachnoid hemorrhage.
- *Cavernous hemangiomas:* Cavernous hemangiomas are greatly distended, loosely organized vascular channels with thin, collagenized walls; they occur most often in the cerebellum, pons, and subcortical regions.
- *Capillary telangiectasias:* Capillary telangiectasias are microscopic foci of dilated, thin-walled vascular channels separated by relatively normal brain parenchyma; they occur most frequently in the pons.

Hypertensive Cerebrovascular Disease
(p. 1368)

In addition to hypertensive hemorrhage and arteriosclerosis, other pathologic processes are related to elevated blood pressures and are discussed in the following paragraphs.

Lacunar Infarcts (p. 1368)

These small (<15 mm), often multiple cystic infarcts result from arteriolar occlusion. These are most frequently seen in the lenticular nucleus, thalamus, internal capsule, deep white matter, caudate nucleus, and pons. Clinically, they can be silent or cause serious impairment. Because of the common involvement of basal ganglia, thalamus, and adjacent white matter, a number of stereotypic syndromes have been described.

Hypertensive Encephalopathy (p. 1369)

This clinicopathologic syndrome is characterized by diffuse cerebral dysfunction (headaches, confusion, vomiting, and convulsions, sometimes leading to coma), with increased intracranial pressure arising in a hypertensive patient. Rapid therapeutic intervention is required because the syndrome often does not remit on its own. Postmortem examination may show an edematous brain with petechiae and necrosis of arterioles.

INFECTIONS (p. 1369)

Five basic categories of infection are based on the time course, etiologic agent, and site of involvement:

- Acute bacterial (pyogenic) or viral (aseptic) infections that involve the leptomeninges and CSF *(meningitis)*
- Acute bacterial infections of the subdural spaces *(subdural empyema)* or CNS parenchyma *(brain abscess)*
- Chronic bacterial infections of the brain and meninges *(meningoencephalitis)*
- Acute, subacute, or chronic viral infection of the brain *(encephalitis)*
- Fungal and parasitic infections

There are four principal routes of entry of organisms into the nervous system:

- *Hematogenous spread*—most common, usually arterial
- *Direct implantation*—usually traumatic
- *Local extension*—from an established infection in an air sinus
- *Axonal transport*—along peripheral nerves (by certain viruses, e.g., in rabies, herpes simplex)

Acute Meningitis (p. 1369)

Acute Pyogenic (Bacterial) Meningitis (p. 1369)

Pathogens differ across age groups:

- Neonates: *Escherichia coli* and the group B streptococci
- Infants and children: *Streptococcus pneumoniae* (*Haemophilus influenzae*, reduced with immunization)
- Adolescents and young adults: *Neisseria meningitidis*
- Elderly: *Streptococcus pneumoniae* and *Listeria monocytogenes*

Morphology

CSF is cloudy or purulent with neutrophils and organisms; meningeal vessels are engorged. Blood vessels become inflamed and occluded, and hemorrhagic infarction of the underlying brain ensues. In chronic or untreated cases, leptomeningeal fibrosis and consequent hydrocephalus may occur.

Clinical Features

Clinical features include meningeal irritation with headache, photophobia, irritability, clouding of consciousness, and neck stiffness. Lumbar puncture shows cloudy or frankly purulent CSF under increased pressure, elevated protein, and a reduced glucose.

Acute Aseptic (Viral) Meningitis (p. 1370)

Enteroviruses (echovirus, coxsackievirus, and poliovirus) are the most commonly isolated pathogens. Viral meningitis is usually self-limited. It is characterized by meningeal irritation, a CSF lymphocytic pleocytosis, moderate protein elevation, and nearly always normal glucose content. Often, there is only a mild to moderate lymphocytic infiltration of leptomeninges.

Acute Focal Suppurative Infections (p. 1371)

Brain Abscess and Subdural Empyema (p. 1371)

Predisposing conditions include acute bacterial endocarditis, cyanotic congenital heart disease, and chronic pulmonary sepsis. Streptococci and staphylococci are the principal organisms. If the subdural space becomes infected, thrombophlebitis may develop in the veins that cross the subdural space (bridging veins), resulting in venous occlusion and brain infarction.

Morphology

There is a central region of liquefactive necrosis and a fibrous capsule surrounded by reactive gliosis. Brain abscess is often associated with marked cerebral edema.

Clinical Features

Brain abscess usually presents with progressive focal deficits and signs of raised intracranial pressure. CSF pressure, cell count, and protein are increased; glucose is normal. A systemic or local source of infection may be apparent. Increased intracranial pressure and progressive herniation can be fatal. Abscess rupture can lead to ventriculitis, meningitis, and sagittal sinus thrombosis.

Chronic Bacterial Meningoencephalitis (p. 1371)

Tuberculosis (p. 1371)

Tuberculous meningitis causes headache, malaise, mental confusion, and vomiting. There is moderate CSF mononuclear cell pleocytosis (occasionally with neutrophils), elevated protein, and moderately reduced or normal glucose. Tuberculous meningitis can cause arachnoid fibrosis, hydrocephalus, and obliterative endarteritis. Infection by *Mycobacterium avium-intracellulare* in patients with acquired immunodeficiency syndrome (AIDS) can cause chronic meningitis, brain abscesses, and rarely diffuse encephalitis or cranial or peripheral neuropathy.

Morphology

The subarachnoid space contains a gelatinous or fibrinous exudate of chronic inflammatory cells and, rarely, well-formed granulomas, most often at the base of the brain, obliterating the cisternae and encasing the cranial nerves. Arteries running through the subarachnoid space may show *obliterative endarteritis,* with inflammatory infiltrates in their walls and marked intimal thickening. Well-circumscribed intraparenchymal masses *(tuberculomas)* can also occur.

Neurosyphilis (p. 1372)

Neurosyphilis represents a tertiary stage of syphilis; it occurs in only about 10% of patients with untreated infections.

- *Meningovascular neurosyphilis* is a chronic meningitis sometimes associated with obliterative endarteritis.
- *Paretic neurosyphilis* is the result of brain invasion by spirochetes, with neuronal loss and proliferation of microglia (rod cells). There is insidious but progressive loss of mental and

physical functions with mood alterations (including delusions of grandeur), terminating in severe dementia.

- *Tabes dorsalis* is the result of spirochete damage to the sensory nerves in the dorsal roots and loss of axons and myelin in the dorsal roots and dorsal columns; impaired joint position sense, locomotor ataxia, loss of pain sensation leading to skin and joint damage (Charcot joints), and other sensory disturbances occur.

Patients with HIV (human immunodeficiency virus) infection are at increased risk for neurosyphilis; moreover, the rate of progression and severity of the disease appear to be accelerated, presumably related to impaired cell-mediated immunity.

Neuroborreliosis (Lyme Disease) (p. 1372)

The causal spirochete *Borrelia burgdorferi* is transmitted by various species of the *Ixodes* tick. Lyme disease may cause aseptic meningitis, encephalopathy, and polyneuropathies. In the CNS, there is proliferation of microglial cells, as well as scattered organisms.

Viral Meningoencephalitis (p. 1372)

Viral encephalitis refers to parenchymal brain infections, almost invariably associated with meningeal inflammation, having a wide spectrum of clinical and pathologic expressions. Characteristic histologic features include perivascular and parenchymal mononuclear cell infiltrate (lymphocytes, plasma cells, and macrophages), microglial nodules, and neuronophagia. The best characterized forms are discussed in the following sections.

Arthropod-Borne Viral Encephalitis (p. 1373)

This form of encephalitis is the cause of most outbreaks of epidemic viral encephalitis; major types include Eastern Equine, Western Equine, Venezuelan, St. Louis, California, and West Nile. All have animal hosts and mosquito or tick vectors. The typical clinical manifestations are seizures, confusion, delirium, and stupor or coma.

Herpes Simplex Virus Type 1 (p. 1373)

Herpes simplex virus type 1 (HSV-1) occurs in any age group but is most common in children and young adults; about 10% have a history of prior labial herpes. Common symptoms are alterations in affect, mood, memory, and behavior. Hemorrhagic, necrotizing encephalitis occurs and is most severe along the inferior and medial regions of the temporal lobes and the orbitofrontal gyri. Cowdry intranuclear viral inclusion bodies may be found in both neurons and glia.

Herpes Simplex Virus Type 2 (p. 1374)

Herpes simplex virus type 2 (HSV-2) causes a generalized, severe encephalitis in up to 50% of neonates born by vaginal delivery to women with primary HSV-2 infection.

Varicella-Zoster Virus (Herpes Zoster) (p. 1374)

Reactivation of latent infection after chickenpox results in a painful vesicular skin eruption in the distribution of a dermatome *(shingles)*. It may cause a granulomatous arteritis or a necrotizing encephalitis in immunosuppressed patients.

Cytomegalovirus (p. 1374)

In utero infection leads to periventricular necrosis, microcephaly, and periventricular calcification. In patients with AIDS, cytomegalovirus is the most common opportunistic viral pathogen, affecting the CNS in 15% to 20% of patients; it causes a subacute encephalitis with microglial nodules or a periventricular necrotizing encephalitis with typical cytomegalic inclusions.

Poliomyelitis (p. 1374)

The virus attacks lower motor neurons and may cause flaccid paralysis with muscle wasting. Death can occur from paralysis of the respiratory muscles and myocarditis. Inflammatory reaction is usually confined to the anterior horns but may extend into the posterior horns. The *post-polio syndrome* typically develops 25 to 35 years after the initial illness and is characterized by progressive weakness associated with decreased muscle bulk and occasional pain. There is no evidence to date for persistence of poliovirus when late symptoms occur.

Rabies (p. 1375)

Rabies is transmitted by the bite of a rabid animal or exposure to bats even without a bite. The virus ascends to the CNS along the peripheral nerves from the wound site. It causes extraordinary CNS excitability, hydrophobia, and flaccid paralysis; death ensues from respiratory center failure. Widespread neuronal necrosis and inflammation, most severe in the basal ganglia, midbrain, and medulla, are present. *Negri bodies* (intracytoplasmic eosinophilic inclusions) are found in hippocampal pyramidal cells and Purkinje cells, sites usually devoid of inflammation.

Human Immunodeficiency Virus (p. 1375)

Up to 60% of patients with AIDS develop neurologic symptoms, and neuropathologic changes have been observed in 80% to 90%. These changes fall into three categories:
- *Opportunistic infections* of the CNS (notably infections with cytomegalovirus, toxoplasma, polyomavirus, varicella-zoster virus, HSV, and cryptococcus)
- *Primary CNS lymphoma*
- *Direct or indirect effects of HIV-1,* expressed as one of the following four syndromes:

  HIV-1 aseptic meningitis occurs within 1 to 2 weeks of seroconversion in about 10% of patients; antibodies to HIV-1 can be demonstrated, and the virus can be isolated from the CSF. Microscopically, there is mild lymphocytic meningitis and some myelin loss in the hemispheres.

  HIV-1 encephalitis manifests as HIV-related cognitive/motor complex, with insidious mental slowing, memory loss, and mood disturbances, later progressing to motor abnormalities, ataxia, bladder and bowel incontinence, and, rarely, seizures. Histologic examination exhibits virus-containing microglial nodules with multinucleated giant cells and myelin damage with gliosis.

Vacuolar myelopathy (found in 20%–30% of patients with AIDS at autopsy) consists of destruction of myelinated fibers and macrophages involving the posterior and lateral columns, resembling subacute combined degeneration (vitamin B_{12} serum levels are normal, however). A disease with some similarities is *tropical spastic paraparesis,* a human T-cell lymphotropic virus (HTLV-1)-related myelopathy.

Cranial and peripheral neuropathies and myopathies include acute and chronic inflammatory demyelinating polyneuropathies, inflammatory myopathy, and a zidovudine-related acute toxic reversible myopathy with *ragged red* fibers and myoglobulinuria.

In children with congenital AIDS, neurologic dysfunction, evident by the first years of life, includes microcephaly with mental retardation and motor developmental delay with long tract signs.

Progressive Multifocal Leukoencephalopathy (p. 1376)

This leukoencephalopathy is an infection of oligodendrocytes by a polyomavirus (JC virus) occurring in immunosuppressed patients. About 65% of normal asymptomatic people have serologic evidence of exposure to JC virus by the age of 14 years. Patients develop multifocal and progressive neurologic manifestations because of irregular regions of myelin destruction. Lesions consist of demyelinated patches, greatly enlarged oligodendrocyte nuclei with viral inclusions, and astrocytes with greatly enlarged atypical nuclei.

Subacute Sclerosing Panencephalitis (p. 1377)

This progressive syndrome of cognitive decline, spasticity, and seizures develops months or years after an early-age acute infection with measles. It represents a persistent but nonproductive infection of the CNS by altered measles virus. There is (i) widespread gliosis and myelin degeneration; (ii) viral inclusions, largely within the nuclei of oligodendrocytes and neurons; (iii) variable inflammation of white and gray matter; and (iv) neurofibrillary tangles.

Fungal Meningoencephalitis (p. 1378)

Fungal and parasitic infections are most frequently encountered in immunocompromised patients. The brain is usually involved only late in the disease, when there is widespread hematogenous dissemination, most often *Candida albicans, Mucor, Aspergillus fumigatus,* and *Cryptococcus neoformans.* In endemic areas, pathogens such as *Histoplasma capsulatum, Coccidioides immitis,* and *Blastomyces dermatitidis* can also involve the CNS after a primary pulmonary or cutaneous infection. There are three basic patterns of infection:

- *Chronic meningitis:* most commonly by *C. neoformans;* may occur in immunocompetent patients

- *Vasculitis:* most frequently seen with *Mucor* and *Aspergillus,* with invasion of blood vessel walls, thrombosis, and hemorrhagic infarction
- *Parenchymal involvement* with granulomas or abscesses, most commonly encountered with *Candida* and *Cryptococcus*

Other Infectious Diseases of the Nervous System (p. 1378)

Other infectious agents that can involve the CNS include protozoa (malaria, toxoplasmosis, amebiasis, and trypanosomiasis); rickettsia (typhus, Rocky Mountain spotted fever), and metazoa (cysticercosis and echinococcosis).

- *Toxoplasma gondii* is one of the most common causes of neurologic symptoms and morbidity in patients with AIDS. Clinical symptoms are subacute and often focal; computed tomography and magnetic resonance imaging studies show multiple ring-enhancing lesions. Abscesses contain both free tachyzoites and encysted bradyzoites. Primary maternal infection with toxoplasmosis, particularly if it occurs early in pregnancy, may be followed by a cerebritis in the fetus and multifocal necrotizing cerebral lesions, which can calcify.
- Among amoebic species, *Naegleria* species cause a rapidly fatal necrotizing encephalitis. A chronic granulomatous meningoencephalitis has been associated with acanthamoeba.

Transmissible Spongiform Encephalopathies (Prion Diseases) (p. 1380)

These diseases are characterized by *spongiform changes* due to intracellular vacuoles in neural cells. These are associated with abnormal forms of a specific protein, termed *prion protein* (PrP). Diseases may be sporadic, infectious, and transmissible, and include:

- Creutzfeldt-Jakob disease (CJD), variant Creutzfeldt-Jakob disease (vCJD), Gerstmann-Straussler-Scheinker syndrome, fatal and sporadic familial insomnias, and *kuru* in humans
- Scrapie in sheep and goats
- Mink transmissible encephalopathy
- Bovine spongiform encephalopathy *(mad cow disease)*
- Chronic wasting disease *(elk, deer)*

Pathogenesis

PrP is a normal 30-kD cellular protein; disease occurs when PrP changes from a native isoform (PrP^c) to an abnormally folded isoform, termed either PrP^{sc} (for PrP *s*crapie) or PrP^{res} (for PrP protease *res*istant). The infectious nature of PrP^{sc} molecules derives from its ability to induce misfolding of PrP^c and thus corrupt the integrity of normal cellular PrP.

Accumulation of PrP^{sc} appears to be the cause of the pathologic changes in these diseases, but the pathways by which this material causes the development of cytoplasmic vacuoles and eventual neuronal death are unknown.

- *CJD:* This disease is a rare cause of rapidly progressive dementia. It is primarily sporadic but may be familial. There are well-established cases of iatrogenic transmission. The disease is uniformly fatal, with an average duration of only 7 months, although a few patients survive for several years. The pathologic finding is a spongiform transformation of the cerebral cortex and, often, deep gray matter structures (such as caudate and putamen). In advanced cases, there is severe neuronal loss, reactive gliosis, and sometimes expansion of the vacuolated areas into cystlike spaces *(status spongiosus)*. No inflammatory infiltrate is present.

- *Variant CJD:* This variant is a CJD-like illness found in a small number of patients, mostly in the United Kingdom, and potentially derived from the bovine spongiform encephalopathy agent. It was distinguished from typical CJD by the following:

   The disease affected young adults.

   Behavioral disorders figured prominently in the early stages of the disease.

   The neurologic syndrome progressed more slowly than what is usually observed in patients with CJD.

   Extensive cortical plaques are present, with a surrounding halo of spongiform change.

- *Gerstmann-Straussler-Scheinker syndrome:* This syndrome is an inherited disease with mutations of the prion protein gene *(PRNP)*; it typically begins with a chronic cerebellar ataxia, followed by a progressive dementia. The clinical course is usually slower than that of CJD, with progression to death several years after the onset of symptoms.

- *Fatal familial insomnia:* This disorder is named, in part, for the sleep disturbances that characterize its initial stages. In contrast to other prion diseases, FFI does not show spongiform pathology; instead the most striking alteration is neuronal loss and reactive gliosis in the anterior ventral and dorsomedial nuclei of the thalamus; neuronal loss is also prominent in the inferior olivary nuclei. Sporadic cases have been reported.

DEMYELINATING DISEASES (p. 1382)

Demyelinating diseases are characterized by myelin damage with relative preservation of axons.

Multiple Sclerosis (MS) (p. 1382)

MS is defined clinically as distinct episodes of neurologic deficit, separated in time and attributable to demyelinating white matter lesions that are separated in space. The natural course of MS is variable; often, it begins as a relapsing and remitting illness in which episodes of neurologic deficits develop over short periods of time (days to weeks) and show gradual partial remission. The frequency of relapses tends to decrease over time. In some patients, there is a steady neurologic deterioration. The cellular basis for symptomatic recovery is unknown.

Cellular immunity directed against myelin components is a strong candidate for the underlying mechanism of multiple sclerosis. Risk is 15-fold higher when the disease is present in a first-degree relative, and the concordance rate for monozygotic twins is approximately 25%.

Morphology

Lesions *(plaques)* are sharply defined areas of gray discoloration of white matter occurring especially around the ventricles but potentially located anywhere in the CNS. *Active plaques* show myelin breakdown, lipid-laden macrophages, and relative axonal preservation. Lymphocytes and mononuclear cells are prominent at the edges of plaques and around venules in and around plaques. *Inactive plaques* lack the inflammatory cell infiltrate and show gliosis; most axons within the lesion persist but remain unmyelinated.

Multiple Sclerosis Variants (p. 1384)

- *Neuromyelitis optica (Devic disease)* is a variant of multiple sclerosis occurring especially in Asians; it is characterized by bilateral optic neuritis and especially destructive demyelinating lesions in the spinal cord.
- *Acute multiple sclerosis* occurs in younger individuals and has a rapid course; the plaques are large, with destruction of myelin and some axonal loss.

Acute Disseminated Encephalomyelitis and Acute Necrotizing Hemorrhagic Encephalomyelitis (p. 1385)

Acute disseminated encephalomyelitis (ADEM) is a monophasic disease (follows viral infection or, rarely, a viral immunization) with headache, lethargy, and coma; there is perivenous demyelination with accumulation of lipid-laden macrophages, a mononuclear infiltrate, and polymorphonuclear leukocytes.

Acute necrotizing hemorrhagic encephalitis (ANHE) is more fulminant than ADEM and includes hemorrhagic necrosis of white and gray matter. There may be a history of a prior viral syndrome.

Other Diseases with Demyelination (p. 1385)

Central pontine myelinolysis is characterized by selective damage to myelin in the basis pontis and portions of the pontine tegmentum, often leading to spastic paresis; it is associated clinically with a rapid correction of a hyponatremic state.

DEGENERATIVE DISEASES (p. 1385)

Degenerative diseases are characterized by:

- Progressive and selective loss of functional neuronal systems
- Onset without any clear inciting event in a patient without previous neurologic deficits
- Empiric grouping according to regions of brain that are primarily affected

Degenerative Diseases Affecting the Cerebral Cortex (p. 1386)

The principal clinical manifestation of degenerative diseases affecting the cerebral cortex is dementia.

Alzheimer Disease (p. 1386)

Alzheimer disease usually begins after age 50, with progressive, insidious impairment of higher intellectual function over the next 5 to 10 years. Most cases are sporadic, although at least 5% to 10% of cases are familial (loci on chromosomes 21 [APP], 14 [PS1], and 1 [PS2]). All patients with trisomy 21 who survive beyond 45 years develop a decline in cognition and the pathologic features of Alzheimer disease. The ε4 allele of apolipoprotein E (chromosome 19) is associated with increased risk for Alzheimer disease (Table 28–2).

Morphology

Gyri are narrowed and the sulci widened, especially in the frontal, temporal, and parietal lobes; hydrocephalus *ex vacuo* follows loss of tissue. Microscopic changes occur:

- *Neuritic plaques:* Spherical, 20 to 200 μm in diameter collections of dilated, tortuous, argyrophilic neuritic processes (dystrophic neurites), with a central amyloid core containing amyloid β-peptide (Aβ), a 40– to 43–amino acid peptide derived from a larger amyloid precursor protein (APP). Plaques are surrounded by microglia and reactive astrocytes. Neuritic plaques occur most often in the hippocampus, amygdala, and neocortex.
- *Neurofibrillary tangles:* These are bundles of argyrophilic paired helical filaments in neuronal cytoplasm, especially in entorhinal cortex, hippocampus, amygdala, basal forebrain, and the raphe nuclei. Neurofibrillary tangles contain hyperphosphorylated tau, MAP2, ubiquitin, and Aβ.

TABLE 28–2 **Genetics of Alzheimer Disease**

Chromosome	Gene	Mutations/Alleles	Consequences
21	Amyloid precursor protein (*APP*)	• Single missense mutations Double missense mutation Trisomy 21 (gene dosage effect)	• Early-onset FAD Increased Aβ production
14	Presenilin-1 (*PS1*)	• Missense mutations Splice site mutations	• Early-onset FAD Increased Aβ production
1	Presenilin-2 (*PS2*)	• Missense mutations	• Early-onset FAD Increased Aβ production
19	Apolipoprotein E (*ApoE*)	• Allele ε4	• Increased *risk* of development of AD Decreased age at onset of AD

AD, Alzheimer disease; FAD, familial Alzheimer disease.

- *Cerebral amyloid angiopathy (CAA):* Vascular wall deposition of Aβ, which occurs in intracortical and subarachnoid vessels, is an almost invariable accompaniment of Alzheimer disease.

These changes can also occur in the brains of elderly nondemented individuals, so the diagnosis of Alzheimer disease requires clinicopathologic correlation.

Frontotemporal Dementias (p. 1389)

This group of disorders was first gathered under a single broad term because they share clinical features (progressive deterioration of language and changes in personality) that correspond to degeneration and atrophy of temporal and frontal lobes. Immunohistochemical, biochemical, and genetic insights are allowing a better understanding of the pathogenesis. Many, but not all, of these diseases, are characterized by tau inclusions.

Frontotemporal Dementia With Parkinsonism Linked to Chromosome 17 (FTD(P)-17) (p. 1389)

This clinical syndrome of a frontotemporal dementia is often accompanied by parkinsonian symptoms; it is linked to mutations in the tau gene. Tau is a microtubule-binding protein; it can have three or four copies of the microtubule-binding domain depending on genetic splicing. Mutations fall into several broad categories: coding region mutations, as well as intronic mutations that affect the splicing of the exon for the additional microtubule-binding domain.

Morphology

Frontal and temporal lobe atrophy is seen in various combinations and to various degrees. The pattern of atrophy can often be predicted in part by the clinical symptomatology. The atrophic regions of cortex are marked by neuronal loss and gliosis as well as the presence of tau-containing neurofibrillary tangles. Nigral degeneration may also occur. Inclusions can also be found in glial cells in some forms of the disease.

Pick Disease (p. 1390)

Pick disease is much rarer than Alzheimer disease; it causes dementia, often with prominent frontal signs. Brains show frontal and temporal lobe atrophy, with sparing of the posterior two thirds of the superior temporal gyrus. Rather than plaques and tangles, there are large ballooned neurons (Pick cells) and smooth argyrophilic inclusions (Pick bodies).

Progressive Supranuclear Palsy (p. 1390)

This progressive striatal syndrome occurs after age 50 and is characterized by loss of vertical gaze, truncal rigidity, dysequilibrium, loss of facial expression, and sometimes progressive dementia. There is widespread neuronal loss and neurofibrillary tangles in the globus pallidus, subthalamic nucleus, substantia nigra, colliculi, periaqueductal gray matter, and dentate nucleus of the cerebellum. Tau pathology can be found in glial cells as well.

Corticobasal Degeneration (p. 1390)

This disease of the elderly is characterized by extrapyramidal rigidity, asymmetric motor disturbances, and sensory cortical dysfunction. Motor, premotor, and anterior parietal cortex show severe loss of neurons, gliosis, and ballooned neurons. The substantia nigra and locus ceruleus show loss of pigmented neurons and argyrophilic inclusions similar to those seen in progressive supranuclear palsy. In addition to neuronal pathology, tau immunoreactivity has been found in astrocytes ("tufted astrocytes") and oligodendrocytes ("coiled bodies").

Frontotemporal Dementias Without Tau Pathology (p. 1391)

Some cases do not show evidence of tau deposition; in such patients, neurons exhibit tau-negative, ubiquitin-positive inclusions in temporal and frontal lobe superficial cortical layers and in the dentate gyrus. Other cases show no specific inclusions but rather have cortical atrophy and some thalamic gliosis. This pattern of injury has been termed *dementia lacking distinctive histology* (DLDH).

Vascular Dementia (p. 1391)

From autopsy analyses of individuals who were carefully studied during life, it has been demonstrated that various types of vascular injury to the brain can result in dementia. Some of the disorders that can cause dementia include:

- Vasculitis
- Combinations of infarctions, including either widespread microinfarcts or strategically located large infarcts (involving hippocampus, dorsomedial thalamus, or frontal cortex, including cingulate gyrus)
- Diffuse white matter injury associated with hypertension (*Binswanger disease*)

Degenerative Diseases of Basal Ganglia and Brainstem (p. 1391)

These diseases are associated with movement disorders, tremor, and rigidity.

Parkinsonism (p. 1391)

Parkinsonism refers to a clinical syndrome characterized by diminished facial expression, stooped posture, slowness of voluntary movement, festinating gait (progressively shortened, accelerated steps), rigidity, and a pill-rolling tremor, associated with decreased function of the nigrostriatal system. A variety of distinct diseases can cause this clinical syndrome. In addition to the three mentioned below, progressive supranuclear palsy (PSP) and corticobasal degeneration (CBD) can have parkinsonism as a prominent component, and are sometimes grouped with the diseases of the basal ganglia.

Parkinson Disease (p. 1391)

This progressive parkinsonian syndrome develops later in life and in some is associated with dementia. There is pallor of the substantia nigra and locus ceruleus with loss of their pigmented, catecholaminergic neurons and gliosis; *Lewy bodies* (intracytoplasmic, eosinophilic inclusions, containing α-synuclein) occur in the remaining neurons. Some autosomal dominant forms are linked to mutations in a gene encoding α-synuclein, while other recessive forms are linked to mutations in the gene for parkin. When there is dementia present, Lewy bodies are often found in cortical regions and the disease is then termed *dementia with Lewy bodies* (DLB). Other patients with Parkinson disease become demented from other diseases, most commonly Alzheimer disease.

Multiple System Atrophy (p. 1393)

This often overlapping group of disorders shares glial cytoplasmic inclusions composed of α-synuclein and includes the following clinical presentations, not commonly seen in the "pure" state:

- *Striatonigral degeneration:* similar to idiopathic Parkinson disease but resistant to L-dopa therapy. There is widespread neuronal loss and gliosis of the caudate and putamen as well as involvement of pigmented neurons of the zona compacta of the substantia nigra, without Lewy bodies.
- *Olivopontocerebellar atrophy:* cerebellar ataxia, with eye and somatic movement abnormalities, dysarthria, and rigidity. Findings include shrinkage of the basis pontis from loss of the pontine nuclei; widespread loss of Purkinje cells, especially in the lateral portions of the hemispheres; and retrograde degeneration in the inferior olives.
- *Shy-Drager syndrome:* parkinsonism and autonomic system failure, with loss of the sympathetic neurons of the intermediolateral column of the spinal cord.

Huntington Disease (p. 1393)

Huntington disease is an autosomal dominant movement disorder that becomes clinically manifest between ages 20 and 50. Affected patients develop chorea, characterized by jerky, hyperkinetic, sometimes dystonic movements affecting all parts of the body; they may later develop parkinsonism with bradykinesia, rigidity, and dementia. There is striking atrophy of the caudate nucleus and, to a lesser extent, the putamen, with severe loss of medium-sized, spiny striatal neurons. Neurons that contain nitric oxide synthase and cholinesterase are spared. The disease is associated with expansion of a trinucleotide repeat encoding a polyglutamine tract in *huntingtin,* the protein encoded by the Huntington disease gene on chromosome 4p.

Spinocerebellar Degenerations (p. 1394)

Spinocerebellar degenerations affect primarily, to a variable extent, the cerebellar cortex, spinal cord, and peripheral nerves (Table 28–3).

Spinocerebellar Ataxias (p. 1394)

Spinocerebellar ataxias (SCAs) are autosomal dominant diseases involving the cerebellum, brain stem, spinal cord, and peripheral nerves. Some forms (SCA1–3, SCA6, SCA7, and SCA17) are caused by unstable expansions of CAG repeats, which encode polyglutamine tracts in different proteins.

TABLE 28–3 Selected Spinocerebellar Ataxias

Disease	Chromosome	Gene Product	Inheritance	Mutation
SCA1	6p23	ataxin-1	AD	CAG in coding region
SCA2	12q24.1	ataxin-2	AD	CAG in coding region
SCA3	14q21	ataxin-3	AD	CAG in coding region
SCA4	16q22.1	?	AD	?
SCA5	11p11–q11	?	AD	?
SCA6	19p13.1–2	α_{1A} voltage-dependent calcium channel subunit	AD	CAG in coding region
SCA7	3p21.1–p12	ataxin7	AD	CAG in coding region
SCA8	13q21	?	AD	Untranslated CTG repeat on antisense strand
SCA10	22q13	ataxin-10	AD	Intronic ATTTC repeat
SCA11	15q14–21	?	AD	?
SCA12	5q31	protein phosphatase 2A	AD	CAG in 5′ UTR region
SCA13	19q13	?	AD	?
SCA14	19q13.4	protein kinase cγ	AD	Point mutations
SCA15	3pter–24.2	?	AD	?
SCA16	8q22.24	?	AD	?
SCA17	6q27	TATA-binding protein	AD	CAG in coding region
FA	9q13–21	frataxin-1	AR	Intronic GAA repeat
Ataxia-telangiectasia	11q22–23	ATM	AR	Point mutations

- *Friedreich ataxia* is autosomal recessive with a male preponderance. The disease develops at around 11 years of age, and symptoms of gait ataxia, dysarthria, depressed tendon reflexes, Babinski signs, and sensory loss evolve progressively over 20 years. Associated findings include pes cavus, kyphoscoliosis, diabetes, cardiac arrhythmias, and myocarditis. The involved gene on chromosome 9q13 usually has expansion of an intronic GAA repeat. Changes include:

  Fiber loss and gliosis in the posterior columns and distal corticospinal and spinocerebellar tracts

  Neuronal loss in Clark column; VIII, X, and XII cranial nerve nuclei; dentate nucleus; Purkinje cells of the superior vermis; and dorsal root ganglion cells

  Peripheral neuropathy

- *Ataxia-telangiectasia:* This autosomal recessive disease presents in childhood with evidence of cerebellar dysfunction and recurrent infections. Telangiectatic lesions are found especially in the conjunctiva. Findings include loss of Purkinje and granule cells, absence of thymus, hypoplastic gonads, and lymphoid malignancy.

Degenerative Diseases Affecting Motor Neurons (p. 1396)

Amyotrophic Lateral Sclerosis (p. 1396)

Amyotrophic lateral sclerosis (ALS) is characterized by loss of lower motor neurons (muscular atrophy, fasciculations, weakness) and upper motor neurons (hyperreflexia, spasticity, and a Babinski reflex); it may have predominantly bulbar manifestations (involvement of motor cranial nerves, sparing those that control the extraocular muscles). Degeneration of the upper motor neurons results in loss of myelinated fibers in the corticospinal tracts; occasionally, there is atrophy of the precentral gyrus. The disease is more common in men, usually with onset after age 50, and is relentlessly progressive, with death from respiratory complications. Approximately 10% of cases show autosomal dominant inheritance; a locus on chromosome 21 is the copper/zinc–binding superoxide dismutase gene.

Bulbospinal Atrophy (Kennedy Syndrome) (p. 1397)

In this X-linked form of spinal muscular atrophy, lower motor neuron loss is associated with gynecomastia, testicular atrophy, and oligospermia. It has been linked to amplification of a trinucleotide repeat in the coding sequence of the androgen receptor gene, with severity of the disease related to the number of repeats present.

Spinal Muscular Atrophy (p. 1397)

This series of diseases are linked to a locus on chromosome 5q. In general, the form with earliest onset (SMA type 1; Werdnig-Hoffmann disease) is a severe autosomal recessive form of lower motor neuron disease, which presents in the neonatal period with hypotonia *(floppy infant)*. Death ensues within a few months from respiratory failure or aspiration pneumonia. Forms with later onset have less aggressive courses.

GENETIC METABOLIC DISEASES (p. 1397)

There are three main groups of inborn errors of metabolism:

- Neuronal storage diseases: mostly related to mutations in genes for synthesis or degradation of sphingolipids, mucolipids or mucopolysaccharides. These diseases result in intraneuronal accumulation of lipid material, typically with eventual neuronal death.
- Leukodystrophies (white matter diseases): selective involvement of enzymes involved in synthesis or turnover of myelin components. These diseases result in hypomyelination, often with storage material in astrocytes or macrophages.
- Mitochondrial encephalomyelopathies: disorders of energy metabolism, which may be linked to either mitochondrial or nuclear genome. They often have systemic involvement targeting high-energy demand tissues (e.g., cardiac and skeletal muscle).

Leukodystrophies (p. 1397)

Krabbe Disease (p. 1397)

Krabbe disease is an autosomal recessive deficiency of galactocerebroside β-galactosidase, the enzyme required for the catabolism of galactocerebroside to ceramide and galactose. The end result is diffuse myelin and oligodendrocyte loss and the aggregation of macrophages around blood vessels as multinucleated cells *(globoid cells)*. These macrophages contain storage material (linear inclusions by electron microscopy).

Metachromatic Leukodystrophy (p. 1397)

Metachromatic leukodystrophy is an autosomal recessive disease with several clinical subtypes (congenital, late infantile, juvenile, and adult), caused by deficiency of arylsulfatase A with an accumulation of sulfatides, especially cerebroside sulfate. Findings include myelin loss and gliosis, with macrophages containing metachromatic material.

Other leukodystrophies include:

- Adrenoleukodystrophy (p. 1398)
- Pelizaeus-Merzbacher disease (p. 1398)
- Canavan disease (p. 1398)

Mitochondrial Encephalomyopathies (p. 1398)

Leigh Syndrome (Subacute Necrotizing Encephalopathy) (p. 1398)

Leigh syndrome is usually an autosomal recessive disorder, with onset at ages 1 to 2 years presenting as arrest of psychomotor development, feeding problems, seizures, extraocular palsies, weakness with hypotonia, and lactic acidemia. Various biochemical abnormalities have been found in the mitochondrial pathway for ATP generation. The brain reveals bilateral regions of destruction with proliferation of blood vessels, usually symmetrically, involving the periventricular gray matter of the midbrain, tegmentum of the pons, and periventricular regions of the thalamus and hypothalamus.

Other Mitochondrial Encephalomyopathies
(p. 1399)

Various other disorders are caused by alterations in mito-chondrial function. These include:

- Diseases caused by point mutations in mtDNA-encoded tRNA (e.g., MERRF [myoclonic epilepsy and ragged red fibers] and MELAS [mitochondrial encephalomyelopathy, lactic acidosis, and stroke-like episodes])
- Diseases caused by deletions of portions of the mtDNA (e.g., Kearns-Sayre ophthalmoplegia)

TOXIC AND ACQUIRED METABOLIC DISEASES
(p. 1399)

Vitamin Deficiencies (p. 1399)

Thiamine (Vitamin B₁) Deficiency (p. 1399)

Beriberi has been discussed (Chapter 9). Thiamine deficiency may also lead to sudden onset of psychosis *(Wernicke encephalopathy)*, which may be followed by a prolonged and largely irreversible disorder of memory *(Korsakoff syndrome)*. The disorder is particularly common with chronic alcoholism but also may follow thiamine deficiency from gastric disease (carcinoma, chronic gastritis, or persistent vomiting). Findings include focal hemorrhage and necrosis, particularly in the mamillary bodies, but also adjacent to the third and fourth ventricles. Lesions in the medial dorsal nucleus of the thalamus are the best correlate of memory disturbance.

Vitamin B₁₂ Deficiency (p. 1399)

Vitamin B₁₂ deficiency causes nervous system symptoms as well as anemia. It usually begins with slight ataxia and numbness and tingling in the lower extremities and may progress rapidly to include spastic weakness of the lower extremities or paraplegia. Recovery from early symptoms may be expected with vitamin replacement; however, if complete paraplegia has developed, recovery is poor. Swelling of myelin layers producing vacuoles affects both ascending and descending tracts (subacute combined degeneration), beginning at the midthoracic spinal cord.

Neurologic Sequelae of Metabolic Disturbances (p. 1400)

Hypoglycemia (p. 1400)

Cellular effects of hypoglycemia are similar to those of oxygen deprivation because the brain requires glucose and oxygen. Neurons that are relatively sensitive to hypoglycemia include large cerebral pyramidal cells, hippocampal pyramidal cells in area CA1, and Purkinje cells. If the level and duration of hypoglycemia are of sufficient severity, there may be a global insult to the neurons of the brain.

Hyperglycemia (p. 1400)

Hyperglycemia is most commonly found in the setting of inadequately controlled diabetes mellitus and can be associated with either ketoacidosis or hyperosmolar coma. The patient becomes dehydrated and develops confusion, stupor, and eventually coma. The fluid depletion must be corrected gradually; otherwise, severe cerebral edema may follow.

Hepatic Encephalopathy (p. 1400)

Cellular response in hepatic encephalopathy is predominantly glial, involving Alzheimer type II cells in the cortex and basal ganglia and other subcortical gray matter regions.

Toxic Disorders (p. 1400)

Carbon monoxide (p. 1400)

Pathology resembles hypoxia, with selective injury of the neurons of layers III and V of cerebral cortex, Sommer sector of the hippocampus, and Purkinje cells. Bilateral necrosis of the globus pallidus may also occur and is more common in carbon monoxide–induced hypoxia than in hypoxia from other causes.

Methanol (p. 1400)

Methanol poisoning may lead to blindness, with degeneration of retinal ganglion cells. Selective bilateral putamenal necrosis also occurs when the exposure is severe. Formate, a major metabolite of methanol, plays a role in the retinal toxicity.

Ethanol (p. 1400)

As many as 1% of patients with a history of long-term high intake of ethanol develop a clinical syndrome of truncal ataxia, unsteady gait, and nystagmus. The early changes are atrophy and loss of granule cells predominantly in the anterior cerebellar vermis. In advanced cases, there is Purkinje cell loss and proliferation of the adjacent astrocytes *(Bergmann gliosis)*.

Radiation (p. 1400)

Injury may develop months to years after irradiation; it can be synergistic with methotrexate. Radionecrosis is composed of large areas of coagulative necrosis in the white matter with adjacent edema. Adjacent to these areas, proteinaceous spheroids may be identified, and blood vessels have thickened walls with intramural fibrin-like material.

TUMORS (p. 1401)

Important features of brain tumors include the following:

- *Consequences of location:* The ability to remove the neoplasm surgically may be restricted by functional anatomic considerations. Benign lesions can have lethal consequences because of their location.
- *Patterns of growth:* Most glial tumors, including many with histologic features of a benign neoplasm, infiltrate entire regions of the brain leading to clinically malignant behavior.
- *Patterns of spread:* Some types of tumor spread through the CSF; however, even the most frankly malignant gliomas (glioblastoma) rarely metastasize outside the CNS.

Tumors of the CNS account for as many as 20% of all cancers of childhood. In this age group, 70% of primary tumors arise in the posterior fossa, whereas in adults, a corresponding proportion arise above the tentorium. Among adults, there is a nearly equal incidence of primary and metastatic tumors.

Gliomas (p. 1401)

Astrocytoma (p. 1401)

Fibrillary (diffuse) astrocytomas represent about 80% of adult primary brain tumors, usually in the cerebral hemispheres, but they may also occur in the cerebellum, brain stem, or spinal cord. All astrocytomas are composed of neoplastic astrocytic nuclei, distributed amid astrocytic processes of varying density; grade is determined histologically.

- Well-differentiated tumors *(astrocytomas)* are poorly defined, gray-white, infiltrative tumors that expand and distort a region of the brain; they show hypercellularity and some nuclear pleomorphism. These are WHO grade II/IV tumors.
- More anaplastic and aggressive tumors *(anaplastic astrocytomas)* reveal increased nuclear anaplasia and the presence of mitoses and vascular cell proliferation. These are WHO grade III/IV tumors.
- Extremely high-grade tumors *(glioblastoma, GBM)* are composed of a mixture of firm, white areas; softer, yellow foci of necrosis; cystic change; and hemorrhage. Increased nuclear density of the highly anaplastic tumor cells along the edges of the necrotic regions is termed *pseudopalisading.* These are WHO grade IV/IV tumors.

Low-grade astrocytomas may remain static or progress only slowly for a number of years. Eventually, however, patients often enter a period of rapid clinical deterioration and rapid tumor growth, corresponding to the appearance of anaplastic features. The prognosis for patients with glioblastoma is poor: mean length of survival after diagnosis is only 8 to 10 months.

- *Pilocytic astrocytomas* (p. 1403) occur in children and young adults, usually in the cerebellum but also in the floor and walls of the third ventricle, the optic nerves, and, occasionally, the cerebral hemispheres. They are often cystic with a mural nodule in the wall of the cyst. The tumor is composed of bipolar cells with long, thin hairlike processes; Rosenthal fibers and microcysts are often present. These tumors are rarely infiltrative and grow slowly. These are WHO grade I/IV tumors.
- *Pleomorphic xanthoastrocytomas* (p. 1404) occur most often relatively superficially in the temporal lobes of children and young adults with a history of seizures. They contain neoplastic astrocytes, sometimes with bizarre forms, abundant reticulin and lipid deposits, and chronic inflammatory cell infiltrates.
- *Brain stem gliomas* (p. 1404) occur mostly in the first 2 decades of life. By the time of autopsy, about 50% have progressed to glioblastomas. With radiotherapy, the 5-year survival rate is 20% to 40%.

Oligodendrogliomas (p. 1404)

Oligodendrogliomas constitute about 5% to 15% of gliomas and are most common in middle life in the cerebral white matter. In general, patients with oligodendrogliomas have a better prognosis than patients with astrocytomas. Current therapies yield an average survival time of 5 to 10 years. Cases of poorly differentiated tumors with increased anaplasia, mitotic activity, cell density, and necrosis have a worse prognosis.

Oligodendrogliomas are well-circumscribed, gelatinous, gray masses, often with cysts, focal hemorrhage, and calcification. The tumor consists of sheets of regular cells with round nuclei containing finely granular chromatin, often surrounded by a clear halo of cytoplasm sitting in a delicate network of anastomosing capillaries. Calcification, present in up to 90% of cases, ranges from microscopic foci to massive deposits.

Ependymoma and Related Paraventricular Mass Lesions (p. 1404)

These tumors arise from the ependymal lining of the ventricular system, including the central canal of the spinal cord. CSF dissemination is a common finding. In the first 2 decades of life, ependymomas typically occur in the fourth ventricle; in middle life, the spinal cord is the most common location.

The tumor cells have regular, round-oval nuclei with abundant granular chromatin; they may form ependymal rosettes (canals) or, more frequently, perivascular pseudorosettes.

- *Myxopapillary ependymomas* are histologically benign lesions arising in the filum terminale of the spinal cord. Cuboidal cells, sometimes with clear cytoplasm, are arranged around papillary cores containing connective tissue and blood vessels. Myxoid areas contain neutral and acidic mucopolysaccharides.
- *Subependymomas* (p. 1405) are solid, sometimes calcified, slow-growing nodules attached to the ventricular lining and protruding into the ventricle. They have clumps of ependymal-appearing nuclei scattered in a dense, finely fibrillar background.
- *Choroid plexus papillomas* (p. 1406) almost exactly recapitulate the structure of the normal choroid plexus, with papillae of connective tissue stalks covered with a cuboidal or columnar ciliated epithelium. Hydrocephalus is common, as a result of either obstruction of the ventricular system or overproduction of CSF. In children, the lateral ventricles are the most common site; in adults, the fourth ventricle is a more frequent site.
- *Colloid cysts of the third ventricle* (p. 1406) are non-neoplastic lesions of young adults; they are located at the foramina of Monro and can result in noncommunicating hydrocephalus, sometimes rapidly fatal. The cyst has a thin, fibrous capsule and a lining of low to flat cuboidal epithelium; the cyst contents are gelatinous proteinaceous material.

Neuronal Tumors (p. 1406)

Ganglion Cell Tumors (p. 1406)

Ganglioglioma is a glial neoplasm with an admixed ganglion cell component of irregularly clustered neurons with apparently random orientation of neurites and frequent binucleated forms. Most occur in the temporal lobe and are slow growing, but occasionally the glial component becomes frankly anaplastic; the tumor then assumes a much more aggressive course. Mature-appearing neurons may constitute the entire population of a tumor, in which case it is termed a *gangliocytoma*.

Other Tumors With Glial and Neuronal Components (p. 1406)

Dysembryoplastic neuroepithelial tumor: A tumor of childhood often presenting as a seizure disorder, with a relatively good prognosis after resection. Features include intracortical location, cystic changes, nodular growth, "floating neurons" in a pool of mucopolysaccharide-rich fluid, and surrounding neoplastic glia without anaplastic features.

Tumors With Only Neuronal Elements (p. 1406)

- *Cerebral neuroblastoma:* This rare, aggressive neoplasm occurs in the hemispheres in children and resembles peripheral neuroblastomas, with small undifferentiated cells and Homer-Wright rosettes.
- *Neurocytoma:* This tumor is found adjacent to the foramen of Monro; evenly spaced, round, uniform nuclei resemble cells of an oligodendroglioma, but ultrastructural and immunohistochemical studies reveal their neuronal origin.

Poorly Differentiated Neoplasms (p. 1407)

Some tumors, although of neuroectodermal origin, express few, if any, of the phenotypic markers of mature cells of the nervous system and are described as poorly differentiated.

Medulloblastomas (p. 1407)

Medulloblastomas account for 20% of childhood brain tumors; they occur exclusively in the cerebellum. Tumors are located in the midline in children, with lateral locations found more often in adults. Rapid growth may occlude the flow of CSF, leading to hydrocephalus. Often well-circumscribed, gray, and friable, they are usually extremely cellular, with sheets of anaplastic cells exhibiting hyperchromatic nuclei and abundant mitoses. The cells have little cytoplasm, and the cytoplasm is often devoid of specific markers of differentiation, although neuronal or glial features may be seen. Extension into the subarachnoid space may elicit a prominent desmoplastic response. Dissemination through the CSF is common.

The tumor is highly malignant, and the prognosis for untreated neoplasm is dismal; however, it is exquisitely radiosensitive. With total excision and radiation, the 5-year survival rate has been reported to be as high as 75%.

Other Parenchymal Tumors (p. 1408)

Primary CNS Lymphoma (p. 1408)

Primary brain lymphomas account for approximately 2% of extranodal lymphomas. One or more dominant masses occur within the brain parenchyma; nodal or bone marrow involvement and involvement outside the CNS are extremely rare late complications. Within the immunosuppressed population (e.g., AIDS), all the neoplasms appear to be of B-cell origin and to contain Epstein-Barr virus genomes within the transformed B cells. Regardless of clinical context, primary brain lymphoma is an aggressive disease with relatively poor chemotherapeutic responses compared with peripheral lymphomas; nevertheless, it is initially responsive to radiotherapy and steroids. The morphology of the neoplastic lymphocytes is nearly always of a high-grade type. The malignant cells diffusely involve the parenchyma of the brain and accumulate around blood vessels, with some vessel walls expanded by multiple layers of malignant cells.

Germ Cell Tumors (p. 1408)

These tumors occur along the midline in adolescents and young adults, with the pineal and suprasellar regions dominating the distribution. Tumors in the pineal region show a strong male predominance, not seen in suprasellar lesions. The histologic appearances of germ cell tumors and their classification are the same as used for other extragonadal sites.

Meningiomas (p. 1409)

Meningiomas are predominantly benign tumors of adults that arise from the meningothelial cell of the arachnoid. They show a moderate (3:2) female predominance within the cranial vault but a 10:1 female-male ratio within the spinal canal. Loss of heterozygosity of the long arm of chromosome 22 is a common finding.

Meningiomas tend to be rounded masses with well-defined dural bases that compress underlying brain but are easily separated from it. Lesions are usually firm to fibrous and lack evidence of necrosis or extensive hemorrhage. Many histologic patterns exist, all with generally comparable favorable prognoses:

- *Syncytial:* clusters of cells in tight groups without visible cell membranes.
- *Fibroblastic:* elongated cells and abundant collagen deposition.
- *Transitional:* features of the syncytial and fibroblastic types.
- *Psammomatous:* abundant psammoma bodies.
- *Papillary tumors:* pleomorphic cells arranged around fibrovascular cores (tend to have a worse prognosis).
- *Malignant meningiomas:* unusual tumors that may be difficult to recognize histologically as being meningothelial; they have abundant mitoses with atypical forms.
- *Sarcomas of the meninges:* uncommon but can include malignant fibrous histiocytomas and hemangiopericytomas.

Metastatic Tumors (p. 1410)

Among general hospital patients, metastatic lesions, mostly carcinomas, account for approximately half of intracranial tumors. Common primary sites are lung, breast, skin (melanoma), kidney, and gastrointestinal tract. The meninges are also a frequent site for involvement by metastatic disease.

Intraparenchymal metastases are sharply demarcated masses, often at the gray-white junction, usually surrounded by a zone of edema. Meningeal carcinomatosis, with tumor nodules studding the surface of the brain, spinal cord, and intradural nerve roots, is an occasional complication particularly associated with small cell carcinoma, adenocarcinoma of the lung, and carcinoma of the breast.

Paraneoplastic Syndromes
(p. 1410; Table 28–4)

Paraneoplastic syndromes are functional and structural changes of the brain in response to malignancy elsewhere in the body. Syndromes may improve with plasmapheresis, immunosuppression, or treatment of the primary neoplasm.

- *Paraneoplastic cerebellar degeneration* is the most common pattern, with loss of Purkinje cells, gliosis, and a mild inflammatory infiltrate associated with an antibody-mediated injury of Purkinje cells.
- *Limbic encephalitis* is a subacute dementia, usually with a prominent component of memory disturbance. Findings are most striking in the anterior and medial portions of the temporal lobe and resemble an infectious process with perivascular inflammatory cuffs, microglial nodules, some neuronal loss, and gliosis.
- *Subacute sensory neuropathy* occurs in association with limbic encephalitis or in isolation, with loss of sensory neurons from dorsal root ganglia, in association with inflammation.

TABLE 28–4 **Paraneoplastic Syndromes**

Syndrome	Target	Tumor	Antigen
Subacute cerebellar degeneration	Purkinje cells	Hodgkin lymphoma Breast, GYN SCLC, neuroblastoma	Tr Yo Hu
Limbic encephalitis; brainstem encephalitis	Various neurons in mesial temporal lobe, brainstem	SCLC, neuroblastoma Testicular, others	Hu Ma
Subacute sensory neuropathy	Dorsal root ganglion neurons	SCLC, neuroblastoma	Hu
Opsoclonus myoclonus	Unknown (presumed brain stem)	Neuroblastoma, Breast	Ri
Retinal degeneration	Photoreceptors	SCLC	Recoverin
Stiff-man syndrome	Spinal intermeurons	Breast	Amphiphysin
Lambert-Eaton myasthenic syndrome	Presynaptic terminals at neuromuscular junction	SCLC	Presynaptic calcium channel

GYN, gynecologic tumors; SCLC, small cell lung carcinoma.

Peripheral Nerve Sheath Tumors (p. 1411)

A large proportion of tumors occurring within the confines of the dura are derived from cells of peripheral nerve; comparable tumors arise along the peripheral course of nerves.

Schwannomas (p. 1411)

Schwannomas are benign tumors of neural crest–derived Schwann cells, most commonly associated with the vestibular branch of the eighth nerve at the cerebellopontine angle (vestibular schwannoma or acoustic neuroma). Spinal tumors mostly arise from dorsal roots; tumors may extend through the vertebral foramen, acquiring a dumbbell configuration. When extradural, schwannomas are most commonly found in association with large nerve trunks. They are well-circumscribed, encapsulated masses, attached to the nerve but separable from it. Axons are excluded from the tumor, although they may become entrapped in the capsule. Tumors show a mixture of two growth patterns:

- *Antoni A:* elongated cells with cytoplasmic processes arranged in fascicles in areas of moderate-to-high cellularity with little stromal matrix
- *Antoni B:* less densely cellular tissue with microcysts and myxoid changes

Electron microscopy shows basement membrane deposition encasing single cells and long-spacing collagen. Malignant change is extremely rare.

Neurofibroma (p. 1412)

Cutaneous neurofibroma and *solitary neurofibroma* occur sporadically and in association with neurofibromatosis type 1 (p. 1413). The skin lesions are evident as nodules, sometimes with hyperpigmentation; these lesions may grow quite large and become pedunculated. The risk of malignant transformation from these tumors is extremely small. Present in the dermis and extending to the subcutaneous fat, these are well-delineated but unencapsulated masses composed of spindle cells in a highly collagenized stroma. Lesions within peripheral nerves are histologically similar. *Plexiform neurofibromas* irregularly expand a nerve as fascicles are infiltrated; in contrast to schwannomas, it is not possible to separate the lesion from the nerve. The lesion has a loose myxoid background with a low cellularity, including Schwann cells, fibroblasts, perineurial cells, and a sprinkling of inflammatory cells, often including mast cells. Axons can be demonstrated within the tumor. A major concern in the care of neurofibromatosis type 1 patients is the difficulty of surgical removal of these tumors from major nerve trunks, combined with their potential for malignant transformation.

Malignant Peripheral Nerve Sheath Tumor (Malignant Schwannoma) (p. 1412)

These highly malignant, locally invasive sarcomas do not arise from malignant degeneration of schwannomas; instead, they arise *de novo* or from transformation of a plexiform neurofibroma. The lesions are poorly defined tumor masses with frequent infiltration along the axis of the parent nerve as well as invasion of adjacent soft tissues. Tumor cells resemble Schwann cells with elongated nuclei and prominent bipolar processes; fascicle formation may be present. Mitoses, necrosis, and nuclear anaplasia are common. Patterns of other sarcoma types may be present.

Familial Tumor Syndromes (p. 1413)

These mostly autosomal dominant disorders are characterized by hamartomas and neoplasms located throughout the body, often prominently involving the nervous system and skin. These syndromes are discussed here.

Neurofibromatosis Type 1 (p. 1413)

This autosomal dominant disorder is characterized by neurofibromas (plexiform and cutaneous), optic nerve gliomas, meningiomas, pigmented nodules of the iris *(Lisch nodules),* and cutaneous hyperpigmented macules *(café au lait spots).* Even in the absence of malignant transformation of neurofibromas, lesions have disfiguring potential and the potential to create spinal deformity, most commonly kyphoscoliosis. Tumors arising in proximity to the spinal cord or brain stem may also have devastating consequences, independent of their histologic grade.

Neurofibromatosis Type 2 (p. 1413)

This distinct autosomal dominant disorder (chromosome 22) has a propensity to develop bilateral eighth nerve schwannomas or multiple meningiomas.

Tuberous Sclerosis (p. 1413)

Tuberous sclerosis is characterized by angiofibromas, seizures, and mental retardation. Hamartomas within the CNS include *cortical tubers* (areas of haphazardly arranged neurons and large cells that express phenotypes intermediate between glia and neurons) and subependymal hamartomas (large astrocytic and neuronal cell clusters beneath the ventricular surface that give rise to a tumor unique to tuberous sclerosis—the subependymal giant cell astrocytoma). In addition, renal angiomyolipomas; retinal glial phakomas; cardiac rhabdomyomas; hepatic, renal, and pancreatic cysts; leathery cutaneous thickenings *(shagreen patches);* hypopigmented areas (ash leaf patches); and subungual fibromas may occur. There is variable expressivity and penetrance, and at least two distinct loci are known, on chromosomes 9 *(hamartin)* and 16 *(tuberin).*

von Hippel–Lindau Disease (p. 1414)

von Hippel–Lindau disease is characterized by

- Capillary hemangioblastomas in the cerebellar hemispheres, retina, and less commonly within the brain stem and spinal cord
- Cysts involving the pancreas, liver, and kidney (with a strong propensity to develop renal cell carcinoma of the kidney)
- Paragangliomas

- Hemangioblastomas containing variable proportions of delicate capillary vessels with stromal cells of uncertain histogenesis and abundant vacuolated cytoplasm between them

They commonly are cystic lesions with a mural node. Polycythemia is an associated finding in about 10% of cases, related to erythropoietin production by the tumor.

CHAPTER 29

The Eye

ORBIT (p. 1423)

Because the orbit (Fig. 29–1) is bounded by bone medially, laterally, and posteriorly, any process that increases orbital contents causes forward eye displacement, or *proptosis*.

Thyroid Ophthalmopathy (p. 1423, Chapter 24)

Proptosis in *Graves disease* is caused by extracellular matrix protein accumulation and fibrosis in the rectus muscles. Severity can be independent of thyroid functional status.

Other Orbital Inflammatory Conditions (p. 1423)

Wegener granulomatosis and extension of maxillary or ethmoid sinus infections can cause proptosis. Idiopathic orbital inflammation *(orbital inflammatory pseudotumor)* is characterized by chronic inflammation and variable fibrosis.

EYELID (p. 1424)

Eyelids are composites of skin externally and mucosa *(conjunctiva)* adjacent to the eye (Fig. 29–2). They cover and protect the eye, as well as generate lipids that retard tear evaporation *(Zeis* and *meibomian* sebaceous glands).

Neoplasms (p. 1424)

Regardless of cause, eyelid neoplasms can distort and impede eyelid closure; subsequent corneal exposure is painful and predisposes to corneal ulceration. Prompt treatment of any lid neoplasm is imperative to preserve vision.

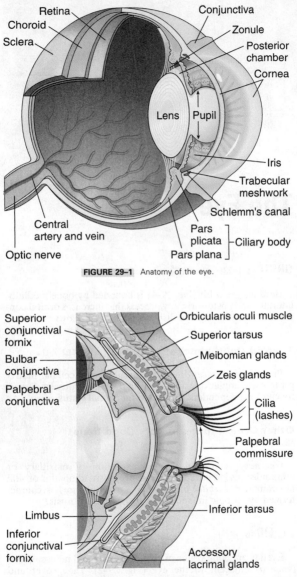

FIGURE 29–1 Anatomy of the eye.

FIGURE 29–2 Anatomy of the conjunctiva and eyelids.

- *Chalazion* is a focus of lipogranulomatous inflammation occurring when sebaceous gland drainage is blocked by chronic inflammation *(blepharitis)* or tumor.
- *Basal cell carcinoma* is the most common malignancy of the eyelid; it has a predilection for lower eyelids and medial canthi.

- *Sebaceous carcinoma* (originating in Zeis or meibomian glands) is the second most common eyelid malignancy. Metastases to regional lymph nodes and pagetoid tumor spread through the epidermis and conjunctiva make resection difficult; overall mortality rate is 22%.

CONJUNCTIVA (p. 1425)

The aqueous component of tear film is generated by accessory lacrimal glands embedded in the eyelid and fornix. Conjunctival goblet cell mucin production is essential for adhering tears to corneal epithelium. Failure of either lacrimal gland (most commonly) or goblet cell production will result in *dry eyes;* when severe, the condition is painful and predisposes to corneal ulceration and opacification.

The conjunctiva has topologic zones (see Fig. 29–2) with distinctive histologic features and disease responses. The *palpebral conjunctiva* is nonkeratinizing stratified squamous epithelium and responds to inflammation by forming minute papillary folds. Conversely, *fornix conjunctiva* is a pseudostratified columnar epithelium rich in goblet cells; its associated lacrimal and lymphoid tissues can be expanded in *viral conjunctivitis* or lymphoid malignancy. Fornix biopsies can yield diagnostic granulomas in 50% of systemic sarcoidosis cases.

Conjunctival Scarring (p. 1425)

Conjunctival scarring will cause goblet cell loss and resulting dry eyes even with adequate aqueous tear film production. Causes of conjunctival scarring include:

- Infections (e.g., *trachoma*)
- Immune-mediated conditions, such as *ocular cicatricial pemphigoid*
- Chemical agents, especially alkalis
- Excessive surgical resection of conjunctival tissue

Pinguecula and Pterygium (p. 1426)

Pinguecula and pterygium are submucosal conjunctival elevations arising from actinic damage; they occur in sun-exposed regions of the conjunctiva (e.g., interpalpebral fissure).

- *Pterygium* is a growth of conjunctival mucosa and fibrovascular connective tissue originating in the limbus and migrating onto the cornea. It does not usually affect vision; resections are performed for irritation or cosmetic reasons, although occult malignancies can occur.
- *Pinguecula* does not invade the cornea, but can affect tear film distribution and result in focal dehydration with corneal depression (a *dellen*); these can also become inflamed due to granulomatous responses to sun-damaged collagen.

Neoplasms (p. 1426)

Neoplasms tend to develop at the limbus, likely related to sun exposure:

- *Squamous cell carcinomas* are associated with human papillomavirus types 16 and 18; they tend to follow indolent courses. *Mucoepidermoid carcinoma* is a substantially more aggressive tumor.

- *Conjunctival nevi* are common and typically benign, rarely invading the cornea or appearing in the fornix. Chronic inflammation with eosinophils may occur during adolescence *(inflamed juvenile nevus)*.
- *Conjunctival melanomas* are unilateral, typically affecting middle-aged fair-complexioned individuals; most arise through an intraepithelial phase termed *primary acquired melanosis with atypia,* roughly analogous to *melanoma in situ.* Conjunctival melanoma will develop in 50% to 90% of these lesions, metastasizing first to the parotid or sub-mandibular lymph nodes with 25% mortality rate. The best treatment is precursor lesion extirpation.

SCLERA (p. 1426)

Sclera is relatively deficient in blood vessels and fibroblasts; thus, wounds and surgical incisions heal poorly. It is thinned physiologically at the limbus, behind the rectus muscle insertions, and near the optic nerve so that blunt force trauma can cause ruptures there. Scleral "blueness" can be due to thinning caused by inflammation, increased intraocular pressure, or defective collagen synthesis (e.g., in *osteogenesis imperfecta*), or may be due to a heavily pigmented nevus in the underlying uvea.

CORNEA (p. 1426)

The cornea and its overlying tear film (and *not* the lens) compose the major refractive eye surface (see Fig. 29–1). The corneal stroma lacks blood vessels and lymphatics, contributing to corneal transparency as well as the success of corneal transplantation. Precise collagen alignment is also necessary to maintain transparency; consequently, scarring or edema markedly affects vision. Anteriorly, the cornea is covered by epithelium overlying a basement membrane and the acellular *Bowman's layer.* Posteriorly, the cornea is bounded by *corneal endothelium* derived from neural crest (and unrelated to vascular endothelium); it sits on a basal lamina *Descemet membrane.* Endothelial loss or malfunction causes stromal edema that can progress to bullous separation of the epithelium *(bullous keratopathy).*

Keratitis and Ulcers (p. 1428)

Bacteria, fungi, viruses (especially herpes simplex and zoster), and protozoa *(Acanthamoeba)* can cause corneal ulceration; corneal stroma dissolution may be accelerated by collagenase activation. Some forms of keratitis have distinctive features (e.g., chronic herpes simplex causes granulomatous responses to Descemet's membrane).

Corneal Degenerations and Dystrophies
(p. 1428)

Degenerations

Degenerations may be uni- or bilateral and are typically nonfamilial.

Band keratopathies (p. 1428)

Calcific band keratopathy, a common complication of chronic uveitis, is characterized by calcium deposition in Bowman's layer. *Actinic band keratopathy* involves UV-induced corneal collagen degeneration.

Keratoconus (p. 1428)

Corneal thinning and ectasia without inflammation or vascularization causes the cornea to become conical (rather than spherical), and distorts vision. Bowman's layer fractures are histologic hallmarks; matrix metalloproteinase activation is etiologically implicated.

Dystrophies

Dystrophies are typically bilateral and are hereditary.

Fuchs Endothelial Dystrophy (p. 1428)

A primary loss of corneal endothelial cells causes the two major clinical manifestations of this entity: *stromal edema* and *bullous keratopathy* (epithelial detachment from Bowman's layer forming bullae). There is blurring and loss of vision.

Stromal Dystrophies (p. 1429)

Stromal deposits (due to specific genetic mutations) form discrete opacities in the cornea, compromising vision; deposits adjacent to epithelium or Bowman's layer can also cause painful erosions or scarring.

ANTERIOR SEGMENT (p. 1430)

The eye is divided into two compartments (Fig. 29–3):

- *Anterior segment* includes the cornea, anterior chamber, posterior chamber, iris, and lens. The ciliary body forms the aqueous humor that enters the posterior chamber, bathes the lens, and circulates through the pupil into the anterior chamber.
- *Posterior pole* (remainder of the eye; see Fig. 29–1).

Cataracts (p. 1431)

Cataracts are congenital or acquired lens opacities. Systemic diseases (e.g., diabetes mellitus, atopic dermatitis), drugs (especially corticosteroids), radiation, trauma, and many intraocular disorders (e.g., uveitis) cause cataracts. Age-related cataracts typically result from lens nucleus opacification. Lens epithelium migration and hyperplasia posterior to the lens can cause *posterior subcapsular cataracts.*

Anterior Segment and Glaucoma (p. 1431)

Glaucoma has distinctive visual field changes and optic nerve cup alterations. It is caused by several diseases; most glaucoma is associated with elevated intraocular pressure (see Fig. 29–3 for normal aqueous flow patterns), although some patients have normal intraocular pressure (*normal-* or *low-tension glaucoma*). There are two major categories of glaucoma:

* *Open angle glaucoma:* This is the most common form of glaucoma. The aqueous humor has complete access to the trabecular meshwork, and intraocular pressure elevations result from increased resistance to outflow in the open angle. Although candidate causal genes and proteins are identified

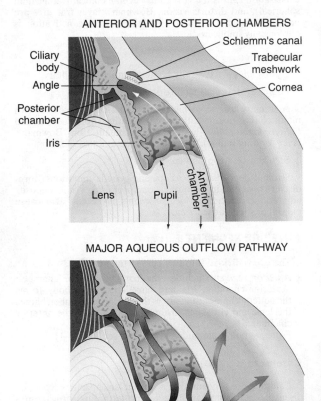

ANTERIOR AND POSTERIOR CHAMBERS

Schlemm's canal

Trabecular meshwork

Ciliary body

Angle

Cornea

Posterior chamber

Iris

Anterior chamber

Lens   Pupil

MAJOR AQUEOUS OUTFLOW PATHWAY

A

FIGURE 29–3 *A,* Normal eye; note the iris surface is highly textured with crypts and folds. Normal aqueous humor flows from the posterior chamber (site of production) through the pupil into the anterior chamber, and through the trabecular meshwork into Schlemm canal; minor outflow pathways through the uveosclera and iris are not depicted.

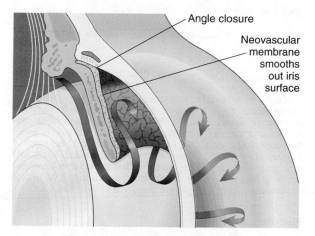

Obstructed flow leads to increased
posterior chamber pressure

Angle closure

Iris bows
forward
(iris bombé)

Pupillary
block

PRIMARY ANGLE CLOSURE GLAUCOMA

Angle closure

Neovascular
membrane
smooths
out iris
surface

NEOVASCULAR GLAUCOMA

B

FIGURE 29–3, cont'd. *B, Top:* Primary angle closure glaucoma occurs in anatomically predisposed eyes by transient iris apposition to the lens blocking aqueous humor passage from the posterior to anterior chambers. Pressure builds in the posterior chamber bowing the iris forward (*iris* bombé) and occluding the trabecular meshwork. *Bottom:* Neovascular glaucoma occurs when a neovascular membrane grows over the iris, smoothing the folds and crypts; contracture of this membrane causes tissue apposition over the trabecular meshwork, blocking aqueous humor outflow and increasing intraocular pressure.

(e.g., *myocilin*) in primary forms of the disease, the etiology remains obscure. Particulate matter (e.g., senescent erythrocytes after trauma, or iris pigment epithelial granules) can also secondarily physically clog the trabecular meshwork.

- *Angle closure glaucoma* (see Fig. 29–3): The peripheral zone of the iris (or associated tissue) adheres to the trabecular meshwork and physically impedes the aqueous outflow from the eye. It may occur as *primary angle closure glaucoma* in eyes with shallow anterior chambers, or may be secondary to neovascular membrane formation (e.g., after trauma) or to ciliary body tumors.

Endophthalmitis and Panophthalmitis
(p. 1432)

Anterior segment inflammation can result from blunt trauma *(traumatic iridocyclitis)*, corneal infections, or uveal inflammation *(uveitis*, see later discussion).

- *Endophthalmitis* is inflammation involving the vitreous in the posterior pole of the eye. The retina does not tolerate endophthalmitis; only a few hours of acute inflammation can irreversibly damage it. Endophthalmitis may be *exogenous* (e.g., following a wound) or *endogenous* (delivered hematogenously).
- *Panophthalmitis* is eye inflammation involving the retina, choroid, and sclera and extending into the orbit

UVEA (p. 1432)

The iris, the choroid, and the ciliary body constitute the *uvea* (see Fig. 29–1).

Uveitis (p. 1433)

Uveitis can be infectious, idiopathic (e.g., *sarcoidosis*), or autoimmune (e.g., *sympathetic ophthalmia*); it can be part of a systemic process, or involve only the eye. Although inflammation in one compartment typically extends into others, uveitis can involve only the anterior segment (e.g., in *juvenile rheumatoid arthritis*). *Sympathetic ophthalmia* exhibits bilateral granulomatous inflammation affecting all uveal components *(panuveitis);* it can complicate penetrating eye injury, developing within 2 weeks (to many years) after the insult.

Neoplasms (p. 1433)

The most common intraocular malignancy in adults is uveal metastasis (typically choroidal) of some other primary tumor. Uveal melanoma is the most common *primary* intraocular adult malignancy. Since uveal nevi (especially choroidal nevi) are common—affecting some 10% of whites—progression of a nevus to melanoma is exceptionally uncommon. Uveal melanomas spread hematogenously (there are no eye lymphatics) and favor the liver—an example of organ-specific metastasis. Although 5-year survival rates approach 80%, cumulative mortality rate is 40% at 10 years, increasing 1% per year thereafter. Prognostic variables include extraocular extension, large basal diameter, location within the eye, cell type, extent of tumor-infiltrating lymphocytes, certain cytogenetic abnormalities, and patterns of extracellular matrix protein deposition *(vasculogenic mimicry).*

RETINA AND VITREOUS (p. 1434)

The neurosensory retina is embryologically derived from the diencephalon, and injury causes gliosis. The retinal architecture explains the ophthalmoscopic appearance of ocular disorders (Fig. 29–4). There are no lymphatics.

Retinal Detachment (p. 1436)

Retinal detachment involves separation of the neurosensory retina from the pigmented epithelium. *Nonrhegmatogenous* versus *rhegmatogenous retinal detachment* is distinguished by the absence or presence of full-thickness retinal defects, respectively.

Retinal Vascular Disease (p. 1436)

Retinal vasculopathy (neovascularization) is a common endpoint of numerous insults; it can occur secondary to vessel occlusion, hypoxia, or primary angiogenic factor production (see causes listed next). Vessel occlusions cause hemorrhages (and changes related to their organization, including retinal detachment), or can result in local ischemia. Retinal hypoxia

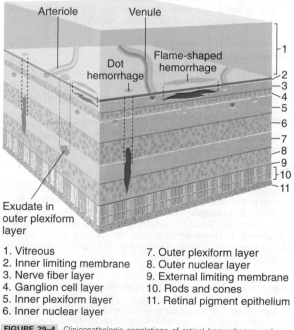

1. Vitreous
2. Inner limiting membrane
3. Nerve fiber layer
4. Ganglion cell layer
5. Inner plexiform layer
6. Inner nuclear layer
7. Outer plexiform layer
8. Outer nuclear layer
9. External limiting membrane
10. Rods and cones
11. Retinal pigment epithelium

FIGURE 29–4 Clinicopathologic correlations of retinal hemorrhages and exudates; location within the retina determines ophthalmoscopic appearance. Hemorrhages of the retinal nerve fiber layer (oriented parallel to the internal limiting membrane) appear flame-shaped. Hemorrhages of the deeper retinal layers (oriented perpendicular to the internal limiting membrane) appear as "dots." Exudates from leaky retinal vessels accumulate in the outer plexiform layer.

causes growth factor production (e.g., VEGF) leading to angiogenesis; subsequent contraction of the neovascular membrane also causes retinal detachment.

Hypertension (p. 1436)

Hypertension results in retinal arteriosclerosis with wall thickening. In malignant hypertension, damaged choroidal vessels may cause choroidal infarcts *(Elschnig spots)* or exudate accumulation between the neurosensory retina and pigmented epithelium (causing retinal detachment). Occlusion of retinal arteries may produce infarcts of the retinal nerve fiber layer, and exudates from damaged retinal vessels accumulate in the outer plexiform layer (see Fig. 29–4).

Diabetes Mellitus (p. 1437)

Diabetes mellitus causes microvascular injury with thickened basement membrane (and physiologic breakdown of the blood-retina barrier with edema and hemorrhage) as well as pericyte loss leading to characteristic microaneurysms.

* *Background (preproliferative) diabetic retinopathy* constitutes a spectrum from structural and functional angiopathic abnormalities to angiogenesis located within the retina (beneath the internal limiting membrane of the retina).
* *Proliferative diabetic retinopathy* reflects new vessels derived from existing vessels (i.e., *retinal neovascularization*) that breach the retinal internal limiting membrane.

Retinopathy of Prematurity (Retrolental Fibroplasia) (p. 1439)

Immature retinal vessels respond to increased oxygen tension (administered to premature infants) by constricting, resulting in local ischemia.

Sickle Retinopathy (p. 1439)

Reduced oxygen tension leads to erythrocyte sickling and microvascular occlusions.

Retinal Artery and Vein Occlusion (p. 1440)

Arterial occlusions due to atherosclerosis or to atheroembolism cause retinal infarction; since onset is typically sudden, there is no prolonged ischemia, and hence no significant neovascularization. Retinal vein occlusion (e.g., due to arteriolar thickening in hypertension that compromises the venous lumen where the vessels cross) typically leads to ischemia and subsequent neovascularization.

Age-Related Macular Degeneration (p. 1441)

Age-related macular degeneration (ARMD) is the most common cause of irreversible visual loss in the United States; the etiology is unclear. ARMD is most commonly (80%–90%) *atrophic* (dry), associated with geographic atrophy of the retinal pigment epithelium. The remainder of ARMD are *exudative* (wet) associated with leaky choroidal neovascular membranes.

Retinitis Pigmentosa (p. 1442)

Retinitis pigmentosa describes a collection of fairly common (1 in 3600 individuals) inherited disorders that affect various aspects of vision including visual cascade and cycle, structural genes, transcription factors, catabolic pathways, and mitochondrial metabolism. Despite the name, these disorders are *not* primarily inflammatory; both rods and cones are lost to apoptosis and there is retinal atrophy, with perivascular retinal pigment accumulation.

Retinoblastoma (p. 1442)

Retinoblastoma is the most common primary intraocular malignancy of children. Prognosis is worsened by extraocular extension, or by optic nerve or choroidal invasion. In 40% of cases, retinoblastoma is associated with a germ-line *RB* mutation; such cases are often bilateral, and are associated with pinealoblastoma ("trilateral" retinoblastoma) with a dismal outcome.

OPTIC NERVE (p. 1443)

Optic nerve pathology is similar to brain pathology; cerebrospinal fluid circulates around the nerve and it is surrounded by meninges. The most common primary neoplasms are gliomas (typically *pilocytic astrocytomas*) and meningiomas.

Anterior Ischemic Optic Neuropathy (p. 1443)

The optic nerve blood supply can be interrupted by vascular inflammation (e.g., temporal arteritis, Chapter 11) or by embolism or thrombosis.

Papilledema (p. 1443)

Optic nerve edema can be due to compression (e.g., by neoplasm) or to elevated cerebrospinal fluid pressure; the latter is typically bilateral and called *papilledema.*

Glaucomatous Optic Nerve Damage (p. 1444)

Glaucomatous optic nerve damage is characterized by atrophy (due to increased intraocular pressures; see earlier discussion) accompanied by optic nerve head cupping.

Other Optic Neuropathies (p. 1445)

Other optic neuropathies can be inherited (e.g., *Leber hereditary optic neuropathy* due to mitochondrial gene mutations) or result from toxins (e.g., methanol) or nutritional deficiency.

THE END-STAGE EYE: PHTHISIS BULBI (p. 1448)

Trauma, intraocular inflammation, chronic retinal detachment, and many other conditions give rise to a small (atrophic) and internally disorganized eye: *phthisis bulbi.*

Index

Note: Page numbers followed by f indicate figures; those followed by t indicate tables.